Part 1 MRCOG Synoptic Revision Guide

Part 1 MRCOG Synoptic Revision Guide

Edited by

Asma Khalil
St George's, University of London

Anthony Griffiths
University Hospital of Wales

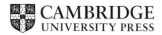
CAMBRIDGE
UNIVERSITY PRESS

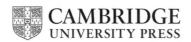

Shaftesbury Road, Cambridge CB2 8EA, United Kingdom

One Liberty Plaza, 20th Floor, New York, NY 10006, USA

477 Williamstown Road, Port Melbourne, VIC 3207, Australia

314–321, 3rd Floor, Plot 3, Splendor Forum, Jasola District Centre, New Delhi – 110025, India

103 Penang Road, #05–06/07, Visioncrest Commercial, Singapore 238467

Cambridge University Press is part of Cambridge University Press & Assessment,
a department of the University of Cambridge.

We share the University's mission to contribute to society through the pursuit of
education, learning and research at the highest international levels of excellence.

www.cambridge.org
Information on this title: www.cambridge.org/9781108714112

DOI: 10.1017/9781108644464

First published 2023

Printed in the United Kingdom by TJ Books Limited, Padstow Cornwall

A catalogue record for this publication is available from the British Library.

Library of Congress Cataloging-in-Publication Data
Names: Khalil, Asma, editor. | Griffiths, Anthony (Anthony N.), editor.
Title: Part 1 MRCOG synoptic revision guide / edited by Asma Khalil, Anthony Griffiths.
Description: Cambridge, United Kingdom ; New York, NY : Cambridge University Press, 2021. |
Includes bibliographical references and index.
Identifiers: LCCN 2021024868 (print) | LCCN 2021024869 (ebook) |
ISBN 9781108714112 (paperback) | ISBN 9781108644464 (ebook)
Subjects: MESH: Obstetrics – methods | Gynecology – methods | Reproductive Medicine – methods |
Study Guide | BISAC: MEDICAL / Gynecology & Obstetrics
Classification: LCC RG101 (print) | LCC RG101 (ebook) | NLM WQ 18.2 | DDC 618.1–dc23
LC record available at https://lccn.loc.gov/2021024868
LC ebook record available at https://lccn.loc.gov/2021024869

ISBN 978-1-108-71411-2 Paperback

Contents

Contributors

Nazar N. J. Amso **FRCOG FHEA PhD**
Emeritus Professor and Consultant, Obstetrics and Gynaecology, School of Medicine, Cardiff University, Cardiff

Balpreet Attilia **BSc MRCOG**
Consultant Obstetrician and Gynaecologist, Musgrove Park Hospital, Taunton

Mary Board **MA DPhil**
Lecturer in Biochemistry, St Hilda's College, University of Oxford, Oxford

Paul Carter **BSc MD FRCS FRCOG**
Head of Anatomical Sciences and Consultant Obstetrician and Gynaecologist, St George's University of London, London

Neil Chapman **PhD SFHEA**
Senior University Teacher (Reproductive Medicine), Academic Unit of Reproductive and Developmental Medicine, University of Sheffield, Sheffield

Raji Ganesan **MD FRCPath CertMedEd**
Consultant Gynaecological Pathologist, Birmingham Women's Hospital, Birmingham

Kelvin F. Gomez **MD FRCSEd MFSTEd**
Clinical Director for Surgery, Aneurin Bevan University Health Board, Newport

Alastair Graham **BPharm**
Clinical Pharmacist, Gloucestershire Royal Hospital, Gloucester

Anthony N. Griffiths **MRCOG FHEA DFFP DipMedEd PGDipMAS**
Consultant Gynaecologist, University Hospital of Wales, Cardiff

Kevin Hayes **FRCOG**
Reader and Consultant Obstetrician and Gynaecologist, St George's University of London, London

Tessa Homfray **FRCP**
Consultant Medical Geneticist, St George's University of London and Harris Birthright Unit, King's College Hospital, London

Jemma Johns **MD FRCOG**
Consultant Obstetrician and Gynaecologist, Early Pregnancy and Gynaecology Assessment Unit, King's College Hospital, London

Sadie Jones **MRCOG PhD**
Obstetrics and Gynaecology Clinical Lecturer, University of Cardiff School of Medicine, Cardiff

Asma Khalil **MD MRCOG MSc**
Consultant and Reader in Obstetrics and Maternal-Fetal Medicine, Fetal Medicine Unit, St George's University of London, London

Erum A. Khan **DFFP MRCOG PGCertClinEd**
Consultant Obstetrician and Gynaecologist, Department of Obstetrics and Gynaecology, Milton Keynes University Hospital, Milton Keynes

Karin Leslie **MRCOG**
Lecturer in Maternal-Fetal Medicine, Fetal Medicine Unit, St George's University of London, London

Sahar Mansour **FRCP**
Consultant and Honorary Professor in Clinical Genetics, St George's University of London, London

Anthony E. Michael **PhD**
Dean for Education, Faculty of Science and Engineering, Queen Mary University of London, London

Laura C. Mongan PhD SFHEA
Senior Lecturer in Medical Education, University of York

Helen Perry MRCOG
Clinical Research Fellow in Obstetrics and Gynaecology, Fetal Medicine Unit, St George's University of London, London

Neil Pugh MSc PhD FInstP CPhys
Consultant Medical Physicist and Head of Ultrasound Physics, University of Cardiff School of Medicine, Cardiff

Taslima Rashid MRCP DipGU-M
Specialty Registrar in Genitourinary Medicine and HIV, 10 Hammersmith Broadway, Chelsea and Westminster Hospital, London

Michael Rayment MA MRCP DipGUM DipHIV
Consultant in Sexual Health and HIV Medicine, 10 Hammersmith Broadway, Chelsea and Westminster Hospital, London

Philip Rice BSc FRCPath
Consultant Virologist, Department of Medical Microbiology, Norfolk and Norwich University Hospital, Norwich

Amy Shacaluga MRCOG
Specialist Registrar in Obstetrics and Gynaecology, University Hospital of Wales, Cardiff

Andrew Sizer BSc MPH MD PhD FRCOG FHEA
Consultant in Reproductive Medicine and Surgery, Royal Shrewsbury Hospital, Shrewsbury and Senior Lecturer, Keele University School of Medicine

Rosemary Townsend MRCOG
Specialist Registrar in Obstetrics and Gynaecology, St George's University of London, London

Archana Vasireddy MRCOG
Clinical Fellow, Early Pregnancy and Gynaecology Assessment Unit, King's College Hospital, London

Josefa E. O. Vella MSc FRCPath
Consultant Gynaecological Pathologist, Birmingham Women's Hospital, Birmingham

Kugajeevan Vigneswaran MRCOG
Specialist Registrar in Obstetrics and Gynaecology, King's College Hospital, London

Ayona Wijemanne BMedSci MRCOG MSc DCRM
Consultant in Obstetrics and Maternal Medicine, St George's Hospital, London

Physiology of Pregnancy and Labour

Asma Khalil

Contents

- Physiology of pregnancy (cardiovascular, respiratory, renal, gastro-intestinal, liver and haematological systems)
- Physiology of onset of parturition, myometrial contractility and cervical dilatation
- Physiology of the third stage of labour
- Lactation and uterine involution

The Cardiovascular System

The cardiovascular changes are illustrated in Figs. 1.1a and 1.1b and Table 1.1.

- Plasma volume ↑ from 2600 ml to 3800 ml
    - Early in pregnancy (6–8 wk)
    - No further ↑ after 32 wk
- Red cell mass ↑ from 1400 ml to 1650–1800 ml
    - Steady ↑ until term
    - Haematocrit and haemoglobin concentration ↓

- Cardiac output (CO) ↑ 40% from 4.5 l/min to ~ 6 l/min
    - Early in pregnancy
    - Plateau at 24–30 wk
    - ↓ to pre-pregnancy level after delivery (variable time)
- Stroke volume ↑ (early)
- Heart rate (HR) ↑ 10% from 80 bpm to 90 bpm (late)
- Supine hypotensive syndrome: If a pregnant woman in the third trimester lies supine, the gravid uterus may compress the inferior vena cava against her spine, impeding venous return which leads to a fall in cardiac output. She may experience a marked fall in blood pressure and may feel faint, dizzy and nauseous. This might also reduce the uterine blood flow, potentially leading to fetal distress in labour. This is known as supine hypotensive syndrome; it is quickly relieved if the woman moves to the lateral position. We also tend to position the mother in a

(a) Maternal Intravascular Volume Changes

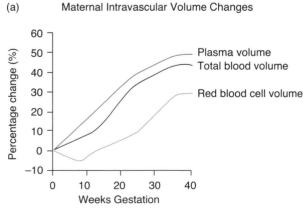

(b) Maternal Cardiovascular Changes

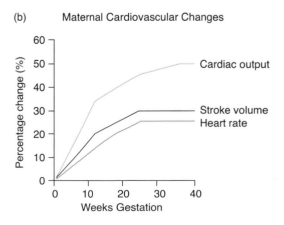

Figure 1.1a Maternal intravascular volume changes
Figure 1.1b Maternal cardiovascular changes

Table 1.1 Maternal cardiovascular changes

	Changes in pregnancy
Blood volume	+30%
Plasma volume	+45%
Red blood cell volume	+20–30%
Cardiac output	+40%
Stroke volume	+ 30%
Heart rate	+10%
Systolic blood pressure	−5 mmHg
Diastolic blood pressure	−10 mmHg
Peripheral resistance	↓
Oxygen consumption	+ 30–50 mL per minute
pCO_2	Falls to 31 mmHg

left lateral position during Caesarean section until delivery for the same reason.

- Oxygen consumption ↑ extra 30–50 ml/min
- Alteration in regional blood flow
  - Uterus
  - Kidney
  - Skin
  - Breasts
  - Skeletal muscles
- During pregnancy, the increase in ventilation is greater than the increase in oxygen consumption. Therefore, the arterio-venous oxygen gradient ↓
- At term, the distribution of the ↑ in CO (1.5 l/min):
  - Uterus 400 ml/min
  - Kidney 300 ml/min
  - Skin 500 ml/min
  - 300 ml/min to gastrointestinal tract (GI), breasts and others
- Early in pregnancy, the extra blood supply shifts mainly to the skin and breasts
- The peripheral vascular resistance ↓
- From 8 to 36 weeks
  - Systolic BP ↓ 5 mmHg
  - Diastolic BP ↓ 10 mmHg
- Other factors which influence the blood pressure include maternal position, uterine contractions, drugs which affect the vascular tone or the cardiac function.

- ECG changes in pregnancy:
  - HR ↑ 10–15%
  - Left axis deviation 15°
  - Inverted T-wave in lead III
  - Q in lead III and AVF
  - Non-specific ST changes
- ECG changes in pregnancy are secondary to:
  - Left ventricular hypertrophy and dilatation
  - No change in the contractility
  - Upward displacement of the diaphragm
  - The apex is shifted anterior and to the left

The Respiratory System

The cardiovascular changes are illustrated in Fig. 1.2.

The lung volumes in a non-pregnant normal individual are shown in Fig. 1.3. These include the tidal

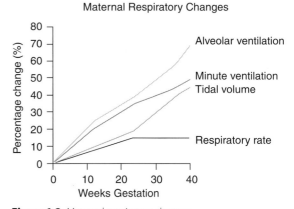

Figure 1.2 Maternal respiratory changes

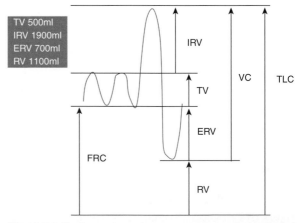

Figure 1.3 The lung volumes in a non-pregnant normal individual

volume (TV), inspiratory reserve volume (IRV), expiratory reserve volume (ERV), residual volume (RV), total lung capacity (TLC), vital capacity (VC) and functional residual capacity (FRC).

- Ventilation ↑ by 40% (from the first trimester)
- Progesterone stimulates respiratory centre both directly (stimulates the respiratory centre) and indirectly (reduce the threshold of the respiratory centre to carbon dioxide)
- Progesterone is a bronchodilator
- Breathing is more diaphragmatic than thoracic
- Airway resistance ↓
- Tidal volume ↑, not respiratory rate
- No change in the vital capacity
- Residual volume ↓ 200 ml
- Expiratory reserve volume ↓
- Both progressively ↓ (by 20% at term)
- IRV ↓ early and ↑ late in pregnancy
- The total lung capacity ↓ 200 ml
- No change in forced expiratory volume 1 (FEV$_1$) or peak flow rate
- Lung compliance is unaffected
- Chest compliance ↓ especially in lithotomy
- 70% of pregnant women experience subjective dyspnoea
- In view of the fact that pregnancy is a pro-coagulant state, the risk of pulmonary embolism is increased
- The oxygen consumption ↑ (50 ml/min at term)
  - Fetus 20 ml/min
  - ↑ CO 6 ml/min
  - ↑ renal work 6 ml/min
  - ↑ metabolic rate 18 ml/min

The changes in the lung volumes during pregnancy in comparison to those in a non-pregnant individual are illustrated in Fig. 1.4. Table 1.2 demonstrates the difference in ventilation in pregnancy, labour and the non-pregnant state.

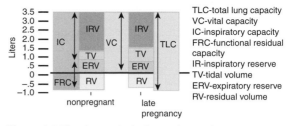

Figure 1.4 The changes in the lung volumes during pregnancy in comparison to those in a non-pregnant individual

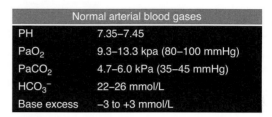

Normal arterial blood gases	
PH	7.35–7.45
PaO$_2$	9.3–13.3 kpa (80–100 mmHg)
PaCO$_2$	4.7–6.0 kPa (35–45 mmHg)
HCO$_3^-$	22–26 mmol/L
Base excess	–3 to +3 mmol/L

Figure 1.5 The normal range of the arterial blood gases

The normal range of the arterial blood gases (ABG) is shown in Fig. 1.5.

- P$_{CO2}$ ↓ to 31 mmHg
- PaO$_2$ ↑ to 14 kPa during the third trimester and then falls to <13.5 kPa at term (↑ CO unable to compensate ↑ oxygen consumption)
- HCO$_3^-$ ↓
- Na ↓
- Osmolarity ↓ 10 mmol/l

A suggested algorithm for the interpretation of the arterial blood gas (ABG) is shown in Fig. 1.6.

The Urinary System

- The kidney size ↑ during pregnancy (1 cm length)
- The ureters become dilated due to:
  - Progesterone is a smooth muscle relaxant
  - Pressure by the gravid uterus

Table 1.2 Ventilation in pregnancy and labour

	Pregnancy	Labour	Non-pregnant
Respiratory rate [per min]	15	22–70	12
Tidal volume [ml]	480–680	650–2000	450
PaCo$_2$ [kPa] (mmHg)	4.1 (31)	2–2.7 (15–20)	5.3 (40)
PaO$_2$ [kPa] (mmHg)	14 (105)	13.5–14.4 (101–108)	13.3 (100)

Table 1.3 The renal function in pregnancy compared to the non-pregnant state

Plasma level	Non-pregnant	Pregnant
Creatinine [micromol per litre]	73	50–73
Urea [mmol per litre]	4.3	2.3–4.3
Urate [mmol per litre]	0.2–26	0.15–0.35
Bicarbonate [mmol per litre]	22–26	18–26

How to interpret ABG?

1. **Assess pH**
2. **Determine respiratory involvement**

acidotic (<7.35) normal (7.35–7.45) alkalotic (>7.45)
PaCO$_2$:
Normal: 35–45 mmHg (4.6–6 kPa)
Respiratory acidosis: >45 mmHg (>6 kPa)
Respiratory alkalosis: <35 mmHg (<4.6 kPa)
HCO$_3$$^-$
Normal: 22–26 mEq/L
Metabolic acidosis: <22 mEq/L
Metabolic alkalosis: >26 mEq/L

3. **Determine metabolic involvement**

BE (Base Excess):
Normal: −2 to +2 mmol/L
Metabolic acidosis: <−2 mmol/L
Mild	−4 to −6
Moderate	−6 to −9
Marked	−9 to −13
Severe	to <−13

Metabolic alkalosis: > +2 mmol/L
Severe	> +13
Marked	9 to 13
Moderate	6 to 9
Mild	4 to 6

4. **Assess for compensation**
5. **Further analysis in cases of METABOLIC ACIDOSIS**

Anion gap $= Na^+ - [CL^- + HCO_3^-]$
Normal anion gap: 12 mmol/L (10–14 mmol/L)
Normal anion gap (hyperchloremic) metabolic acidosis
Increased anion gap metabolic acidosis

Figure 1.6 A suggested algorithm for the interpretation of arterial blood gases

- These changes lead to pregnant women being prone to urinary tract infection
- The renal blood flow ↑ from 1.2 l/min to 1.5 l/min (from the first trimester)
- The glomerular filtration rate (GFR) ↑ to 140–170 ml/min
- Both the renal blood flow and the GFR are 50–60% higher at term
- The blood urea level ↓ from 4.3 to 3.1 mmol/l
- The creatinine serum level ↓ from 73 to 47 μmol/l
- Both the urate and HCO$_3$$^-$ ↓
- Mild glycosuria and proteinuria
- The plasma osmolarity ↓ due to the effect of:
  - Progesterone
  - Renin-angiotensin-aldosterone pathway

Table 1.3 demonstrates the renal function in pregnancy compared to the non-pregnant state.

The Gastrointestinal Tract

The following changes are seen during pregnancy:

- Gastric relaxation
- Delayed gastric emptying
- Relaxation of the gastro-oesophageal sphincter
- Reflux of gastric acid
  - 80% of pregnant women experience heartburn at term
- Pregnant women are prone to gastric aspiration
- Slower bowel peristalsis; therefore, constipation is common in pregnancy

- Changes affecting the liver
  - Alkaline phosphatase ↑ 3 times the normal level (produced from the placenta)
  - Cholecystokinin release ↓
  - Gall bladder contractility ↓
  - Pregnant women are prone to gallstones
- The following occurs in obstetric cholestasis:
  - Interaction between inherited and acquired abnormalities in bile salt transporters
  - Itching in pregnancy
  - ↑ liver enzymes and bile salts
  - Similar reaction to the combined oral contraceptive pill
  - Associated with intrauterine death and fetal distress in labour

The daily requirements of a number of vitamins are shown in Table 1.4.

The Haematological System

The following changes are seen in pregnancy:

- ↑ erythropoiesis from early pregnancy (due to ↑ erythropoietin and placental lactogen)
- Physiological anaemia due to the fact that the increase in the plasma volume is more than the increase in the red cell volume

- WBC ↑ and peaks after delivery. This rise is primarily in neutrophils.
- The effect of pregnancy on the platelet count is debated, but in some women, there may be a modest decline by term, perhaps by as much as 25%. This fall is believed to be due to increased destruction of platelets not caused by immune factors (as happens in gestational thrombocytopenia).
- ↑ iron demand
  - Total requirement 700–1400 mg extra
  - Overall requirement 4 mg/day (from 2.8 mg/day in non-pregnant to 6.6 mg/day by the end of pregnancy)
- The normal range of the ferritin level in the maternal serum is 15–300 µg/l (considered as an indicator of the iron stores)
- ↑ iron absorption (erythroid hyperplasia)
- The amount absorbed depends on
  - Iron stores
  - Dietary content
  - Iron supplements
- Evidence that iron absorption ↑ in the latter half of pregnancy
- Still not enough for the needs in pregnancy and puerperium
- Iron deficiency anaemia

Table 1.4 The daily requirements of a number of vitamins

Vitamin	Non-pregnant woman	Pregnant woman	Lactation
A (µg)	800	1000	1200
B$_1$ (mg)	1	1.3	1.3
B$_2$ (mg)	1.5	1.8	2
Niacin (mg)	15	20	20
B$_6$ (mg)	2	2.5	2.5
Pantothenic acid (mg)	5	10	10
B$_{12}$ (mg)	2	3	3
Folic acid (µg)	200	500	400
C (mg)	30	60	80
D (µg)	10	10	10
E (mg)	10	12	11
K	None	None	None

Table 1.5 A list of the clotting factors

I Fibrinogen	VIII Anti-hemophilic factor A
II Prothrombin	IX Anti-hemophilic factor B or Christmas factor
III Tissue factor	X Stuart-Prower factor
IV Calcium	XI Plasma thromboplastin antecedent
V Proaccelerin (labile factor)	XII Hageman factor
VII Proconvertin (stable factor)	XIII Fibrin-stabilizing factor

	Non-pregnant Adult	First Trimester	Second Trimester	Third Trimester
PT(sec)	12.7 - 15.4	9.7 - 13.5	9.5 - 13.4	9.6 - 12.9
APTT(sec)	26.3 - 39.4	24.3 - 38.9	24.2 - 38.1	24.7 - 35.0
Platelet (x 10^9/L)	165 - 415	174 - 391	155 - 409	146 - 429

Figure 1.7 The normal range of the coagulation screening

- Commonest haematological problem in pregnancy
- Symptoms: dyspnoea, tiredness, faintness (which overlap with common symptoms of pregnancy)
- Serum iron <12 µmol/l
- Total iron-binding capacity (TIBC) saturation < 15%
- Haemostasis in pregnancy
  - ↑ coagulation factors, all except XI and XIII (from the first trimester)
    - VII
    - VIII
    - X
    - Fibrinogen
      - ↑ erythrocyte sedimentation rate (ESR)
      - The level reaches double of the non-pregnant level near the end of the pregnancy
- A list of the clotting factors is shown in Table 1.5.
- ↑ platelet production but count ↓ (dilution)
- Platelet function remains normal
- Routine coagulation screening is essentially normal (Fig. 1.7)
- The fibrinolytic system
  - Remains low in labour
  - Returns to normal within one hour of delivery of the placenta
- Evidence that the inhibition of fibrinolysis is mediated through the placenta (plasminogen activator inhibitor 2)
- What stops bleeding after delivery of the placenta?
  - Uterine contraction
  - Pro-coagulant state during pregnancy
  - Fibrin mesh covering the placental site

Implications of Maternal Physiological Changes on Therapeutic Drug Administration

Absorption of drugs from the gastrointestinal tract may be impaired by:

- Gastric stasis
- Poor gut motility
- Lower gastric pH (for some drugs)

The increase in plasma volume means that the volume of distribution of the drug increases, so the concentrations may be lower than expected. This is particularly important in women taking antiepileptic drugs or thyroxine. Because of the increased glomerular filtration rate, excretion of drugs mainly excreted by the kidneys will be accelerated. These changes often require doses of a drug given during pregnancy to be adjusted.

Physiology of Lactation

- Fourteen days' exposure to oestrogen followed by stimulation by prolactin is enough to establish milk production.
- Prolactin is a long chain polypeptide hormone and is essential for successful lactation.
- In early pregnancy, there is hyperplasia of the alveolar cells and lactiferous ducts, followed in later pregnancy by alveolar cell hypertrophy and the initiation of secretion. These changes are stimulated by the increased levels of prolactin and human placental lactogen (HPL).
- During pregnancy, the high levels of oestrogen and progesterone hold this process in check, full milk production achieved only after delivery, when progesterone and oestrogen levels fall rapidly.
- Milk production averages 500–1000 ml per day and is highly dependent on continued suckling (which causes the release of both prolactin and oxytocin).

- In women who do not suckle, milk production gradually falls and may persist for 3–4 weeks postpartum.
- In breast-feeding mothers, equilibrium is reached after around 3 weeks.
- Mothers who are breast-feeding twins produce twice as much milk, i.e. ≥ 2 litres/day.

The Suckling Stimulus

- The suckling stimulus sends afferent impulses to the hypothalamus, which leads to a surge of prolactin release.
- This surge reaches a peak around 30 minutes after the baby is put to the breast and gradually declines to basal levels by 120 minutes.
- The control of prolactin release from the anterior pituitary is primarily via prolactin inhibitory factors (PIF) from the hypothalamus which are secreted into the pituitary portal blood system.
- The most important PIF is dopamine. Therefore, dopamine agonists, such as bromocriptine and cabergoline, can be used in the early puerperium to suppress milk production.
- Conversely, dopamine antagonists such as metoclopramide increase prolactin levels and are sometimes used in breast-feeding women to stimulate milk production.
- Thyrotropin-releasing hormone (TRH) may also play a role in stimulating prolactin production.
- After the sixth postpartum week, both basal prolactin levels and the peak level following suckling gradually decline; the greater the frequency and duration of suckling, the slower the decline.
- Suckling also stimulates oxytocin (octapeptide) release through afferent impulses to specialised neurons in the supraoptic and paraventricular nuclei of the hypothalamus.
- The release is from the posterior pituitary.
- The release of oxytocin, which typically occurs in short, one-minute bursts, may begin even before the baby is put to the breast (neuroendocrine reflex can also be initiated by the mother hearing her baby cry or even thinking about breast-feeding).
- Oxytocin binds to specific receptors on the myoepithelial cells which surround the alveolar (milk-producing) cells in the breasts, and which are longitudinally arranged in the walls of the milk ducts.

- Contraction of these myoepithelial cells forces the milk into the ducts; contraction of the longitudinally arranged cells in the duct walls causes them to dilate, allowing milk to flow more easily toward the nipple.
- Both prolactin and oxytocin are necessary for successful breast-feeding; prolactin stimulates the *production* of milk while oxytocin stimulates its *ejection/let down.*

The Composition of Breast Milk

The composition of breast milk is listed in Table 1.6.

- After delivery, the colostrum (or early milk) has a high concentration of protein relative to the concentration of lactose.
- The concentration of lactose ↑ sharply and the concentration of protein ↓ over the following few days.
- The main reason for this ↓ in protein concentration is dilution (in order to maintain ionic equilibrium, water is drawn into the breast, causing an ↑ in milk volume), and the total amount of protein in the milk is relatively unchanged.
- The main carbohydrate in human milk is lactose. In the baby's intestine, it is broken down by the enzyme lactase into galactose and glucose.
- 40% of the protein in human milk is casein, compared with 80% of cow's milk. Other proteins include immunoglobulins and lactoferrin.
- Triglycerides are the main fat found in milk and are its most variable component, which means that the estimated energy content of 75 kcal/100 mL is only an approximation.
- Fat also carries the fat-soluble vitamins: A, D, E and K.
- Vitamin D deficiency can lead to rickets

Table 1.6 The composition of the breast milk

Energy (kcal/100 mL)	75
Protein (g/100 mL)	1.1
Casein (%)	40
Whey protein (%)	60
Lactose (g/100 mL)	6.8
Fat (g/100 mL)	4.5
Sodium (mmol)	7
Chloride (mmol)	11

- Vitamin K deficiency can lead to haemorrhagic disease of the newborn.
- Compared with cow's milk, human milk has approximately one-third the concentrations of sodium and chloride. This is advantageous in babies with diarrhoea because a high solute load can exacerbate diarrhoea.
- There is little iron in breast milk.
- The major immunoglobulin in breast milk is IgA, with smaller amounts of IgM and IgG.
- The IgA in breast milk is poorly absorbed so most stays in the baby's intestinal tract where it protects against infection. When a mother encounters a specific pathogen in her own GI tract, plasma cells migrate from her gut to breast where they release into breast milk a specific IgA against that pathogen, thus protecting her baby.
- The composition of the breast milk varies from woman to woman, over time in an individual woman and even differs between the beginning and end of the same feed.
- The most important factor is the time postpartum, suggesting that the milk is adapted in a very sensitive way to the changing needs of the baby.
- Any statements about the composition of human breast milk are at best averages.

Calorie Intake Required for Breast-Feeding

A breast-feeding woman requires 2950 kcal a day.

The recommended daily calorie intake is 2700 kcal (2200 kcal for the non-lactating non-pregnancy requirement plus 500 kcal toward the energy requirement of the milk).

An extra 250 kcal per day should come from the maternal fat stores.

Pregnancy during Breast-Feeding

If a woman conceives during lactation, the rapidly rising levels of oestrogen and progesterone will suppress milk production, despite the effects of the baby's suckling.

High prolactin levels during breast-feeding tend to suppress ovulation and therefore cause amenorrhoea.

Breast-feeding is not a reliable form of contraception; at the end of a year of exclusive breast-feeding, 10% of women who do not use another form of contraception will have fallen pregnant.

Uterine Involution

- Immediately after delivery of the placenta: the uterus weighs around 900 g
- By seven days postpartum: the uterus weighs half that
- By six weeks: almost returned to its pre-pregnancy size and weight of around 100 g
- Uterine water, weight, muscle, protein and collagen all ↓ in the same proportions
- Result from the rapid withdrawal of placental hormones after delivery
- Three days postpartum: the superficial decidual layer becomes necrotic (shed with the lochia)
- Within a week: the uterine cavity has a new endometrial layer, with the exception of the placental bed; this takes around three weeks to establish an endometrial cover
- The lochia gradually ↓ over 3–6 weeks, changing in turn from red (lochia rubra) to pink (lochia serosa) to yellowish-white (lochia alba)

The Third Stage of Labour

- The time from delivery of the baby until delivery of the placenta and membranes
- Soon after delivery of the baby, the uterus has a strong and sustained contraction.
    - ↓ the surface area of the placental bed, thus shearing off the placenta
    - Helps to control bleeding from the vessels of the placental bed
- It is likely that prostaglandin F2α play a major role here, as oxytocin levels do not change significantly during this time.

The Onset of Labour, Myometrial Contractility and Cervical Dilatation

- The precise mechanism of the onset and maintenance of labour is still poorly understood.
- During pregnancy, myometrial quiescence is maintained by pro-pregnancy factors (mainly progesterone).
- Progesterone suppresses the formation of myometrial gap junctions and the effect of interleukin 8 (which causes cervical ripening).

- Progesterone also decreases uterine sensitivity to oxytocin.
- Antiprogesterones such as mifepristone (RU4A6) cause cervical ripening and increase myometrial contractility.
- Catecholamines and relaxin also play a role in the maintenance of uterine quiescence.
- During the third trimester, maternal oestrogen and corticotrophin-releasing hormone (CRH) gradually ↑. Oestradiol ↑ the concentration of oxytocin receptors in the myometrium and also ↑ oxytocin synthesis in the uterus.
- CRH increases prostaglandin synthesis and may stimulate myometrial contractility.
- The concentration of myometrial gap junctions increases as labour approaches.
- Oestrogen promotes the formation of gap junctions.
- CRH also promotes an inflammatory-type mechanism by increasing the expression of inflammatory cytokines, such as interleukin 1β and interleukin 8, and cyclo-oxygenase type II (Cox-2).
- It is possible that there is a 'functional withdrawal' of progesterone.
  - It happens only locally within the fetal membranes.
  - Close to term, the dominant progesterone receptor within the uterus changes from type 1 to type 2.
- Nitric oxide does not play a significant role in the onset of labour.
- Neither does oxytocin; there is no significant rise in maternal oxytocin concentration immediately prior to labour (or indeed during labour).
- A marked increase in oxytocin *receptors* in the myometrium as term approaches, so it seems certain that oxytocin plays an important role in labour, probably in combination with prostaglandins.
- Nevertheless, oxytocin does not seem to be the trigger for the onset of labour.
- The fetus also secretes some oxytocin (the concentration in the umbilical artery is twice that in the umbilical vein), but it is not certain if this plays a role in labour.
- It is possible that the fetus triggers labour through increased cortisol release which can stimulate placental CRH synthesis.

- There is a rapid rise in the activity of Cox-2 and other inflammatory cytokines at the onset of labour, leading some to compare labour to an inflammatory process.
- Increased Cox-2 activity leads to an increase in prostaglandin synthesis.
- The amnion and chorion secrete primarily PGE2 while the decidua favours PGF-2α.
- Prostaglandin synthase inhibitors such as indomethacin may thus be used in the management of preterm labour.
- Prostaglandins act on the myometrium in the uterine body to cause contractions.
- Toward the end of pregnancy and in early labour, under the influence of prostaglandins and interleukin 8 (and perhaps in combination with relaxin and oestrogen), neutrophils are attracted into the cervix, where they release collagenase. This leads to gradual proteolysis of the collagen fibres in the cervix, leading to cervical ripening.
- Contraction of the myometrium results from the interaction of actin and myosin. This interaction is controlled by a calcium modulated protein kinase. Communication between myometrial cells through gap junctions facilitates the coordinated contraction of the uterus.
- Drugs which reduce available calcium, such as beta-agonists (e.g. ritodrine, salbutamol), thus cause uterine relaxation.
- Magnesium sulphate, which inhibits calcium influx into myometrial cells, inhibits the action of myosin light chain kinase, thus causing uterine relaxation.
- Calcium channel blockers also inhibit calcium influx through the cell membrane and are used for tocolysis.
- Once labour has started, there are multiple feedback mechanisms which further increase prostaglandin and cytokine activity; this process is currently poorly understood.

The organs and the mechanisms involved in the physiology of labour, as well as the feto-maternal interaction, are shown in Figs. 1.8 and 1.9.

Further Reading

1. Chapter 31: Physiology of Pregnancy and Labour. *MRCOG Part One*. Fiander and Thilaganathan. RCOG 2010.

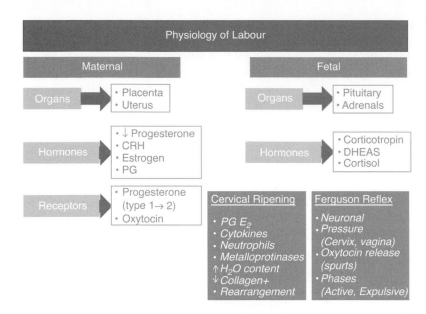

Figure 1.8 The organs and the mechanisms involved in the physiology of labour

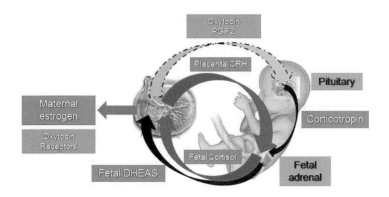

Figure 1.9 The feto-maternal interaction involved in the physiology of labour

2. Williams DJ. Physiology of Healthy Pregnancy. In: Warrell DA, Cox TM, Firth JD, editors. *Oxford Textbook of Medicine*, 4th ed. Oxford: Oxford University Press, 2003. pp. 383–385.

3. Buchan AS, Sharwood-Smith GH. Physiological Changes in Pregnancy. In: Buchan AS, Sharwood-Smith GH, editors. *The Simpson Handbook of Obstetric Anaesthesia*. Edinburgh: Albamedia on Behalf of the Royal College of Surgeons of Edinburgh, 1999

4. de Swiet M, Poston L, Williams D. Physiology. In: de Swiet M, Chamberlain G, Bennett P, editors. *Basic Science in Obstetrics and Gynaecology, A Textbook for MRCOG Part 1*, 3rd ed. Churchill Livingstone: Elsevier, 2002. pp. 173–231.

5. Hunter S, Robson SC. Adaptation of the maternal heart in pregnancy. *Br Heart J.*1992;**68**:540–3.

6. de Swiet M. *Medical Disorders in Obstetric Practice*, 4th ed. Oxford: Blackwell Publishing, 2002.

7. Coustan DR. Maternal Physiology. In: Coustan DR, Haning RV, Singer DB, editors. *Human Reproduction: Growth and Development*. Boston: Little, Brown, 1995. pp. 161–81.

8. Cunningham FG, MacDonald PC, Gant NF, Leveno KJ, Gilstrap LC. Maternal adaptations to pregnancy. In: *Williams Obstetrics*, 19th ed. Norwalk: Appleton and Lange, 1989. pp. 209–46.

9. Catherine NP. *Obstetric Medicine*, 3rd ed. London: Informa Healthcare, 2006.

10. Burrow G, Ferris T. *Medical Complications During Pregnancy*, 4th ed. Philadelphia: Saunders, 1984.

11. Cruikshank DP, Hays PM. Maternal Physiology in Pregnancy. In: Gabbe SG, Niebyl JR, Simpson JL, editors. *Obstetrics Normal and Problem Pregnancies*, 2nd ed. New York: Churchill-Livingstone, 1991. pp. 125–46.

12. Chamberlain G and Pipkin FB. *Clinical Physiology in Obstetrics*, 3rd ed. Oxford: Blackwell Science, 1998.

Single Best Answer Questions

1. What is the physiological change in total lung capacity in pregnancy?

   a. Decreased by 100 ml
   b. Decreased by 200 ml
   c. Increased by 100 ml
   d. Increased by 200 ml
   e. No change

2. What is the change in forced expiratory volume (FEV1) in pregnancy?

   a. +10%
   b. +20%
   c. −10%
   d. −20%
   e. No change

3. Which lung volume is increased in pregnancy?

   a. Expiratory reserve volume
   b. Inspiratory reserve volume
   c. Respiratory dead volume
   d. Tidal volume
   e. Total lung capacity

4. Which coagulation factors are not increased during pregnancy?

   a. III, IV
   b. IX, X
   c. V, VII
   d. XI, XII
   e. XI, XIII

5. What is the increase in oxygen consumption in pregnancy at term?

   a. 10 ml/min
   b. 20 ml/min
   c. 50 ml/min
   d. 100 ml/min
   e. 200 ml/min

6. At what gestational age does the maximum physiological anaemia occur?

   a. 12 weeks
   b. 24 weeks
   c. 32 weeks
   d. 38 weeks
   e. 42 weeks

7. How many multiples of the normal range is alkaline phosphatase increased in pregnancy?

   a. No increase
   b. 3
   c. 8
   d. 10
   e. 12

Chapter 2

Fetal Physiology

Helen Perry and Asma Khalil

This chapter will be split into two parts in line with the exam curriculum and blueprint:

1. A system-by-system review of fetal physiology throughout pregnancy and its development with fetal growth.
2. Fetal physiology, in late pregnancy and during labour, including methods of assessment of fetal wellbeing.

Part 1: Fetal Physiology throughout Pregnancy and Its Development with Fetal Growth

1.1 Cardiovascular Physiology

- The myocardium grows by hyperplasia until birth and by hypertrophy after birth.
- Fetal myocytes have less contractile tissue than adult myocytes (30% vs. 60%) and there are less fetal myofibrils, with those present arranged randomly, rather than as parallel fibres. The fetal heart is also less compliant (stiffer) than the adult heart. These factors mean that stroke volume is maximal with little capacity to be increased. An increase in heart rate is therefore required to increase cardiac output.
- The adult heart uses long-chain fatty acids as the main source of fuel, but the fetus lacks the enzyme required to transport them into the mitochondria and thus uses lactate and carbohydrate as its primary fuel source instead.

Fetal Circulation

- The fetal circulation differs from the adult circulation in that it is arranged in a parallel rather than a series system due to the presence of three shunts (ductus venosus, foramen ovale and ductus arteriosus), which close after birth.
- Before birth, the pulmonary circulation is at high resistance owing to compression of the capillaries

by collapsed lung and the vasoactive effects of the low PO_2. Conversely, systemic circulation is at low resistance owing to the large placental bed. These factors, along with the presence of shunts, allow blood to be diverted from the lungs to the placenta.

- Oxygenated blood leaves the placenta via the umbilical vein and enters the liver. Here, 20–30% of umbilical blood is shunted through the ductus venosus to the inferior vena cava (IVC). The remainder supplies the hepatic-portal system.
- The ductus venosus has a narrow diameter, causing acceleration in blood velocity. This high-velocity blood flow allows preferential streaming of the oxygenated blood by exerting pressure on the flap valve of the second shunt, the foramen ovale. The highly oxygenated blood flows anteriorly and to the left within the IVC.
- The foramen ovale is a communication between the right and left atria and is formed from the overlap of the septum secundum over the septum primum. High pressure in the right atria ensures the valve is maintained open allowing right-to-left flow. As the blood enters the right atrium from the IVC it is divided into two streams by the crista dividens; the high-velocity oxygenated blood is shunted left, through the foramen ovale into the left atrium and the lower velocity, less oxygenated blood is shunted to the right, mixing with blood from the superior vena cava and the coronary sinus.
- This results in the blood in the left ventricle being more highly-oxygenated that the blood in the right ventricle.
- Blood from the left ventricle is pumped into the ascending aorta. 90% flows to the coronary arteries, left carotid and subclavian veins. 10% flows to the descending aorta.
- Blood from the right ventricle is pumped through the third shunt; the ductus arteriosus. This allows blood to bypass the lungs, with only about 13% of

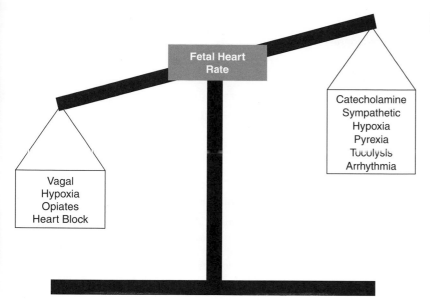

Figure 2.1 The fetal heart rate modulators

the cardiac output entering the pulmonary circulation. Blood from the ductus arteriosus enters the descending aorta, from which a third returns to the placenta via the umbilical arteries.

- The patency of the ductus arteriosus is maintained by vasodilatory effects of prostaglandins, prostacyclins and reduced fetal oxygen tension.

Fetal Heart Rate

- The fetal heart rate (FHR) is determined by depolarisation of the SA node, under sympathetic influence and inhibited by parasympathetic stimulation.
- Other factors that influence the fetal heart rate are epinephrine and norepinephrine from the adrenal medulla, maternal drugs, temperature and autonomic control from baroreceptors and chemoreceptors, which are sensitive to changes in blood pressure and partial oxygen pressures.
- The normal FHR is between 100 and 160 bpm and declines with increasing gestation owing to the maturation of the parasympathetic nervous system.
- The autonomic nervous system is also responsible for beat-to-beat variability within the FHR, defined as fluctuation in the FHR of at least 2 cycles per minute. Normal variability is considered between 5 and 25 bpm. Variability is reduced in hypoxia as well as fetal sleep, prematurity, CNS depressant drugs (including magnesium sulphate) and underlying neurological abnormality.

- Accelerations in FHR are defined as a rise of 15 bpm for at least 15 seconds. They are usually caused by fetal movement or stimulation and reflect a non-hypoxic fetus.
- Decelerations in FHR are defined as a decrease of 15 bpm for at least 15 seconds and are classified as early, late or variable. These are described in more detail in part 2.
- The modulators of the fetal heart rate are shown in Fig. 2.1.

1.2 Respiratory Physiology

- The five stages of lung development are summarised in Table 2.1.
- Fetal breathing movements start from the end of the first trimester and increase in strength and frequency with advancing gestation. They are increased in acidosis and with hyperglycaemia (e.g. after maternal meal). They are decreased in hypoxic states and after consumption of alcohol or sedative drugs. Breathing movements are crucial for adequate lung development and ablation of the phrenic nerve in animal studies resulted in lung hypoplasia.
- Lung fluid is mainly formed of alveolar epithelial cell secretions. It forms a small proportion of amniotic fluid. Lung hypoplasia can occur if levels of lung fluid or amniotic fluid are decreased.

Table 2.1 Stages of lung development

Stage	Gestation	Developments
Embryonic	0–7 weeks	Main bronchi and bronchopulmonary segments form
Pseudoglandular	7–17 weeks	Branching of airways and blood vessels
Canalicular	17–27 weeks	Formation of acini (gas-exchange areas)
Saccular	28–36 weeks	Enlargement of peripheral airways, thinning of airway walls to form peripheral sacs
Alveolar	36 weeks- 2 years	Formation of definitive alveoli

- Surfactant is a lipoprotein produced by type II pneumocytes and has a major role in pulmonary function. Its primary function is to reduce surface tension to allow normal lung compliance and inflation. It also prevents lung collapse at the end of expiration.
- 90% of surfactant is lipid, of which 2/3 is dipalmitoylphosphatidylcholine (DPPC). The remaining 10% is composed of proteins, including surfactant proteins A–D. DPPC regulates surface tension while surfactant proteins B and C allow surfactant spread over the alveolar surfaces. Surfactant proteins A and D aid innate immunity.

1.3 Renal Physiology

- Urine production begins at 9–10 weeks, reabsorption in the Loop of Henle begins at 12 weeks, and from 16–18 weeks, fetal urine becomes the primary component of amniotic fluid. Before 16 weeks, most amniotic fluid is produced by the placenta and fetal skin.
- The fetal kidney only receives 2–3% of the cardiac output (adult kidneys receive 20%), so fluid and electrolyte balance is mainly under the control of the placenta.
- The fetal kidney has a limited ability to concentrate urine, although this increases with advancing gestation.
- From 34 weeks, the number of nephrons is similar to in adults, but they are not functionally mature until postnatal life.
- After birth, renal blood flow increases to about 10% of cardiac output by 4 days of age. Glomerular filtration rate doubles by 2 weeks of age.
- The composition of the amniotic fluid is shown in Fig. 2.2.

Clinical Significance

Reduced amniotic fluid from mid-gestation can reflect reduced urine production and is seen in fetal growth restriction.

Preterm infants are less able to maintain fluid and electrolyte balance due to their immature nephrons.

1.4 Gastrointestinal Physiology

- Swallowing movements start from 12 weeks and increase to 250 ml/day at term, meaning swallowing is an important component of amniotic fluid balance.
- Stomach motility and secretions start from 20 weeks.
- Intestinal villi begin developing at 7 weeks and are well developed by 20 weeks. Peristalsis is mature by the third trimester.
- Intestinal transport of amino acids develops at 14 weeks, glucose transport develops at 18 weeks and fatty acid absorption develops from 24 weeks.
- Meconium is present from as early as 12 weeks and slowly moves to the colon by 16 weeks. 98% of newborns pass meconium within 48 hours of birth.

1.5 Neurological Physiology

- Neurons proliferate from 8–20 weeks, with peak activity from 12–16 weeks.
- Neurons migrate from the periventricular germinal areas in a radial fashion into areas where grey matter is established. This begins at 8 weeks, and by 20 weeks the cortex has acquired the majority of neurons. In the cerebellum, proliferation and migration continue until 1 year postnatally.

Table 2.2 Fetal haematopoiesis

Period of haematopoiesis	Gestation	Features
Mesoblastic	14 days–12 weeks	In the yolk sac
Hepatic	6 weeks, peaking at 10–18 weeks	
Myeloid	8 weeks–adult life	Blood cells develop from stem cells and migrate from the yolk sac to fetal tissues, where they give rise to primitive cells, followed by definitive cells.

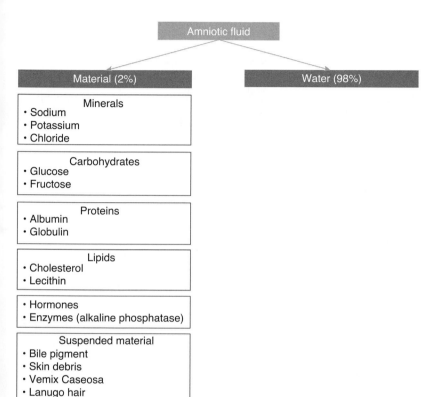

Figure 2.2 The composition of the amniotic fluid

- Synapse formation begins at 12 weeks and peaks in the third trimester.
- Myelinisation begins around 24 weeks, peaks at birth and continues throughout childhood.
- Biochemical activity in the brain is evident from 16 weeks.
- Electroencephalographic activity starts around 20 weeks and is synchronised at 26 weeks. Wake/sleep cycles are seen from 30 weeks.

1.6 Haematological Physiology

Table 2.2 outlines the stages of haematopoiesis in the fetus.

- Fetal red blood cell production is regulated by fetal erythropoietin (EPO), which is produced by the liver and kidneys and increases from 20 weeks onwards. Production is also increased in hypoxic conditions.
- Fetal white blood cells are produced in the liver from 6 weeks and are also produced in the spleen, thymus and lymphatic system.
- Platelet production occurs in the yolk sac from 6 weeks and in the liver from 8 weeks.
- The differences in adult and fetal haemoglobin are summarized in Table 2.3. The differences in O_2 affinity are due to the fact that adult haemoglobin binds with 2, 3-diphosphoglycerate (2, 3-DPG), reducing its O_2 affinity, whereas fetal haemoglobin does not bind with 2, 3-DPG.

Table 2.3 Differences between adult and fetal haemoglobin

	Adult haemoglobin (HbA)	Fetal haemoglobin (HbF)
Composition	2 alpha and 2 beta globulin chains	2 alpha and 2 gamma globulin chains
Predominance	Present from 10 weeks' gestation in small amounts, rapid increase in the third trimester, becomes predominant between birth to 12 weeks postnatally	Predominant from 10 weeks' gestation, provides 90% of haemoglobin at 32 weeks, declining to 60–80% at birth, present until 3–6 months postnatally
Oxygen affinity	P_{50}=4.8 kPa (lower O_2 affinity)	P_{50} = 3.6 kPa (higher O_2 affinity, O_2 saturation curve shifted to left)

- The immune system precursors develop in the yolk sac in the embryonic life before migrating to the liver, spleen, bone marrow and thymus.
- Lymphoid stem cells give rise to B lymphocytes (from the liver) and T cells (from the thymus). Mature B cells are present in the blood from 12 weeks and T cells from 14 weeks.
- Placental transfer of maternal IgG increases in the second trimester. IgM cannot cross the placenta.
- The fetal immune system is fairly inactive and immature until 32 weeks of gestation when production increases.
- Normal values for a term newborn: Hb 14–21 g/dl, Haematocrit 40–65%, WCC 20–40 × 10^9/L, platelets 150–400 × 10^9/L. Platelet activity is reduced in the neonate, increasing the risk of bleeding and coagulopathy.

Clinical Significance: Any increase in IgM is fetal in origin and may be due to intrauterine infection. The immature immune system is an important consideration of care for premature babies. Vitamin K is offered to all newborns to counteract the low levels.

Part 2: Fetal Physiology in Late Pregnancy and Labour

2.1 Assessment of Fetal Wellbeing during Labour

- During labour, the fetus is subjected to a prolonged period of repetitive intermittent compression and temporary reduction in placental blood flow during contractions.
- While most healthy-term fetuses have enough reserve to cope with this, there is a risk of fetal hypoxia and metabolic acidosis, and several methods have been developed to detect this based on fetal physiology.

2.1.1 Methods of Fetal Monitoring

Intermittent Auscultation

- The National Institute for Health and Care Excellence (NICE) recommends offering 'low risk' women intermittent auscultation during labour. It can be performed with a Pinard or Doppler device and is recorded as a single rate.
- Recordings should be documented every 15 minutes for 1 minute after a contraction in the first stage of labour and every 5 minutes in the second stage of labour.
- It is not possible to determine variability using intermittent auscultation. An abnormal baseline rate or the detection of decelerations warrants a cardiotocograph.

Electronic Fetal Monitoring

- NICE recommends the use of continuous CTG in any 'high-risk' labour.
- CTGs are classified using four features: baseline rate, variability, presence of accelerations and presence of decelerations. It also records the frequency of contractions.
- The NICE classification of these four features and the action recommended are displayed in Tables 2.4 and 2.5. Baseline rate, variability and accelerations were described previously.
- Early decelerations are due to head compression and characterised by being uniform in shape, size and duration. They are seen in about 5% of cases.
- Late decelerations start after the contraction has started and finish after the contraction has finished. They are not common but are indicative of fetal hypoxia and are mediated by

Table 2.4 NICE classification of CTG features

Description	Feature		
	Baseline (bpm)	Variability (bpm)	Decelerations
Normal	110–160	5–25	• None or early • Variable decelerations with no concerning characteristics* for less than 90 minutes
Non-reassuring	100–109† or 161–180	Less than 5 for 30 to 50 minutes OR More than 25 for 15 to 25 minutes	Variable decelerations with no concerning characteristics* for 90 minutes or more **OR** Variable decelerations with any concerning characteristics* in up to 50% of contractions for 30 minutes or more **OR** Variable decelerations with any concerning characteristics* in over 50% of contractions for less than 30 minutes **OR** Late decelerations in over 50% of contractions for less than 30 minutes, with no maternal or fetal clinical risk factors such as vaginal bleeding or significant meconium
Abnormal	<100 or >180	Less than 5 for more than 50 minutes OR More than 25 for more than 25 minutes OR Sinusoidal	Variable decelerations with any concerning characteristics* in over 50% of contractions for 30 minutes (or less if any maternal or fetal clinical risk factors [see above]) **OR** Late decelerations for 30 minutes (or less if any maternal or fetal clinical risk factors) **OR** Acute bradycardia, or a single prolonged deceleration lasting 3 minutes or more.

* Concerning characteristics: lasting more than 60 seconds; reduced baseline variability within the deceleration; failure to return to baseline; biphasic (W) shape; no shouldering.

† continue normal care if there is normal baseline variability and no variable or late decelerations.

chemoreceptors in response to fetal hypoxaemia, hypercarbia and acidosis.

• Variable decelerations are the most common and are due to cord compression. They are variable in size and shape. Whilst short variable decelerations are a normal response to cord compression, a widening and deepening of variable decelerations (>60 seconds long and > 60 bpm deep) is reflective of an evolving hypoxia.

Fetal Blood Sampling

• Fetal blood sampling (FBS) has been used as an additional test of fetal wellbeing for many years. It works on the principle that during hypoxia, a fetus changes from aerobic metabolism to anaerobic metabolism and produces lactic acid as a by-product. Lactate can be measured directly or pH can be measured to identify metabolic acidosis secondary to hypoxia.

• The NICE classification of FBS results are shown in Table 2.6.

Fetal Electrocardiogram (ECG)

• The ECG represents the electrical activity of the heart. It can be recorded for a fetus (>36 weeks gestation) during labour by application of a scalp electrode.

• As in an adult ECG, a waveform is produced with P, Q, R, S and T patterns. The P wave is caused by atrial depolarisation, the QRS complex is caused by ventricular depolarisation and the ST segment and the T wave represent ventricular repolarisation.

• In a hypoxic environment, there are metabolic changes that can alter the waveform, and this

Table 2.5 NICE management based on CTG interpretation

Category	Definition	Management
NORMAL	All 3 features are reassuring	• Continue CTG and normal care. Talk to the woman and her birth partner about what is happening. • If CTG was started because of concerns arising from intermittent auscultation, remove CTG after 20 minutes if there are no non-reassuring or abnormal features and no ongoing risk factors unless the woman asks to stay on continuous cardiotocography.
SUSPICIOUS	1 non-reassuring feature and 2 reassuring features (but note that if accelerations are present, fetal acidosis is unlikely)	• correct any underlying causes, such as hypotension or uterine hyperstimulation • perform a full set of maternal observations • start one or more conservative measures • inform an obstetrician or a senior midwife • document a plan for reviewing the whole clinical picture and the cardiotocography findings • talk to the woman and her birth companion(s) about what is happening and take her preferences into account.
PATHOLOGICAL	1 abnormal feature **OR** 2 non-reassuring features	• obtain a review by an obstetrician and a senior midwife • exclude acute events (for example, cord prolapse, suspected placental abruption or suspected uterine rupture) • correct any underlying causes, such as hypotension or uterine hyperstimulation • start one or more conservative measures • talk to the woman and her birth companion(s) about what is happening and take her preferences into account. • If the cardiotocograph trace is still pathological after implementing conservative measures: • obtain a further review by an obstetrician and a senior midwife • offer digital fetal scalp stimulation) and document the outcome. If the cardiotocograph trace is still pathological after fetal scalp stimulation, consider: • fetal blood sampling **or** • expediting the birth Take the woman's preferences into account.
NEED FOR URGENT INTERVENTION	Acute bradycardia or a single prolonged deceleration for 3 minutes or more	• Urgently seek obstetric help • if there has been an acute event (for example, cord prolapse, suspected placental abruption or suspected uterine rupture), expedite the birth. • correct any underlying causes, such as hypotension or uterine hyperstimulation • start one or more conservative measures • make preparations for an urgent birth • talk to the woman and her birth companion(s) about what is happening and take her preferences into account • expedite the birth if the acute bradycardia persists for 9 minutes. • If the fetal heart rate recovers at any time up to 9 minutes, reassess any decision to expedite the birth, in discussion with the woman.

Table 2.6 NICE interpretation of FBS

Lactate (mmol/L)	pH	Interpretation	Management
≤ 4.1	≥7.25	Normal	Repeat 1 hour later if CTG not improved (sooner if deteriorates)
4.2–4.8	7.21–7.24	Borderline	Repeat 30 mins later if CTG not improved
≥4.9	≤7.20	Abnormal	Immediate delivery

forms the basis of the use of fetal ECG as a means of assessing fetal wellbeing

2.1.2 Types of Hypoxia

Gradually Evolving Hypoxia

- This is seen in labour due to repeated episodes of umbilical cord occlusion, inadequate placental reserve or inadequate placental function. These changes may cause decelerations as described previously.
- There is a stepwise pattern of changes as the fetus conserves energy and oxygen. The first change is loss of accelerations. This is followed by a rise in the baseline rate in order to increase cardiac output. This is caused by a surge in catecholamine which also causes peripheral vasoconstriction to redirect blood flow (and oxygen) to the brain and heart. If oxygen requirements are not met, the fetus will prioritise perfusion of the myocardium and a loss of variability may reflect hypoxia of the autonomic nervous system. If there is no intervention, there will be a stepwise decline in FHR and eventually fetal death.

Chronic Hypoxia

- Refers to a long-standing hypoxia present before the onset of labour. The characteristic features on CTG are due to the direct effect of the chronic hypoxia on the vasomotor centre. Thus there is reduced variability and a higher baseline rate. In late chronic hypoxia, the baseline rate may be normal as the vasomotor centre is further damaged and unable to autoregulate and increase the baseline rate in response to the hypoxia. It is also common to see shallow decelerations, particularly with the onset of contractions.
- A fetus with chronic hypoxia will not withstand the further stress of labour, and deterioration will occur much quicker with rapid onset of metabolic acidosis.
- Causes include maternal conditions including diabetes, smoking and recreational drug use, fetal

growth restriction, infection, anaemia, prematurity and congenital abnormalities.

Acute Hypoxia

- This can be due to reversible (maternal hypotension, epidural top-up, uterine hyperstimulation) or non-reversible (cord prolapse, placental abruption, and scar dehiscence) causes and is usually reflected as a prolonged deceleration lasting greater than 3 minutes.
- After exclusion of a non-reversible cause, measures should be taken to resolve reversible causes and observe the response, particularly if the fetal monitoring was normal prior to the prolonged deceleration. If the baseline rate has not recovered by 9 minutes, delivery should be expedited by the safest method.

Sub-acute Hypoxia

- In order to maintain adequate perfusion of the brain and heart, the fetal heart must beat at an optimum rate to provide adequate cardiac output.
- In sub-acute hypoxia, there are repetitive decelerations, with inadequate time spent at the optimum baseline rate required to replenish oxygen and excrete carbon dioxide.

2.2 Transitional Physiological Changes around Birth

2.2.1 Cardiovascular Changes

- After birth, the systemic resistance doubles due to loss of the placenta circulation. Pulmonary vascular resistance falls as the lungs expand with inhalation of air during the first breath.
- These pressure changes dramatically reduce blood flow through the ductus arteriosus, and it closes after a couple of days of postnatal life.
- The ductus venosus closes 1–3 weeks after birth.

- The foramen ovale closes functionally with the increase in left atrial pressure and is anatomically closed by 1 year of age.

2.2.2 Respiratory Changes

- Toward term, lung fluid starts to decline.
- From the first breath, pulmonary fluid continues to be replaced by air, and most has been absorbed within 2 hours of life.

Further Reading

1. Chapter 32: Fetal Physiology. *MRCOG Part One.* Fiander and Thilaganathan. RCOG 2010.
2. *Oxford Handbook of Neonatology.* Fox, Hoque, Watts. Oxford University Press 2010.
3. NICE Intrapartum Care Guidance 2014.

Single Best Answer Questions

1. What proportion of fetal cardiac output enters the pulmonary circulation?

   a. 3%
   b. 10%
   c. 13%
   d. 20%
   e. 30%

2. Which statement is most accurate?

   a. Fetal haemoglobin binds with 2, 3-diphospho-glycerate (2, 3-DPG), increasing its O_2 affinity.
   b. Fetal haemoglobin binds with 2, 3-diphospho-glycerate (2, 3-DPG), decreasing its O_2 affinity.
   c. Adult haemoglobin binds with 2, 3-diphospho-glycerate (2, 3-DPG), increasing its O_2 affinity.
   d. Adult haemoglobin does not bind with 2, 3-diphosphoglycerate (2, 3-DPG), increasing its O_2 affinity.
   e. Fetal haemoglobin does not bind with 2, 3-diphosphoglycerate (2, 3-DPG), increasing its O_2 affinity.

3. Which of these is not a non-reassuring feature of cardiotocograph monitoring?

   a. Variable decelerations with no concerning characteristics for 90 minutes or more.
   b. A baseline rate of 100–109 bpm.
   c. Variability of more than 25 for 30 to 50 minutes.
   d. Late decelerations in over 50% of contractions for less than 30 minutes, with no maternal or fetal clinical risk factors such as vaginal bleeding or significant meconium.
   e. Variable decelerations with any concerning characteristics in more than 50% of contractions for less than 30 minutes.

4. At what stage post-natally does the ductus venosus close?

   a. With the first breath
   b. 1–3 hours
   c. Within 24 hours
   d. 1–3 days
   e. 1–3 weeks

5. Select the correct statement:

   a. 90% of surfactant is protein, of which 2/3 is dipalmitoylphosphatidylcholine (DPPC).
   b. 90% of surfactant is protein, of which 1/3 is dipalmitoylphosphatidylcholine (DPPC).
   c. 90% of surfactant is lipid, of which 1/3 is dipalmitoylphosphatidylcholine (DPPC).
   d. 90% of surfactant is lipid, of which 2/3 is dipalmitoylphosphatidylcholine (DPPC).
   e. 30 % of surfactant is lipid, of with 1/3 is dipalmitoylphosphatidylcholine (DPPC).

6. Which of these statements regarding fetal renal physiology is not correct?

   a. Before 16 weeks, most amniotic fluid is produced by the placenta and fetal skin.
   b. Urine production begins from 16 weeks.
   c. Amniotic fluid is composed of 98% water.
   d. The fetal kidney receives 2–3% of the cardiac output, which increases to 10% within 4 days of postnatal life.
   e. From 34 weeks gestation, the number of nephrons is similar to in an adult.

Acid-Base Balance

Kelvin F. Gomez

Acid-Base Terminology

Proton (H⁺)

The secret to understanding the principles of acid-base balance is hydrogen, or more specifically, a positively charged hydrogen atom that has lost its circulating electron – the proton (H^+). H^+ is an extremely reactive cation and tiny changes in its concentration can significantly affect the body's pH.

pH

This is a given value which corresponds to the 'negative logarithm to base 10 of hydrogen ion concentration' within a solution.

pH Scale

The pH scale is a numeric scale used to specify the acidity or alkalinity (basicity) of an aqueous solution. The pH scale commonly uses ranges from 0–14, with a pH equal to 7 classified as neutral, pH less than 7 classified as acid and a pH greater than 7 classified as alkali. However, as pH itself is a dimensionless concept, values less than 0 and greater than 14 are possible.

A pH of 7 = 100 nmol/l H^+

p$_a$CO$_2$ (usually written as pCO$_2$)

This is the partial pressure of carbon dioxide in arterial blood. Arterial pCO_2 has a normal range of 4.5–6.0 kPa.

Hco$_3$-

The bicarbonate ion is an anion that plays an important role in maintaining physiological homeostasis.

Acid

An acid is a substance which increases the hydrogen ion concentration when dissolved. It acts as a proton donor. Acids are characterised by a sour taste (origin of the word acid is from the Latin word for sour – *acidus*) and can turn litmus paper red.

Acidosis

This is the process by which acid is allowed to accumulate, leading to a lowered blood pH. It is said to have occurred when the blood pH falls below 7.35.

Base (Alkali)

A base is a substance that accepts protons from any proton donor. They turn litmus paper blue and are characterised by a bitter taste. They react with acids to form salts.

Alkalosis

This is the process by which the concentration of H^+ ions is reduced within blood. It is said to have occurred when the blood pH rises above 7.45.

Buffer

A buffer is a solution, consisting of a mixture of a weak acid and its conjugate base, which resists an overall change in pH, when either an acid or base is added to it.

Cation

This is any positively charged ion (+).

Anion

This is any negatively charged ion (−).

Weak and Strong Acids

A weak acid is one that incompletely dissociates, releasing only some of its protons into a solution, while a strong acid releases all of its protons into any given solution.

Metabolic Acid / Fixed Acid

A metabolic acid or fixed acid describes any acid produced in the body from sources other than CO_2. These acids are not excreted by the lungs and must be excreted by the kidneys, almost always against a concentration gradient. They are produced mainly from incomplete metabolism of carbohydrates, fats or proteins (e.g. lactic acid, sulphuric acid).

Volatile Acid

This describes any acid produced by CO_2. Carbonic acid (H_2CO_3) is the main volatile acid in acid-base metabolism. The CO_2 component of H_2CO_3 is excreted via the lungs. The rate of excretion is proportional to the ventilation rate which is controlled by pCO_2 and the respiratory centre in the medulla. The rate of alveolar ventilation is inversely related to pCO_2 and directly proportional to total body CO_2 production. Therefore, excess CO_2 can be 'blown off' by increasing the respiratory rate.

Anion Gap

Under normal circumstances, the number of cations (+) and anions (−) are in equilibrium.

Historically, blood tests measure mostly cations, with sodium (Na^+) being the primary measured cation. $HCO3^-$ and Cl^- are the primary measured anions. Adding the measured cations and anions leaves a natural gap – which reflects the unmeasured anions (e.g. albumin, lactate, phosphate).

The anion gap is calculated using the following formula:

$$Na^+ - (HCO3^- + Cl^-)$$

A normal anion gap ranges between 8–16 mmol/l.

Note: Some hospital laboratories include K^+ when calculating the anion gap. When K+ is included in the cation calculation, the normal range is 12–20 mmol/l.

Base Excess

This is defined as 'The quantity of base or acid needed to titrate 1 litre of blood to a pH of 7.4 with the pCO_2 held constant at 5.3 kPa (40 mmHg)'. It only reflects the metabolic component of an acid-base disturbance. A typical reference range for base excess is −2 to +2 mEq/l.

In metabolic acidosis base excess is negative.

In metabolic alkalosis the base excess is positive.

Compensation

The action taken by the body to correct any acid-base imbalance. Usual compensatory measures include:

- Buffers – rapid response (minutes)
- Ventilatory response – minutes to hours
- Renal response – more long-term solution

Achieving Homeostasis

Human physiology has evolved to attempt to maintain equilibrium at a pH of 7.4. It has been shown that the majority of human enzymes function optimally when the pH lies between 7.35–7.45. There are of course some enzymes (e.g. gastrin, glutaminase) that function at the extreme ends of the pH scale; however, these usually are organ specific and have a targeted role.

The aim of all acid-base homeostatic processes, therefore, is to keep the H^+ concentration stable. Acid is produced during both aerobic and anaerobic metabolism and when amino acids are oxidised. Ironically, the greatest potential for acid formation in the body occurs as a by-product of aerobic metabolism.

CO_2 in itself is not an acid, as by definition it cannot donate a proton in solution. However, the CO_2 produced during aerobic metabolism reacts rapidly with water to form carbonic acid (H_2CO_3). Carbonic acid is a weak acid and a key component in acid-base maintenance because:

a) it dissociates rapidly and readily
b) its dissociation and ionisation products are usually in equilibrium

At equilibrium,

$$[CO_2] + [H_2O] = H_2CO_3 = [H^+] + [HCO3^-]$$

Under basal conditions, the average 70 kg adult produces 13,000 mmol of CO_2 per day (approximately

300 litres). CO_2 is excreted by the lungs at a rate of 9 mmol per minute (200 ml/min); therefore small changes in either ventilation rate or efficiency can have a significant effect on pH.

For every 500 mmol of CO_2 present in solution, there is 1 mmol of H_2CO_3.

For every 4000 mmol of H_2CO_3 present in solution, there is 1 mmol of H^+.

90% of the CO_2 within blood is transported as HCO_3^-. Carbamino compounds (CO_2 bound to haemoglobin or other proteins) account for a further 5% and CO_2 dissolved directly into plasma the final 5%.

For the body to remain in equilibrium the amount of acid excreted per day must equal the amount of acid produced daily. The lungs excrete CO_2, which reduces the potential for acid production. The kidneys are involved in excreting all metabolic acids.

To deal with the approximately 100 mmol of H^+ from metabolic acid production daily, the renal acid-base system actively secretes H^+ ions, usually against a concentration gradient, into both the proximal and distal collecting tubules of the kidney. This allows relatively large amounts of H^+ to be excreted without the compensatory need for large volumes of urine. The kidneys are essential to acid-base maintenance, as there is no other way to excrete metabolic acids from the body.

Buffering Systems

a) Bicarbonate (HCO₃-)

Bicarbonate (HCO_3^-) is found in high concentrations within extracellular fluid (ECF) and accounts for approximately 80% of the body's extracellular buffering capability. HCO_3^- is freely filtered at the renal glomerulus, and if there was no active reabsorption of almost all filtered HCO_3^- (85% at the proximal convoluted tubule, 10% at the distal convoluted tubule and 4% within the collecting ducts), the buffering ability of blood would be severely depleted.

b) Protein Buffers (Haemoglobin and Plasma Proteins)

In addition to its O_2 carrying capacity, haemoglobin (Hb) acts as another important ECF buffer for CO_2. Hb is found at a much higher concentration (120-150 g/l in women) compared to the other plasma proteins (70 g/l) – with albumin being the most abundant plasma protein (50 g/l).

Hb is six times more efficient than the other plasma proteins combined at maintaining the plasma pH because it has three times more histidine residues on its molecular structure. It is these histidine residues that provide the actual buffering capability of proteins.

Deoxygenated Hb is a weaker acid than oxygenated Hb and therefore has a greater affinity for CO_2. This means the buffering ability of Hb is at its greatest when it is most required. CO_2 combines with Hb to form carbaminohaemoglobin, which is transported into the lungs, where the CO_2 is then released down a concentration gradient into the alveoli before being exhaled.

c) Phosphate (PO₄³⁻)

The concentration of phosphate in the blood is so low that it is quantitatively unimportant as an ECF buffer. Its importance as a buffer lies intracellularly and as part of renal acid excretion where its concentration is higher.

Phosphate (PO_4^{3-}) is freely filtered at the renal glomerulus. It can then combine with up to 3 H^+ ions (in exchange for Na^+ ions) to form phosphoric acid (H_3PO_4), which is excreted via renal tubules. Energy for this process is provided by Na^+K^+ATPase and helps maintain the Na^+ concentration gradient in the renal tubular system.

d) Ammonia (NH₃)

Ammonia (NH_3) is formed in renal tubular cells by the action of glutaminase on the amino acid glutamine. Glutaminase is one of those organ-specific enzymes that functions at a low pH; therefore more ammonia is produced during periods of acidosis, which then improves the buffering ability of urine.

Ammonia crosses into the renal tubule down a concentration gradient, where it combines with H^+ to form ammonium (NH_4^+) and is excreted in urine.

The ability of the renal system to excrete extra H^+ ions by combining these with ammonia (NH_3) to create ammonium (NH_4^+) creates an important degree of flexibility to renal acid-base regulation. The rate of NH_4^+ production and excretion can be rapidly regulated in response to the constantly changing acid-base requirements of the body.

(Compare this to the phosphate buffering system, where any increase in its capacity to act as a buffer must come from a dietary change, and is therefore a long-term process.)

e) Bone

The important role of bone as a buffer is often over-looked in discussions about acid-base physiology, but the carbonate and phosphate salts in bone act as a long-term supply of buffer, especially during prolonged periods of metabolic acidosis.

Approximately 40% of the buffering of an acute acid load occurs within bone (after both the intracellular and ECF buffers have been used up), and bone contains 80% of the body's total CO_2 stores (as CO_2, HCO_3^- or CO_3^{2-})

The uptake of H^+ in bone is at the expense of surface Na^+ and K^+, which can cause bone mineral dissolution. Chronic metabolic acidosis causes progressive bone lysis and in children, can lead to growth retardation.

Arterial Blood Gas (ABG)

When discussing an ABG result, the question that must always be foremost in your mind is 'Why did this patient warrant a doctor putting a needle in their wrist (or groin) to obtain an arterial sample?' because without a clinical context, data interpretation of this sort is a meaningless academic exercise. The commonest reasons for an ABG being taken are:

a) To check for any acid-base disturbance
b) Monitor oxygenation – the arterial pO_2 provides information about the efficiency of gas exchange
c) Diagnose and establish the severity of any respiratory failure – the arterial pCO_2 provides information on ventilation
d) Guide therapeutic options – e.g. in the treatment of chronic obstructive pulmonary disease (COPD) or diabetic ketoacidosis

Among the many variables found within an ABG, the most important for discovering the source and consequence of an acid-base disturbance are:

	Normal range
Arterial pCO2	4.5–6.0 kPa
Arterial pO$_2$	11.0–13.0 kPa
HCO$_3^-$	22–28 mmol/l
Base excess	−2 to +2 mEq/l
Anion gap	8–16 mmol/l

The simplified Henderson-Hasselbalch equation for determining the pH of blood is

$$pH = 6.1 + + \log_{10} \frac{[HCO_3\text{-}]}{[0.03 \times pCO_2]}$$

If you remove the constants, you will notice that pH is a ratio of the concentration of bicarbonate to carbon dioxide:

$$pH \approx \frac{[HCO_3\text{-}]}{[CO_2]}$$

If you extrapolate this knowledge and include the organs that deal with the regulation of both of these components, you will find that

$$pH \approx \frac{[HCO_3\text{-}]}{[CO_2]} \approx \frac{Base}{Acid} \approx \frac{Kidneys}{Lungs} \approx \frac{Metabolic\ cause}{Respiratory\ cause}$$

Once you grasp this concept, the complexities of trying to interpret the causes of a metabolic disturbance from an ABG result become much simpler.

How to Interpret an ABG

When the blood gas results are being conveyed down the phone to you, the first step is DO NOT PANIC!

Using the method described in this chapter, you will soon be able to discuss ABG results with either the respiratory registrar on call or the consultant anaesthetist in ITU without feeling out of your depth. The # (hashtag) symbol will grow to be your friend, not only when you are tweeting but also when deciphering an ABG.

To diagnose an acid-base imbalance properly one needs to ask three pertinent questions:

1) Does the pH indicate acidosis or alkalosis?
2) Is the cause of the pH imbalance metabolic or respiratory?
3) Is there compensation for this imbalance?

The best way to understand any system is to work through examples, so let's begin.

Example 1

Mrs Jones is a 30-year-old insulin-dependent diabetic with a poor compliance record. She is 12-weeks pregnant and gets admitted to the ward after she collapses in the Early Pregnancy Assessment Unit. The on-call doctor performs an ABG as part of her blood work-up.

These are her results:

pH	7.26
PaCO$_2$	5.1 kPa
HCO$_3^-$	17 mmol/l

Step 1: Draw a large hashtag!

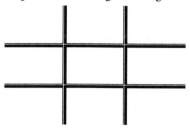

Step 2: Label the three columns Acid, Normal and Alkali. The acid column is on the left as acids have a lower pH, and on a sequential scale, lower numbers would be on the left.

ACID	NORMAL	ALKALI

Step 3: Place the pH, PCO$_2$ and HCO$_3^-$ values into the appropriate columns.

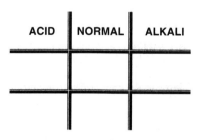

Normal Ranges: ABGs	
• Arterial pCO$_2$	4.5–6.0 kPa
• Arterial pO$_2$	11.0–13.0 kPa
• HCO$_3^-$	22.0–28.0 mmol/l
• Base express	–2.0 to +2.0
• Anion gap	8.0–16.0 mmol/l
• Chloride	98.0–107.0 mmol/l

Mrs Jones' ABG results are as follows:

pH	7.26
PaCO$_2$	5.1 kPa
HCO$_3^-$	17 mmol/l

Important Points

- The column that the **pH** is in determines whether this is acidosis or alkalosis.
- The relative positions of all three parameters will reveal the origin of any acid-base imbalance.
- If the **pH** and **HCO$_3^-$** fall in the same column, the problem is **metabolic**.
- If the **pH** and **PaCO$_2$** fall in the same column (other than normal), the problem is **respiratory**.
- Look for the third parameter not associated with the pH. If this is in the 'normal' column, there is no evidence of compensation.

Based on the data presented herein, Mrs Jones is suffering acute metabolic acidosis (Table 3.1), with no evidence of compensation.

Example 2

Mrs Patel is a 74-year-old lady with a long history of COPD who underwent a laparotomy for a large ovarian mass three days ago. The ward nurses have informed you that she has a pyrexia with productive green sputum.

Her ABG results are:

pH	7.24
PaCO$_2$	6.9 kPa
HCO$_3^-$	34 mmol/l

Table 3.1 Causes of metabolic acidosis

Increased endogenous acid production	• **Ketoacidosis**
	a) **alcohol**
	b) **poorly controlled diabetes**
	c) **starvation**
	• **Lactic acidosis**
	a) **From impaired tissue oxygenation – increased lactate from anaerobic tissue metabolism / hypoperfusion**
	b) **Despite normal tissue oxygenation – impaired lactate metabolism from liver failure**
Increased exogenous acid exposure	• Methanol
	• Ethylene glycol (antifreeze)
	• Aspirin
Inability to excrete acid	• Chronic renal failure

Table 3.2 Causes of respiratory acidosis

Central depression of the respiratory drive	• **Drugs** a) **opioids** b) **benzodiazepines** c) **anaesthetics** • **Central nervous system trauma, infarct / haemorrhage or tumours**
Neuromuscular complications	• Motor neurone disease • Guillain-Barré syndrome • Muscular dystrophy • Myaesthenia gravis • Toxins (e.g. snake venom, organophosphates)
Airway causes	• Obstructive sleep apnoea • Laryngospasm • Bronchospasm / Severe asthma attacks
Lung and thoracic cage abnormalities	• Hypoventilation of obesity (e.g. Pickwickian syndrome) • Kyphoscoliosis • Significant chest trauma (e.g. flail chest, large contusions, haemothorax) • Adult respiratory distress syndrome (ARDS) • Pulmonary oedema • Aspiration • COPD

ACID	NORMAL	ALKALI
pH		HCO_3^-
pCO_2		

Normal Ranges: ABGs
• Arterial pCO_2	4.5–6.0 kPa
• Arterial pO_2	11.0–13.0 kPa
• HCO_3^-	22.0–28.0 mmol/l
• Base express	−2.0 to +2.0
• Anion gap	8.0–16.0 mmol/l
• Chloride	98.0–107.0 mmol/l

Note: HCO_3^- is not lying within the 'normal' column, which indicates that there exists partial compensation for the acid-base disturbance. If the compensation had been complete, the pH would have been in the 'normal' column too. Based on the data provided, Mrs Patel has respiratory acidosis (Table 3.2) with partial compensation.

Example 3

Eliza is an 18-year-old brought to A&E after a road traffic accident. She was the passenger in a small car that was rear-ended by a bus. The airbags did not deploy, but she has been hyperventilating since the accident and now feels faint.

Her ABG results are:

pH	7.49
$PaCO_2$	3.8 kPa
HCO_3^-	23 mmol/l

ACID	NORMAL	ALKALI
	HCO_3^-	pH
		pCO_2

Normal Ranges: ABGs
• Arterial pCO_2	4.5–6.0 kPa
• Arterial pO_2	11.0–13.0 kPa
• HCO_3^-	22.0–28.0 mmol/l
• Base express	−2.0 to +2.0
• Anion gap	8.0–16.0 mmol/l
• Chloride	98.0–107.0 mmol/l

Based on the data provided, Eliza has acute respiratory alkalosis (Table 3.3) with no evidence of compensation.

Example 4

Dr Smith is a 32-year-old obstetric trainee who is 12 weeks pregnant with twins. She presents to A&E with intractable vomiting.

Her ABG results are:

pH	7.43
$PaCO_2$	6.5 kPa
HCO_3^-	30 mmol/l

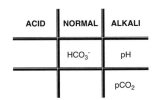

ACID	NORMAL	ALKALI
pCO_2	pH	HCO_3^-

Normal Ranges: ABGs
• Arterial pCO_2	4.5–6.0 kPa
• Arterial pO_2	11.0–13.0 kPa
• HCO_3^-	22.0–28.0 mmol/l
• Base express	−2.0 to +2.0
• Anion gap	8.0–16.0 mmol/l
• Chloride	98.0–107.0 mmol/l

Table 3.3 Causes of Respiratory Alkalosis

Central causes (direct effect on the respiratory centre)	• **Pain**
	• **Hyperventilation**
	• **Anxiety / panic attacks**
	• **Head injury**
	• **Cerebrovascular accidents (CVAs)**
	• **Tumours**
	• **Drugs / Endogenous compounds**
	
	  a) **Salicylates**
	  b) **Progesterone during pregnancy**

Hypoxia	• High altitude sickness • Severe anaemia
Pulmonary causes	• Asthma • Pulmonary embolism • Pneumonia • Pulmonary oedema

Table 3.4 Causes of metabolic alkalosis

Loss of H^+ ions	1.	Gastrointestinal
		  • Prolonged vomiting (through loss of acidic gastric juice)
		  • Nasogastric suctioning

	2.	Renal • Diuretics (Loop or Thiazide)
Loss of K^+ ions	•	Conn's syndrome • Cushing's disease • Severe diarrhoea
Loss of Cl^- ions	•	Prolonged vomiting (through loss of acidic gastric juice) • Diuretics • Post-hypercapnia

Important Note

If the pH lies within the 'normal' range but the other parameters are not, then this represents a case of complete compensation.

In this situation, you will need to perform an extra step to reveal the origin of the acid-base imbalance.

Using both decimal places of any given pH value, the exact midpoint of the normal range is determined to be 7.40. It is then assumed that any pH value <7.40 indicates an acidosis, while a pH value >7.40 indicates an alkalosis. These compensated pH values are given the label pH(c).

In this example, the pH is 7.43; therefore the pH(c) should be placed in the 'alkali' column.

ACID	NORMAL	ALKALI
pCO_2	pH	HCO_3^-
		pH(c)

ACID	NORMAL	ALKALI
pCO_2	pH	HCO_3^-
		pH(c)

Therefore, based on the data provided, Dr Smith has metabolic alkalosis (Table 3.4) with complete compensation.

When it comes to acids and bases, the difference between prolonging life or hastening death comes down to balance. The body will do all that it can, via the organs of homeostasis and using all available buffering mechanisms, to correct any acid-base imbalance such that it remains in equilibrium.

The priority of deciphering ABG results must be to allow the causes of these acid-base disturbances to be readily diagnosed so that treatment can be initiated. Prompt correction of the underlying cause will lead to a rapid return of the underlying pH to normality.

One should never however allow the interpretation of ABG results to occur in isolation or to overshadow the importance of a full patient history and thorough clinical assessment when prioritising interventions.

External Sources of Information and References

www.wfsahq.org/archive-update-in-anaesthesia/update-in . . . /download

(article by Stephen Drage and Douglas Wilkinson)

www.acid-base.com/history.php

(website by Alan Grogono, Emeritus Professor, Tulane University Department of Anaesthesia)

http://cjasn.asnjournals.org/content/early/2015/11/22/CJN.07400715.full

(article by L Lee Hamm, N Nakhoul and KS Hering-Smith)

www.nejm.org/doi/full/10.1056/NEJMra1003327

(article by K Berend, APJ de Vries and ROB Gans, *N Engl J Med* 2014; 371:1434–1445)

Female Reproductive Physiology

Chapter 4

Ayona Wijemanne

Introduction

The female reproductive system is designed to enable a number of processes that permit fertility in the adult female. These consist of the following:

- Production and storage of ova
- Folliculogenesis
- Selection of a dominant follicle and oocyte
- Regular spontaneous ovulation
- Preparation of the endometrium
- Fertilisation
- Support of the fertilised oocyte prior to implantation

1 Production and Storage of Ova

- Migration of primordial germ cells occurs during embryonic life, from the hindgut to the gonadal tissue
- In the absence of the SRY gene, the following occurs:
  - Gonad develops into an *ovary*
  - Primordial germ cells become *oogonia*
- Rapid mitosis of oogonia → Several million oogonia → Oogonia become surrounded by granulosa cells to become primordial follicles→ Primordial follicles enter first meiotic division and become arrested
- Many primordial follicles lost through atresia in second trimester → Less than one million primordial follicles by puberty

2 Folliculogenesis

- The activation of the hypothalamo-pituitary-gonadal axis at puberty results in the activation of the primordial follicles

- The earliest stages of follicular growth are not dependent on the follicle-stimulating hormone (FSH; Fig. 4.1)
- Follicular growth and differentiation involve (Fig. 4.2):
  - Mitosis of granulosa cell layer (avascular)
    - Cells directly surrounding the oocyte are *cumulus granulosa cells*
    - Cells adjacent to basal lamina are *mural granulosa cells*
  - Production of basal lamina by granulosa cells, which acts as a protective layer
  - Differentiation of a second cell layer external to the basal lamina, called the *theca cell* layer
    - Vascular
    - Produces nutrients for the growing follicle
  - Creation of an antrum (fluid-filled space) within the follicle

- During this process, follicular diameter increases 1000-fold from 0.02 mm to 20–50 mm
- The total length of the process is around 80–90 days

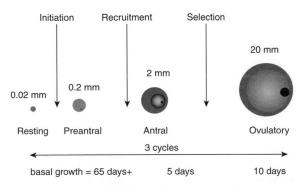

Figure 4.1 Stages of follicle growth

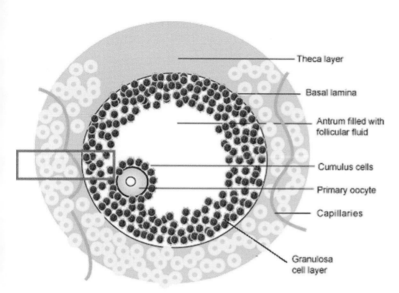

Figure 4.2 Structure of an ovarian follicle

Theca layer

Basal lamina

Antrum filled with
follicular fluid

Cumulus cells

Primary oocyte

Capillaries

Granulosa
cell layer

○ There are 65 days between the initiation of growth to recruitment and the menstrual cycle

○ Many follicles are lost through atresia before the recruitment stage

3 Selection of Dominant Follicle and Ovulation

• Latter stages of folliculogenesis are dependent on the hormonal changes of the menstrual cycle

• The antral phase onwards is dependent on FSH

• The different cell types within the follicle respond to and produce different hormones (Fig. 4.3):

○ Granulosa cells

▪ Contain FSH receptors

▪ FSH drives aromatization of androgen to estradiol

○ Theca cells

▪ Contain luteinizing hormone (LH) receptors

▪ LH drives conversion of cholesterol to androgen

▪ Express CYP17, which encodes for the enzymes needed for androgen production

· 17-alpha-hydroxylase

· 17,20-lyase

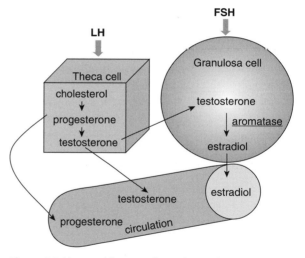

Figure 4.3 Hormonal function of granulosa and theca cells

3.1 Hormonal Changes during the Menstrual Cycle

• In terms of what is happening inside the ovary, the menstrual cycle can be split into two phases:

○ *Follicular phase:* Predominant steroid hormone *estradiol*

○ *Luteal phase:* Predominant steroid hormone *progesterone*

• Fluctuations in both steroid hormones have varying feedback effects on the hypothalamo-pituitary-gonadal axis (Fig. 4.5)

29

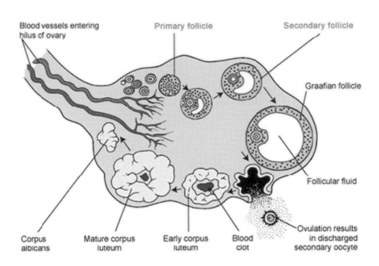

Figure 4.4 Folliculogenesis within the ovary

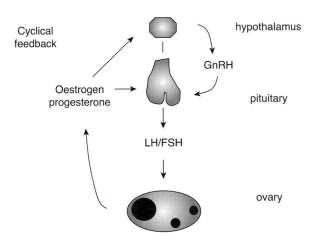

Figure 4.5 The hypothalamic-pituitary-ovarian axis

3.1.1 Phase A (Late Luteal / Early Follicular Phase; Fig. 4.6)

- Death of corpus luteum → ↓ estradiol

  ↓ progesterone

  Shedding of endometrium

- Low levels of steroid hormone → Removal of negative feedback effect on pituitary → ↑ FSH levels for 3 days (*intercycle rise*)
- On day 1 of the menstrual cycle, there are approximately 4–6 antral follicles within the ovary
  - The intercycle rise in FSH results in the selection of the dominant follicle

3.1.2 Phase B (Mid-follicular Phase)

- Rapid increase in the size of the dominant follicle
- Increase in number of granulosa cells in dominant follicle → Increased levels of estradiol → Negative feedback effect on pituitary → ↓ FSH levels
- Action of FSH on dominant follicle results in the induction of LH receptors on the theca cells
  - Enables survival of the dominant follicle when FSH levels fall
- The increased LH levels result in a rapid increase in estradiol levels

3.1.3 Phase C (Mid-cycle: Ovulation)

- Once estradiol levels have been >300 nmol/l for 2–3 days, feedback on the pituitary switches from negative to positive
  - This results in a massive release of LH from the pituitary (*LH surge*)
- LH surge results in a cascade of events:
  - Increased permeability of the capillaries within the theca layer results in a rise in fluid pressure within the antrum
    - Enables protrusion of follicle from ovarian surface
  - Cascade of local enzymes → Breakdown of follicle wall → Extrusion of oocyte and cumulus cells under pressure

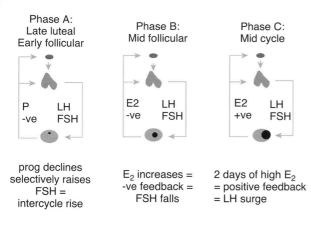

Figure 4.6 Phases of the menstrual cycle

- Oocyte completes first meiotic division to become *secondary oocyte*
  - Surplus chromosomes are packed within the first polar body
  - Secondary oocyte enters second meiotic division but becomes arrested
  - Oocyte-cell complex is collected by the fimbrial end of the uterine tube
- Ovulation occurs 18 hours following the peak of the LH surge

3.1.4 Phase D (Mid-luteal Phase)

- Immediately after ovulation, the remaining follicle collapses
  - Theca cell layer vessels invade the centre, creating a clot
  - Dramatic fall in steroid production
- The corpus luteum forms from the remaining mass of cells, and steroid production resumes
- Progesterone levels rise to a greater extent and exert a negative feedback effect on the pituitary, resulting in low levels of FSH and LH
- Because the corpus luteum is the only source of significant levels of progesterone during the menstrual cycle, it serves as an ideal marker for ovulation

4 Transport of Oocyte to Uterus

- The oocyte is passed along the uterine tube by two actions:
  - Peristalsis of uterine tube
  - Action of cilia

- Estradiol production by the dominant follicle results in differentiation in the cells of the uterine tube
  - Growth in cilia on surface of ciliated cells
  - Secretion of products from glandular cells that will
    - Support the oocyte
    - Provide an environment for sperm capacitation
- Once the oocyte has passed into the uterus, progesterone levels increase, causing changes that prevent any further oocytes from passing through the uterine tube:
  - Retraction of cilia
  - Shortening of glandular cells

5 Fertilisation

- Fertilisation, which tends to occur in the ampulla of the uterine tube, results in a cascade of events:
  - Completion of second meiotic division of oocyte to form a second polar body and female pronucleus (which combines with male pronucleus)
  - Penetration of oocyte by sperm → Migration of cortical granules to outer edge of oocyte → Hardening of oocyte membrane and prevention of further penetration (*cortical reaction*)
  - Mitosis of fertilised oocyte to form blastocyst
    - Blastocyst produces beta-hCG, which rescues the corpus luteum from demise

Changes in the Ovary & Endometrium during the menstrual cycle

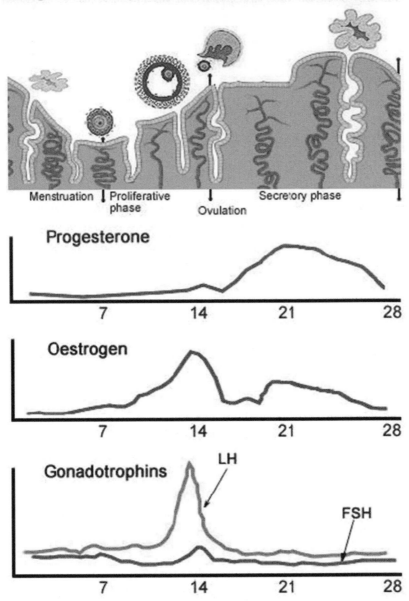

Figure 4.7 Summary of hormonal changes in the menstrual cycle

6 Cyclical Changes in Uterus, Cervix and Vagina

6.1 Uterus

- Endometrium contains:
  - ○ Glandular cells
  - ○ Vessels supplied by the uterine arteries

- Following menstruation, the myometrium is covered by a basal layer of endometrium
- The changes occurring within the endometrium during the menstrual cycle can be divided into two phases:
  - ○ *Proliferative phase*
    - ▪ Analogous to follicular phase in the ovary

- Estradiol is the predominant steroid hormone and causes
  - Rapid division of the endometrial cells (endometrial thickness is a good bioassay of estradiol levels)
  - Growth of glandular cells
  - Vascular growth
  - Induction of progesterone receptors
  - *Secretory phase*
    - Analogous to the luteal phase in the ovary
    - Progesterone is the predominant steroid hormone and causes
      - Reduction in the rate of cell division
      - Increased oedema within endometrium (measures approximately 6 mm at this point)
      - Increased coiling and permeability of spiral arterioles
      - Increase in size and tortuosity of glands
  - Secretion of glycoproteins
    - Maintenance in quiescence of myometrial layer
- The demise of the corpus luteum following failed fertilisation of the oocyte results in
  - Withdrawal of steroid hormones
  - Release of prostaglandins, causing
    - Constriction, then dilatation of the spiral arterioles, resulting in bleeding
    - Hypoxia, causing tissue necrosis
      - Accelerated by the release of proteolytic enzymes
  - Shedding of outer layer of endometrium
    - 50% is shed within the first 24 hours
    - Approximately 80 ml of blood is shed

6.2 Cervix

- Proliferative phase (estradiol dependent)
  - Increase in vascularity and oedema
  - Watery mucous
    - Glycoproteins align themselves to form microscopic channels through which sperm can pass
- Secretory phase (progesterone dependent)

  - Reduction in oedema
  - Thickening of mucous
    - Glycoproteins form mesh
      - Act as a barrier to sperm
      - One mechanism of action of the progesterone-only pill (POP)

6.3 Vagina

- Lined with stratified non-keratinised squamous epithelium
  - Layers constantly shed downwards
- Lubricated by
  - Cervical secretions
  - Transudate from vaginal epithelium
- Secretions generally acidic in order to provide antimicrobial protection

7 Systemic Effects of Steroid Hormones

7.1 Oestrogen

- Maintenance of vascular tone
- Maintenance of bone density
- Lipoprotein effects:
  - Increased high-density lipoprotein (HDL) levels
  - Reduced low-density lipoprotein (LDL) levels
- Alteration in clotting factors

7.2 Progesterone

- Increase in aldosterone production → Retention of salt and water → Oedema
- Increase in appetite
- Smooth muscle relaxant

Further Reading

Fiander A, Thilaganathan B. *Your Essential Revision Guide: MRCOG Part One: The Official Companion to the Royal College of Obstetricians and Gynaecologists Revision Course.* London: RCOG Press, 2010.

Swiet M. *Basic Science in Obstetrics and Gynaecology: A Textbook for MRCOG, Part 1.* 2nd ed. Edinburgh: Churchill Livingstone, 1992.

Single Best Answer Questions

1. Regarding folliculogenesis:

   a. Follicular diameter increases 100-fold
   b. The earliest stages are dependent on FSH
   c. Theca cells contain LH receptors which drive the aromatisation of androgen to estradiol
   d. The antral phase onwards is dependent on FSH
   e. Prior to puberty, the primordial follicles have completed the first meiotic division

2. Regarding the menstrual cycle:

   a. Progesterone is only released during the luteal phase
   b. The intercycle rise in FSH enables the selection of the dominant follicle
   c. Rising levels of progesterone during the follicular phase cause the LH surge
   d. The oocyte completes the second meiotic division at ovulation
   e. The corpus luteum is maintained by high levels of LH in the luteal phase

3. Regarding the corpus luteum:

   a. It contains a large number of FSH receptors
   b. It only produces progesterone
   c. It must be removed in order to initiate a new menstrual cycle
   d. It has a finite lifespan of 7 days if fertilisation does not occur
   e. If fertilisation occurs, it is rescued from death by beta-hCG, which acts on FSH receptors

4. Regarding the endometrium:

   a. Progesterone is the predominant hormone during the proliferative phase
   b. Maximal cell division occurs during the secretory phase
   c. Progesterone inhibits cell division
   d. All layers are shed during menstruation
   e. The proliferative phase is analogous to the follicular phase in the ovary

5. Regarding hormone production within the ovarian follicle:

   a. The theca cells produce progesterone, which is converted to oestrogen in the granulosa cells
   b. The granulosa cells produce androgen, which is converted to oestrogen in the theca cells
   c. The theca cells produce androgen, which is converted to progesterone in the granulosa cells
   d. The theca cells produce androgen, which is converted to oestrogen in the granulosa cells
   e. Both the theca and granulosa cells produce oestrogen, androgen and progesterone

6. Regarding oestrogen:

   a. It reduces HDL levels
   b. It increases the coiling and permeability of the spiral arterioles within the endometrium
   c. It is the predominant steroid hormone during the follicular phase
   d. It increases appetite
   e. It causes the glycoproteins within cervical mucous to form a mesh during the secretory phase

7. Regarding ovulation:

   a. It occurs 18 hours after the peak of the LH surge
   b. It occurs as a result of the LH surge, which results from positive feedback effects of rising progesterone levels
   c. The oocyte completes the first meiotic division to become a primary oocyte
   d. The oocyte is collected by the fimbrial end of the uterine tube and is moved by peristalsis as a result of raised progesterone levels
   e. The oocyte does not enter the second meiotic division

Male Reproductive Physiology

Ayona Wijemanne

Introduction

- Spermatogenesis is a complex process involving:
  - ○ Mitosis
  - ○ Meiosis
  - ○ Structural change
- Infertility affects 6% of men in the UK
  - ○ 90% have errors in spermatogenesis
- Errors of mitosis and meiosis contribute to chromosomal abnormalities in:
  - ○ 9% of all conceptions
  - ○ 0.7% of live births

1 The Male Reproductive System

1.1 Testes

- 3.5–5.5 cm long and 2–3 cm wide (total volume 15–30 ml)
- Ellipsoid, glandular organs
- Functions:
  - ○ Sperm production and storage
  - ○ Production of testosterone

- Lie outside the body in scrotum (sac-like structure made of skin and muscle):
  - ○ Keeps testes 1.5–2.5°C below body temperature, which is optimal temperature for spermatogenesis
  - ○ If too warm, smooth muscles of scrotum relax to move testes away from body
  - ○ Overheating reduces sperm count
- Rich vascular and nerve supply
- 90% of testis is made up of tightly coiled seminiferous tubules
  - ○ Tubules coiled in groups of lobules
- Lobules connect to form area called rete testis, which leads to epididymis and vas deferens
- Each seminiferous tubule consists of:
  - ○ Sertoli (supporting) cells
    - Tall columnar cells which sit on basement membrane
    - Equivalent of granulosa cells in female
    - Responsible for nourishment of spermatozoa
    - Bound by tight junctions, which:

Figure 5.1 Male reproductive tract

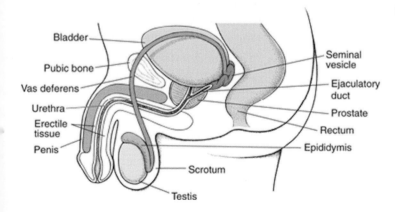

35

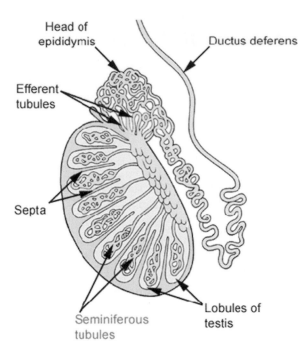

Head of epididymis

Ductus deferens

Efferent tubules

Septa

Seminiferous tubules

Lobules of testis

Figure 5.2 Internal structure of testis

· Divide tubule into luminal and adluminal compartments

· Open to allow passage of spermatozoa

· Enable enclosed environment for spermatogenesis

▪ Contain FSH receptors

▪ Produce antimullerian hormone (AMH), inhibin and androgen binding protein (ABP)

○ Spermatogonia (primary germ cells) lying between Sertoli cells on basement membrane

- Leydig cells lie in spaces between seminiferous tubules:

○ Equivalent of theca cell in female

○ Produce testosterone which controls spermatogenesis

○ Contain LH receptors

1.2 Epididymis

- Tube of 5 m in length, coiled on superior and posterior surface of testis

- Passage of sperm through epididymis takes 8–14 days

- Sperm are stored and undergo final stages of maturation

- The ducts of the individual tubules join to form the vas deferens

2 Spermatogenesis

- Production of haploid male gametes

- 300 million mature spermatozoa produced per day (3500 per second)

- Entire process takes 74 days

○ New wave every 16 days

- Takes place in seminiferous tubules

○ Self-contained environment providing necessary nutrients and protecting developing sperm from immune attack

- Can be split into three stages:

○ **Spermatogenesis** (production of haploid gametes- secondary spermatocytes)

○ **Spematidogenesis** (production of spermatids)

○ **Spermiogenesis** (maturation of spermatid to spermatazoan)

2.1 Spermatogenesis

- Spermatogonia (primordial germ cells – diploid) are located on basement membrane of seminiferous tubules

- Mitotically inactive until the peripubertal period

○ Increased gonadotrophin production from Leydig cells induces large mitotic proliferation

- Spermatogonia enter meiosis and differentiate into primary spermatocytes (diploid). They will then do one of two things:

○ Divide mitotically to form more primary spermatocytes

○ Complete meiosis I to form secondary spermatocytes (haploid)

▪ Tight junctions between Sertoli cells part to allow movement into adluminal compartment

2.2 Spermatidogenesis

- Secondary spermatocytes complete meiosis II to form four spermatids (haploid)

- Marked reduction in cytoplasmic volume

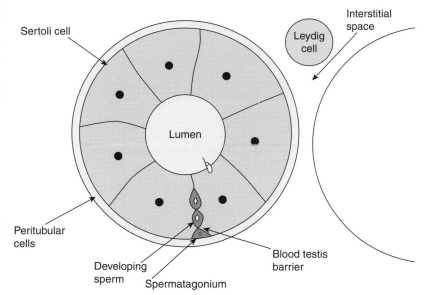

Figure 5.3 Section through seminiferous tubule

Sertoli cell

Interstitial space

Leydig cell

Lumen

Peritubular cells

Developing sperm

Spermatagonium

Blood testis barrier

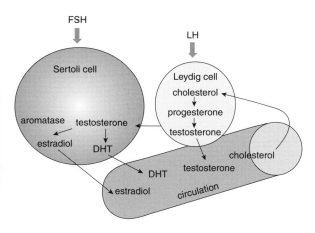

FSH = follicle stimulating hormone.   LH = luteinizing hormone.
DHT = dihydrotestosterone.

Figure 5.4 Hormonal function of Sertoli and Leydig cells

- Spermatids remain connected by a syncytium (membrane), which breaks down once the spermatozoa leave the space between the Sertoli cells

2.3 Spermiogenesis

- Maturation of round spermatids into mature spermatozoa (haploid)
- Controlled by testosterone

- Involves the following changes:
  - Elongation to produce tail and components of tail
  - Nuclear hypercondensation
  - Morphogenesis of head into spatulate shape
  - Removal of excess cytoplasm and cellular contents (phagocytosis by neighbouring cells)
- As spermatids mature and develop, they move away from basement membrane toward lumen of seminiferous tubule
- Once fully differentiated and mature, spermatozoa are released from cytoplasmic bridges in the Sertoli cells and bud off into lumen of tubules
- These spermatozoa are still not motile, so are transported to the epididymis for storage and further maturation by peristaltic action of the seminiferous tubules

2.4 Final Maturation and Storage of Spermatozoa (Epididymis)

- Mature sperm collect in rete testis and pass into epididymis, where they are stored and undergo further maturation within the three areas of epididymis:

Several generations of mitosis by germ line stem cells

Figure 5.5 Spermatogenesis

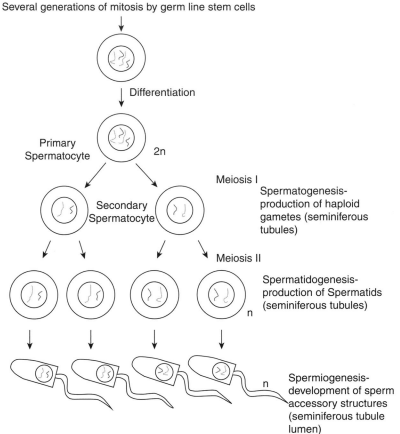

Differentiation

Primary Spermatocyte

2n

Meiosis I

Secondary Spermatocyte

Spermatogenesis- production of haploid gametes (seminiferous tubules)

Meiosis II

n

Spermatidogenesis- production of Spermatids (seminiferous tubules)

n

Spermiogenesis- development of sperm accessory structures (seminiferous tubule lumen)

TAIL   MIDPIECE   HEAD

Figure 5.6 Mature spermatozoan

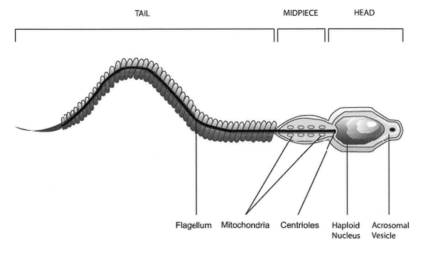

Flagellum   Mitochondria   Centrioles   Haploid Nucleus   Acrosomal Vesicle

○ Caput (head): Maturation begins

○ Corpus (body): Maturation completed and sperm become motile

○ Cauda (tail): Mature sperm stored until release (some stored in ampulla of vas deferens)

• Spermatozoa stored in epididymal fluid

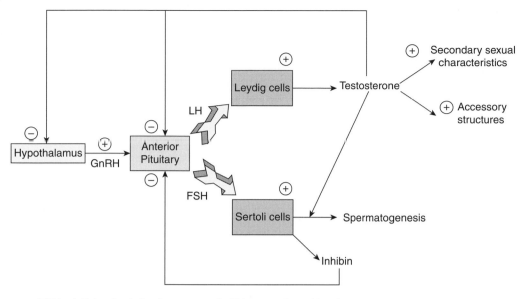

FSH = follicle stimulating hormone.   GnRH = gonadotrophin releasing hormone.
LH = luteinizing hormone.

Figure 5.7 Hormonal control of spermatogenesis

2.5 Hormonal Control of Spermatogenesis

- FSH initiates spermatogenesis at the onset of puberty

  o Estradiol exerts a negative feedback on release at both the hypothalamic and pituitary level

  o Testosterone also exerts a negative feedback effect, but to a lesser extent

- LH stimulates testosterone production within the Leydig cells

  o Testosterone exerts a negative feedback effect on release by:

    ▪ Inhibition of GnRH release

    ▪ Reducing sensitivity of pituitary to GnRH

  o Estradiol also exerts a negative feedback effect, but to a lesser extent

- Testosterone stimulates spermatogenesis and the development of secondary sexual characteristics
- Testosterone is produced by Leydig cells under the influence of LH from the anterior pituitary gland
- Testosterone is converted into its active form, dihydrotestosterone, within the Sertoli cells. Dihydrotestosterone controls spermatogenesis within the Sertoli cells.

- Testosterone is also aromatised to oestradiol within the Sertoli cells
- Oestradiol, testosterone and dihydrotestosterone are all released into the peripheral circulation from Sertoli and Leydig cells
- Testosterone secretion by the Leydig cells in the fetal testes is under the control of beta-hCG in early pregnancy, which acts on LH receptors

3 Erection and ejaculation

3.1 Erection

- Neurovascular event triggered by sexual stimuli

  o Afferent limb carried by internal pudendal nerves

  o Efferent outflows carried by:

    ▪ Parasympathetic pelvic nerve

    ▪ Sympathetic hypogastric nerve

    ▪ Somatic pudendal nerve

- Sexual stimulation causes release of neurotransmitters and relaxation factors from endothelial cells causing smooth muscle relaxation in arteries and arterioles supplying erectile tissue

- This causes the corpus cavernosum to fill with blood, increasing rigidity
- Expansion of the penile blood volume results in compression of the subtunical venules by the outer tunica albuginia, causing obstruction of venous outflow and erection

3.2 Ejaculation

- Activation of autonomic nervous system causes coordinated contractions of vas deferens and glands
- Sympathetic stimulation
  - Moves sperm into epididymis, vas deferens and penile urethra
  - Causes expulsion of glandular secretions from seminal vesicles, prostate and bulbourethral glands
- Ejaculate consists of:
  - Secretions from above glands and epididymal fluids
  - Approximately 120 million sperm
    - Average volume of ejaculate 3–5 ml
    - Normal concentration 40–100 million sperm/ml
- Most sperm expelled in first half of ejaculate
  - 99.9% lost before reaching egg
  - Only 120,000 get close to egg
- Concentration of less than 20 million sperm/ml is considered oligospermic

4 Fertilisation

4.1 Passage of Sperm through the Vagina and Cervix

- Coagulation of seminal fluid in vagina
  - Prevents loss of seminal fluid
  - Neutralises acidic pH of vagina
- Changes in cervical mucus
  - Glycoprotein arrange in parallel lines
  - Micelles vibrate to aid passage of motile sperm
- Non-aligned sperm form reservoir in cervical crypts
- Uterus contracts in order to aid the passage of sperm
- Some sperm stored at utero-tubal junction

4.2 Capacitation

- Initiated by cervical mucus, uterine and uterine tube fluid
- Removal of the surface glycoprotein initiates a whiplash movement of the tail (sperm become hyperactive)
- Enables sperm to reach and penetrate the oocyte

4.3 Acrosome Reaction

- After ovulation, the oocyte is surrounded by a layer of cumulus cells and a hyaluronic acid matrix
- Receptors on the plasma membrane of the sperm bind to a component of the zona pellucida surrounding the oocyte
- This creates multiple fusion points between the plasma membrane and the outer acrosomal membrane (the acrosome reaction)
- This results in exposure of the inner acrosomal membrane to the extracellular matrix resulting in the release of several enzymes
  - Hexosaminidase B prevents further sperm binding to zona pellucida
  - Other membrane proteins enable further binding to the zona pellucida

4.4 Fertilisation

- Head of sperm taken into oocyte by phagocytosis
- Cortical reaction
  - Migration of cortical granules to edge of oocyte and fusion with zona pellucida
  - Fusion of the oocyte plasma membrane with zona pellicida, causing it to become impenetrable
- Transformation of sperm nucleus into male pronucleus
- Completion of meiosis II in oocyte to form:
  - Female pronucleus
  - Second polar body
- Pronuclei come together and membranes fuse and break down
- The resultant 23 pairs of chromosomes align on a mitotic spindle and the first cleavage occurs, forming a zygote
  - Spermatozoon only provides DNA

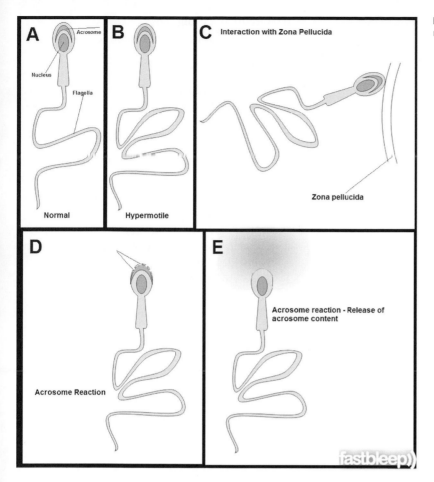

Figure 5.8 Capacitation and acrosome reaction

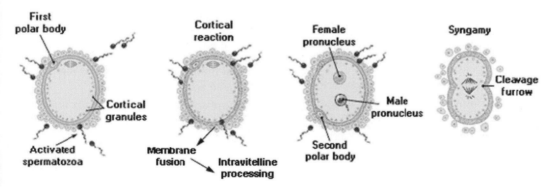

Figure 5.9 Fertilization

- ○ Oocyte provides machinery required for cell division (mitochondria and cell membrane)
- Zygote passes into the uterus after a few days aided by action of cilia

- At 8–16 cell stage, blastocyst becomes morula
  - ○ Cell mass becomes polarised into
    - ▪ Outer trophoblast (develops into chorion)
    - ▪ Inner cell mass (develops into embryo)

○ Beta-hCG from the syncytiotrophoblast prevents demise of corpus luteum
○ Implantation begins

Further Reading

Fiander A, Thilaganathan B. *Your essential revision guide: MRCOG Part One: The official companion to the Royal College of Obstetricians and Gynaecologists revision course.* London: RCOG Press; 2010

Sofikitis N, Giotitsas N, Tsounapi P, Baltogiannis D, Giannakis D, Pardalidis N. Hormonal regulation of spermatogenesis and spermiogenesis. *The Journal of Steroid Biochemistry and Molecular Biology.* 323–30

Swiet M. *Basic science in obstetrics and gynaecology: A textbook for MRCOG, Part 1.* 2nd ed. Edinburgh: Churchill Livingstone; 1992

Single Best Answer Questions

1. In the testis:

   a. 70% of the volume is composed of seminiferous tubules
   b. Sertoli cells contain LH receptors
   c. Leydig cells are the equivalent of theca cells in the female
   d. Sertoli cells lie in the spaces between seminiferous tubules
   e. Fully mature spermatozoa enter the epididymis

2. Regarding spermatogenesis:

   a. The entire process takes 16 days
   b. It is stimulated by testosterone produced by the Sertoli cells
   c. All spermatogonia become spermatocytes
   d. One spermatogonium produces four secondary spermatocytes
   e. One spermatogonium produces four spermatids

3. Spermiogenesis:

   a. Produces fully motile spermatozoa
   b. Is the maturation of round spermatids to diploid spermatozoa
   c. Involves the removal of excess cytoplasm and cellular contents

   d. Occurs in Leydig cells
   e. Is not controlled by testosterone

4. Regarding the ejaculate:

   a. It is 5–10 ml in volume
   b. Approximately 12,000 spermatozoa get close to the egg
   c. It is composed of fluid from the epididymis
   d. It contains approximately 120 million sperm
   e. Normal concentration is 20–40 million sperm/ml

5. Regarding fertilisation:

   a. Capacitation enables penetration of the zona pellucida of the egg by the sperm
   b. Sperm undergo capacitation followed by the acrosome reaction
   c. The acrosome reaction occurs in the uterus
   d. The cortical reaction causes the zona pellucida to become penetrable
   e. The egg completes meiosis I

6. Regarding spermatogonia:

   a. There is a finite supply
   b. They cannot divide mitotically
   c. One spermatogonium divides meiotically to produce two primary spermatocytes
   d. They lie on the basement membrane of Leydig cells
   e. One spermatogonium produces four spermatids

7. Following ejaculation:

   a. Seminal fluid alters the pH of the vagina from alkaline to acid
   b. Passage of sperm through the cervix is aided by the arrangement of glycoprotein molecules to form a mesh
   c. Most sperm are ejaculated in the second half of the fluid
   d. Seminal fluid coagulates in the vagina to prevent loss of sperm
   e. 50% of sperm are lost before reaching the egg

Correct answer: d

The Pituitary, Adrenal, Thyroid and Pancreas

Erum A. Khan

Pituitary Gland

- The master gland
- Pea-size

Structure of the Gland

- Anterior (adenohypophysis) lobe
- Posterior (neurohypophysis) lobe
- A small intermediate lobe

Embryology

Anterior pituitary: Formed by the ventral ridges of the primitive neural tube, which are pushed forward by the developing Rathke's pouch

Intermediate lobe: A small part of anterior pituitary adjacent to posterior pituitary becomes the intermediate lobe.

Posterior pituitary: Formed by the invagination of the diencephalon called the infundibulum

Anatomical Relations

It occupies the bony space within the skull called *Sella turcica*.

- Anteriorly and inferiorly: Sphenoid sinus
- *Laterally*: Cavernous sinus (has internal carotid arteries and sixth cranial nerve travelling through it)
- *Posteriorly*: Clinoid processes of the sphenoid bone
- *Superiorly*: The pituitary stalk anterior to which is the optic chiasm

Blood Supply

- *Superior hypophyseal artery:* It forms a primary plexus in the base of the hypothalamus. This then converts in portal vessels that travel to the anterior pituitary to form the secondary plexus.
- *Inferior hypophyseal artery*: It supplies the posterior pituitary.
- Both of these arteries are driven from the carotid arteries

Products of the Pituitary Gland

- *Anterior pituitary*: It consists of cells that can be differentiated according to their staining affinities with stains; eosin and haematoxylin
  - *Acidophils:* Secrete prolactin (PL) and growth hormone (GH)
  - *Basophils:* Secrete gonadotrophins (FSH and LH), thyroid stimulating hormone (TSH) and ACTH
  - *Chromophobes*: Likely resting but chromophobe adenomas can secrete gonadotrophins subunits
- *Posterior pituitary*: It contains the nerve terminals of the paraventricular and the supraoptic nuclei, which pass down the pituitary stalk to reach it. The nuclei synthesize and release oxytocin and vasopressin.

Function of the Products of the Pituitary Gland

Tables 6.1 and 6.2 list the functions of the pituitary hormones.

Dysfunction of the Pituitary Gland

The function of the pituitary can be affected by an excessive or underproduction of associated hormones or by a mass effect of a tumour (Table 6.3).

Table 6.1 Functions of the anterior pituitary hormones

Cells	Hormones	Role
Acidophils	GH	Stimulates hepatic IGF-11 synthesis & release
	PL	Stimulates lactation
Basophils	LH	ovarian hormone synthesis & oocyte release
	FSH	Follicle maturation
	TSH	Stimulates thyroid hormone release
	ACTH	Stimulates cortisol synthesis in the adrenal gland

Table 6.2 Function of the posterior pituitary hormones

Hormone	Source	Role
Oxytocin	Lateral & superior paraventricular & supraoptic nuclei	Stimulates the contraction of: • Myoepithelial cells of breast • Uterine myocytes in labour
Vasopressin	Lateral & superior paraventricular & supraoptic nuclei	• Retains water by altering permeability of collecting ducts in kidneys • Cardiovascular regulation • Enhances CRH-stimulated ACTH release

Adrenal Gland

These are the two glands; adjacent to either kidney, responsible for our flight or fight response.

Structure of the Gland

It consists of two parts:

- *Cortex:* Is further subdivided into an outer (zona glomerulosa), middle (zona fasciculate) and inner (zona reticularis) layers
- *Medulla*

Embryology

- *Adrenal cortex*: Mesoderm
- *Adrenal medulla*: Neural crest cells

Anatomical Relations

The adrenal glands are retroperitoneal and are also called suprarenal glands as they lie on top of the kidneys.

Blood Supply

- *Arterial blood supply:* Branches of aorta, renal and inferior phrenic arteries
- *Venous blood drainage:* Inferior vena cava from right adrenal gland and renal vein from the left gland

Products of the Adrenal Gland

Cortex

- *Zona glomerulosa*: Aldosterone
- *Zona fasciculate and zona reticularis:* Androgens and cortisol. Both of these zones are controlled by adrenocorticotrophic hormone (ACTH).

Medulla: Produces adrenaline and noradrenaline, also known as catecholamines

Function of the Products of the Adrenal Gland

Cortisol is essential for life, as it:

- Stimulates:
  - Gluconeogenesis
  - Fat breakdown
  - Mobilisation of amino acids

Dexamethasone is the most potent synthetic steroid at the glucocorticoid receptor.

Aldosterone is a mineralocorticoid steroid hormone which:

- Increases reabsorption of sodium and water by the kidney
- Stimulates secretion of potassium and H+ ions in the kidney

Condition	Clinical features	Diagnosis	Management	Effects on pregnancy
Prolactinoma • Micro <10 mm • Macro >10 mm	• Infertility • Galactorrhoea • Amenorrhoea • Frontal headache • Diabetes insipidus • Visual field defects	• CT or MRI of the pituitary gland • Raised serum level of PL (outside pregnancy)	• Dopamine-receptor agonists (Bromocriptine/cabergoline). • Discontinue if pregnant unless used to stop tumour expansion. • Formal visual field testing if macroprolactinoma or symptomatic • Surgery or radiotherapy in rare cases but delayed till after delivery • In pregnancy, review once in each trimester	• 15% risk of expansion of macroprolactinomas especially in third trimester in comparison to 1.6% for micro • Above risk is reduced (2–3% for macro) if it is treated prior to pregnancy • 40 % of women will have remission following pregnancy and lactation • There are no associated congenital abnormalities or adverse pregnancy outcome
Diabetes insipidus (DI)	• Excessive thirst • Polyuria	• Low ADH levels • If plasma osmolality (>295 mOsmol/kg) or serum sodium (>145 mmol/L) is inappropriately raised in the presence of polyuria and a low urine osmolality (<300 mOsmol/kg) • Administration of dDAVP (synthetic vasopressin) will cause concentration of urine in cranial DI	• dDAVP is safe to use in pregnancy • Check serum electrolytes and plasma osmolality	• If treated, there is no adverse effect on pregnancy or labour • If untreated or undiagnosed, severe dehydration along with electrolyte imbalance can occur
Acromegaly	• Gross enlargement of tongue, hands or feet • Coarse facial features • Headache, sweating • Can be infertile with hyperprolactinaemia	• Difficult in pregnancy • Insulin growth factor-1 used outside pregnancy	• Treatment prior to pregnancy with surgery and/or radiotherapy • Bromocriptine or Cabergoline only work in 50% of cases • Somatostatin analogues are used outside pregnancy	• Increase risk of gestational diabetes and macrosomia • Less commonly expand and can cause visual field changes on expansion
Sheehan's syndrome	• Infertility • Amenorrhoea • Inability to lactate • Hypothyroidism • Loss of axillary and pubic hair • Low blood sugar, hypotension	• Diagnosis is suspected in the presence of history of postpartum haemorrhage • Diagnostic evaluation of pituitary hormones	• Replacement of the deficient hormones	• Occurs post partum
Cushing's disease	• Increased truncal obesity • Purple striae • Diabetes mellitus • HTN • Headache • Proximal myopathy • Bitemporal hemianopsia with central visual defects.	• CT/MRI of pituitary • Dexamethasone suppression test will suppress cortisol level to less than 50% of baseline.	• Surgery • Hormonal replacement	• Increased risk of fetal loss and prematurity • Risk of adrenal insufficiency in the neonate • Severe pre-eclampsia • Wound infection

Effects of Catecholamines

Dysfunction of the Adrenal Gland

These can be related to the cortex or medulla.

Tables 6.4 and 6.6 outline the main causes of hyperadrenalism and hypoadrenalism. Table 6.5 lists the features of Cushing syndrome.

Congenital Adrenal Hyperplasia (CAH)

CAH is rare and is autosomal recessive.

Pathogenesis

- 90% are due to 21-alpha-hydroxylase deficiency
- 10% are due to 11-βhydroxylase deficiency

Table 6.4 Main causes of hyperadrenalism

	Primary hyperadrenalism	**Secondary hyperadrenalism**
Causes	Conn's syndrome Bilateral adrenal hyperplasia Adrenal carcinoma	Renal artery stenosis Renin secreting tumour
Biochemical abnormalities	Hypokalaemia Suppressed Renin activity High plasma aldosterone	Increased renin (renin secreting tumour) Hypokalaemia High plasma aldosterone
Clinical Features	Hypertension	Hypertension (poorly controlled)
Diagnostic tests	U/S scanning of the adrenal glands Biochemical findings as above	Angiography U/S or CT Renal vein sampling (renin secreting tumour)
Treatment	Antihypertensive treatment Amiloride Surgery	Angioplasty Revascularisation Pharmacologic agents: Calcium channel blocking agents (to optimise renal perfusion)

Table 6.5 Features of Cushing syndrome

Pathogenesis	- 65–70% due to pituitary adenomas (Cushing disease) - 10–15% by Ectopic ACTH or CRH production - 20% due to adrenal adenoma, nodular hyperplasia or carcinomas
Clinical features	- Hypertension - Diabetes mellitus - Central obesity - Moon facies - Purple striae - Buffalo hump - Easy bruising - Acne - Proximal myopathy - Menstrual abnormalities - Osteoporosis
Diagnosis	*High dexamethasone dose suppression test*: - Low ACTH & high cortisol level if adrenal causes - High ACTH & no effect on cortisol if ectopic ACTH producing tumours - Low cortisol if pituitary causes - U/S, CT or MRI of the adrenal or the pituitary glands
Effects on pregnancy	- Increased risk of fetal loss, prematurity & perinatal mortality - Risk of severe preeclampsia, gestational diabetes, wound infection and maternal mortality and morbidity
Management	- Surgery is the usual treatment - Limited experience in pregnancy with ketoconazole, cyproheptadine and metyrapone

Table 6.6 Main causes of hypoadrenalism

	Primary hypoadrenalism	Secondary hyporadrenalism
Causes	Addison's disease	Disorder of hypothalamus or pituitary (irradiation, metastatic cancer, infection or infarction)
Biochemical abnormalities	• Low aldosterone • Hyponatraemia • Hypoglycaemia • Hyperkalaemia • Raised blood urea	• Reduced ACTH levels • Decreased cortisol and androgens • Normal or near-normal aldosterone • No marked hyponatremia and hyperkalaemia
Clinical features	• Weight loss • Postural hypotension • Weakness • Hyperpigmentation	Hyperpigmentation is lacking
Diagnostic tests	• There will be a loss of cortisol response to synthetic ACTH (Synacthen) • 09:00 AM cortisol level will be low • Raised ACTH level	There is a prompt rise in plasma cortisol levels when ACTH is administered
Treatment	Both hydrocortisone (25–30 mg/day orally in divided doses) and fludrocortisone (0.1 mg/day) are required	Treat the cause

Clinical Features

- Female fetus can present with ambiguous genitalia (due to androgen excess).
- Male fetus may experience salt-losing crisis (due to mineralocorticoid deficiency).
- Precocious puberty in a male
- Features of adrenal androgen excess (e.g. hirsutism or anovulation, infertility, psychological sequel and premature menopause in females)

Management

Mineralocorticoid and steroid replacement

Pheochromocytoma

Pheochromocytoma is a tumour of the adrenal medulla.

Pathogenesis

10% is an important figure to remember pertaining to pheochromocytoma, as 10% are bilateral, 10% extra adrenal and 10% malignant

Clinical Features

- Paroxysmal hypertension
- Excessive perspiration
- Anxiety
- Pallor
- Tremor
- Headache
- Palpitations

Diagnosis

- Raised levels of plasma catecholamines
- 24 hours of urinary excretion of VMA
- CT/MRI/US for tumour localisation

Management

- α-blockade with phenoxybenzamine or prazosin
- β-blockade for control of tachycardia
- Surgical removal cures it
- Maternal and fetal mortality is high
- Labour, vaginal or abdominal delivery can precipitate fatal hypertensive crises
- α-blockade must be given at least 3 days prior to surgery
- Expert anaesthetist care is required

Thyroid Gland

It is the first endocrine gland to develop in a fetus.

Embryology

- Develops as a diverticulum from the root of the tongue called foramen caecum

- Develops between the first and second pharyngeal arches
- Travels down to settle in front of tracheal cartilages
- Fourth pharyngeal arch forms the ultimobranchial body that forms the c cells of the thyroid gland

Structure of the Gland

- It weighs 20 g.
- It is 4 cm long.
- It has two lobes and an interconnecting isthmus.
- It sometimes has a small pyramidal lobe.

Anatomical Relations

- *Medially*: Inferior thyroid artery. Recurrent laryngeal nerve, trachea, larynx, oesophagus
- *Posteriorly*: Trachea, parathyroids, carotid sheath, prevertebral fascia
- *Anteriorly*: Pretracheal fascia, sternohyoid, sternothyroid, venous arch

Blood Supply

- *Arterial blood supply*: Superior thyroid artery; branch of external carotid and the inferior thyroid artery; branch of subclavian artery
- *Venous blood supply*: Superior and middle thyroid veins drain into the internal jugular vein and the inferior thyroid vein drains into the brachiocephalic vein

Products of the Thyroid Gland

- The thyroid gland is made of more than a million follicles.
- Each follicle has a central colloid that is surrounded by a layer of follicular cells.
- *Follicular cells*: Secrete thyroxine (T4) and tri-iodothyronine (T3) in colloid, where these are stored in thyroglobulin.
- *Para follicular cells (C-cells)*: Synthesize and secrete calcitonin and reside in the connective tissue adjacent to the thyroid follicles.

Physiology of the Thyroid Hormones

- *Iodide trapping*: Iodide is actively taken up into the follicular cells by the iodide and sodium pump against the concentration gradient.

- *Iodine oxidation*: It is converted to iodine by the enzyme peroxidase.
- Iodine combines with tyrosine to form mono iodotyrosine (MIT) or diiodotyrosine (DIT).
- Coupling of these can result in T3 or T4, which are stored in the colloid in the form of thyroglobulin.
- This is phagocytised by the follicular cells and broken down to free T3 and T4 which diffuse into the blood.
- 20 times more T4 than T3 released into the blood.
- T3 is four times more potent than T4. Cells convert T4 to T3 by deiodination.

Function of the Thyroid Gland

General

- Tissue growth
- Brain maturation

Metabolism

- Increased heat production and oxygen consumption
- Increase in glucose and amino acid transport
- Stimulates lipolysis, glycolysis, gluconeogenesis, absorption of glucose and the metabolism of insulin and cortisol

Gut

Increases gut motility

Bones

Increases bone resorption

CNS

- Maintains the normal hypoxic and hypercapnic drives to the respiratory centre
- Increases in expression of β-receptors in the heart, skeletal muscle and the adipose tissue

The Thyroid Axis

- The hypothalamus secretes thyrotropin-releasing hormone (TRH), which acts on the anterior pituitary gland to secrete thyroid-stimulating hormone (TSH).
- TSH then stimulates the thyroid gland to produce T3, T4 and when the levels rise sufficiently, the

Table 6.7 Salient points of hyperthyroidism

Causes	• Graves' disease (80% of cases) • Toxic multinodular goitre • Toxic adenoma • Thyroiditis • TSH secreting tumour • Thyroid follicular carcinoma
Clinical features	• Heat intolerance • Tachycardia, palpitations • Palmer erythema • Goitre • Vomiting • Weight loss • Tremor • Lid lag • Exophthalmos
Diagnosis	• Raised free T4 or free T3 • TSH is low
Effect on pregnancy	• Thyrotoxicosis improves in the second and third trimester • If untreated, risk of miscarriage, fetal growth restriction, preterm labour and perinatal mortality. *Note in relation to pregnancy:* • Stimulation of the thyroid by HCG • Reduced plasma iodine concentration • Increase in thyroid-binding globulin – Less free I4
Management	• Carbimazole 15-40 mg or propylthiouracil 150-400 mg for 4–6 weeks • Dose then reduced to 5–15 mg for carbimazole and 50–150 mg for PTU • Beta-blockers • Surgery • Radioactive iodine (contraindicated in pregnancy and breastfeeding)

release of TRH and TSH is suppressed in a negative feedback loop.

• If T3 and T4 levels are suppressed, the persistent stimulation of the thyroid gland by TSH results in a goitre.

Dysfunction of the Thyroid Gland

Dysfunction of the thyroid gland can result in excessive thyroid hormones called hyperthyroidism (Table 6.7) or a deficiency in thyroid hormones, resulting in hypothyroidism (Table 6.8).

Causes of Primary Hypothyroidism

• Hashimoto's disease (commonest cause in pregnancy)
• Primary (atrophic) hypothyroidism
• Radio iodine therapy
• Thyroid surgery
• Thyroiditis
• Genetic defect resulting in impaired T4 synthesis
• Anti-thyroid drugs

• Loss-of-function mutation in the gene encoding the TSH receptor
• Thyroid hormone resistance

Causes of Secondary Hypothyroidism

• Hypopituitarism caused by tumour, surgery or radiotherapy
• Impaired thyroid synthesis

Causes of Tertiary Hypothyroidism

Hypothalamic changes

Pancreas

Embryology

Pancreas is developed from two buds arising from the caudal part of the foregut:

• *Ventral bud*: Uncinate process, inferior part of the head of pancreas, main pancreatic duct

Table 6.8 Salient points of hypothyroidism

Clinical features	• Weight gain • Lethargy • Hair loss • Dry skin • Constipation • Goitre • Cold intolerance • Slow pulse rate • Delayed relaxation of tendon reflexes • Oligomenorrhoea • Menorrhagia • Infertility • In children results in cretinism
Diagnosis	• Low level of free T4 • TSH is raised • Thyroid autoantibodies in 20–30%
Effect on pregnancy	• Pregnancy has no effect on hypothyroidism • If untreated, increased risk of miscarriage, anaemia, fetal loss, pre-eclampsia and low birth weight infant
Management	• Dose of thyroxine between 100–200 micrograms, depending on the TFT results • If increased in pregnancy, ensure to check in puerperium

- *Dorsal bud*: Upper part of the head, body and tail of the pancreas, as well as the distal part of duct

Structure of the Gland

- It weighs 80 g.
- Is divided into head, uncinate process, neck, body and tail.
- The parenchyma is derived from the endoderm of the pancreatic bud.
- The pancreatic islets develop from the pancreatic parenchyma.

Anatomical Relations

The pancreas is retroperitoneal.

- Anteriorly: Stomach
- Posteriorly: Vena cava, aorta

Blood Supply

Arterial Supply

- Celiac trunk
- Superior mesenteric artery

Venous Supply

- Superior pancreaticoduodenal veins drain in the portal vein

- Inferior pancreaticoduodenal vein drains into the superior mesenteric vein

Products of the Pancreas (Table 6.9)

Dysfunction of the Pancreas

The most significant is diabetes mellitus. The main types are as follows:

- Type 1
- Type 2
- Gestational diabetes

Type 1 DM: No or too little insulin production. It occurs in 10% of the people with diabetes.

Risks

- Surgery
- Alcohol
- Disease
- Destruction of the beta cells of the pancreas

Type 2 DM: The body does not respond to insulin levels as normal and develops insulin resistance. The body cannot produce enough insulin to overcome this resistance. It occurs in 90% of the people with diabetes.

Risks

- Age >40 years
- Weight BMI > 30 kg/m^2

Table 6.9 Products of the pancreas

	Cells of origin	Function	Stimulated by	Inhibited by
Insulin	Beta cells of islets of Langerhans	Transport of glucose and amino acids across cell membranes	Glucose, basic amino acids, ketones, free fatty acids, glucagon, growth hormone, gut hormones	Hypoglycaemia, adrenaline, somatostatin
Glucagon	Alpha cells	Inhibits glucose and amino acid uptake, enhances lipolysis, hepatic glycogen lysis, gluconeogenesis, ketone production	Hypoglycaemia, basic amino acids, gut hormones, exercise, adrenaline	Hyperglycaemia, ketones, free fatty acids, insulin, somatostatin
Pancreatic somatostatin	Sigma cells	Regulates stomach motility, inhibits insulin, glucagon, gastrin, secretin	Increased level of glucose and amino acid	Low levels of the hormones that it regulates
Pancreatic polypeptide (PP)	PP cells	Regulation of digestion	Protein meal, exercising, fasting	Somatostatin and IV glucose

- Ethnicity
- Genetics

Gestational diabetes: Diabetes occurring in pregnancy as the pancreas may not produce sufficient insulin to manage high blood glucose levels in pregnancy.

Risks
- As Type 2 plus history of previous GDM

References

1. *Handbook of Obstetric Medicine.* 5th edition. 2015 Catherine Nelson Piercy.

2. *Basic Science in Obs & Gynae: A Textbook for MRCOG Part 1.* 4th edition. 2010. Phillip Bennett, Catherine Williamson.

3. *Medical Problems in Pregnancy.* 1st edition. 2007. Ian A Greer. Catherine Nelson-Piercy, Barry Walters.

4. *Pathologic Basis of Disease.* 5th edition. Cotran, Kumar, Robbins.

Single Best Answer Questions

1. A 25-years-old female presented with headaches, galactorrhoea and amenorrhoea for 4 months. Her likely diagnosis is:

   a. Thyroid nodule
   b. Prolactinoma
   c. Conn's syndrome
   d. Diabetes mellitus
   e. Pancreatic pseudocyst

2. A 28-year-old woman failed to establish lactation following the birth of her third child. The only complication of her delivery was a massive postpartum haemorrhage. She also had persistent amenorrhoea with nausea, vomiting and hypotension. The likely diagnosis is:

   a) Postpartum thyroiditis
   b) Diabetes insipidus
   c) Sheehan's syndrome
   d) Optic neuroma
   e) Conn's disease

3. In a woman with Addison's disease, you will find the following biochemical abnormalities:

   a) Low aldosterone, hyponatraemia, hypoglycaemia, hyperkalaemia
   b) Low aldosterone, hyponatraemia, hyperglycaemia, hyperkalaemia
   c) High aldosterone, hyponatraemia, hypoglycaemia, hyperkalaemia
   d) Low ACTH, hyponatraemia, hyperglycaemia, hyperkalaemia
   e) Low aldosterone, hyponatraemia, hypoglycaemia, hypokalaemia

4. A 16-year-old girl at 9 weeks in her first pregnancy came for a routine check-up. She had no recorded high B/P except incidentally, on a couple of separate occasions at the GP when the values were

190/120 and 180/110. Her mother has neuro-fibromatosis.

On arrival, she complained of excessive sweating. Her observations were:

B/P: 180/110 mmHg repeat reading (without medication) 110/60 mmHg

Pulse: 115 bpm

O_2 saturation: 100% on air

R/R: 12/min

Temp: 36.5°C

Urine dipstick: Blood: negative
                   Leucocytes: negative
                   Protein: negative

The diagnosis is:

a) White-coat syndrome
b) Pituitary apoplexy
c) Severe pre-eclampsia
d) Pheochromocytoma
e) Hypothyroidism

5. A 30-year-old woman presented with menorrhagia. She complained of heat intolerance and increase appetite associated with weight loss. On examination: She looked anxious and had a tremor.

Pulse: 105 bpm

B/P: 110/70 mmHg

What is your diagnosis?

a) Hypothyroidism
b) Malignancy
c) Anxiety disorder

d) Hyperthyroidism
e) Parkinson's

6. A 32-year-old woman at 12 weeks of her first pregnancy, attends the ANC. She is known hypothyroid and is currently on 50 micrograms of thyroxine. Her TFTs are as follows:

TSH: 4.5 mIU/L

T4: 6 µg/dL

How are going to manage her?

a) Decrease thyroxine
b) Increase thyroxine
c) Stop thyroxine
d) Start propylthiouracil
e) Start carbimazole

7. A 21-year-old, 28-weeks pregnant woman presented in A&E with nausea, vomiting, feeling lethargic, thirsty and frequently passing urine. Investigations:

Arterial pH: < or = 7.30

Bicarbonate level: < or = 18 mEq/l

Blood glucose: 20 mmol/l

Urine dipstick: ++++ ketones

What is your diagnosis?

a) Migraine
b) Addison's disease
c) Diabetic ketoacidosis
d) Gastric ulcer
e) Insulinoma

Congenital Infections

Philip Rice

Lists

List 1: Infective agents predominantly transmitted in utero

List 2: Infective agents predominantly transmitted peri-partum

List 3: Classifications of viral agents capable of causing maternal illness and/or fetal infection

List 4: Modes of transmission

List 5: Incubation periods, infectious periods and transmission risks

List 6: Prophylaxis available for specific infectious agents

List 7: Antenatal screening (country-specific)

List 8: Travel associated infections posing a risk to the fetus

List 9: Vaccinations recommended and/or used in pregnancy if the risk of infection justifies the use

List 10: Tests recommended for pregnant women in contact with specified infective agents

List 11: Clinical features of maternal illness with specified infections (% asymptomatic)

List 12: Clinical clues in maternal history and examination to help identify possible infective agents

List 13: Risk factors associated with increased risk of transmission

List 14: Incidence of infection in pregnancy

List 15: Risk of fetal transmission by trimester of maternal primary infection

List 16: Risk of long-term sequelae or adverse pregnancy outcome by trimester of maternal infection

List 17: Clinical findings in newborns with symptomatic congenital infection

List 18: Investigation of suspected symptomatic maternal infection

List 19: Investigations in cases of suspected congenital infection by fetal and maternal testing

List 20: Persistence of organism-specific IgM after symptom onset in pregnant women

List 21: Infections associated with a more severe outcome if acquired in pregnancy

List 22: Treatments available for congenital/ perinatal infection

Range of Infective Organisms – List 1

A wide range of organisms are capable of infecting the developing fetus. They range in size from the smallest viruses, e.g. parvoviruses, through to bacteria such as Treponema pallidum and protozoal parasites, namely Toxoplasma gondii. Many of these agents are, or once were common childhood infections, but if infection is delayed until adulthood, the fetus may be put at risk. Vaccination has almost eliminated the burden of disease in the case of rubella and hepatitis B, but significant problems remain with CMV and parvovirus, where neither effective vaccines nor safe anti-virals are yet available to prevent fetal infection and/or pregnancy loss.

List 1: Infective Agents Predominantly Transmitted In Utero	
Cytomegalovirus (CMV)	Fig. 7.1
Varicella-Zoster virus (VZV)	Fig. 7.1
Rubella virus	
Parvovirus B19	
Toxoplasma gondii	
Treponema pallidum (syphilis)	
Listeria monocytogenes	

Transmission in Pregnancy

Prevention of maternal infection remains the mainstay of efforts to reduce fetal morbidity caused by these organisms. However, this may be difficult or almost impossible for those viruses which are shed

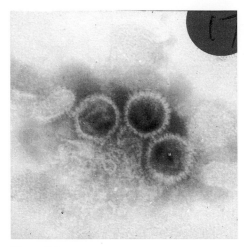

Figure 7.1

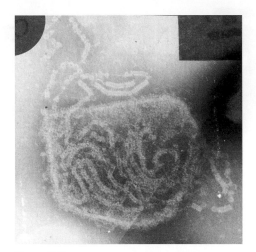

Figure 7.2

List 2: Infective Agents Predominantly Transmitted Peri-Partum

Herpes simplex virus (1 + 2)
Human immunodeficiency virus (HIV-1 and HIV-2)
Human papillomavirus (HPV)
Enteroviruses (e.g. Coxsackie B3)
Hepatitis B virus
Listeria monocytogenes
Group B streptococcus

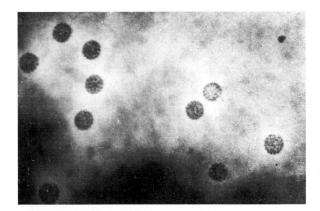

Figure 7.3

List 3: Classifications of Viral Agents Capable of Causing Maternal Illness and/or Fetal Infection (see Figs. 7.2. and 7.3)

Virus	Virus type	Nucleic envelope acid		Latency (L)/ chronic (C)	Subtypes/ strains	Vaccine
CMV	Herpes	DNA	Yes	Yes (L)	Multiple	No
HSV-1	Herpes	DNA	Yes	Yes (L)	No	No
HSV-2	Herpes	DNA	Yes	Yes (L)	No	No
VZV	Herpes	DNA	Yes	Yes (L)	No	Yes (live)
Rubella togavirus	RNA	Yes	No	No	Yes (live)	
Parvo	Erythrovirus	RNA	No	No (C*)	No	No
HPV	Papillomavirus	DNA	No	Yes (C)	>100	Yes (recombinant)
Measles morbillivirus	RNA	Yes	Yes (rarely, C)	No	Yes (live)	

List 3: (cont.)

Virus	Virus type	Nucleic envelope acid		Latency (L)/ chronic (C)	Subtypes/ strains	Vaccine
HAV	Hepatovirus	RNA	No	No	Yes	Yes (killed)
HBV	Hepadnavirus	DNA	Yes	Yes (L,C)	Yes	Yes (recombinant)
HCV	Hepacivirus	RNA	Yes	Yes (C)	Yes	No
HEV	Hepevirus	RNA	No	Yes (C*)	Yes[#,@]	Yes[@]

HAV = hepatitis A virus; HBV = hepatitis B virus; HCV = hepatitis C virus; HEV = hepatitis E virus.

* In immune compromised

\# Genotype 1 has a mortality of c. 15–25% in pregnancy

@ Genotype 1 only

silently, cause asymptomatic infection (e.g. CMV and parvovirus B19) and especially where a licensed vaccine is not yet available (namely parvovirus, HSV and CMV).

It is important to understand the mode of transmission since educating pregnant women, ideally pre-conception, should reduce the infection risk. Indeed, some infections are largely avoidable by adhering to such advice (e.g. dietary and hygienic practices for T. gondii and Listeria), while others are realistically preventable only by childhood immunisation (e.g. rubella, measles and varicella). Antenatal testing is also an essential component of the prevention strategy, e.g. in prevention of mother to child transmission (MTCT) of HIV, hepatitis B and syphilis. The nature of antenatal screening evolves over time, however, as has recently been demonstrated in the UK. Antenatal rubella testing has recently been dropped from the national programme for two linked reasons: since 2013 the number of confirmed rubella cases in England is between one and three cases annually, and this rarity has led to errors or delay in pre-natal diagnosis when pregnant women have been exposed to or developed a rash illness. Consequently, the UK antenatal rubella antibody screening programme has been replaced by assessing the evidence for pre-pregnancy rubella immunisation. If two doses of a rubella-containing vaccine have been received pre-conception, immunity is assumed. Testing after exposure to or upon the development of, a rubella-like rash may still take place, but the

List 4: Modes of Transmission and Infective Agents

Modes of transmission	Infective agents
Sexual	HSV-1, HSV-2, CMV, T. pallidum, HIV, HPV
Droplet	Measles, rubella, varicella, enterovirus
Close/kissing contact	CMV, HSV-1, HSV-2, parvovirus B19
Fomites	CMV
Nosocomial	Measles, rubella, HSV, VZV
Faeco-Oral	Hepatitis A and E, enteroviruses, T. gondii, listeria

results of previous rubella antibody tests will be interpreted alongside the vaccination history.

If exposure to an infection occurs which could, if contracted, pose a risk to the mother or the developing fetus, the following list gives advice on how to proceed with assessment of the woman's immunity to infection.

Features Suggesting a Specific Clinical Diagnosis

The acronym TORCH is often used as a shorthand, umbrella term for the diagnosis of suspected congenital infection. However, it is often used too widely and indiscriminately, and it should be abandoned. The early detection of specific infections in pregnant

List 5: Incubation Periods, Infectivity Periods and Transmission Risks of Organisms Capable of Causing Fetal Infection or Loss

Virus	Incubation period	Infectivity[#]	Risk of transmission (% and/or R_0) Median days (range) (pre & post rash)
VZV	14 days (10–21)	−2* to + 5	Household 90%+ in temperate zone, 15–25% tropics[§]
CMV	4–6 weeks	Shed intermittently;	0.5–10% per year[$] saliva, urine and genital tract
Rubella	14 days (12–20)	−7 to + 2	$R_0 = 6$
Measles	12 days (7–18)	−4 to +4	90+% ($R_0 = 12–18$)
HSV	3–7 days	Shed intermittently;	1–5% per year in discordant
		c.1–2 episodes/100	couples days
Parvovirus	16 days (13–20)	−6 to −2 pre rash	Up to 50% in outbreaks Household: 20–30%

\# = The phase of illness during which the virus may be transmitted

R_0 = The number of secondary cases from an index case in a non-immune population

§ = This difference is due to virus inactivation in the skin lesions by UV radiation

$ = The wide range reflects the low background risk, with the higher rate reflecting different occupational or risk groups, e.g. nursery workers, teenagers

---

List 6: Prophylaxis Available for Specific Infectious Agents Capable of Causing Congenital or Peri-Partum Infection

Pre-exposure Vaccination

Rubella vaccine (as part of MMR)
Varicella vaccine
CMV recombinant glycoprotein B vaccine – investigational (not yet licensed)

Pre-exposure Anti-virals

Aciclovir (ACV) in HSV sero-discordant couples – c. 50–60% efficacy in preventing infection
Tenofovir in HIV discordant couples

Post-exposure Prophylaxis

Varicella zoster immune globulin (VZIG) for protection against chickenpox in pregnancy

List 7: Antenatal Screening (Country-Specific)

HIV – universal; consider re-testing later in pregnancy only if at high risk of primary infection, e.g. new or concurrent STI diagnosis, multiple or frequent partner change
HBV – universal – HBsAg
T. pallidum – universal
Rubella – universal; dropped from UK programme in 2016
CMV – selective – Israel and eight European countries (France, Belgium, Spain, Italy, Germany, Austria, Portugal, and the Netherlands), Australia, USA
T. gondii – Austria, France, some Brazilian states

With the arrival and now global spread of the Zika virus, it is timely to examine the organisms which pose a risk to pregnant women contemplating travel or living/ working overseas. Many vaccines, for obvious reasons, are not subjected to clinical trials in pregnancy, yet are safe to give in pregnancy and would be recommended depending on the degree of risk.

List 8 outlines infective agents which pose a risk to the developing fetus during travel overseas, and List 9 lists the organisms for which vaccination may be justifiable and/or recommended in pregnancy.

women helps decision making about pre-natal diagnosis and the eventual outcome of the pregnancy. Some clinical clues aid this process by directing the clinician to request the most appropriate tests. However, as this diagnostic area is often complex, it is essential that expert interpretive advice is sought from a consultant microbiologist or virologist or clinical scientist as appropriate. The following lists highlight some of the clinical features, elements of the

maternal history and risk factors which should act as triggers for diagnostic testing.

List 8: Infections Posing a Risk to the Fetus Associated with Travel to Developing Countries

CMV	Commonly associated with travel; no recommendations for testing after return home; testing advised if maternal symptoms or fetal signs of infection
Rubella virus	At risk only if not previously adequately immunised
Measles virus	At risk only if not previously adequately immunised
Yellow fever	Vaccination advised if at high risk of infection or local outbreak
Zika virus	No vaccine available; testing and/or serial fetal ultrasound scans recommended after travel to an endemic country
Hepatitis A/B	If at significant risk, vaccination recommended before travel

List 9: Vaccinations Recommended and/or Used in Pregnancy If Risk Justifies Use

Virus/organism	Type of vaccine	Risk to fetus
Hepatitis A	Inactivated vaccine	Theoretical
Hepatitis B	Recombinant sAg	Theoretical
		Vaccination advised if woman has > 1 sexual partner in past 6 months, has been treated recently for an STI, has recent or current injecting drug use or has an HBsAg positive partner
HPV	Recombinant VLP*	Not recommended; no need for fetal investigations if immunised while pregnant
Influenza	Inactivated	Recommended
Influenza	Live attenuated	Contraindicated
MMR	Live attenuated	Contraindicated#
Meningococcal	Polysaccharide	May be used if indicated$
Polio	Inactivated	Should be avoided on theoretical grounds but if at risk may be justified
Smallpox	Live attenuated	Contraindicated (Global eradication 1979)
Tetanus	Toxoid	May be given if requires immediate protection
Pertussis¥	Acellular/inactivated	Recommended to prevent neonatal whooping cough
Varicella vaccine	Live attenuated	Contraindicated; no proven link with fetal infection
Yellow fever	Live attenuated	Precaution; vaccinate if at significant infection risk, e.g. travel to country with outbreak
Zoster vaccine	Live attenuated	Contraindicated; no data on risk to fetus

* VLP = Virus-like particle
# = No cases of congenital rubella syndrome have been attributed to inadvertent rubella vaccination in pregnancy
$ = Applies only to ACWY vaccine; no information on Men B vaccine
¥ = Whooping cough

Incidence of Infection in Pregnancy and In Utero Transmission Rate

The risk of maternal infection in pregnancy for many infections is low, though the potential for fetal harm can still be considerable, especially for those infections where prophylaxis is not available, i.e. CMV and parvovirus B19.

The determinant of the fetal outcome is a complex interplay between the specific infective agent, the trimester at which maternal infection is acquired, the gestational age at which fetal infection takes place and

List 10: Procedure for Pregnant Women in Contact with Specified Infective Agents

Varicella/shingles exposure	Test maternal booking or current blood for VZV IgG:
	VZV IgG >100 miu/ml – VZIG not required
	VZV IgG <100 miu/ml – VZIG recommended within 10 days of exposure. (There is evidence that a level of VZV IgG between 50 and 100 miu/ml is indicative of past infection and thus protective)
Measles exposure	Take history of (H/O) measles infection and vaccination and year of birth:

Born before 1970:
    H/O measles infection: assume immune
    No H/O measles infection: assume immune
Born between 1970 and 1990:
    H/O measles infection: assume immune
    No H/O measles infection: test for measles IgG
Born after 1990:
    1 dose of measles vaccine: test for measles IgG
    2 doses of measles vaccine: assume immune
    Unvaccinated: test for measles IgG *
    * If not able to test within 6 days, issue HNIG

Parvovirus B19	Test maternal booking or current clotted blood sample
	If IgG is detected and IgM not detected at booking, this indicates immunity
	If IgG and IgM are not detected at booking or in a current sample, the woman is susceptible and should be advised to have another sample 4 weeks after the last exposure
	If a current sample is tested and IgG is detected but IgM is negative, test the booking blood to exclude recent infection and a transient IgM response from asymptomatic infection
	If IgG and IgM are both detected in a current sample, test the booking blood to demonstrate sero-conversion
CMV	If an 'exposure' to CMV occurs, do not test the woman but offer to discuss with a virologist to decide the best course of action
	Exposures to CMV are common, as a large proportion of infants/toddlers shed virus in urine and saliva, and sexual transmission is also a common mode of spread

* HNIG = Human Normal Immune Globulin

List 11: Clinical Features of Maternal Illness Caused by Different Infectious Agents (% without Symptoms during the Primary Infection)

CMV	Pyrexia of unknown origin (PUO), glandular fever-like illness, biochemical hepatitis (50%)
HSV	Symptomatic genital herpes if never before infected; recurrent genital ulcers; recurrent meningitis (Mollaret's; 30–70%; Fig. 7.4)
VZV	Chickenpox, primary infection (0%); shingles/zoster, reactivation (0%)
HIV	Sero-conversion illness (flu/glandular-fever illness with rash; 10–20%)
Rubella	Morbilliform rash, arthralgia, occipital lymphadenopathy (20–50%; Fig. 7.5)
Measles	Morbilliform rash with prodromal illness (cough, coryza, conjunctivitis; 0%; Fig. 7.6)
	Parvovirus B19 Pruritic maculo-papular rash, slapped cheeks, widespread arthralgia (Fig. 7.7)
Enterovirus	Maculo-papular rash, coryza, pharyngitis, oral ulcers, mild febrile illness (50%; Fig. 7.8)
T. Pallidum	Painless oral/genital ulcer(s), maculo-papular rash, generalised lymphadenopathy
T. gondii	Asymptomatic (75%); isolated cervical lymph node, rarely more generalised
Zika virus	Fever, rash, conjunctivitis, arthralgia (70–80%)

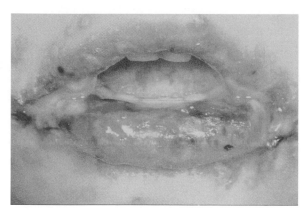

Figure 7.4

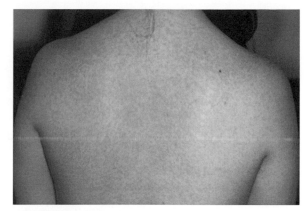

Figure 7.5

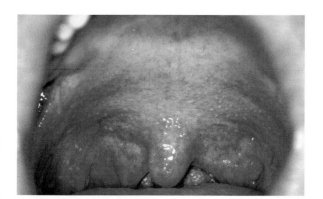

Figure 7.6

Figure 7.7

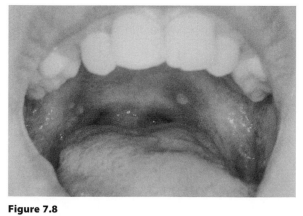

Figure 7.8

List 12: Key Elements of Maternal History, Clinical Signs and Infective Agents to Consider

Rash	Parvovirus B19, rubella, measles, varicella, primary HIV, enterovirus (EV), secondary syphilis, Zika/dengue (CMV, EBV – esp. if received amoxicillin)
Arthralgia	Parvovirus B19, rubella, Zika, chikungunya, dengue (EV, CMV, EBV)
Animal exposure	Cats, esp. kittens (toxoplasma, [Bartonella, Coxiella burnetii]
Undercooked meat/raw/unwashed uncooked veg/salad cat faeces; gardening without gloves	} } } Toxoplasma gondii } }

List 13: Risk Factors Associated with an Increased Risk of Infection	
CMV	Travel overseas, first child at home attending day-care, teenage pregnancy, multiple sexual partners, nursery/day-care worker
Rubella	Unimmunised, travel overseas
Measles	Unimmunised, travel overseas especially to countries/areas with outbreak
VZV	Born in tropics; no history of previous chickenpox; no siblings
T. gondii	Exposure to cats/kittens and their litter, consumption of under-cooked fresh (not previously frozen) meat, unwashed vegetables/salad, gardening without gloves
T. pallidum	Multiple sexual partners, unprotected sexual intercourse (UPSI)
HIV	Untested partner, multiple or frequent partner change, UPSI
HSV	Multiple or frequent partner change, UPSI, no H/O cold sores
HPV	Firstborn, vaginal delivery, aged <20 yrs, active genital warts
Parvovirus	Ongoing community-wide outbreak

List 14: Incidence of Selected Infections in Pregnancy	
CMV	0.5–2%
Rubella	<0.1%
T. gondii	0.01–0.1%
Measles	<0.1%
Parvo	c. 1% (up to 10% in epidemic years)
VZV	c. 0.3% (higher in Tropics)
HSV	c. 1–3%

List 15: Approximate Risk of Transmission to Fetus According to Trimester When Primary Infection Occurs

	First	Second	Third
CMV	35%	45%	70%
Rubella	90%	25–35%	50%
Parvovirus	15%	20–40%	50–60%
VZV	5%	10%	>25%
T. gondii	9%	27%	60%

whether there is any evidence of pre-existing maternal infection. One virus infection exemplifies this perfectly, namely CMV. In general, as the pregnancy advances, although the risk of the fetus being infected increases, the risk of the fetus being affected decreases.

Details of this risk are outlined in List 15.

The risks of the fetus being affected in some way, from minor unilateral sensori-neural hearing loss (SNHL) through to multi-system disease, are outlined in List 16.

Specifically for CMV, the 20th week of gestation appears to be a hard cut-off in terms of the risk of long-term sequelae from infection in the developing CNS. It is well established that the risk of a poorer outcome is increased if infection occurs before 20 weeks, with approximately 25–30% having CNS abnormalities compared with just 6% when infection occurs after 20 weeks. CMV is also unique, perhaps, in that the risk of the fetus being affected is not diminished by a previous infection. Re-infection with CMV is thought to pose the same risk to the developing fetus.

The same 20-week gestation rule applies to chickenpox in pregnancy, where the risk of a fetus being affected when maternal infection occurs after week 20 is almost negligible. Part of the reason for this must lie with the ability of the fetus to control virus reactivation, since this is believed to be the mechanism by which fetal damage ensues. The current theory regarding the development of varicella embryopathy is as follows:

Maternal viraemia with chickenpox rash

↓

Virus crosses placenta and fetus develops varicella

↓

Fetus recovers without apparent sequelae

↓

VZV establishes latent infection

↓

Virus reactivates down nerve axons in utero

↓

List 16: Risk of Long-Term Sequelae or Adverse Pregnancy Outcome by Trimester of Maternal Infection

	First	Second	Third
CMV	20–25%	10%	2–5%
Rubella	90%	6–17%*	1–2%§
Parvovirus	9%	9%	<1 3%
VZV	0.5%	1.4%	0%
T. gondii	80%	15–20%	10%

* Up to the 20th week; § After the 20th week

List 17: Clinical Findings in Newborns with Symptomatic Congenital Infection

CMV	Microcephaly, symmetrical fetal growth restriction (FGR), rash, hepatosplenomegaly, jaundice, respiratory difficulties, cerebral palsy, SNHL
Rubella	Cataracts (uni-/bilateral), retinopathy, microphthalmia, patent ductus arteriosus (PDA), pulmonary artery stenosis, ventricular septal defect (VSD), myocarditis, microcephaly, symmetrical FGR, hepatosplenomegaly, thrombocytopenia with purpura, pneumonitis
Parvovirus B19	None recognised; a possible persisting anaemia if transfused in utero
VZV	Skin scarring, skin hypo-/hyper-pigmentation, hypoplastic limbs, muscle wasting, retinopathy, microphthalmia
Measles	None
T. gondii	Microcephaly, hydrocephalus, FGR, hepatosplenomegaly, convulsions, chorioretinitis, cataracts
Enteroviruses	Acute fatal myocarditis (most often due to Coxsackie B3), sepsis-type syndrome
HPV	None; later develops recurrent, respiratory papillomatosis (RRLP)
T. pallidum	Failure to thrive, fever, snuffly with nasal discharge, irritability, oro-genital and skin rash, saddle nose

List 18: Investigation of Suspected Symptomatic Maternal Infection

Virus	Samples and recommended testing methods
CMV	Clotted blood for CMV specific IgG and IgM
	Perform IgG avidity if CMV IgM detected. (If low avidity CMV IgG detected, a primary infection is confirmed. May also be able to show a rise in the CMV IgG titre or even a rise in avidity from high to even higher in cases of re-infection.) NB symptomatic re-infection is likely to carry just as great a risk to fetal development as a primary infection.
	EDTA blood for CMV DNA PCR – NB viraemia may be low level or undetectable. If CMV IgM is detected, interpret a negative CMV PCR result cautiously – does not necessarily exclude infection, primary of re-infection
Rubella	Clotted blood for rubella specific IgG and IgM; NB if blood is taken ≤3 days after rash onset IgG and IgM are often undetectable – a repeat sample is required. If virus-specific IgM is detected, confirm with IgG avidity. Check for stored samples taken before rash
Parvovirus	Clotted blood for parvovirus specific IgG and IgM. If IgG is low and IgM is negative, collect a repeat sample as, rarely, IgM may appear after the IgG response in acute infection. If IgM is

detected, check for earlier samples, e.g. booking to try and demonstrate an IgG sero-conversion

Measles	Collect urine/throat swab for measles RNA PCR if rash onset is <7 days; collect clotted blood for measles specific IgG and IgM if rash onset > 3 days
HIV	Clotted blood for 4th generation HIV-1/HIV-2 antigen/antibody (Ag/Ab) test; consider HIV RNA testing if results are inconclusive and a repeat clotted sample 3–5 days after first sample for repeat Ag/Ab testing
Zika	EDTA blood for viral PCR if duration of illness is < 7 days; clotted blood for virus-specific IgG and IgM (cross-reacting antibodies can occur with previous yellow fever vaccine or dengue virus infection)

List 19: Recommended Investigations in Cases of Suspected Congenital Infection by Testing the Pregnant Woman, Fetus or Newborn

Infective agent	Samples and recommended testing methods
CMV	Pregnant woman: current and booking sera tested for CMV IgM and IgG and IgG avidity; locate pre-pregnancy samples if possible; consider CMV DNA PCR on maternal blood (unknown sensitivity)
	Newborn: urine/ naso-pharyngeal aspirate (NPA)/saliva in first 2–3 weeks of life for virus detection – c. 100% sensitive; CMV IgM 70% sensitive; IgG avidity is uninterpretable because of interference by maternal antibody. However, if CMV IgG is not detected in newborn and they are delivered at >34 weeks gestation, congenital infection is extremely unlikely as maternal Ab should be detectable
	Fetus: amniotic fluid ≥ 6 weeks after maternal diagnosis/illness for CMV DNA PCR
	There is a risk of a false negative PCR result before 6 weeks and rarely after this time period has passed
Rubella	Pregnant woman: undertake investigation only if vaccination history not known or known to have *not* received two doses of rubella vaccine; booking blood should be available for testing retrospectively
	Newborn: serum for rubella IgM; urine/NPA for rubella RNA RT-PCR; persistence of rubella IgG at 1 year of life (pre-MMR vaccine) confirms in utero infection
Fetus:	amniotic fluid for RT- PCR; fetal blood for virus-specific IgM ≥23 weeks gestation
Parvovirus B19	Pregnant woman: booking and current blood tested in parallel for virus-specific IgG and IgM (NB maternal IgM may be negative at time of fetal hydrops diagnosis)
	Fetus: fetal blood and/or amniotic fluid for B19 DNA PCR
VZV	Pregnant woman: always confirm the diagnosis by either a lesion swab for VZV PCR or demonstration of VZV IgG sero-conversion using the booking blood. NB VZV IgG is not detectable if blood is taken within 3 days of rash onset
	Fetus: if abnormal scan findings, consider amniocentesis for VZV DNA PCR; good negative, but poor positive predictive value; persistence of VZV IgG at a year of life confirms in utero infection
Toxoplasma	Pregnant woman: test current and booking sample if available for IgG and IgM by EIA. If IgG and/or IgM are detected, confirmation with the Sabin-Feldman dye test is required
	Newborn: serum for Toxoplasma IgM and IgA by EIA and ISAGA*. False negatives may occur so repeat samples may be necessary. Test infant over 3 months to monitor for reduction in Toxoplasma dye test titre. If CNS is involved, PCR on CSF is useful.
	Fetus: amniotic fluid for T. gondii DNA PCR
Syphilis	Pregnant woman: test current sample to look for sero-conversion when compared with booking, or increase in RPR/VDRL titre if acute infection or fetal infection suspected
	Newborn: test for T. pallidum IgM and compare RPR/VDRL antibody titre with maternal sample. Monitor for reduction in RPR/VDRL titre and appearance of IgM, as this may occasionally be delayed. Look for loss of antibody at a year of life to exclude congenital infection

| HIV | Test maternal and newborn EDTA blood for HIV provirus and/or HIV RNA by PCR. Monitor infant for loss of HIV antibody; NB HIV antibody may take >18 months to disappear completely |

*ISAGA – Immuno-sorbent agglutination assay
RT-PCR= Reverse transcriptase-polymerase chain reaction

It is important to liaise closely with the laboratory undertaking testing to give exact dates of samples and onset of xsymptoms or signs. This is because testing, with either molecular or serological methods, is complex and the significance of positive or negative results is heavily dependent upon correct information.
List 20 outlines the usefulness of organism-specific IgM as a means of confirming or refuting infection.

List 20: Duration of Organism-Specific IgM Results

Infective agent	Common duration of IgM (range)
CMV	2 months (3 weeks–>1 year)
T. gondii	6 months (6–18 months)
Parvovirus	1–2 months (1–3 months)
Rubella	1–2 months (2 weeks–3 months)
Measles	1–2 months (1–3 months)
HEV	1–2 months (1–3 months)

List 21: Infections Associated with a More Severe Maternal Outcome If Acquired in Pregnancy

Virus	Complications	Mortality % or RR
Influenza virus	Pneumonia, sepsis syndrome	2 fold (Fig. 7.9)
Varicella	Pneumonia; bacterial sepsis	No increased risk*
Hepatitis A/B	Liver failure	No increased risk
Hepatitis E (GT1)	Liver failure	20–30%
Lassa fever	Multi-organ failure	30–50%
Ebola virus	Multi-organ failure	90%

* Potential for an increased risk of varicella pneumonia in the late third trimester

Motor units may die as a result, leading to loss of digits/limb hypoplasia and skin scars in a dermatomal distribution.

Parvovirus B19 infection follows a similar pattern; after 20 weeks there is no risk of fetal loss, presumably because the fetus receives passive maternal parvovirus specific IgG which helps limit virus replication so that severe anaemia is uncommonly seen after 20 weeks.

As congenital infection with a specific organism is a life-long diagnostic label, and the clinical features in the fetus or newborn are non-specific and often overlap with regard to individual pathogens, it is essential to either confirm or refute a specific diagnosis either in the fetus or in a pregnant woman. Moreover, as it is unknown what the long-term effects may or may not be, laboratory confirmation of even a simple clinical diagnosis, such as chickenpox, in pregnancy is necessary and advisable.

Maternal infection can sometimes be exacerbated by pregnancy. While there is a risk from over-reporting bias, some infections do pose a risk to life in pregnant women. They are shown in List 21.

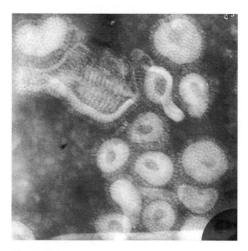

Figure 7.9

Once infection has been confirmed, treatment is possible, but this is not always effective in reducing the extent of disease in the newborn.

References

1. Enders G, Bäder U, Lindemann L, Schalasta G, Daiminger A. Prenatal diagnosis of ongenital cytomegalovirus infection in 189 pregnancies with known outcome. *Prenat Diagn* 2001;**21**(5):362–377.

2. Pass RF, Fowler KB, Boppana SB, Britt WJ, Stagno S. Congenital cytomegalovirus infection following first trimester maternal infection: symptoms at birth and outcome. *J Clin Virol* 2006;**35**(2):216–220.

3. Leruez-Ville M, Ghout I, Bussières L, et al. In utero treatment of congenital cytomegalovirus infection with valacyclovir in a multicenter, open-label, phase II study. *Am J Obstet Gynecol* 2016;**215**(4):462.e1–462.e10.

4. Rice PS. Ultra-violet radiation is responsible for the differences in global epidemiology of chickenpox and the evolution of varicella-zoster virus as man migrated out of Africa. *Virol J* 2011, 189

5. Miller E, Fairley CK, Cohen BJ, Seng C. Immediate and long term outcome of human parvovirus B19 infection in pregnancy. *Br J Obstet Gynaecol* 1998; **105**: 174–8

6. Enders M, Weidner A, Zoellner I et al. Fetal morbidity and mortality after acute human parvovirus B19 infection in pregnancy: Prospective evaluation of 1018 cases. *Prenat Diagn* 2004; **24**: 513–18

7. Enders G. Management of varicella-zoster contact and infection in pregnancy using a standardized varicella-zoster ELISA test. *Postgrad Med J* 1985; **61**: (Suppl 4), 23–30

Data Interpretation in Obstetrics

Rosemary Townsend and Asma Khalil

Module 1: Clinical Skills

- Principles of fluid and electrolyte and acid-base balance.
- Interpret results of investigations including microbiology swabs, haematological tests and electrolyte levels.

Fluid Balance

- Fluid balance charts make an easy question for examiners
- Normal fluid outputs: urine (0.5–1 ml/kg/hr), insensible losses (850 ml) and faeces (100 ml)
- Likely clinical scenarios are peri-operative gynaecology patients or pre-eclamptic obstetric patients
- Oliguria is <400 ml/day
- Be aware of the importance of avoiding fluid overload in pre-eclampsia. NICE recommends limiting fluid intake to 80 ml/hr (1)

Routine Blood Tests

- Candidates will be familiar with full blood count, urea and electrolytes, liver function tests and coagulation profiles from routine medical practice
- Normal ranges are usually supplied in the MRCOG paper but candidates should be aware of values that may differ in pregnant from non-pregnant patients (Table 8.1).

Module 3: IT, Clinical Governance and Research

- Understand the accuracy of tests used in diagnosis.

Sensitivity and Specificity

- Candidates must be familiar with 2×2 tables of diagnostic testing and the calculation of sensitivity, specificity and positive and negative predictive value (Table 8.2).

Table 8.1 Common Biochemical Test Results

Test	Normal range (non-pregnant)	Change in pregnancy
Haemoglobin	115–135 g/L (2)	Dilutional anaemia occurs during pregnancy giving a normal range of 95–150 by the end of the third trimester (3)
White blood cells (WBC)	5.5–15.5 10^9/L	WBC may be mildly elevated in pregnancy, particularly in the puerperium when the normal range may extend to 16.9 (3). The rise is largely driven by a neutrophilia.
Creatinine	55–100 μmol/L	Be aware that eGFR increases in pregnancy and creatinine levels are typically lower. A rise from baseline may be significant even within the normal range.
Alkaline phosphate	50–120 U/L	Levels rise in pregnancy and may be up to 3 times higher than normal by the end of the third trimester
Albumin	35–50 g/L	Albumin levels fall by 20–40% in pregnancy and may be even more so in sepsis and pre-eclampsia. The normal range by the end of pregnancy is 23–42 (3)

Table 8.2

	Condition present	Condition absent	Total
Test positive	TP	FP	TP + FP
Test negative	FN	TN	FN + TN
Total	TP + FN	FP + TN	All patients

Sensitivity	The percentage of cases with the condition that have a positive test	TP/(TP + FN)
Specificity	The percentage of cases without the condition that have a negative test	TN/(TN + FP)
Positive predictive value	Chance of having the condition if test is positive	TP/(TP+FP)
Negative predictive value	Chance of not having the condition if the test is negative	TN/(TN + FN)

Forest Plots

- The graphical representation of meta-analysis of multiple randomized controlled trials.
- The left-hand column lists the studies analysed while the right-hand column plots the measured effect on that trial as a box with confidence intervals expressed as horizontal lines.
- The vertical line represents no effect, and confidence interval lines that cross the line show a non-significant result.
- The size of each box represents the weight of the study in the analysis.
- The overall effect seen by meta-analysis is expressed as a diamond, where the width of the diamond corresponds to the confidence interval (Fig. 8.1).

Module 5: Core Surgical Skills

- Methods of measurement and interpretation of clinically important physiological variables as applied to surgical practice.

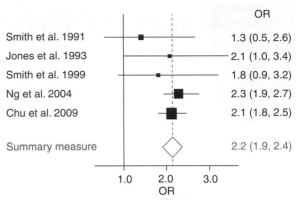

Figure 8.1 Meta-analysis (James Grellier, CC BY-SA 3.0, https://commons.wikimedia.org/w/index.php?curid=10253357)

Spirometry

- Spirometry values include forced vital capacity (FVC, total volume of air the patient can forcibly exhale in one breath), forced expiratory volume in 1 second (FEV_1, volume of air exhaled in the first second of forced expiration) and their ratio (Fig. 8.2) (4). FVC, tidal volume and peak expiratory flow reportedly increase during pregnancy while the FRC (functional residual capacity) is decreased (5).

ECG Interpretation

- ECG interpretation is covered in detail in numerous textbooks. Clinical scenarios presented in the MRCOG are unlikely to be complex, but candidates would be expected to recognise atrial fibrillation and flutter, supraventricular tachycardia and ischaemic changes.
- ECG changes in pregnancy include increased heart rate, Q waves in leads III and aVF and T wave inversion in lead III. The cardiac axis may be deviated by up to 15 degrees secondary to elevation of the diaphragm (Fig. 8.3).

Arterial Blood Gas Analysis

- Candidates will be expected to identify respiratory and metabolic acidosis and alkalosis on blood gas analysis.
- Remember that a degree of hyperventilation is normal in pregnancy so the $PaCO_2$ will tend to low/normal.

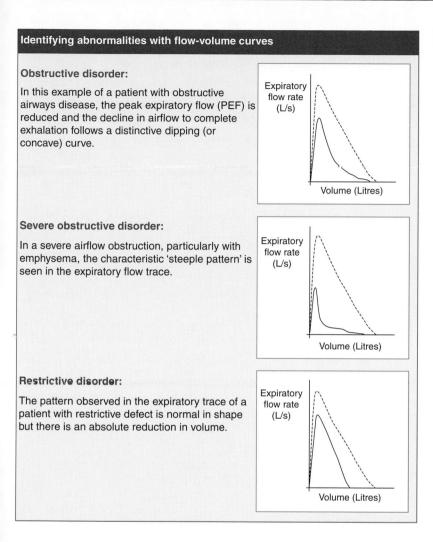

Figure 8.2 Identifying abnormalities with flow-volume curves (Taken from (4))

Identifying abnormalities with flow-volume curves

Obstructive disorder:

In this example of a patient with obstructive airways disease, the peak expiratory flow (PEF) is reduced and the decline in airflow to complete exhalation follows a distinctive dipping (or concave) curve.

Severe obstructive disorder:

In a severe airflow obstruction, particularly with emphysema, the characteristic 'steeple pattern' is seen in the expiratory flow trace.

Restrictive disorder:

The pattern observed in the expiratory trace of a patient with restrictive defect is normal in shape but there is an absolute reduction in volume.

Module 8: Antenatal Care

- Interpret commonly performed tests in pregnancy, including screening tests.

Interpret Data on Maternal Mortality

Screening Tests

- The majority of tests performed in antenatal care are screening tests, and candidates should be familiar with timing of the tests in routine UK antenatal care and the appropriate follow-up for positive or high-risk results (Table 8.3).
- It is important to grasp that screening tests are not mandatory and are not diagnostic. Follow-up testing is usually required before making management decisions.

Maternal Mortality Statistics

- You may also be asked to interpret or comment on maternal mortality data. It is helpful to be familiar with the common indices and normal ranges for these (Table 8.4).
- Maternal deaths may be direct, indirect or coincidental.
- The MBRRACE-UK annual report releases data on maternal mortality up to 12 months postpartum in the UK in the preceding triennium.

Module 9: Maternal Medicine

- Interpret commonly performed tests used in maternal medicine

Table 8.3 Screening tests

Timing of test	Test	Condition screened for	Follow-up management
Booking and 28 weeks	FBC	Anaemia	Haematinics or haemoglobinopathy screening
Booking	Syphilis, HIV, hepatitis B and rubella	Vertically transmissible infections	Confirmatory testing and postnatal vaccination if non-rubella immune while treatment in pregnancy can improve outcome in syphilis, HIV and hepatitis B.
After 10 weeks	Cell-free fetal DNA (cffDNA) also known as non-invasive prenatal testing (NIPT)	Trisomies 21, 13 and 18	Highly sensitive for T21 and T18, less so for T13. False positives and negatives are possible and the sample may not give results if <4% fetal DNA. Confirmatory invasive testing is required.
11–14 weeks	Combined test (nuchal translucency, bHCG and PAPP-A)	Trisomies 21, 13 and 18	Amniocentesis or chorionic villus sampling. Non-invasive prenatal testing may be an option.
15–20 weeks	Quadruple test (bHCG, PAPP-A, AFP, inhibin A)	Trisomies 21, 13 and 18	Amniocentesis or chorionic villus sampling. Non-invasive prenatal testing may be an option.
18–22 weeks	Anomaly scan	Multiple congenital abnormalities	Amniocentesis, fetal MRI for certain anomalies, detailed fetal echocardiography.
Booking, 28 and 34 weeks	Group and screen	Red blood cell antibodies (alloimmunisation)	Antibody titres at regular intervals, fetal blood sampling if suggestion of fetal anaemia on scan.
Every visit	Blood pressure	Hypertension	Blood pressure profile or 24-hour monitoring. Be aware that blood pressure varies through pregnancy with a nadir in normal pregnancy at around 20–22 weeks and then a steady rise until the end of pregnancy.
Every visit	Urine dip	Proteinuria, urinary tract infection	Spot protein creatinine ratio or 24-hour urine collection (gold standard) for proteinuria. Send a sample for microscopy and culture if suggestive of infection and consider empirical treatment if symptomatic.

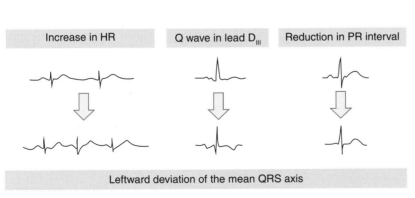

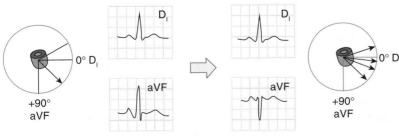

Figure 8.3 ECG changes in pregnancy (From Angeli et al. 2015 (6))

Table 8.4 Maternal mortality statistics

Statistic	What is it?	UK	Sierra Leone
Maternal mortality ratio (MMR)	Number of maternal deaths/100,000 births* in 1 year	8.5 (7)	1360 (8)
Perinatal mortality rate (PNMR)	Number of stillbirths and neonatal deaths before 7 days/1000 births	5.92 (9)	30.8 (10)

* Including termination, miscarriage or ectopic pregnancies

Table 8.5 Diagnostic criteria for gestational diabetes after OGTT

Diagnostic criteria for gestational diabetes after OGTT	
Fasting plasma glucose	>5.6 mmol/litre
2-hour plasma glucose	>7.8 mmol/litre

Diabetes

- The two-hour 75 g oral glucose tolerance test (OGTT) is used to test for gestational diabetes in women with risk factors. HbA1c, glucose on urine dipstick, random or fasting plasma glucose should not be used to identify women at risk of gestational diabetes (Table 8.5) (11).
- Glycosuria is common in pregnancy due to increased GFR and reduced tubular reabsorption. Repeated glycosuria should prompt investigation for gestational diabetes.

Thyroid Disease

- In hypothyroidism, most women will require an increase in dose of thyroxine with the aim of maintaining good control of the TSH levels, particularly in the first half of pregnancy.
- Target TSH should be <2.5 μU/ml in the first trimester and <3 μU/ml in the second and third trimesters in patients with known hypothyroidism (12).
- If the TSH is subnormal in pregnancy, this can be because of the suppressive effect of bHCG and is often noted in cases of hyperemesis gravidarum. Hyperthyroidism may be suggested by a history of autoimmune diseases or the presence of goiter or TSH receptor autoantibodies.
- Thyroid peroxidase antibodies (anti-TPO) are primarily associated with Hashimoto's thyroiditis.

TSH receptor antibodies (TRAb) are present in Graves' disease.

Renal Disease in Pregnancy

- GFR increases by 50% and therefore urea and creatinine fall to around 10 micromol/L below pre-pregnancy levels
- Physiological hydronephrosis, particularly in the right kidney may be observed on ultrasound.
- Uric acid falls in the first trimester and then rises by term. Levels may be increased in pre-eclampsia, twin pregnancies and in acute fatty liver of pregnancy.

Liver Disease in Pregnancy

- Obstetric cholestasis is characterized by itching of palms and feet in association with raised transaminases and bile acids.
- Gall bladder disease may still occur in pregnancy and the typical obstructive pattern of abnormal liver function tests may be observed. A raised alkaline phosphatase can be normal in pregnancy but in conjunction with a raised gamma glutamyl transferase (GGT), and symptoms of biliary colic can reflect gall bladder pathology.
- HELLP syndrome is the conjunction of haemolysis, elevated liver enzymes and low platelets, and is a variant of pre-eclampsia. The clinical picture may change rapidly, and the condition is potentially life-threatening.
- Acute fatty liver of pregnancy (AFLP) is a rare but very serious diagnosis. Hypoglycaemia is classically present in AFLP, and glucose testing should be performed in any unwell pregnant woman with deranged liver function tests.

Haematology in Pregnancy

- Thrombocytopenia may be physiological, idiopathic, drug-induced or related to HELLP or other microangiopathic diseases.
- Physiological thrombocytopenia usually presents with levels $>100 \times 10^9$/L.
- There is an increase in several clotting factors: Factors V, VII, VIII, IX, X, XII, fibrinogen, vWF, antithrombin III, protein C and protein S.

Module 10: Management of Labour

- Interpret commonly performed tests in labour, including fetal blood sampling.

Cardiotocography (CTG)

- If asked to interpret a CTG, candidates should use the NICE 2014 classification until a new guideline is issued (Fig. 8.4) (13).

- In this classification, the CTG may be normal (all features reassuring), non-reassuring requiring conservative measures (one non-reassuring feature) or abnormal needing either further testing (one abnormal or two non-reassuring features) or urgent delivery (severe abnormalities like a prolonged fetal bradycardia) (Fig. 8.5).

Partograph

- Candidates could reasonably be asked to interpret and act on the documentation in a partogram.
- Partograms vary from unit to unit, but all show cervical dilatation, descent of the presenting part, contractions and fetal heart rate over time. Maternal observations, fluid balance and drugs administered are all often documented on the partogram (Fig. 8.6).

NICE National Institute for Health and Care Excellence

Description	Feature		Decelerations
	Baseline (beats/minute)	Baseline variability (beats/minute)	
Normal/reassuring	100–160	5 or more	None or early
Non-reassuring	161–180	less than 5 for 30–90 mintues	Variable decelerations: • dropping from baseline by 60 beats/minute or less **and** taking 60 seconds or less to recover, • present for over 90 minutes • occurring with over 50% of contractions **OR** Variable decelerations: • dropping from baseline by more than 60 beats/minute **or** taking over 60 seconds to recover • present for up to 30 minutes • occurring with over 50% of contractions **OR** Late decelerations: • present for up to 30 minutes • occurring with over 50% of contractions
Abnormal	Above 180 or below 100	Less than 5 for over 90 minutes	Non-reassuring variable decelerations (see row above): • still observed 30 mintues after starting conservative measures • occurring with over 50% of contractions **OR** Late decelerations • present for over 30 minutes • do not improve with conservative measures • occurring with over 50% of contractions **OR** Bradycardia or a single prolonged deceleration lasting 3 minutes or more
Abbreviation: CTG, cardiotocography.			

Intrapartum care: NICE guideline CG190 (December 2014).

Figure 8.4 NICE CTG guidelines

Fetal Blood Sampling (Table 8.1)

- Fetal scalp blood sampling is frequently performed as additional testing of fetal wellbeing in the presence of an abnormal CTG.
- A small incision is made on the fetal scalp and blood is collected via capillary tube for analysis.
- pH, lactate and base excess values can be used to inform clinical decision making. pH is most commonly used, but lactate can be obtained from a smaller sample and therefore also has clinical utility.

Table 8.1 Fetal blood sampling

Classification	Lactate	pH
Normal	<4.1	>7.25
Borderline	4.2–4.8	7.21–7.24
Abnormal	>4.9	<7.2

(From NICE CG190 (14))

Module 11: Management of Delivery

- Interpret cord blood samples.

Umbilical Cord Acid-Base Balance

- Umbilical cord acid-base balance is usually tested after any intervention at delivery or where the neonate is delivered in poor condition.
- Testing paired umbilical arterial and venous samples can give information on the timing and degree of hypoxic insult and has some prognostic value for the child's outcome.
- Base excess represents the metabolic component of any acidosis present and can help distinguish between respiratory and metabolic acidosis.
- A sharp difference between the pH in the two samples reflects a more acute event.

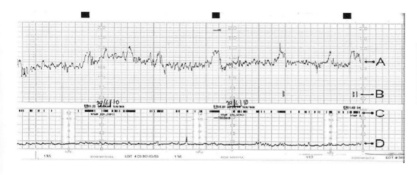

Normal CTG featuring normal variability, accelerations, and a baseline of 130 bpm.

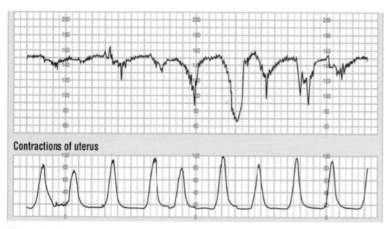

Variable decelerations >60 bpm deep and >60s long. If continuing this CTG would be classified as non-reassuring and then abnormal if persisting even after conservative measures.

Figure 8.5

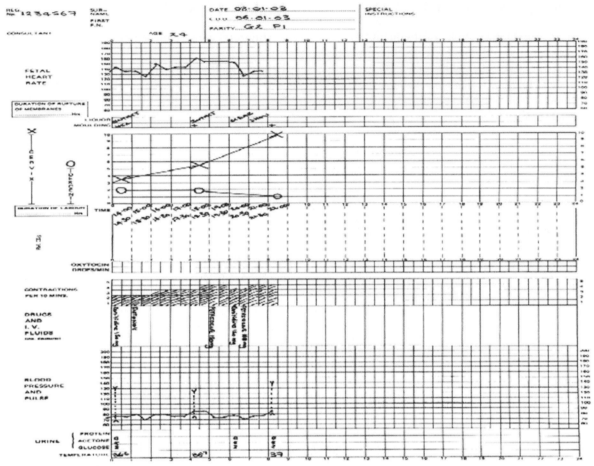

Figure 8.6 Partograph

APGAR Scores (Table 8.2)

- The five component APGAR score out of 10 is calculated at 1 and 5 minutes of life at all births.
- The APGAR score was primarily designed to guide resuscitation rather than predict long term outcomes, but lower scores are associated with a higher risk of long-term sequelae.

Module 15: Sexual and Reproductive Health

- Interpret results of investigations for genital tract infection.

Microbiology Swab Results (Table 8.3)

- Interpreting vaginal, cervical or anal swab culture reports is a common question. Candidates should be familiar with the microbiology of common sexually transmitted infections.

Hepatitis B

- Testing for hepatitis B infection and immunity is routinely done in pregnancy, and candidates should be able to interpret antibody and antigen results.
- Hepatitis B vaccination is offered to newborns whose mothers have chronic hepatitis B infections but are not acutely infectious. Babies born to highly infective mothers may also be given immunoglobulins to prevent vertical transmission (Table 8.3).

Table 8.2 APGAR scores

Parameter	0	1	2
Appearance (colour)	Blue/pale	Blue extremities only	Pink
Pulse rate	Absent	<100 bpm	>100 bpm
Grimace (reflexes/irritability)	No response	Grimace/weak cry	Good cry/sneeze
Activity (muscle tone)	No tone	Some flexion	Good flexion of arms and legs
Respiration	Absent	Weak effort	Good cry

Table 8.3 Microbiology swab results

Disease	Causative organism	Microbiological findings
Gonorrhoea	*Neisseria gonorrhoeae*	Gram negative, bean-shaped diplococci
Chlamydia	*Chlamydia trachomatis*	Obligate intracellular bacterium Gram negative, ovoid
Trichomoniasis	*Trichomonas vaginalis*	Anaerobic flagellated protozoa
Bacterial vaginosis	*Gardnerella vaginalis* (other species are also associated with BV)	Small, gram variable coccus, seen covering epithelial cells which are then termed 'clue cells' Elevated pH and a fishy smell
Group B streptococcal infection	*Streptococcus agalactiae*	Gram positive coccus, seen in chains, beta-haemolytic and catalase positive

Syphilis

- Syphilis is routinely screened for in pregnancy by serological testing.
- VDRL testing is non-specific and can have false positives including other treponemal infections (yaws or pinta), other systemic infections, auto-immune diseases and pregnancy itself. Positive tests should always be followed up with a treponemal antibody test – for example, *T. pallidum* particle agglutination assay (TPPA)

References

1. NICE. Hypertension in Pregnancy CG107. *Guidance and Guidelines*. NICE 2010

2. WHO. *Iron Deficiency Anaemia: Assessment, Prevention and Control*. World Health Organization 2015

3. Abbassi-Ghanavati M, Greer LG, Cunningham FG. Pregnancy and Laboratory Studies.*Obstet Gynecol*. 2009 Dec **114** (6): 1326–31

4. Booker R, Connellan S, Halpin D, Holt K, Jennings J, Wiltshire L. *Spirometry in Practice: A Practical Guide to Using Spirometry in Primary Care*. British Thoracic Society 2005

5. Grindheim G, Toska K, Estensen M-E, Rosseland L. Changes in Pulmonary Function during Pregnancy: A Longitudinal Cohort Study. *BJOG*. 2012 **119**: 94–101

6. Angeli F, Angeli E, Verdecchia P. Electrocardiographic Changes in Hypertensive Disorders of Pregnancy. *Hypertens Res* 2014 Nov **37** (11): 973–5.

7. Knight M, Nair M, Tuffnell D, Kenyon S, Shakespeare J, Brocklehurst PKJ. *Saving Lives, Improving Mothers' Care: Surveillance of Maternal Deaths in the UK 2012–14 and Lessons Learned to Inform Maternity Care from the UK and Ireland Confidential Enquiries into Maternal Deaths and Morbidity 2009–14*. MBRRACE-NPEU 2016

8. WHO. Trends in Maternal Mortality 1990 to 2015: Estimates by WHO, UNICEF, UNFPA, World Bank Group and the United Nations Population Division. 2015

9. Manktelow BN, Smith LK, Seaton SE, Hyman-Taylor P, Kurinczuk JJ, Field DJ, Smith PW, Draper ES. MBRRACE-UK Perinatal Mortality Surveillance Report, UK Perinatal Deaths for Births from January to December 2014. MBRRACE-NPEU 2016

10. Save the Children. *Ensuring Every Baby Survives: Ending Newborn Deaths*. 2014

11. NICE. Diabetes in Pregnancy: Management from Preconception to the Postnatal Period. *Guidance and Guidelines*. NICE 2015

12. Abalovich M, Amino N, Barbour LA et al. Management of Thyroid Dysfunction during Pregnancy and Postpartum: An Endocrine Society Clinical Practice Guideline. *J Clin Endocrinol Metab*. 2007 Aug **92** (8 supp): s1–47

13. NICE. Interpretation of Cardiotocograph Traces. In: *Intrapartum Care for Health Women and Babies* CG190. 2014

14. NICE. Intrapartum Care for Healthy Women and Babies. *Guidance and Guidelines*. NICE 2014

Single Best Answer Questions

1. Table 8.4 shows the results of a new test for the detection of Down's syndrome.

Table 8.4 Test results

		Baby affected by Down's syndrome	
Test		Affected	Not affected
	Positive	A	B
	Negative	C	D

How would you calculate the sensitivity of this new test?

a. a/a+d
b. a/a+c
c. b/b+c
d. b/b+d
e. d/a+b+c

2. A woman sees her midwife for a routine antenatal check at 24 weeks of gestation. A urine dipstick is performed with the following result:

Protein	+
Ketones	−
Nitrites	+
Glucose	−

What is the appropriate course of action?
a. Admit to hospital for IV antibiotics
b. Arrange a 24-hour urine collection
c. Commence oral antibiotics

d. Reassure and do nothing
e. Send urine for culture and microscopy

3. An anxious pregnant 38-year-old undergoes a combined test for Down's syndrome screening. The risk comes back as 1 in 1000. What is the appropriate course of action?

a. Advise that diagnostic tests are not indicated
b. Amniocentesis
c. Chorionic villus sampling
d. Inform the woman that the baby does not have Down's syndrome
e. Termination of pregnancy

4. Caucasian woman with type II diabetes attends the obstetric endocrine clinic at 16 weeks gestation, complaining of lethargy, weight gain and constipation. Thyroid function tests gave the following results:

TSH 10.2
Free T4 0.4
Thyroid peroxidase antibodies: Positive
Thyroid receptor antibodies: Negative
What is the most likely diagnosis?
a. Iodine deficiency
b. Graves' disease
c. Hashimoto's thyroiditis
d. Previous treatment with radioactive iodine
e. Sheehan's syndrome

5. A 27-year-old primigravida has failure to progress in the first stage of labour and is commenced on a Syntocinon infusion. The midwife calls the registrar because of a suspicious CTG. The woman is found to be 6 cm dilated, and the registrar performs fetal blood sampling. The sample has a pH of 7.15. What is the appropriate course of action?

a. Perform an instrumental delivery
b. Perform an immediate caesarean section
c. Reassure the woman that all is well and the labour can continue
d. Repeat the fetal blood sampling in 1 hour
e. Repeat the fetal blood sampling in 2 hours

6. What is the WHO definition of perinatal mortality?

a. Number of stillbirths per year
b. Number of stillbirths per 1000 births
c. Number of neonatal deaths per 1000 births

d. Number of stillbirths and early neonatal deaths per 1000 births

e. Number of stillbirths and early neonatal deaths per 10,000 births

7. A semi-conscious pregnant woman is admitted to the labour ward presenting with dry skin, hyperventilation and a rapid pulse rate. Her blood gas result is as follows. What is the most likely diagnosis?

pH 7.14

pCO_2 30 mmHg

HCO_3 14 mmol/l

Na^+ 140 mEq/l

K^+ 4.5 mEq/l

Glucose 12 mmol/l

a. Metabolic acidosis

b. Metabolic acidosis with respiratory compensation

c. Metabolic alkalosis

d. Respiratory acidosis

e. Respiratory alkalosis

8. A 32-year-old Asian woman presents at 36 weeks of gestation with abdominal discomfort, 2+ proteinuria and a blood pressure of 140/90 mmHg. She has blood tests in accordance with the NICE guideline for the management of hypertension in pregnancy. The midwife asks you to review the following blood results.

What do these results suggest?

Urea 2.8 mmol/l

Creatinine 67 micromol/l

Sodium 138 mmol/l

Potassium 4.2 mmol/l

Urate 0.37 mmol/l

Albumin 32 g/l

Alkaline phosphatase 198 iu/l

Alanine transferase 33 iu/l

Bilirubin 5 mmol/l

a. Acute fatty liver of pregnancy

b. Cholecystitis

c. HELLP syndrome

d. Normal blood results for 36 weeks of pregnancy

e. Pre-eclampsia

9. An Asian woman books in for her third pregnancy at 12 weeks of gestation. She has recently moved to the UK from Thailand to be with her new husband. After pre-test counselling, with the aid of an interpreter, she agrees to hepatitis B virus (HBV) screening. The results return as follows. What is the significance of these results?

HBsAg POSITIVE

Anti-HBc POSITIVE

Anti-HBc IgM NEGATIVE

HBeAg NEGATIVE

Anti-HBe POSITIVE

HBV DNA 203 iu/ml

a. Acute HBV infection

b. Chronic infection (immune control phase)

c. Natural HBV immunity (resolved infection)

d. Occult HBV infection

e. Post vaccination

10. A woman attends for a pre-operative review in preparation for gynaecological surgery. Routine blood tests are performed, including a full blood count. One of the clinic nurses remarks that the patient looks mildly jaundiced. Later that day, the laboratory informs the following results:

Haemoglobin 7.6 g/l

White cell count 2.5×10^9/l

Platelets 275×10^9/l

MCV 109 fl

MCHC 30 fl

Haematocrit 21%

Reticulocytes >15%

The blood film shows polychromasia with numerous microspherocytes and occasional normoblasts. There is a slight increase in neutrophils. What is the most likely diagnosis?

a. Acute myeloid leukaemia

b. Aplastic anaemia

c. Haemolytic anaemia

d. Iron-deficiency anaemia

e. Pernicious anaemia

11. A midwife asks the obstetric registrar to review a primigravida in labour who has progressed to 6 cm dilatation with an abnormal CTG. She has been monitored by continuous electric fetal monitoring because of suspected fetal growth restriction. The CTG has been normal up to 30 minutes previously.

The registrar reviews the patient and confirms that the CTG has a baseline heart rate of 150 bpm with a baseline variability of 4 for the last 30 minutes.

There were no accelerations but variable decelerations were present. What would be appropriate management with these CTG findings?

a. This is a normal CTG and no intervention required
b. This is a non-reassuring CTG and requires continued obstetric review
c. This is an abnormal CTG and fetal blood sampling is required
d. This is an abnormal CTG and urgent delivery is required
e. This is a non-reassuring CTG and fetal blood sampling is required

12. A CTG is performed in labour following normal pregnancy. The reading has a baseline rate of 120 bpm, a variability of 5 bpm, no decelerations and no accelerations. A fetal blood sample has been performed and the pH is 7.25. What is the most appropriate management?
a. Delivery is indicated
b. Do not repeat the fetal blood sample unless the CTG deteriorates
c. If the CTG remains the same, repeat the fetal blood sample in 30 minutes
d. Maternal oxygen therapy and repeat the fetal blood sample in 20 minutes
e. Repeat the fetal blood sample in 30 minutes regardless of the CTG

13. A 34-year-old woman has just returned to the UK following missionary work in the northern parts of South America. She is delighted to be pregnant and presents for booking at 12 weeks of gestation. After counselling, she agrees to have routine blood investigations, including screening for syphilis. The results are returned as follows:
Venereal Disease Research Laboratory (VDRL) test REACTIVE
Treponema pallidum particle agglutination (TP-PA) test NON-REACTIVE
Fluorescent treponemal antibody absorption (FTA-Abs) test NON-REACTIVE
What is the most likely appropriate interpretation of these results?

a. Consistent with treponemal infection at some time
b. Diagnostic of latent syphilis
c. Indicative of early primary syphilis
d. Likely biological false positive
e. Suggests a past treated infection

14. A 24-year-old woman presents with heavy vaginal bleeding at 12 weeks of gestation. She passes products of conception. Her blood pressure is 70/40 mmHg and her pulse is 110 bpm.
Her full blood count is as follows:
Haemoglobin 5.2 g/dl
White blood cell count 9.5 g/dl
Mean corpuscular volume 85
Platelet count 258
Which management option is the most appropriate?
a. Blood transfusion with 2 units of blood
b. Colloid infusion
c. Iron tablets 200 mg daily for 1 month
d. Iron tablets 200–300 mg two to three times daily for 2 months
e. Parenteral iron infusion

15. A patient with two previous caesarean sections presents at 35 weeks of gestation with a painless vaginal blood loss of 400 ml. She is 'unbooked' – that is, she has not presented for any previous antenatal appointments so far in this pregnancy.
Clinical findings are as follows:
Blood pressure 120/75 mmHg
Pulse 78 bpm
No clinical evidence of hypovolaemia
Urinalysis: Normal
Examination: Abdominal mass is soft, not tender, with a transverse lie
Cardiotocography: Normal
What is the most likely cause of the blood loss?
a. Cervical fibroid degeneration
b. Likely abruption
c. Likely placenta praevia
d. Likely vasa praevia
e. Show

Clinical Management in Obstetrics

Rosemary Townsend and Asma Khalil

Module 1. Clinical Skills

- Analyse an obstetric and gynaecological history.
- Understand the principles underpinning clinical examinations.
- Be aware of Fraser competence issues.

Obstetric History

- Gravida: only if currently pregnant
- Parity: every live birth or pregnancy that passes 24 weeks of gestation
- Twins = Para 2

Fraser and Gillick Competence (Table 9.1)

- The Gillick case gave rise to the concept of Gillick competence which applies broadly to the competence of children under the age of 16 to consent to medical treatment.
- The Fraser principles (Table 9.2) were prepared by one of the judges in the Gillick case and specifically apply to the prescription of contraceptive advice and treatment to minors (under 16) without parental consent.

Table 9.1 Gillick competence

The child understands the problem and its implications.
The child understands the risks and benefits of treatment.
The child understands the consequences of not treated, any alternatives and the likely effect on their family.
The child is able to retain information, weigh the pros and cons, and communicate their reasoned decision.

Table 9.2 Fraser guidelines

The patient understands your advice
The patient is very likely to continue having sexual intercourse
The patient's health is likely to suffer without contraception
The patient's best interests require contraceptives

Module 3. Core Surgical Skills

- You will be expected to demonstrate knowledge of the principles underpinning fluid and electrolyte balance and coagulation.
- You will be expected to demonstrate knowledge of the basic clinical skills in core surgical practice.

Surgical Considerations in Pregnancy

- After 24 weeks, the supine position causes aorto-caval compression in pregnancy, so all operative procedures should be carried out with a left lateral tilt to the operating table.
- Obesity increases the difficulty of surgical access and risk of postoperative infection and venous thromboembolism.
- Risk of adhesions and invasive placenta increases with multiple uterine surgeries.
- Tubal ligation can be performed at Caesarean section and should be offered to any woman who considers that her current pregnancy completes her family and is planning delivery by CS.

Anaesthesia in Pregnancy

- The anaesthesia of choice for surgical procedures in the puerperium (including Caesarean section, trial of instrumental delivery, complex perineal repairs and manual removal of placenta) is spinal anaesthetic.
- Complications of spinal anaesthesia include sympathetic block, high spinal, postdural puncture headache.
- Labour analgesia may be provided with transcutaneous electric nerve stimulation (TENS), opioid analgesics, inhaled Entonox, water or epidural anaesthetics.

Table 9.3 Surgical infection control considerations

Reducing the risk of surgical site infections (NICE CG74(1))		
Pre-operative	**Intra-operative**	**Post-operative**
Shower or bathe before surgery	Operative team should wash their hands using an antiseptic surgical solution and make sure they are visibly clean	Use non-touch technique for changing dressings
Use electric clippers if hair has to be removed	Sterile gowns and gloves	Patients can shower 48 hours post-op
All staff to wear specific non-sterile theatre wear	Skin preparation with antiseptic	Use interactive dressings to manage wounds healing by secondary intention
Prophylactic antibiotics should be given before all clean-contaminated surgery (the majority of obstetric and gynaecological surgery)	Diathermy should not be used for skin incision	Early mobilisation may reduce infections
	Maintain patient temperature, oxygenation and perfusion	
	Cover wound with dressing	

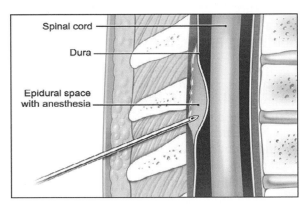

Figure 9.1 Insertion of epidural anaesthetic

- For epidural analgesia a larger dose of drug is infiltrated into the epidural space with a slower onset of action but longer duration than a spinal anaesthetic (Fig. 9.1).
- Epidural injection may be performed anywhere along the vertebral column and inserting an indwelling catheter allows top-ups to prolong the analgesic effect during labour and to provide analgesia for surgical procedures in the puerperium.
- Performing a pudendal block may provide adequate analgesia for operative vaginal delivery or perineal repair. Local anaesthetic is infiltrated around the pudendal nerve trunk as it enters the lesser sciatic foramen. The appropriate site for infiltration may be identified 1 cm inferior and medial to the attachment of the sacrospinous ligament to the ischial spines.

Module 4: Postoperative Care

- You should be able to show understanding of the management surrounding surgical complications, infection, and infection control.

Infection Control

- All staff at all times should observe strict hand hygiene according to the WHO protocols.
- See Table 9.3 for surgical infection control considerations.

Module 5: Surgical Procedures

- Principles of procedures used in surgical practice

Caesarean Section: Abdominal Wall

- Layers of the anterior abdominal wall: skin, fat, rectus sheath, rectus abdominis and parietal peritoneum
- Rectus sheath closure (Fig. 9.2): the length of the incision increases by 30% post-operatively, so adequate suture length must be used in closure. A ratio of 4:1 is recommended, so stitches should be taken 1 cm apart and 1 cm from the fascial edge.

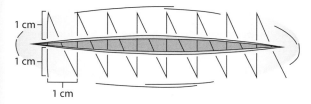

Figure 9.2 Closure of the rectus sheath

Table 9.4

Absorbable sutures	Non-absorbable sutures
Lower risk of sinus formation or buttonhole hernia Less wound pain	Less tissue reaction More resistance to infection May need to be removed (if using non-absorbable skin sutures)
Polydioxanone (PDS, monofilament, slowly absorbable) Polyglyconate (Vicryl, braided)	Polypropylene (Prolene) Nylon Polyethylene (Ethibond) Polyamide (Ethilone)

- The abdominal wall may take up to 140 days to regain 93% of pre-operative strength

Caesarean Section: Uterus

- The standard for uterine entry is low transverse lower segment incision, which carries the lowest risk of future uterine rupture. Intra-operative blood loss, is lower because the lower segment is less vascular and more fibrous and the risk of post-operative infection is lower.
- A vertical (or 'classical') incision on the uterus may be necessary in extreme preterm gestations where the lower segment is not yet formed, in a placenta praevia or accreta where the intention is to leave the placenta in situ or where uterine fibroids obstruct the lower segment and prevent lower segment incision. A vertical incision carries a greater risk of uterine rupture in subsequent pregnancies, particularly in labour, and a repeat Caesarean is usually recommended.
- Uterine repair in two layers carries a lower risk of uterine rupture but a higher risk of morbidly adherent placenta

General Surgical Principles

- Continuous repair is faster, distributes tension evenly, uses less suture material and is therefore cheaper. Both continuous and interrupted stitches carry the same risk of incisional hernia formation but continuous closures have a higher bursting strength and therefore resistance to rupturing (Table 9.4).

Perineal Repair

- Continuous technique is preferred, minimizing knots associated with perineal pain post-delivery

- For repair of the external anal sphincter overlapping or end-to-end techniques have similar long-term outcomes. Slowly absorbed sutures should be used for repair of the anal sphincter complex (2).
- For repair of the anorectal mucosa in fourth-degree tear, a fine braided absorbable suture is preferred to minimise tissue reaction and risk of sinus formation.

Module 6: Antenatal Care

- Principles underlying the management of common disorders of pregnancy

Hyperemesis Gravidarum

- Severe nausea and vomiting leading to >5% weight loss in pregnancy
- Rare and potential serious complication of pregnancy
- Management revolves around rehydration, anti-emetics and supplementation of vitamin B1 (thiamine) because of the risk of Wernicke's encephalopathy. Appropriate venous thromboembolism prophylaxis is also an important consideration.
- Diagnosis of Wernicke's encephalopathy requires the triad of mental confusion, ophthalmoplegia and ataxia.

Anaemia

- The most common cause of anaemia in pregnancy is dilution from the physiological expansion in plasma volume.
- Iron deficiency anaemia is also common. Supplementation with iron reduces anaemia

and incidence of postpartum haemorrhage at delivery. Vitamin C enhances iron absorption, and women should be advised to take their iron tablets with foods rich in vitamin C (e.g. orange juice).

- Other causes of anaemia to be considered in pregnancy include vitamin B12 and folate deficiency.

Gastric Reflux

- Reflux is a common symptom in pregnancy and may be managed with simple antacids or H2 receptor antagonists like ranitidine.
- Red flags include sudden deterioration in symptoms, severe and unremitting epigastric pain or haematemesis.

Module 7: Maternal Medicine

- Principles underlying the management of common medical disorders of pregnancy or pregnancy complicated by maternal disease

Hypertension/Pre-eclampsia

- Many antihypertensive drugs are contraindicated in pregnancy, including ACE inhibitors (potentially teratogenic), diuretics and beta-blockers (fetal growth restriction; Table 9.5).
- Induction of labour at term reduces the risk of maternal complications and Caesarean section in pregnancies complicated by gestational hypertension or pre-eclampsia (3).
- Magnesium sulphate may be used in the prophylaxis and treatment of eclamptic seizures. There is no role for diazepam.

Gestational Diabetes

- Pregnancy is a diabetogenic state because the syncytiotrophoblast produces human placental lactogen which has anti-insulin properties. This polypeptide is similar to growth hormone and facilitates energy supply to the fetus but also predisposes to gestational diabetes.
- Glycaemic control can be achieved with diet, metformin or insulin. Good control reduces the risk of macrosomia, stillbirth and neonatal hypoglycaemia.

Table 9.5 Antihypertensive drugs that are suitable for use in pregnancy

Antihypertensive drugs that are suitable for use in pregnancy	
Methyldopa	Alpha2-adrenergic receptor agonist that competitively inhibits DOPA decarboxylase and inhibits presynaptic sympathetic nervous system. May be associated with depressive side effects, so advised to stop postnatally
Labetalol	Mixed alpha/beta-adrenergic antagonist, reduces peripheral vascular resistance
Hydralazine	Direct-acting smooth muscle relaxant, works by increasing cGMP levels decreasing the phosphorylation of smooth muscle myosin light chains. Requires endothelium to provide nitric oxide (NO)
Nifedipine	Calcium channel blocker. Side effects of tachycardia, flushing and headache

Thyroid Disease

- Women with pre-existing hypothyroidism commonly need an increase in thyroxine dosage in pregnancy to maintain the euthyroid state.
- Women with known anti-thyroid antibodies (anti-TPO) are at particular risk of postpartum thyroiditis, which can present up to one year postpartum.

Obstetric Cholestasis

- Bile acids are synthesized from cholesterol and play a role in the digestion of dietary fats.
- The mechanism of rising bile acids in obstetric cholestasis is unknown but is almost certainly hormonal.
- Obstetric cholestasis symptoms may be improved with the use of ursodeoxycholic acid, but this has no apparent effect on the risk of stillbirth, and therefore induction of labour at term is an important component of management.

Epilepsy

- Epilepsy is the most common neurological problem encountered in obstetric patients.
- Some anticonvulsants are potentially teratogenic, and women planning a pregnancy should have pre-conception counselling in order to select the

safest combination that provides adequate symptom control.

- Sodium valproate in particular is associated with a specific syndrome (fetal valproate syndrome), with characteristic facies in the child (a vertical fold of skin on either side of the nose that forms a groove under the eye [epicanthal folds]; a small, upturned nose with a flat bridge; a small mouth [microstomia]; a long, thin, upper lip; a downturned mouth; and/or minor abnormalities of the ears), congenital anomalies and associated neurological impairment.

Module 8: Management of Labour

- Understand principles of management of labour

Induction of Labour

- Induction of labour refers to starting the process of labour in a patient with no current features of labour.
- Augmentation of labour refers to intervening in the ongoing process of labour for a medical indication – for example, using rupture of membranes or oxytocin in a non-progressive labour or oxytocin to start uterine contractions where the membranes have ruptured spontaneously but contractions have not yet commenced.
- Induction of labour can be for maternal or fetal disease, or planned to ensure delivery in hospital at a specific time (e.g. for a baby likely to need early neonatal surgery).

- The choice of induction agent and timing of induction of labour will depend on the clinical scenario and the wishes of the mother. See Table 9.6 for commonly used induction agents.

Obstetric Anatomy

- The anatomy of the pelvis determines the ease of rotation and descent of the fetal head during labour.
- There is no evidence for any form of pelvic assessment prior to labour to predict obstructed labour but the finding of a narrower than expected pelvis in conjunction with a non-progressive labour may point to relative cephalopelvic disproportion.
- Candidates should be familiar with the pelvic diameters and able to relate them to fetal head anatomy (Fig. 9.3).

Anatomy of Fetal Head (Fig. 9.4)

- The position of the fetal head relative to the pelvis may determine the possibility of vaginal delivery.
- Persistent brow presentation is unlikely to deliver vaginally.
- Although mento-anterior face presentation can deliver vaginally, mento-posterior cannot.

Module 9: Management of Delivery

- Understand principles of operative delivery and perineal repair

Table 9.6 Induction agents (4, 5)

Prostaglandin E2 (Dinoprostone)	Available in tablets, gels and pessaries and administered vaginally Softens the cervix and induces expression of oxytocin receptors in the myometrium Risk of hyperstimulation
Prostaglandin E1 analogues (Gemeprost, Misoprostol)	Highest risk of hyperstimulation, but has the shortest interval to delivery Administered orally or vaginally Can also be used as an abortifacient, and in the management of obstetric haemorrhage
Intracervical balloon (e.g. Cook's balloon)	Mechanical stretching of the cervix causes dilatation and autologous prostaglandin release Lowest risk of hyperstimulation but increases risk of infections morbidity
Synthetic oxytocin (Syntocinon)	Synthetic nonapeptide that stimulates uterine contractions. Theoretically increases the risk of amniotic fluid embolism if used with intact membranes
Artificial rupture of membranes (ARM)	Can only be performed if the cervix is sufficiently favourable May require additional oxytocin after ARM in order to trigger active labour contractions

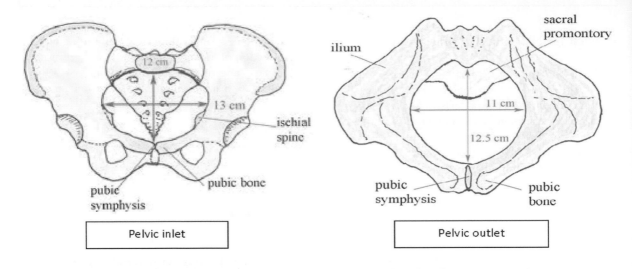

Pelvic diameters	Inlet	Mid cavity	Outlet
Anterior-posterior	11 cm	12 cm	13 cm
Transverse	13 cm	12 cm	11 cm
Oblique	12 cm	12 cm	12 cm

Figure 9.3 Pelvic diameters

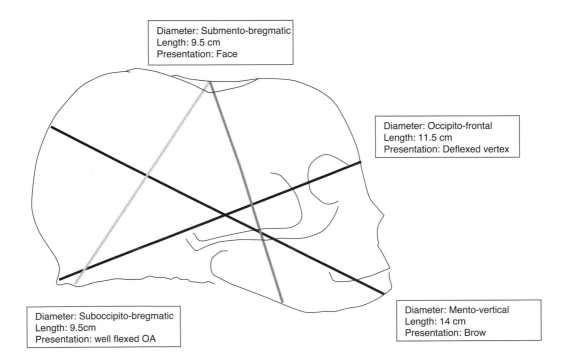

Diameter: Submento-bregmatic
Length: 9.5 cm
Presentation: Face

Diameter: Occipito-frontal
Length: 11.5 cm
Presentation: Deflexed vertex

Diameter: Suboccipito-bregmatic
Length: 9.5cm
Presentation: well flexed OA

Diameter: Mento-vertical
Length: 14 cm
Presentation: Brow

Figure 9.4 Anatomy of the fetal head

Operative Vaginal Delivery

- Operative vaginal delivery may be indicated for delay in the second stage of labour, maternal exhaustion, fetal distress or to electively limit the length of pushing.
- The choice of instrument depends on the clinical scenario and the operator's skill and experience (Table 9.7).

Perineal Trauma

- Perineal trauma to some degree occurs in most vaginal deliveries.
- Appropriate classification allows appropriate repair and minimizes the risk of long term complications.
- First-degree tears involve only the perineal skin and vaginal mucosa.
- Second-degree tears involve only the perineal muscles and not the anal sphincter complex.
- Third-degree tears involve the anal sphincter complex and carry a risk of long term sequelae,

including faecal incontinence and urgency. Surgical repair in theatre, prophylactic antibiotics and pelvic floor physiotherapy can reduce the risk of long term complications. See Table 9.8 for classification (2).

Module 10: Postpartum Problems

- Understand the principles of management of postpartum problems, including haemorrhage.

Physiology of the Postpartum Period

- The postpartum period classically lasts for up to 6 weeks after delivery as the physiological adaptations of pregnancy gradually return to the non-pregnant state.
- Uterus involutes at 1 cm/day by autolysis of structural proteins, and should not be palpable above the symphysis pubis by 10–12 days post-delivery.

Table 9.7 Choice of instruments for operative vaginal delivery

	Ventouse	Forceps
Varieties	Kiwi cup Silastic cup Metal cup	Outlet forceps Long-handled traction forceps Kielland's rotational Pipers forceps for breech deliveries
Application	Median flexing – applied over the flexion point, which is 2 cm anterior to the posterior fontanelle	Sagittal suture directly in the midline and perpendicular to the shanks, posterior fontanelle 1 cm above shanks and fenestration admitting no more than one finger
Advantages	Can be used to rotate or on asynclitic heads if appropriately placed Lower risk of severe perineal trauma	Not dependent on maternal effort
Disadvantages	Higher risk of failure to achieve delivery	Rotational delivery carries higher risks
Maternal risks	Perineal and vaginal trauma	Perineal and vaginal trauma, including occult levator ani trauma
Fetal risks	Superficial lacerations and bruising, cephalohaematoma, intracranial haemorrhage	Superficial lacerations and bruising; skull fracture, facial nerve palsy, intracranial haemorrhage

Table 9.8 Classification of perineal trauma

Classification	Description
3a	<50% of external anal sphincter torn
3b	>50% of external anal sphincter torn
3 c	Both external and internal anal sphincter torn
4th degree tear	Injury involves both anal sphincter complex and anorectal mucosa

Breastfeeding

- The high levels of progesterone and oestrogen during pregnancy suppress lactation.
- After delivery lactation is stimulated by oestrogen and prolactin.
- In women not planning to breastfeed for medical reasons (e.g. HIV infection) or where the fetus was stillborn, lactation can be suppressed by dopamine agonists (Cabergoline or Bromocriptine) that directly inhibit the pituitary lactotroph cells.

Postpartum Haemorrhage (PPH)

- Every obstetric practitioner must be fully conversant with the management of PPH, the most common cause of maternal death worldwide.
- The common causes of PPH are summarized in the four Ts (tone, tissue, thrombin, trauma).
- Active management of the third stage reduces the risk of PPH by 50–76% and should be offered to all women (6).
- Active management includes the administration of prophylactic oxytocics and controlled cord traction. Umbilical cord clamping should be delayed for at least 1 minute unless there are any contra-indications, even with active management (Table 9.9).

Peripartum Cardiomyopathy

- Cardiac mortality is the leading cause of maternal mortality in the UK, and 18% of deaths secondary to cardiac disease are due to cardiomyopathies (7). Peripartum cardiomyopathy may occur even in women with no known cardiac history.

Table 9.9 Management of PPH

Medical	Surgical
Oxytocin	Manual removal of placenta
Ergometrine	Balloon tamponade
Misoprostol	B-lynch suture
Carboprost (Haemabate)	Ligation of uterine and ovarian arteries
Uterine artery embolization	Ligation of internal iliac arteries
	Hysterectomy

- Patients may present with breathlessness on exertion and orthopnoea. Patients are often misdiagnosed with pulmonary embolism on presentation.

References

1. Surgical Site Infections: Prevention and Treatment. *Guidance and Guidelines.* NICE. 2008

2. RCOG. *The Management of Third-and Fourth-Degree Perineal Tears. Green-top Guideline No. 29.* 2015

3. Koopmans CM, Bijlenga D, Groen H, Vijgen SMC, Aarnoudse JG, Bekedam DJ, et al. Induction of labour versus expectant monitoring for gestational hypertension or mild pre-eclampsia after 36 weeks' gestation (HYPITAT): A multicentre, open-label randomised controlled trial. *Lancet* 2009 Sep 19 **374** (9694):979–88.

4. Mozurkewich EL, Chilimigras JL, Berman DR, Perni UC, Romero VC, King VJ, et al. Methods of induction of labour: A systematic review. *BMC Pregnancy Childbirth.* 2011 Dec 27 **11**(1):84.

5. Alfirevic Z, Keeney E, Dowswell T, Welton N, Medley N, Dias S, et al. Methods to induce labour: A systematic review, network meta-analysis and cost-effectiveness analysis. BJOG 2016 **123**(9):1462–70.

6. RCOG. Postpartum Haemorrhage, Prevention and Management. *Green-top Guideline No. 52.* 2016

7. Knight M, Nair M, Tuffnell D, Kenyon S, Shakespeare J, Brocklehurst PKJ. *Saving Lives, Improving Mothers' Care: Surveillance of Maternal Deaths in the UK 2012–14 and Lessons Learned to Inform Maternity Care from the UK and Ireland Confidential Enquiries into Maternal Deaths and Morbidity 2009–14.* 2016

Single Best Answer Questions

1. What is the recommended suture length to wound length ratio?

   a. 1:1
   b. 1:5
   c. 1:2
   d. 1:4
   e. 1:3

2. Which compound is useful in the prophylaxis and treatment of eclampsia?

   a. Magnesium hydroxide
   b. Magnesium chloride

c. Magnesium sulphate

d. Potassium chloride

e. Potassium hydroxide

3. A 25-year-old primigravida presents at 34 weeks of pregnancy with intense itching, which is worse on the palms of her hands and soles of her feet.

A set of liver function tests are requested, with the following results:

Albumin	29 g/l	(35–50)
Serum alkaline phosphatase	279 u/l	(40–120)
Alanine transaminase	80 u/l	(0–45)
Gamma GT	50 u/l	(0–45)
Bilirubin	19 umol/l	(0–21)

What other blood test would you request at this stage?

a. Bile acids

b. Calcium and phosphate levels

c. Full blood count

d. Urea and electrolytes

e. Viral hepatitis screen

4. A midwife calls the obstetric registrar to review a labouring woman. The partogram shows no progress of cervical dilatation for the past 4 hours. The cervix is currently 7 cm dilated, and the membranes are intact. The midwife is also concerned that the CTG is suspicious.
What is the next course of action?

a. Advise the woman to mobilise and review again in 2 hours

b. Arrange a Caesarean section

c. Commence a Syntocinon infusion

d. Perform artificial rupture of membranes

e. Perform fetal blood sampling

5. Following a forceps delivery, a woman is found to have extensive vaginal and perineal tears. When she is examined in theatre by the obstetric registrar, it is noted that approximately 40% of the external anal sphincter is torn, although the internal anal sphincter is intact.
How would you classify this tear?

a. 2

b. 3a

c. 3b

d. 3c

e. 4

6. Following a water birth, a woman elects *not* to have oxytocics for the management of the third stage of labour. Thirty minutes later, she is brought to the consultant unit with a postpartum haemorrhage due to an atonic uterus.
If she had received standard oxytocic management for the third stage of labour, by what amount would she have reduced her risk of a postpartum haemorrhage?

a. 10%

b. 20%

c. 30%

d. 60%

e. 90%

7. A primigravid woman presents in spontaneous labour at 39 weeks of gestation. At 18:00 h, her cervical dilatation is 6 cm. A further vaginal examination at 22:00 h reveals that cervical dilatation is still at 6 cm. At 02:10 h, the fetus is in the occipitoposterior position; uterine activity is present and dilatation is still 6 cm.
What is the most appropriate action?

a. Amniotomy

b. Commence intravenous oxytocin

c. Membrane sweep

d. Repeat vaginal examination after 2 hours

e. Repeat vaginal examination after 4 hours

8. While you are attending to a patient in the antenatal ward, the patient collapses and becomes unresponsive. You open their airway but they are not breathing.
What should you do next?

a. Commence artificial ventilation

b. Commence cardiac compressions

c. Get help

d. Give a precordial thump

e. Left lateral tilt

9. You answer an emergency call for a postpartum haemorrhage. The midwife estimates that the patient has lost approximately 1 l of blood.
What should you be your first action?

a. Assess the patient's airway, breathing and circulation and administer oxygen at a rate of 15 l/min

b. Bimanual compression of the uterus

c. Catheterise the bladder

d. Obtain blood for cross match of 4 units

e. Site two large-bore intravenous cannulae

10. You answer an emergency call for a postpartum haemorrhage. The midwife estimates that the patient has lost approximately 500 ml of blood. What is the most likely cause of the bleeding?

    a. Cervical trauma

    b. Coagulopathy

    c. Retained placenta tissue

    d. Uterine atony

    e. Vaginal tear

11. You are asked to assess a patient who is receiving magnesium sulphate infusions for severe pre-eclampsia. She has passed only 5 ml urine in the last 2 hours. Tests demonstrate that her deep tendon reflex is absent.
    What other observation should you take?

    a. Blood pressure

    b. Glasgow coma score

    c. Pulse rate

    d. Respiratory rate

    e. Temperature

12. A nulliparous woman presents with spontaneous rupture of membranes at 41 weeks of gestation, draining clear liquor.
    At 11:00 h, her cervical dilatation is 3 cm. A further vaginal examination at 15:00 h reveals that her cervical dilatation is still 3 cm. At 17:15 h, the fetus is in the occipitoanterio position; uterine activity is present and the vaginal examination findings are unchanged.
    What is the most appropriate action?

    a. Administer prostaglandin per vaginam

    b. Caesarean section

    c. Commence intravenous oxytocin

    d. Membrane sweep

    e. Repeat vaginal examination after 4 hours

Concise Anatomy of the Urinary, Intestinal and Reproductive Tracts within the Pelvic Cavity

Paul Carter

The Kidneys

- Situated, retro-peritoneally, on the posterior abdominal wall – 12 cm long, 6 cm wide and 3 cm thick, weighing 100 g. Right kidney is lower than the left.
- Set back in the para-colic gutters such that that the *hilum* faces antero-medially.
- Surrounded by a *renal capsule* and then fat within the *peri-nephric space*, which, itself, is surrounded by the *peri-nephric fascia*.
- Possess upper and lower poles, anterior and posterior surfaces, a lateral convex border and a medial concave border (hilum) at L1.
- Posterior relations are similar on both sides.
- The diaphragm separates the upper pole from the *costo-diaphragmatic recesses* of pleural cavity and 11th and 12th ribs.
- Surgical approach may be *trans-thoracic* and *penetrating wounds* to the thorax may injure the kidneys.
- Below this (from medial to lateral), the kidney lies on psoas major, quadratus lumborum (with the sub-costal nerve and artery, iliohypogastric and ilio-inguinal nerves) and, more laterally, on transversus abdominis.
- Situated anterior to the right kidney are adrenal gland, descending duodenum, right colic flexure and coils of small intestine.
- Situated anterior to the left kidney are adrenal gland, spleen, stomach, left colic flexure and coils of small intestine with the pancreatic tail and splenic vessels crossing the hilum.
- From anterior to posterior, at the hilum, are the *renal vein*, *renal artery* and *ureter*.
- Blood supply is from renal arteries, arising from aorta at the level of L1.

- Renal veins drain into the IVC. Left renal vein receives left gonadal vein, left supra-renal vein and left inferior phrenic vein (embryological reasons).
- The nerve supply is from the coeliac plexus. Vagus nerves (para-sympathetic) and from T12 and L1 (sympathetic).
- Internally, the kidney consists of an outer *cortex* and an inner *medulla*. The cortex extends towards the renal pelvis, as the *renal columns*, between the triangular *pyramids* of the medulla. The apices of several pyramids open into a *renal papilla*.
- The cortex contains the glomeruli and convoluted tubules and the medulla contains loops of Henle and collecting tubules are in the medulla.
- The collecting tubules unite and drain into the renal papillae. The papillae open into a number of *minor calyces* which, in turn, open into 2-3 *major calyces*, which coalesce to form the *renal pelvis* located within the *renal sinus*.

The Ureters

- Narrow, muscular tubes, 25 cm long, conveying urine from kidneys to bladder along the posterior abdominal wall.
- They are retroperitoneal, descending on psoas major, crossing the genito-femoral nerve.
- May be absent or duplicated. Important to determine pre-operatively.
- Radiologically, the ureters are located at the tips of the transverse processes of the lumbar vertebrae.
- Crossing the right ureter are the descending duodenum, right colic and ileo-colic vessels, ovarian vessels and the root of the mesentery.
- Crossing the left ureter are the left colic and ovarian vessels and the root of the sigmoid meso-colon.

- Ureters enter pelvis anterior to the sacro-iliac joint, crossing the bifurcation of common iliac artery and descend on the pelvic side wall to the ischial spine.
- Then travels, medially, in the root of the broad ligament and is crossed, superiorly, by the uterine artery before passing lateral to the vaginal fornix before entering bladder.
- Ureteric obstruction leads to hydro-ureter and hydro-nephrosis. May be obstructed by pelvic mass/ fibrosis or inadvertent ligation, during surgery.
- During pelvic surgery the ureters are at risk of injury, at three points:
  a) During oophorectomy due to proximity to gonadal vessels
  b) During hysterectomy due to proximity to uterine vessels
  c) During hysterectomy due to proximity to upper vaginal angles (laterally)
- During surgery, they can be easily identified due to visible 'vermiculation' and a characteristic feel when pinched between forefinger and thumb.
- Blood supply to ureters is taken from different levels:
  1) Renal artery
  2) Ovarian artery
  3) Inferior vesical artery

The Urinary Bladder

- A hollow, muscular, dilatable organ covered, superiorly, by peritoneum with a capacity of 1 litre.
- Pyramidal shape (and extra-peritoneal) when empty – ovoid (and intra-peritoneal) when full. The apex of the pyramid is antero-superior.
- Formed from smooth (detrusor) muscle, lined by transitional epithelium forming folds when empty.
- It has a posterior base, a superior surface and two infero-lateral surfaces.
- The trigone fixes the base and the urethra exits, inferiorly.
- Ureters enter the postero-lateral angles of the trigone.
- They are separated by the inter-ureteric bar (2.5 cm apart).
- The trigone is firmly adherent, posteriorly, to the cervix and anterior vaginal fornix.
- The median umbilical ligament (remnants of the urachus) attaches the apex to the umbilicus.

- The medial umbilical ligaments (obliterated umbilical arteries) are lateral to the bladder. Visible at laparoscopy. Important landmark in pelvic lymphadenectomy.
- The uterus lies posteriorly and the symphysis pubis is anterior (separated by retro-pubic space).
- Bladder must be mobilized from anterior aspect of uterus, cervix and upper vagina during hysterectomy and from the uterus during abdominal delivery of a fetus.
- The proximity of the vagina to the bladder important in vesico-vaginal fistula (surgery, radiation, malignancy, compression from presenting part of fetus).
- Blood supply is from superior and inferior vesical arteries from the internal iliac artery (anterior division).
- Venous drainage to vesical plexus → internal iliac veins.
- Lymphatic drainage to internal and external iliac nodes.
- Sympathetic supply is from the pelvic plexus (L1,2) – motor to sphincter and inhibitory to detrusor.
- Parasympathetic supply (motor to detrusor and inhibitory to sphincter) is from pelvic splanchnic nerves (S2,3,4).

The Urethra

- Muscular tube 3.5-4 cm long, which pierces the perineal membrane. Catheterization easier in women than men.
- Lined by transitional epithelium throughout.
- Prolapse of mucosa of terminal urethra is a urethral caruncle.
- Mainly longitudinal muscle in wall of urethra.
- Surrounded by compressor urethrae and sphincter urethra-vaginalis muscles (external urethral sphincter).
- Some proximal, para-urethral (Skene's) glands (homologous with prostate).
- Supplied by the perineal nerve.

The Intestinal Tract

The Caecum and Appendix

- Blind end of the large intestine, situated in RIF (5-7 cm in length).

- Terminal ileum opens into it and ascending colon arises from it.
- Lies on iliacus and psoas major muscles with gonadal vessels, femoral, lateral femoral cutaneous nerve of thigh and genito femoral nerves intervening.
- Mobile structure, almost completely surrounded by peritoneum, and may lie in the lesser pelvis.
- Ileo-caecal orifice opens into the medial aspect of caecum as a horizontal slit, invaginating the caecum and creating two folds (*ileo-caecal valve*), which meet, laterally, as the *frenulum* of the valve.
- In adults, the lateral wall has grown disproportionately compared to the medial wall and bulges down, inferior to appendix, such that it comes to lie postero-medial to the caecum.
- Peritoneal attachments to iliac fossa, frequently form a retro-caecal peritoneal recess (often containing the appendix).
- The *appendix* arises as a blind ending tube (6–9 cm), from the point at which the taeniae coli fuse, 2 cm below ileo-caecal valve.
- Variable position for apex but often, retro-ileal.
- Suspended from the ileum by a mesentery (*meso-appendix*).
- Small fold of peritoneum extends from the ileum to the anterior surface of meso-appendix (*ileo-caecal fold*).
- Caecal blood supply is from the *ileo-colic artery* (superior mesenteric).
- Its inferior branch gives *appendicular artery* (end artery).
- Thrombosis of the artery leads to gangrene of the appendix.

The Sigmoid Colon

- The sigmoid colon commences at the termination of the descending colon, in the left para-colic gutter, at the pelvic brim. It demonstrates an 'S' shaped curve.
- It turns medially onto the anterior aspect of the sacrum and then makes a sharp turn, downwards, as it becomes the rectum, at the level of S3.
- Suspended on a mesentery (risk of volvulus) and variable in length (average 45 cm).
- Sigmoid meso-colon has a ∧ shaped attachment to the posterior abdominal wall.

- The ureter crosses the apex of the ∧.
- The *inferior mesenteric artery* divides near the apex of the meso-colon and the *superior rectal artery* enters the medial limb of the ∧ while branches to the sigmoid enter the left limb.
- Like the remainder of the colon, the longitudinal muscle is restricted to 3 longitudinal bands (*taeniae coli*). These widen as rectum is approached.
- *Diverticuli* and *appendices epiploicae* are frequent in the sigmoid colon.
- Nerve supply is from *hypogastric nerve* (sympathetic) – L10-S2 and the *pelvic splanchnic nerves* (parasympathetic (S2-4).

The Rectum

- Terminal portion of the alimentary canal from the sigmoid colon (S3) to the anus.
- Rectus (Latin) = straight. Approximately 12 cm long but not straight in humans.
- The rectum has no mesentery.
- The upper 1/3 is covered anteriorly and laterally by peritoneum, the middle 1/3 has a peritoneal covering anteriorly only, and the lower 1/3 is extra-peritoneal.
- The peritoneal reflection, from the anterior surface, passes to the posterior aspect of the vagina (*recto-uterine pouch of Douglas*).
- The rectum (unlike the colon) has a complete coat of longitudinal muscle.
- Therefore, unlike the colon, there are no diverticuli or appendices epiploicae.
- The rectum follows the curve of the sacrum and has three lateral *rectal curves* (upper & lower, convex to the right, and the middle, convex to the left).
- The corresponding grooves, between the curves, are the *rectal valves*.
- Inferior to the recto-uterine pouch, the rectum is separated from the vagina by the *recto-vaginal fascia (of Denonvillier)*, which terminates in the perineal body.
- The *ano-rectal junction* is pulled anteriorly by the sling of the pubo-rectalis component of the pubo-coccygeus muscle.
- Blood supply from two arteries: *superior rectal* (from inferior mesenteric) and the *middle rectal* (from the internal iliac).
- Note that it is not supplied by the inferior rectal artery (from the pudendal) as this supplies the anus.

- The sympathetic nerve supply (inhibitory to muscle) is from fibres accompanying the arteries and from the hypogastric plexus.
- The para-sympathetic supply is from the pelvic splanchnic nerves (S2,3,4) via the hypogastric plexus (motor to rectal muscle).

The Anus

- Terminal 4 cm of alimentary canal.
- Muscular tube of circular muscle forming *internal* and *external* anal sphincters.
- The ano-rectal junction is at the pelvic floor, with the pubo-rectalis sling pulling it forwards such that the anal canal passes postero-inferiorly to the perineum.
- Blood supply is, mainly, from the *inferior rectal artery* but with a contribution from the superior rectal artery.
- Provides anastomosis between portal and systemic circulations and can be significant in cases of portal hypertension.
- The muscle arrangement is that of a 'tube' (internal sphincter) within a 'funnel' (levator ani and external anal sphincter).
- The *external sphincter* is a continuous tube with *deep, superficial* and *sub-cutaneous components*. Its upper portion blends with the pubo-rectalis muscle.
- The middle part is connected to the coccyx by the ano-coccygeal ligament.
- The middle part contributes to perineal body
- The *internal sphincter* is the thickened continuation of the circular muscle of the rectum and extends 3/4 along the anal canal.
- Between the two sphincters is the continuation of the outer longitudinal muscle of rectum, which combines with fibres of the levator ani muscle to form the *conjoined longitudinal muscle*.
- Below the level of the internal sphincter, this conjoined muscle curves medially beneath it and, within the lumen, creates the *inter-sphincteric groove*.
- The upper 1/3 of the canal is lined with mucous membrane, arranged into longitudinal ridges (*anal columns*) and joined, inferiorly, by horizontal folds (*anal valves*), creating small pockets (*anal sinuses*).
- Below the level of the anal valves (*pectinate line*), the lining is smooth *non-keratinised* epithelium

(*pecten*) and extends to the level of the inter-sphincteric groove.
- Superior to the pecten, the mucosa is derived from the hind gut, but inferior to this, it is *cloacal* in origin.
- Below the inter-sphincteric groove, the lining is *keratinized* and extends to the anus.
- Sub-mucous masses form anal cushions in upper part of the canal and can become enlarged (*haemorrhoids*).
- The upper part is supplied by the superior rectal vessels (*portal system*).
- The lower part is supplied by the inferior rectal vessels (*systemic system*).
- The nerve supply is from the *inferior rectal nerve* from the pudendal nerve.
- The sympathetic supply is from the pelvic plexus (L1,2) → contraction.
- The para-sympathetic supply is from the pelvic splanchnic nerves (S2,3,4) → relaxation.

The Reproductive Tract

The Uterus

- Formed by a fusion of the *para-mesonephric ducts* (meso-dermal).
- Intra-peritoneal organ (8 cm × 5 cm × 3 cm) equivalent in size and shape to a pear.
- Hollow organ with a thick muscular wall, consisting of an upper *corpus uteri* (2/3) and a lower *cervix uteri*. (Proportions are reversed in post-menopausal women.)
- The *fundus* is that part of the uterine corpus superior to the *uterine tubes*.
- *Version* refers to the angle made between the axis of the vaginal canal with the axis of the cervical canal, and 80% of women have a uterus that is 'ante-verted'.
- *Flexion* refers to the angle made between the axis of the corpus uterus with the cervix uterus. The majority of women have an 'ante-flexed' uterus.
- *There can be any of the four variations between version and flexion, ante and retro.*
- The organ is covered by peritoneum passing, laterally, to the pelvic side wall as the *broad ligament* and, anteriorly, as the *utero-vesical pouch*.

- *The intra-uterine cavity is lined by endometrium (to the level of the internal os).*
- The *internal os* separates the corpus uterus from the cervix uterus.
- The cervix has *supra-vaginal* and *intra-vaginal* components.
- The supra-vaginal portion of cervix is surrounded by the *para-metrium*.
- *Thickenings in the para-metrium form three pairs of 'ligaments'.*
- The *round ligament* passes from the anterior junction of the uterine tube and fundus to the deep inguinal ring. Minimal role in uterine support.
- The *cardinal ligaments* extend from the base of the broad ligament to the pelvic side wall and provide support for the uterus.
- The *utero-sacral ligaments* extend from the posterior aspect of the cervix to the anterior aspect of the sacrum and provide support for the uterus.
- Blood supply is from the *uterine arteries* (internal iliac).
- Nerve supply is from the *inferior hypogastric plexus*. Uterine pain (labour) is conveyed to sympathetic chain (L1,2) and hence to the spinal cord (T11,12).

The Cervix (Uteri)

- The cervix uterus has an upper, *supra-vaginal*, portion and a lower (1/3) *intra-vaginal* portion projecting into the upper vagina and creating the *vaginal fornices*.
- *Posterior vaginal fornix* is immediately anterior to the *recto-uterine pouch* and allows access to the peritoneal cavity (oocyte retrieval/drainage of a collection).
- The intra-vaginal portion is covered with non-keratinising squamous epithelium. The posterior fornix is the deepest and is covered, posteriorly, by peritoneum.
- The cervix consists of stromal tissue, surrounding a central canal. The *endo-cervical canal* is lined with glandular epithelium.
- Endo-cervical canal extends from isthmus (*internal os*) to the opening into the vagina (*external os*).
- The base of the bladder lies anteriorly.
- The ureters lie lateral to the supra-vaginal portion.
- The nerve supply is from the *nervi erigentes* (pelvic splanchnic nerves).

- Cervical pain is conveyed via pelvic splanchnic nerves (S2,3,4).
- The *latent phase of labour* involves effacement of the cervix, whereby it loses its length, softens and dilates to approximately 3 cm. The *active phase of labour* involves the fully effaced cervix becoming fully dilated.

The Uterine Tubes (of Fallopius)

- Developed from the unfused portions of the para-mesonephric ducts.
- The ducts retain their intra-peritoneal openings as the open *fimbrial* ends.
- They are intra-peritoneal structures and situated in the superior border of the broad ligament, suspended from the round ligament by the *meso-salpinx*.
- 10 cm long and lined by ciliated epithelium. Easily damaged by infection.
- Infection can result in tubes dilated by fluid (*hydro-salpinx*) or pus (*pyo-salpinx*).
- Lined with a thick mucous layer with longitudinal folds, surrounded by a muscular coat of smooth muscle and an outer serosal layer.
- Consists of four portions: *intra-mural* (narrowest), *isthmus, ampulla* and *infundibulum*.
- Fertilisation generally occurs in the ampullary region (which is also the commonest site for *ectopic pregnancies*).
- Blood supply is from uterine and ovarian arteries.
- Sympathetic nerve supply from pelvic plexus.

The Ovary

- Develops high on the posterior abdominal wall and, like the testes, descend but only to the level of the pelvic brim.
- Intra-peritoneal, almond shaped organs, 3 cm long with medial and lateral surfaces and tubal and uterine poles.
- They lie posterior to the broad ligament, attached to the round ligament by fold of peritoneum (*mesovarium*). The ovary, itself, is not invested by peritoneum.
- Situated medial to the pelvic side wall and attached by the *infundibulo-pelvic 'ligament' (suspensory ligament of the ovary)* containing the ovarian vessels.
- Obturator nerve passes, lateral to the ovary, in the pelvic side wall and can be irritated by ovarian pathology.

- *Uterine pole of ovary* is attached to the posterior aspect of the uterus, at the junction of tube and fundus, by the *ovarian ligament*.
- *Tubal pole* is attached to uterine tube by *tubal fimbriae*.
- Blood supply is from the ovarian artery, from the aorta (level of L2).
- Ovarian veins drain to IVC (Rt) and *left renal vein* (Lt).
- Nerve supply is from sympathetic fibres from T10 segment via the aortic plexus.
- Lymphatic drainage follows arteries to the *para-aortic nodes* which may be involved in ovarian malignancy.

The Vagina

- An expandable fibro-muscular tube, 10 cm long, passing upwards and posteriorly, at an angle of 60° to the horizontal.
- Lined by squamous epithelium, and contains no glands. It is lubricated by cervical secretions.
- The upper 2/3 develops from a fusion of para-mesonephric ducts.
- The lower 1/3 develops from the uro-genital sinus.
- The vagina has an acidic pH from lacto-bacilli during reproductive years.
- The opening (introitus) has an antero-posterior plane, but the canal has horizontal plane. Important in clinical examination/speculum insertion.
- The *vestibule* is the space between the labia minora.
- The vestibule contains the *urethral meatus*, openings of *greater* and *lesser vestibular glands,* and the *hymenal remnants* (surrounding the *introitus*).
- The urethra opens into the anterior aspect of the vestibule.
- The vagina is posterior to the bladder, urethra and intra-vaginal cervix.
- The vagina is anterior to the rectum and anus.
- It is inferior to the recto-uterine pouch, separated from the rectum by a thin septum (the fascia of Denonvilliers).
- Upper end expands to receive cervix-surrounded by a sulcus (fornix) – anterior, posterior and lateral.
- The ureter is lateral to the lateral fornix and passes anterior to the anterior fornix to the bladder.

- The posterior wall is longer than the anterior, and the upper part is covered by the peritoneum of the recto-uterine pouch.
- The vagina descends between pubo-vaginalis part of levator ani, through the uro-genital diaphragm and perineal membrane.
- The greater vestibular (Bartholin's) glands are postero-lateral to the lower 1/3 of the vagina, with the ducts opening postero-lateral to the hymen.
- The lesser vestibular (Skene's) glands open between the urethral meatus and the introitus.
- The blood supply is from the anterior division of the internal iliac artery, via the vaginal artery (supplemented by branches from uterine, middle rectal and inferior vesical arteries).
- Lymphatic drainage is to pelvic node (upper) and inguinal nodes (lower).
- The nerve supply is from the pudendal nerve, via the perineal and posterior labial branches (sensory) and from the hypogastric plexus (autonomic).

Arterial Supply of the Pelvic Organs

- The aorta divides into two *common iliac arteries* (CIA) at the level of L4.
- The CIA descends downwards and laterally and divides into *internal* and *external* iliac arteries, anterior to the sacro-iliac joint but posterior to the ureter.
- Common iliac veins lie posterior and to the right of the arteries.
- The ureter crosses the bifurcation of the CIA, anteriorly.
- The left CIA is crossed, anteriorly, by the superior rectal artery and the root of the sigmoid meso-colon.
- Posteriorly, both arteries are crossed by the sympathetic trunk, obturator nerve and lumbo-sacral trunk.
- The external iliac artery extends from the sacro-iliac joint to the mid-inguinal point.
- The external iliac artery lies anterior to psoas major and lateral to the external iliac vein. It is crossed, anteriorly by the ovarian artery and, more distally, the round ligament.
- Distal to the inguinal ligament, it becomes the femoral artery.
- The external iliac artery only has two branches – *inferior epigastric* and *deep circumflex iliac*.

- The deep circumflex iliac artery passes, superiorly, around the iliac crest. It gives an *ascending branch* which may be injured by the insertion of laparoscopic ports.
- *Inferior epigastric artery* passes medial to the deep inguinal ring to enter the inferior part of rectus abdominis. It raises a fold of peritoneum, the *lateral umbilical fold.*

The Internal Iliac Artery

- This artery originates anterior to the sacro-iliac joint and descends on the posterior wall of the pelvis to the greater sciatic notch.
- The ureter is anterior and the lumbo-sacral trunk (L4,5) is posterior.
- The external iliac vein and obturator nerve are lateral.
- It divides into *anterior* and *posterior* divisions.
- The *visceral* branches are all from the *anterior division.*
- *Parietal* branches arise from both anterior and posterior divisions.
- The posterior division gives parietal branches, only: *ilio-lumbar, lateral sacral* and *superior gluteal arteries.*
- The anterior division gives *obturator, umbilical (superior vesical & obliterated umbilical), middle rectal, uterine, vaginal, inferior vesical* and *inferior gluteal arteries,*
- It continues as the *internal pudendal artery*, into the perineum and divides into *inferior rectal* and *perineal* branches.
- In summary, the 12 branches of the internal iliac artery are as follows: 3 arise from the posterior division. Of the 9 branches arising from the anterior division, 3 are related to the bladder (umbilical, superior & inferior vesicle), 3 are related to viscera (uterine, vaginal & middle rectal) and 3 are destined for the body wall (obturator, inferior gluteal & internal pudendal).

The Ovarian Artery

- The ovarian arteries arise below the renal arteries at L2.
- They slope downwards and laterally, on psoas major, and the genito-femoral nerve.

- The ovarian artery crosses the ureter and (on the right) the IVC. It is at risk during oophorectomy.
- It is crossed by the *colic vessels* (Rt and Lt), *duodenum* (third part) and the *root of the mesentery* (Rt), and *inferior mesenteric vein* (Lt).
- It reaches the pelvic brim halfway between the sacro-iliac joint and the inguinal ligament.
- It crosses the external iliac vessels to enter the *suspensory ligament of the ovary.*
- The right ovarian vein drains into the IVC and the left into the left renal vein.

Anatomy of the Fetal Skull and Vaginal Delivery

- Maximum dimension of fetal skull is antero-posterior.
- Maximum dimension of pelvic inlet is transverse.
- Fetal head must enter pelvic cavity in a transverse position.
- Determining factor becomes the widest part of the transverse aspect of the fetal head (i.e. the bi-parietal diameter).
- Maximum diameter of the pelvic outlet is antero-posterior.
- Fetal head must, therefore, rotate 90° as it descends through pelvic cavity.
- Ideally, the *occiput* rotates, anteriorly, as it meets the pelvic floor.
- Fetal skull composed of the following bones:
  - *Frontal* separated from each other by the *frontal suture*
  - *Parietal* – separated from each other by the *sagittal suture* and from
  - *Frontal* bones by the *coronal suture*
  - *Occipital* – separated from the parietal bones by the *lambdoid suture*
- Between the bones are the *anterior* and *posterior* fontanelles – important in determining the position of the *presenting part.*
- Anterior fontanelle is diamond-shaped and is between the frontal and parietal bones.
- The (smaller) posterior fontanelle is situated between the parietal bones and the occipital bone.
- The *vertex* is the part of the skull between the two fontanelles.
- The ideal diameter to present for a successful vaginal delivery is the *sub-occipito-vertical*

(10 cm), as found in the *occipito-anterior* position.

- An *occipito-posterior position* involves deflexion of the fetal head such that the presenting diameter is *sub-occipito-frontal diameter* (11 cm).
- Further deflexion of the head results in an *occipito-frontal diameter*, which is a *brow presentation* (12 cm).
- Still further deflexion results in a *sub-mento/vertical* presentation (diameter 10 cm) and is a *face presentation* that can deliver, vaginally, if in the mento-anterior position, as the delivered head can flex.

The Central Nervous System (as Relevant to Obstetrics and Gynaecology)

The Hypothalamus

- Functions as centre for homeostasis and controls the *autonomic nervous system*.
- Located in the ventral part of the *diencephalon*.
- Like the thalamus, above it, it is situated in the walls of the *third ventricle*, but below the *hypothalamic sulcus*.
- It also forms the floor of the third ventricle and has the *pituitary gland* inferiorly.
- The anterior border is the *lamina terminalis*.
- Composed of a collection of nuclei and their fibre tracts.
- In the sagittal plane, it can be divided into *peri-ventricular, medial and lateral zones*.
- Of particular importance are the *supra-optic* and *para-ventricular nuclei*.
- These send axons into the *pituitary stalk* to the *posterior lobe* of the pituitary gland.
- They deliver neuro-secretions to the posterior pituitary gland (*neuro-hypophysis*): *oxytocin* from the *para-ventricular nucleus* and *anti-diuretic hormone* from the *supra-optic nucleus*.
- The peri-ventricular nucleus (lateral to third ventricle and medial to the para-ventricular nucleus) produces releasing and inhibiting factors which are released into the *hypothalalamo-pituitary portal system* and reach the anterior part of the pituitary gland (*adeno-hypophysis*).

The Pituitary Gland

- Consists of *anterior* and *posterior* lobes, with separate developmental origins.
- Anterior lobe (*adeno-hypophysis*) develops from *Rathke's pouch* (an ecto-dermal outgrowth of the stomodeum) and consists of the *pars anterior, pars tuberalis* and the *pars intermedia*.
- Posterior lobe is a neuro-ectodermal downgrowth of the hypothalamus and consists of the *pars posterior, infundibular stalk* and *median eminence*. Connects to the hypothalamus via a stalk.
- The gland lies within the *pituitary fossa* (sella turcica).
- The *cavernous sinus* is lateral and the *optic chiasm* is superior and the *sphenoid sinus*, inferiorly such that a trans-nasal surgical approach is possible.
- Enlargement (adenoma) of the anterior pituitary can compress the optic chiasm and damage the nasal fibres of the retina, producing a *bitemporal hemi-anopia*.
- The anterior part (75%) of the gland consists of *chromophobes* (50%), *acidophils* (35%) and *basophils* (15%).
- Acidophils secrete growth hormone and prolactin.
- Basophils produce ACTH, TSH, FSH and LH.
- The posterior part consists of approximately 100,000 nerve fibres whose cell bodies are in the supra-optic and para-ventricular nuclei of the hypothalamus.
- Blood supply: from the internal carotid artery via a single *inferior hypophyseal artery* and several *superior hypophyseal arteries*. These form a hypothalamo-hypophyseal-portal system connecting the hypothalamus with the adeno-hypophysis.
- The various hormones are secreted into these vessels.

The Meninges of the Central Nervous System

- The CNS (brain and spinal cord) is covered by three *meninges*: *dura mater, arachnoid mater* and *pia mater*.
- Pia mater adheres to the surface of the neural tissue.
- The arachnoid mater adheres to the inner surface of the dura mater.

- The space between the pia mater and arachnoid mater is the *sub-arachnoid space* and contains *cerebro-spinal fluid (CSF)*.
- This space is the site of a *spinal block* (or lumbar puncture).
- The dura mater is adherent to the bone of the skull but separated from the vertebral bone by a fat filled space.
- This *epidural space* is external to the dura mater and the location of an *epidural block*.

Single Best Answer Questions

1. A 24-year-old woman, undergoing a laparoscopy for right-sided pelvic pain is unexpectedly found to have appendicitis and she needs an appendicectomy. The appendicular artery needs to be ligated. From which artery does this arise?

   a. Ileo-colic
   b. Inferior mesenteric
   c. Left colic
   d. Middle colic
   e. Right colic

2. A 35-year-old woman is experiencing severe headaches after an epidural. Which is the most likely position that the tip of the anaesthetist's needle found itself?

   a. Between the arachnoid mater and the pia mater
   b. Between the dura mater and the arachnoid mater
   c. Between the ligamentum flavum and the dura mater
   d. Between the pia mater and the spinal cord

   e. Within the spinal cord

3. A 26-year-old nulliparous woman has a delayed second stage of labour due to the foetus being in the occipito-posterior position. With respect to the anatomy of the foetal skull, which diameter is presenting?

   a. Mento-vertical
   b. Occipito-frontal
   c. Submento-bregmatic
   d. Sub-occipito-bregmatic
   e. Sub-occipito-frontal

4. Of the branches of the anterior division of the internal iliac artery, which one is only present in 20–30% of the population?

   a. Inferior gluteal
   b. Inferior vesical
   c. Middle rectal
   d. Obturator
   e. Vaginal

5. A 33-year-old woman presents with amenorrhoea and hypothyroidism. She also has a visual field defect (bi-temporal hemi-anopia). Which nerve fibres, in the visual pathway, are being affected?

   a. All fibres of the optic nerve
   b. All fibres of the optic tract
   c. Fibres from both halves of the retina
   d. Fibres from the nasal half of both retinas
   e. Fibres from the temporal half of both retinas

Concise Anatomy of the Pelvic Floor and Perineum

Paul Carter

- The *pelvic floor* is formed by the anterior facing, gutter shaped sheet of muscle (*levator ani*) which slings around the three tracts traversing the pelvic cavity.
- The pelvic floor/diaphragm supports the pelvic viscera, directs the fetal head anteriorly, counteracts increased intra-abdominal pressure, and relaxes to allow the expulsion of effluents or fetus.

Levator Ani Muscle

- Consists of *pubo, ilio* and *ischio coccygeus* components.
- The *pubo-coccygeus* arises from the anterior ½ of the tendinous arch and the posterior aspect of the body of the pubis (on pelvic surface of ilio-coccygeus).
- Its most anterior fibres loop around the *ano-rectal junction* (*pubo-rectalis*) and fuse with the *external anal sphincter*. Even more medial fibres loop around the posterior vaginal wall (*pubo-vaginalis*). Some insert to the *perineal body*.
- *Ilio-coccygeus* arises from posterior ½ of the tendinous arch and the pelvic surface of the ischial spine. It overlaps ischio-coccygeus, anteriorly.
- This muscle inserts into the coccyx and midline *ano-coccygeal raphe*.
- The *ischio-coccygeus* muscle arises from the ischial spine, and fans out to its insertion into the coccyx and lower sacrum.
- Note that the gluteal surface of ischio-coccygeus is the sacro-spinous ligament.
- Nerve supply – sacral plexus (S3 and S4), perineal branch of S4 and branch from inferior rectal nerve (pudendal).

Ano-Coccygeal Ligament

- A midline musculo-tendinous structure between the anal canal and the caudal part of the vertebral column.
- From superior to inferior, it consists of:
  - Pre-sacral fascia
  - Tendinous plate of pubo-coccygeus
  - Muscular raphe of ilio-coccygeus
  - Posterior parts of pubo-rectalis and external anal sphincter

The Perineum

- Defined as the part of trunk which is caudal to the pelvic diaphragm.
- A diamond-shaped area divided into a smaller *anterior (uro-genital) triangle* and a larger *posterior (anal) triangle* by a line joining the anterior parts of the ischial tuberosities.
- The anterior margins are the ischio-pubic rami and the posterior margins are the sacro-tuberous ligaments.
- The anal triangle contains the *anus* and the *ischio-rectal fossae*.
- The ischio-rectal fossa is a fat-filled, wedge-shaped space, lateral to the anal canal. Its apex is where the levator ani attaches to the tendinous line on the fascia of obturator internus. The base is on the skin of the perineum. The medial wall is the levator ani musculature (superiorly) and the external anal sphincter (inferiorly). The lateral wall is the obturator internus muscle, superiorly, and the ischial tuberosity, inferiorly. This space can become infected (ischio-anal abscess).
- The *pudendal canal* is a tunnel in the lower lateral wall of the ischio-rectal fossa, on the medial side of

the ischial tuberosity and on the medial surface of the obturator internus muscle.

- It contains the *pudendal nerve* and the *internal pudendal vessels* which exit the greater sciatic foramen, wind around the ischial spine to enter the perineum via the lesser sciatic foramen (the nerve is medial to the artery).

The Uro-Genital Triangle

- *Vulva*: The vulva contains the following structures:

  Mons pubis

  Labia majora – join anteriorly and posteriorly as anterior and posterior commissures. The space between the labia majora is the *pudendal cleft*.

  Labia minora – split, anteriorly, into the prepuce and frenulum of the clitoris

  Clitoris – crura (covered by ischio-cavernosus muscle) and corpora cavernosa

- *Vestibule*: The space between the labia minora and containing:

  Urethral meatus

  Ducts of the greater and lesser vestibular glands

  Hymen surrounding the introitus

  Bulbs of vestibule (covered by the bulbo-spongiosus muscle)

  Greater vestibular (Bartholin's) glands and lesser vestibular (Skene's) glands

- *Perineal body*: Central tendon of perineum:

  A midline, fibro-muscular ring between anal canal and vagina

  Gives attachment to: External anal sphincter (posteriorly)

  Recto-vaginal septum (superiorly)

  Superficial and deep transverse perineal muscles (laterally)

  Bulbo-spongiosus (antero-laterally)

  Pubo-vaginalis (anteriorly)

  Perineal membrane (inferiorly)

- Contributes to support and integrity of the levator ani muscle.

- *Perineal membrane*: Separates deep from superficial perineal spaces:

  A triangular ligament attached to pubic rami, laterally

  Gives attachment to the crura of clitoris (covered by ischio-cavernosus muscle)

  Gives attachment to bulb of vestibule (covered by bulbo-spongiousus muscle)

  The bulb of vestibule is medial to the crus of clitoris

  Bounded, posteriorly, by deep transverse perinei muscles and the perineal body

- *Deep perineal space*:

  Inferior boundary is the perineal membrane

  Superior boundary is the superior fascia of the uro-genital diaphragm Traversed by urethra and vagina

  Contains three muscles: deep transverse perineal

  Sphincter urethra-vaginalis

  Compressor urethra

  Contains the pudendal nerve and the internal pudendal artery

- *Superficial perineal space*:

  Inferior boundary is the *superficial perineal (Colle's) fascia*.

  Superior boundary is the perineal membrane.

  Contains three muscles:

  superficial transverse perineal

  bulbo-spongiosus

  ischio-cavernosus

  Contains greater and lesser vestibular glands, bulb of vestibule and crura of clitoris.

- *Nerve supply*:

  Uro-genital part (anterior 1/3 labium majus) – *ilio-inguinal nerve* (L1)

  Uro-genital part (posterior 2/3 labium majus – *perineal (pudendal) nerve* (S3)

  Clitoris – *dorsal branch of pudendal nerve* (S2)

  Contribution from genital branch of genito-femoral nerve, anteriorly and from the *posterior femoral cutaneous nerve of the thigh*, laterally.

- *Anal part*: Inferior rectal nerve (pudendal), S3, 4 and perineal branch of S4

Nerve Supply within Pelvis: Lumbar Plexus

- Forms in the psoas major muscle from the *anterior rami* of L1–L4. Gives the following branches:
- *Ilio-hypogastric nerve* (L1) – supplies supra-pubic skin and skin of upper buttock.
- *Ilio-inguinal nerve* (L1) – enters the inguinal canal to supply the skin of the mons pubis and anterior 1/3 of the labia majora.

- *Genito-femoral nerve* (L1, 2) runs on surface of psoas to supply skin of external genitalia- genital branch (passes through inguinal canal) and skin of femoral triangle (femoral branch). Care to preserve during pelvic lymphadenectomy.
- *Lateral femoral cutaneous nerve of the thigh-* descends on iliacus, passing lateral to inguinal ligament to the skin on lateral side of thigh. May be irritated by the gravid uterus (meralgia paraesthetica).
- *Femoral nerve: posterior* divisions of L2, 3, 4 and descends in the groove between psoas and iliacus and passes deep to the inguinal ligament into femoral triangle, lateral to femoral artery. Supplies iliacus, *quadriceps femoris*, pectineus and sartorius muscles.
- The *obturator nerve* (L2, 3, 4), discussed as follows.
- The *lumbo-sacral trunk* (L4, 5) – a branch to the sacral plexus trunk which emerges from the medial aspect of psoas major and descends. It passes above the superior gluteal vessels.

The Obturator Nerve

- Part of lumbar plexus formed in substance of psoas from *anterior* divisions of L2, 3, 4 and emerges from its medial aspect.
- Descends medial to psoas and enters pelvis lateral to origin of internal iliac artery.
- Passes along pelvic side wall, superior to *obturator artery* and lateral to the ovary.
- May be irritated by pathology of the ovary.
- Runs along medial surface of obturator internus muscle on side wall of pelvis.
- Enters thigh through obturator foramen.
- Supplies skin of medial thigh and gives branches to knee joint.
- Supplies *obturator externus, gracilis* and *adductor muscles of thigh*.
- Needs to be identified in dissections of lymph nodes in obturator fossa.

Nerve Supply within Pelvis: Sacral Plexus

- A triangular-shaped plexus on the anterior surface of piriformis muscle.
- Anterior to the sacrum and converges toward the greater sciatic notch.

- Consists of the lumbo-sacral trunk (L4, L5) and the *ventral rami* of S1-S4.
- The main *lateral* nerve is the *sciatic nerve* (L4, 5, S1, 2, 3).
- The main *medial* nerve is the *pudendal nerve* (S2, 3, 4).
- The *superior gluteal nerve* (L4, 5 and S1) – passes above piriformis, through the greater sciatic notch to supply glutus medius, gluteus minimus and the tensor fascia lata muscles.
- The *inferior gluteal nerve* (L5 S1, 2) – passes below piriformis, through the greater sciatic notch, to supply the gluteus maximus muscle.
- *Nerve to obturator internus* (L5, S1, S2).
- *Nerve to quadratus lumborum* (L4, 5, S1). Nerve to *levator ani*.

Sacral Plexus – The 'P' Nerves

- There are a number of branches from the sacral plexus beginning with 'P'.
- *Perforating cutaneous nerve* (S2, 3) – supplies the skin of lower medial buttock.
- *Posterior femoral cutaneous nerve* (S1, 2, 3) – supplies the skin from buttock to calf.
- *Perineal branch of S4-* supplies the muscles of the pelvic floor (levator ani).
- *Piriformis (nerve to)* S1, 2.
- *Pelvic splanchnic nerves* (S2, 3, 4) – sacral parasympathetic outflow, passing to inferior hypo-gastric plexus. Motor to bladder and bowel, from the splenic flexure. Supplies clitoris. Receive afferents from bladder, cervix, colon and rectum. (Not to be confused with *sacral splanchnic nerves* from the sympathetic trunk.)
- *Pudendal nerve* (S2, 3, 4 – discussed later).

The Pudendal Nerve

- The main medial nerve is the pudendal (S2, 3, 4) which leaves the pelvis through the greater sciatic notch, curves around the ischial spine and sacro-spinous ligament.
- The nerve is medial to the internal pudendal artery, at the ischial spine – important for pudendal nerve blocks.
- The nerve enters the *pudendal canal* and supplies the pelvic floor and perineum.

- Branches: *inferior rectal nerve* – supplies external anal sphincter and peri-anal skin.
- *Perineal branch* supplies posterior 2/3 of labia majora, urethra, vagina and perineal muscles (ischio-cavernosus, bulbo-spongiosus and transverse perineal)
- *Terminal branches are the* perineal *and* dorsal nerve of clitoris.
- Note that the anterior 1/3 labia majora is supplied by the ilio-inguinal nerve, from the lumbar plexus, and a *caudal block* will not anaesthetise this.

Single Best Answer Questions

1. A 28-year-old woman is having an episiotomy repair. Which is the most likely muscle to have been transected?

   a. Bulbo-spongiosus
   b. Deep transverse perineal
   c. External anal sphincter
   d. Ischio-cavernosus
   e. Superficial transverse perineal

2. A 40-year-old woman is undergoing a radical hysterectomy and pelvic node dissection for a cervical carcinoma. When removing the external iliac chain of nodes, which structure, on the surface of the psoas major muscle, should be preserved?

   a. Femoral nerve
   b. Genito-femoral nerve
   c. Ilio-hypogastric nerve
   d. Ilio-inguinal nerve
   e. Obturator nerve

3. The vestibule is best described as:

   a. The space between the clitoris and perineum
   b. The space between the labia majora
   c. The space between the labia minora
   d. The space between the mons pubis and the perineum
   e. The space circumvented by the hymen

4. The perineal body is important in maintaining the support and integrity of the pelvic floor and receives the attachment of several muscles. Which perineal muscle does not insert into the perineal body?

   a. Bulbo-spongiousus
   b. Deep transverse perineal
   c. External anal sphincter
   d. Ischio-cavernosus
   e. Superficial transverse perineal

5. Cysts/abscesses of the Bartholin's gland are a common gynaecological problem? In which compartment is the gland found?

   a. Deep perineal space
   b. Ischio-anal fossa
   c. Reteo-oubic space
   d. Superficial perineal space
   e. Vestibule

99

Chapter 12

Concise Anatomy of the Pelvic Girdle

Paul Carter

Components

- The pelvic girdle is a part of the appendicular skeleton.
- It consists of the two *coxa (hip) bones (os innominatum)* and the *sacrum* and coccyx.
- The coxa bones articulate with each other, anteriorly, at the *pubic symphysis* (a secondary cartilaginous joint).
- The coxa bones articulate with sacrum, posteriorly, at the *sacro-iliac joint* (synovial joint).

Differences between the Sexes

- Smaller, lighter and thinner in the female.
- Oval pelvic inlet (female) and heart-shaped in the male.
- Larger pelvic outlet in female (everted ischial tuberosities).
- Pelvic cavity is wider and more shallow in the female.
- The pubic arch is wider and larger in females.
- The greater sciatic notch is wider in females.
- The sacrum is shorter and wider in females.
- The obturator foramen is oval (round in males).

Innominate/Hip (Coxa) Bone: Ilium, Pubis and Ischium

- Consists of these three bones, fused in a Y-shaped epiphysis, in the *acetabulum.*
- The acetabulum provides the socket for the head of the *femur.*
- The pelvic girdle is inclined, forwards, such that, in the anatomical position, the *pubic tubercle* and the *anterior superior iliac spine* (ASIS) lie in the same vertical plane and the pubic symphysis and *ischial spine* lie in the same horizontal plane.

- The plane of the ilium is at right angles with the ischium and pubis and, thus, the coxa bone is similar to a propeller where the two blades are separated by a hub (acetabulum). The larger blade is the ilium and the smaller blade (ischium and pubis) is perforated by a hole (*obturator foramen*).
- The pubis and ischium form an incomplete bony wall for the pelvic cavity and provide attachment for the muscles of the thigh.
- The ilium forms the 'wing' above the pelvic brim (*greater or 'false' pelvis*).
- The *pelvic brim* separates the 'true' (lesser) pelvis from the 'false' (greater) pelvis.
- From anterior to posterior, the *pelvic brim* consists of: *symphysis pubis,* superior border of the *pubic crest, pectineal line, arcuate line, ala of the sacrum* and the superior border of sacrum (*sacral promontory*).
- The plane of the pelvic brim (inlet) is 60° to the horizontal (*angle of inclination*) while the plane of the outlet is 25° to the horizontal.
- The cavity of the pelvis (Latin: basin) has a long posterior wall (sacrum) and a short anterior wall (body of pubic bone). The *pelvic axis* is the curved axis that is taken by the descending presenting part of a fetus passing through the pelvic cavity.
- Note that the pelvic cavity protrudes, posteriorly, into the *gluteal region.*

The Iliac Bone

- Forms the portion of the pelvic brim between the hip joint and the sacro-iliac joint.
- The anterior 2/3 forms the *iliac fossa* – part of the posterior abdominal wall and contains the iliacus muscle (nerve supply: femoral nerve).
- The posterior 1/3 forms the *auricular surface* to articulate with the sacrum.

- The outer surface has the posterior, anterior and inferior *gluteal lines* between which arise the *gluteal muscles* (maximus, medius and minimus) of the buttocks).
- The convex upper margin (anterior to posterior superior iliac spines) is the *iliac crest*, and is easily palpable. It is only 4 cm from the lowest part of the thorax (L3).
- The most lateral part is the *tubercle* at the level of L5, (5 cm posterior to the ASIS).
- The highest part is a further 2.5 cm posterior, at the level of L4 (level at which lumbar puncture/ epidural injections are sited).
- The posterior border is a rounded bar between *posterior superior iliac spine* (PSIS), at the level of S2, and *the posterior inferior iliac spine* (PIIS), at the level of the ischial spines.
- The posterior border is concave, anteriorly and forms the majority of the greater sciatic notch.
- The *inguinal (Poupart's) ligament* (lower edge of external oblique muscle) runs from the ASIS to the pubic tubercle.
- The junction with superior ramus of the pubis is the *ilio-pubic eminence.*
- The iliacus muscle arises from the upper 2/3 down to the level of the AIIS.
- The *psoas major muscle* passes along the pelvic brim to cross the ilio-pubic eminence. Inserts (with iliacus) into the *lesser trochanter* of the femur.

The Pubic Bone

- Consists of the *body, superior* and *inferior pubic rami.*
- The superior pubic rami form the anterior portion of the *pelvic brim.*
- The rami diverge from the symphysis and create the *sub-pubic arch.*
- The inferior pubic ramus fuses with the ischium, inferior to the obturator foramen.
- The pubic bones unite at the symphysis by a secondary cartilaginous joint.
- A prominence (*pubic tubercle*) lies lateral to the symphysis into which the medial end of the inguinal ligament inserts.
- Two ridges diverge from the tubercle: the upper is the pectineal line, and the lower is the *obturator crest.*
- The upper border of the superior ramus (pectineal line) forms the anterior part of the pelvic brim, between the pubic tubercle and the ilio-pubic eminence.

- Below the obturator crest is the *obturator groove* for the obturator nerve and vessels which exit the pelvic cavity through the obturator foramen, to the thigh.
- The inferior ramus joins the ischial ramus halfway between the tuberosity and crest.
- The inferior ramus is below the pelvic diaphragm, i.e. in the perineum.
- The *conjoint tendon* (discussed later) inserts into the pubic crest as the *pectineal ligament*, along the *pectineal line.*
- The pectineal line also gives attachment to the *lacunar (Gimbernat's) ligament.*

The Ischial Bone

- An L shaped bone with the *ischial tuberosity* at the angle. It supports the body weight in the sitting position.
- The thick upper portion forms the lower portion of the *greater sciatic foramen.*
- The lower, thinner, part forms the ischial ramus and the lower border of the obturator foramen.
- The ischial spine projects medially and separates the *greater sciatic notch* from the *lesser sciatic notch* and, also, receives the *sacro-spinous ligament.*
- With the *sacro-tuberous ligament*, this converts the greater and lesser sciatic notches into *greater* and *lesser sciatic foramina.*
- The *pudendal nerve* lies on the sacro-spinous ligament, medial to the ischial spine (*internal pudendal* vessels are more lateral). This anatomical relationship is important for pudendal nerve blocks.
- The obturator foramen is ringed by the margins of the pubic rami and ischium.
- The foramen is filled by the *obturator membrane* (apart from the obturator canal, superiorly). The *obturator internus muscle* arises from the pelvic surface of the membrane, and the surrounding bone.
- The *levator ani muscle* arises from the *tendinous line* on the fascia on the medial surface of the obturator internus muscle.

The Sacrum

- An inverted triangular-shaped bone, concave toward the pelvis, consisting of a fusion of five progressively smaller vertebrae and their costal elements.

- It carries the whole body weight – through ligaments rather than bone.
- It articulates with the ilium forming the posterior boundary of the pelvic brim.
- The upper surface of S1 slopes anteriorly, 30° to the horizontal.
- The anterior surface has four transverse ridges where the five bodies fuse.
- Lateral to the ridges are the four *anterior sacral foramina* which transmit the anterior rami of the upper four sacral nerves. (S5 exits through the *sacral hiatus*, inferiorly.)
- The bar of bone above the first sacral foramen is continuous with the arcuate line of the ilium and forms the posterior part of the pelvic brim and, medially, forms the *sacral promontory*.
- The lateral mass of bone, lateral to foramina, represents the fused costal elements.
- The *ala* are crossed by the *sympathetic trunk, lumbo-sacral trunk, ilio-lumbar artery* and *obturator nerve* (from medial → lateral).
- The *piriformis muscle* arises from the anterior surface of the sacrum (with the sacral plexus on its anterior surface) and exits the pelvis through the greater sciatic foramen. This muscle is the 'key structure' to the region.
- The retro-peritoneal part of the rectum lies on the lower three bodies of the sacrum.
- The posterior surface is irregular and rough, giving rise to strong ligaments, especially, the *posterior sacro-iliac ligaments*.
- The posterior surface is closed in the midline by a fusion of adjacent laminae with the dorsal protrusion of the fused spinous processes (*median sacral crest*).
- The fusion of the articular processes forms the *articular (intermediate) crest* and the fusion of transverse processes forms the *lateral sacral crest*.
- The four posterior foramina, between the articular and lateral sacral crests, allow the exit of the *dorsal rami* of the sacral nerves.
- The *erector spinae muscles* lie in the groove between median and lateral crests.
- The body of S1 is narrower in the female and the ala are wider than the body.
- The sacro-iliac joint (synovial) is between the cartilage of auricular surface of ilium and the ala of the sacrum (occupying the length of two vertebrae).

- The stability of the sacro-iliac joint depends on ligaments as the bony surfaces diverge from the midline and the body weight forces the sacrum downwards between the iliac bones.
- The *anterior sacro-iliac ligament* is weak and the main strength is provided by the strong *posterior sacro-iliac ligaments* which support the weight of the body and prevent the sacrum from being forced between the iliac bones.
- The sacro-iliac joint is stabilised by accessory ligaments such as the *ilio-lumbar ligament* from the transverse process of L5 to the iliac bone.
- The sacro-tuberous ligament (strong) is attached to the posterior border of the ilium (between PSIS and PIIS) and the transverse tubercles of sacrum and then slopes inferiorly to the medial surface of the ischial tuberosity to a ridge of bone (*falciform process*), inferior to the *pudendal canal*.
- The *sacro-spinous* ligament lies on the pelvic aspect of the sacro-tuberous ligament. It has a broad base, arising from lower sacrum, narrowing to an apex, attached to the ischial spine. The *ischio-coccygeus* muscle is on its pelvic surface.
- The sacro-tuberous ligaments resist the weight of the body forcing the sacrum to rotate, around a horizontal axis, between the sacro-iliac joints.

The Pelvic Cavity

- The pelvic cavity projects posteriorly from the abdominal cavity toward the gluteal region and the buttocks.
- The pelvic inlet is bounded by the pelvic brim which is oval in shape (transverse diameter greater than the antero-posterior).
- The pelvic outlet is diamond shaped and bounded by the symphysis pubis, inferior pubic rami, ischial rami, ischial tuberosities, sacro-tuberous ligaments and the coccyx. The antero-posterior dimension is greater than the transverse.
- The true pelvis contains pelvic organs (genital, urinary and intestinal tracts). They are not accessible to palpation, per abdomen. Clinical examination must be per vaginam or per rectum.
- The key structure in the gluteal region is the piriformis muscle which leaves the pelvis, through the greater sciatic foramen, to insert into the *greater trochanter* of the femur.

- The only structures exiting the pelvis, above piriformis, are the *superior gluteal artery and nerve*. The nerve supplies gluteus medius and minimus.
- Structures leaving the pelvic cavity, through the greater sciatic foramen, below the piriformis muscle, include:

  Sciatic nerve

     Posterior cutaneous nerve of thigh

     Nerve to quadratus femoris

     Inferior gluteal nerve and artery

     Nerve to obturator internus

  Pudendal nerve

     Internal pudendal artery

- The latter three structures then wind around the ischial spine to enter the perineum, through the lesser sciatic foramen, below the pelvic diaphragm (the pudendal nerve being the most medial).
- The only structure to leave the pelvic cavity, through the lesser sciatic foramen, is the *tendon of the obturator internus muscle*, which inserts into the greater trochanter of the hip.

Single Best Answer Questions

1. A 52-year-old woman presents with acute bowel obstruction from a strangulated femoral hernia. Which structure is occluding the blood supply of the small bowel?

   a. Conjoint tendon
   b. Femoral sheath
   c. Inguinal ligament
   d. Lacunar ligament
   e. Pectineal ligament

2. Which is the only structure to leave the pelvic cavity through the lesser sciatic foramen?

   a. Inferior gluteal nerve
   b. Piriformis muscle
   c. Pudendal nerve
   d. Sciatic nerve
   e. Tendon of obturator internus

3. There has been a recent resurgence in performing the 'Burch' colposuspension for women with stress incontinence. Having opened the retro-pubic space and elevated the vagina, to which structure is it then attached?

   a. Inguinal ligament
   b. Lacunar ligament
   c. Obturator membrane
   d. Pectineal ligament
   e. Symphysis pubis

4. A 30-year-old woman who is 37 weeks pregnant, experiences pubic symphysial diastasis.
   What type of joint is the pubic symphysis?

   a. Fibrous
   b. Primary cartilaginous
   c. Secondary cartilaginous
   d. Syndesmosis
   e. Synovial

5. The weight of the upright body tends to force the vertebral column between the two iliac bones. Which ligament is most important in resisting this?

   a. Anterior sacro-iliac
   b. Ilio-lumbar
   c. Posterior sacro-iliac
   d. Sacro-spinous
   e. Sacro-tuberous

Chapter 13

Concise Anatomy of the Abdominal Walls

Paul Carter

- For descriptive and clinical examination purposes, the anterior abdominal wall is divided into nine regions by four lines (Fig. 13.1).
- It consists of skin, sub-cutaneous fat, *Scarpa's fascia*, muscles (and their aponeuroses), *transversalis fascia* and *parietal peritoneum*.
- Laterally, are three muscles *(external oblique, internal oblique, transversus abdominis)* which become aponeurotic, ventrally. Below the *arcuate line*, all three aponeuroses pass anterior to the rectus abdominis forming the *rectus sheath*. The arcuate line is 2.5 cm below the umbilicus.

- The *neuro-vascular plane* is between the internal oblique and transversus abdominis muscles and is the plane for regional anaesthesia.
- The *rectus abdominis muscles* consist of two parallel muscles, arising from a medial head (anterior to pubic symphysis) and a lateral head, on upper border of pubic crest. Its insertion is onto the anterior aspects of the 5th–7th *costal cartilages*.
- The two bellies are separated by the *linea alba*. Above the arcuate line, the muscle is enclosed by both *anterior* and *posterior* leaves of the rectus sheath as a result of a splitting of the aponeurosis

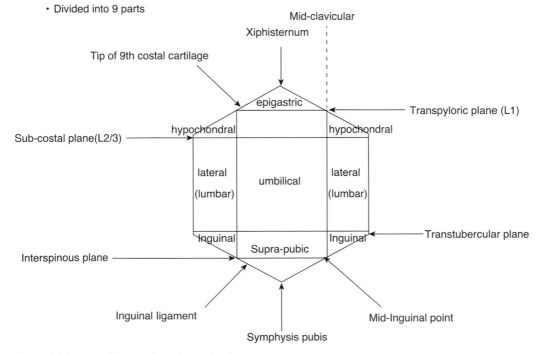

Figure 13.1 Areas of the anterior abdominal wall

of the internal oblique, around the rectus abdominis, such that aponeurosis of external oblique passes anteriorly and that of transversus abdominis passes posteriorly.

- 2.5 cm below umbilicus all three aponeuroses pass anterior to the rectus abdominis, creating a free lower margin of posterior sheath (*arcuate line/ semi-circular fold*).

- Blood supply – branches of the *superior* and *inferior epigastric arteries* (from *internal thoracic* and *external iliac arteries*, respectively).

- Below the umbilicus, there is a blood supply from branches of the *femoral artery*: *superficial circumflex iliac, superficial epigastric* and from the *ascending branch of the deep circumflex iliac artery* (external iliac artery). These may be at risk when inserting lateral laparoscopic ports.

- Nerve supply is segmental T7–T12 (lateral and anterior branches of their ventral rami) and a contribution from the *ilio-hypogastric nerve*, inferiorly (L1), as discussed later.

The External Oblique Muscle

- The external oblique muscle arises from digitations from the lower eight ribs at their anterior angles.

- The upper four interdigitate with the *serratus anterior* muscle; the lower four with the *latissimus dorsi* muscle.

- It fans out to a wide, aponeurotic insertion. Fibres passing down and forwards.

- There are three free borders (posterior, superior and inferior).

- The upper border passes from 5th rib to the *xiphisternum*.

- The lower border forms *inguinal (Poupart's) ligament*.

- Inferior insertion is to anterior half of iliac crest, inguinal ligament and pubic tubercle.

- Medially, its aponeurosis passes anterior to the rectus abdominis to the linea alba.

- The inguinal ligament passes from the ASIS→pubic tubercle. Its edge is rolled to form a gutter, the lateral part of which gives partial origin to the internal oblique and transversus abdominis muscles.

- Nerve supply: segmentally, from T7–T11.

Internal Oblique and Transversus Abdominis Muscles

- The internal oblique arises from the *thoraco-lumbar fascia* (posteriorly), the anterior 2/3 of the iliac crest and lateral 2/3 of the inguinal ligament. Its fibres run upwards and medially to insert into the costal margin.

- Medially, the aponeurosis passes anterior to rectus muscle, inferiorly (i.e. below the arcuate line) but splits around it, above the arcuate line.

- Inferiorly, it has a free lower border, arching over inguinal canal as the *conjoint tendon* (with transversus abdominis), which inserts into the *pectineal line* of the pubic bone as the *pectineal ligament*.

- The transversus abdominis arises from the costal cartilages of T7–T12, the thoraco-lumbar fascia (posteriorly), the anterior 1/2 of the iliac crest and the lateral 1/2 of the inguinal ligament.

- The fibres arising from the costal cartilages (inside the thoracic cage) interdigitate with fibres of the *diaphragm*.

- The muscle becomes aponeurotic, medially, passing anterior to the rectus abdominis, inferiorly, but passing, posteriorly, above the arcuate line.

- Some lower fibres join similar fibres of the internal oblique muscle to form the conjoint tendon which arches (from anterior to posterior) over the inguinal canal.

- Both have a segmental nerve supply from T7–12 and L1. Note that the L1 fibres supply the conjoint tendon and are carried by the ilio-inguinal nerve.

- Actions: Depress ribs, move trunk, compress abdomen and support the viscera.

The Inguinal Canal

- An oblique intra-muscular passage (4 cm) passing through anterior abdominal wall.

- Extending from the *deep ring* (superior to mid-point of inguinal ligament) to the *superficial ring* (above pubic tubercle).

- The inferior epigastric artery marks the medial border of deep ring and, anatomically, distinguishes between direct and indirect inguinal hernias.

- The anterior wall is the aponeurosis of the external oblique reinforced, laterally, by the internal oblique muscle.
- The posterior wall is composed of transversalis fascia, laterally, and the conjoint tendon, medially.
- The floor is the grooved surface of the inguinal ligament, and its pectineal part (lacunar ligament), curving upwards to the pectineal line.
- The roof is the arched lower borders of the internal oblique and transversus abdominis muscles (conjoint tendon) passing from anterior to posterior.
- It contains the *round ligament* in females (spermatic cord in males).
- In the female, it contains three nerves – ilio-inguinal, genital branch of the *genito-femoral nerve* and *sympathetic fibres*.

The Femoral Triangle and Femoral Ring

- Boundaries: inguinal ligament (superiorly), medial border of the *sartorius muscle* (laterally) and the lateral border of the *adductor longus muscle* (medially).
- From medial to lateral, the floor is composed of adductor longus, *pectineus* and *ilio-psoas muscles*. The roof is from the *fascia lata* of the thigh, sub-cutaneous fat and skin.
- Contents: (medial→lateral): *Femoral vein* (and *long saphenous vein*), *femoral artery* (and branches) and the femoral nerve. (Vein posterior to artery at apex of the Δ.)
- The vessels are surrounded by a funnel-shaped prolongation of the *transversalis fascia (femoral sheath)*.
- The medial part of the femoral sheath surrounds the femoral canal which is entered via the femoral ring.
- Femoral ring: boundaries are the inguinal ligament (anterior), pectineal ligament (posterior), lacunar ligament (medial) and femoral vein (lateral).
- The lacunar ligament is the medial border of the femoral canal (can cause ischaemia of herniating bowel in cases of 'strangulated' femoral hernia).
- The femoral ring continues, inferiorly, as the femoral canal.
- The canal allows the femoral vein to expand during increased venous return.

- Femoral canal contains *Cloquet's node* and lymphatics (including those from the clitoris).
- Femoral ring is bounded anteriorly, medially and posteriorly by the femoral sheath.

The Posterior Abdominal Wall

Thoraco-Lumbar Fascia

- Covers the three muscles of the posterior abdominal wall and comprises the lumbar part of the thoraco-lumbar fascia.
- The three layers enclose two muscle compartments, the anterior occupied by *quadratus lumborum* and the posterior occupied by the erector spinae muscle.
- The anterior layer extends from the ilio-lumbar ligament and iliac crest to the 12th rib. The medial attachment is to the anterior surface of the transverse processes of the lumbar vertebrae. Laterally, it blends with the middle layer along the lateral border of quadratus lumborum.
- The middle layer extends from the ilio-lumbar ligament and iliac crest to the 12th rib. The medial attachment is to the tips of the transverse processes of the lumbar vertebrae. Laterally, it blends with the anterior and posterior layers.
- The posterior layer extends from the sacrum to the neck. It covers the mass of erector spinae muscle and is reinforced by the origin of latissimus dorsi muscle. The medial attachment is to the tips of the spinous processes of T12–S5. Laterally, it blends with the anterior and middle layers. The lateral margin extends along the transverse tubercles of the sacrum to the posterior aspect of the iliac crest to the 12th rib and the angles of all higher ribs.

Posterior Abdominal Wall Musculature

- Consists of the *crura of the diaphragm* and the *para-vertebral gutters* (created by protrusion of vertebral column into abdominal cavity and accentuated by the lumbar lordosis) – with psoas major and quadratus lumborum, above the iliac crest, and iliacus, below the iliac crest.
- Psoas major arises from the inter-vertebral discs of L1–L5 and the intervening fibrous arches. It inserts, with iliacus, into the lesser trochanter of

femur. Covered, anteriorly by psoas fascia. Nerve supply: lumbar plexus.

- The *lumbar plexus* (L1–L5) is embedded within psoas major muscle (discussed later).
- A thickening of the psoas fascia, from L1 (body) → L1 (transverse process), forms the *medial arcuate ligament*. It gives origin to fibres of the diaphragm and has the *sympathetic chain* posterior to it.
- Psoas major muscle is supplied by L1, L2, L3. It is a lateral flexor of the trunk and, with the opposite side, is an anterior flexor.
- The quadratus lumborum muscle: a flat sheet of muscle, lateral to psoas major and medial to transversus abdominis (and in series with it as the innermost muscle layer of body wall).
- It arises from the transverse process of L5, ilio-lumbar ligament and the adjoining iliac crest. It inserts into the transverse process of L4 and inferior border of the 12th rib.
- The fascia on the anterior surface is thickened from transverse process L1 →12th rib *(lateral arcuate ligament)* and gives rise to fibres of the diaphragm.
- Action: lateral flexor of spine, depresses 12th rib and prevents its elevation, by the diaphragm, during inspiration. Nerve supply from T12, L1–L3
- *Iliacus muscle*: Δ shaped muscle arising from the upper 2/3 of the iliac fossa and the anterior surface of the anterior sacro-iliac ligament. Fibres converge medially toward psoas major.
- Passes, with psoas major, beneath the inguinal ligament, to the lesser trochanter of the femur.
- Nerve supply: femoral nerve (L2, L3). Action: flexor and medial rotator of hip (flexor of trunk, if limb is fixed)

The Diaphragm

- A musculo-tendinous septum separating the thorax from the abdomen.
- A derivative of the innermost (transversus) muscles of the body wall.
- The *central tendinous portion* is adherent to the *pericardium* (embryological).
- The peripheral muscular portion has sternal, costal and vertebral components.
- Sternal – from two muscular slips on the posterior surface of the *xiphisternum*.

- Costal – from inner surfaces of the lower six costal cartilages.
- Vertebral
  a) Right crus from bodies of L1–L3 – surrounds oesophageal opening
  b) Left crus from bodies of L1 and L2
  c) Medial arcuate ligament
  d) Lateral arcuate ligament
- Inferiorly are: liver, kidney and adrenal gland (right), stomach, spleen, kidney and adrenal gland (left). The heart and lungs are superior. Posteriorly are the lungs and costo-diaphragmatic pleural recesses.
- Opening for the *inferior vena cava* (with *right phrenic nerve*) is in central tendon at the level of T8.
- Opening for the *oesophagus* (with *anterior* and *posterior vagus nerves*) is at T10.
- Opening for the *aorta* (with the *thoracic duct and azygous vein*) is at T12.
- Blood supply from lower five *inter-costal arteries* and *subcostal artery*.
- Right and left *phrenic arteries* supply crura (on abdominal surface).
- Nerve supply from right and left phrenic nerves (C3,4,5).
- Peripheral sensory branches are from inter-costal nerves.
- Crura supplied by lower inter-costal nerves.
- *Splanchnic nerves* pierce the crura (left phrenic nerve pierces the left dome).
- Sympathetic trunk passes posterior to the medial arcuate ligament.
- Subcostal nerve and vessels pass posterior to the lateral arcuate ligament.
- Superior epigastric vessels pass between the sternal and costal portions.

Abdominal Aorta

- Abdominal aorta passes down the posterior abdominal wall from T12 to L4.
- Note that, at L4, it may only be 3–4 cm from the anterior abdominal wall, especially, in slim women and is at risk from injury by the insertion of laparoscopic ports
- Enters the abdomen posterior to the *median arcuate ligament* (T12).

- Gives three anterior branches to the gut (*coeliac, superior and inferior mesenteric*).
- Gives three paired parietal branches (*inferior phrenic, lumbar, sacral*)
- Gives three paired visceral branches (*supra-renal, renal and gonadal*).
- Anterior relations – *lesser sac, pancreas, splenic vein, left renal vein*, and *duodenum* (3rd part).
- Divides into right and left *common iliac arteries* at L4.
- The IVC is on the right side and the left sympathetic trunk on the left side.

Inferior Vena Cava (IVC)

- The IVC forms at L5 from a confluence of the *common iliac veins*, posterior to the *right common iliac artery*. It pierces the central tendon of the diaphragm at T8.
- It is anterior to the right *renal artery, right supra-renal artery, inferior phrenic artery* and the *coeliac artery*.
- It is posterior to the root of the *mesentery, right gonadal artery, 3rd part of the duodenum* (infracolic).
- It is posterior to the *portal vein, pancreas, bile duct, epiploic foramen* and the *bare area of liver* (supracolic).
- Note that its tributaries are not identical to the branches of the aorta.
- Note that there are no tributaries equivalent to the three arterial branches to the gut.
- In ascending order, the tributaries are: 3rd and 4th lumbar veins, right gonadal vein, renal veins, right supra-renal vein, right and left inferior phrenic veins and the hepatic veins

Single Best Answer Questions

1. A 30-year-old woman, undergoing a laparoscopy, suffers an injury to the aorta, during the insertion of the trocar. In a woman with a BMI in the normal range, how far is the aorta from the umbilicus (before any insufflation of gas)?

   a. 2 cm
   b. 4 cm
   c. 6 cm
   d. 8 cm
   e. 10 cm

2. A 32-year-old woman develops a haematoma in a lateral port site, following a laparoscopy. Which artery is most likely to have been injured?

   a. Deep circumflex iliac
   b. Inferior epigastric
   c. Obliterated umbilical
   d. Superficial circumflex iliac
   e. Superficial epigastric

3. A patient is experiencing pain at the umbilical port site, following a laparoscopy. Which dermatome supplies the umbilicus?

   a. L1
   b. L2
   c. T8
   d. T10
   e. T12

4. During a routine laparotomy for a pelvic procedure, the triangular-shaped pyramidalis muscle is exposed at the lower end of the incision. What is the nerve supply of this muscle?

   a. Genito-femoral
   b. Ilio-hypogastric
   c. Ilio-inguinal
   d. Obturator
   e. Sub-costal

5. An anaesthetist is inserting a 'TAP' block (transversus abdominus plane) under ultrasound guidance to provide post-operative analgesia after a laparoscopic procedure. In which plane are the nerves found?

   a) Between the external oblique and the internal oblique muscles
   b) Between the internal oblique and transversus abdominus muscles
   c) Between transversalis fascia and parietal peritoneum
   d) Between transversus abdominus muscle and transversalis fascia
   e) Superficial to the external oblique muscle

Chapter 14

Early Embryonic Development

Laura C. Mongan

Introduction

Put in the broadest terms, the events taking place during the first four weeks of development following fertilisation lay the foundations for the development of the structures of the body (i.e. organ systems). Early embryonic development encompasses some key developmental events and processes that result in the production of sufficient cells, of the right type in the right place to ensure that structural development of the organs can proceed. These events and processes are linked and inter-dependent and can be conceptualised as a cascade of events where a given event primes the succeeding event.

The study of embryology is not only of interest in its own right but has significant importance to the development of a deep understanding of the anatomy of the human body, allowing explanation of those anatomical peculiarities that appear to defy logic and/or normal rules. In addition, an understanding of the developmental journey of the various structures of the human body allows for insight into the aetiology and explanation of congenital malformations, both commonly seen and those rarely described.

Taking fertilisation as a given, what follows is the creation of a *morula* from the *zygote* though the process of cleavage. Compaction and cavitation together create a *blastocyst*, the developmental stage that must be reached before *implantation* can be initiated. The *inner cell mass* of the blastocyst undergoes differentiation, creating a *bilaminar embryonic disk*. *Gastrulation* within the bilaminar disk creates an embryo comprised of the three key *germ layers* necessary to begin the processes leading to the structural development of the organ system. A further consequence of gastrulation is the definition of the axes of the body, initiating the establishment of a body plan. The development of arguably the most complex system of the body, the central nervous system, gets underway shortly after gastrulation with the

establishment of *neurulation*. A simple body plan is in place at the end of the fourth week with the development of *body segments* and *folding* of the embryonic disk.

The First Week of Development: Zygote, Morula and Blastocyst

The zygote undergoes cell division to produce a two-cell stage which is normally achieved approximately 30 hours following fertilisation. Thereafter follows a series of mitotic cell divisions which result in the formation of a cluster of identical cells (blastomeres). Because at this stage the zona pellucida is still intact, the daughter cells become increasingly small. This process results in compaction, and the cells of the morula become tightly packed. Tissue fluid begins to pass through the zona pellucida and accumulates, creating a fluid-filled space through cavitation. This space, the blastocoele, is enclosed by a population of cells forming an outer shell (outer cell mass), and a second population of cells (inner cell mass) clusters at one pole. The conceptus is now termed a blastocyst (Fig. 14.1).

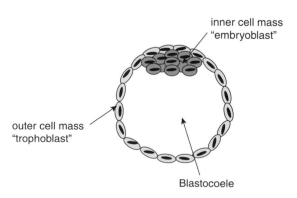

inner cell mass
"embryoblast"

outer cell mass
"trophoblast"

Blastocoele

Figure 14.1 Schematic diagram of blastocyst organization

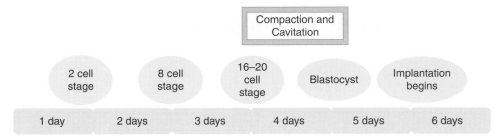

Figure 14.2 Summary timeline of the major events in the first week following fertilization

The blastocyst hatches from the zona pellucida allowing the cells of the outer cell mass, the trophoblast, to interact with the uterine epithelium to initiate implantation. The events in the first week after fertilisation are summarized in Fig. 14.2.

For clarity, the timeframe referred to in this chapter is that based on fertilisation age, that is, time since fertilisation. Gestational age, used clinically, is time since last menstrual period. Therefore, based on a standard 28-day menstrual cycle, gestational age is equal to fertilisation age plus 14 days.

In assisted reproductive techniques, fertilisation of the oocyte occurs in vitro, and the embryo is maintained in culture until the eight-cell stage (morula) is achieved before transfer to the uterus. Those embryos that undergo division quickly after fertilization have better prospects for subsequent development, that is, achieve development to the blastocyst stage required at implantation (Fenwick, J., et al. 2002).

The formation of the blastocoele marks a significant event in early development with the formation of the first embryonic cavity. Cavities are of huge significance in early development as these provide the spaces into which the embryo will grow.

Progression of development into the second week sees differentiation within the two cell populations of the blastocyst. The outer cell mass or trophoblast differentiates into two discrete cell layers: an outer syncytiotrophoblast and an inner cytotrophoblast layer. Similarly, the inner cell mass, or embryoblast, differentiates into a two-layered, bilaminar disk, comprised of epiblast and hypoblast (Fig. 14.3).

Spaces appear between the cells of the epiblast, which coalesce to form the amniotic sac. The hypoblast of the bilaminar disk migrates and lines the blastocoele creating the primitive yolk sac, from which the definitive yolk sac is ultimately formed. Finally, a large supporting sac, the chorionic sac, is formed as the yolk sac membrane is separated from

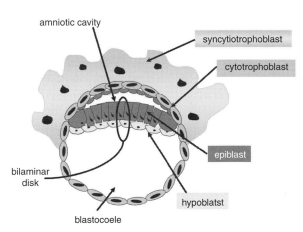

Figure 14.3 The embryo in the second week of development, the 'week of twos'. Note development of a pair of tissue layers in each of the trophoblast and embryoblast, and two embryonic cavities.

the cytotrophoblast layer by a layer of extraembryonic mesoderm. Spaces appear within the extraembryonic mesoderm, which coalesce to form a space, the chorionic cavity.

By the end of the second week of development, the conceptus has begun the process of implantation. The embryo (bilaminar disk) and its two spaces, the amniotic and yolk sacs, are suspended by a condensation of extraembryonic mesoderm, termed a connecting stalk, in an outer supporting chorionic sac.

Implantation

Human implantation is interstitial; that is to say that the uterine epithelium is breached in an invasive process and the conceptus implants within the endometrium and consequently has access to endometrial glands and capillaries for support. Human placentation is defined as haemomonochorial. Placental classification is on the histological basis of which maternal tissue makes contact with the chorion. In humans, maternal

Table 14.1 Derivatives of the germ layers

Ectoderm derivatives	Mesoderm derivatives	Endoderm derivatives
Nervous system Epidermis of skin	Muscles, cartilage, bone, dermis of skin, vascular system include heart and great vessels	Epithelial lining of gastrointestinal tract, respiratory tract and parts of the urinary and reproductive tracts Parenchyma of glands associated with the primitive gut tube

blood bathes the chorion and its specialisations, the chorionic villi. The early stages of implantation set in place the steps required to establish the uteroplacental circulation. This allows for haemotrophic support of the conceptus, which quickly becomes too large to be supported by diffusion alone. The process of implantation begins in the second week of development but is not complete until the end of the first trimester. Detailed consideration of the cellular interactions required to establish healthy implantation is beyond the scope of this chapter.

Gastrulation

'It is not birth, marriage or death that is truly the most important time in your life, it is gastrulation', so Lewis Wolpert, eminent developmental biologist, is often quoted as saying in 1986.

Gastrulation is the process that establishes the three germ layers from which all of the tissues of the body are derived. Gastrulation in the bilaminar embryonic disk creates a new trilaminar embryonic disk comprised of ectoderm, mesoderm and endoderm.

The onset of gastrulation is marked by the appearance of a distinct feature on the surface of the epiblast layer, the primitive streak. At the primitive streak, cells of the epiblast layer undergo a process of migration and invagination through the streak to spread widely. The hypoblast is displaced by newly formed endoderm. The mesoderm formed at gastrulation spreads laterally and cephalad, separating the endoderm now lining the yolk sac from the uppermost ectoderm layer. There are two locations, one cranially and one caudally, where no mesoderm lies between endoderm and ectoderm. These are the buccopharyngeal and cloacal membranes, respectively.

The molecular control of this process and the patterning that follows is beyond the scope of this chapter, but suffice to say that control and regulation of this process are complex (Sutherland, AE 2015).

From three simple germ layers, an extensive array of tissue types will differentiate. Ectoderm gives rise to

tissues that maintain contact with the environment; mesoderm gives rise to 'middle' tissues or supporting tissues, while endoderm gives rise to internal structures (Table 14.1).

A further significant structure is formed as a consequence of gastrulation. A discrete population of cells undergoing gastrulation form a solid rod of cells within the mesoderm layer (Stemple, DL 2005, Annona, G et al 2015). This *notochord* runs in the midline, creating the axis of the embryo and has an important signalling role. The axial skeleton forms around it from the mesoderm surrounding it. Once the process of neurulation has been established by it, the notochord regresses. The vestigial remnant of the notochord is seen as the nucleus pulposus of the intervertebral disks.

Neurulation

The neural plate forms as ectoderm overlying the notochord differentiates into neuroectoderm. This neural plate thickens, and the edges of the plate rise until the edges of the plate curl toward each other in the midline fusing to create a tube (Hill, MA 2016). The neural tube represents the primordium of the nervous system, the first system of the body to begin development, and is also the last to complete development.

Body Segments

Development is now in the third week and has been characterised by key events such as initiation of the development of the nervous system and establishment of the body axis. The mesoderm formed at gastrulation begins to organise itself into discrete zones. At the lateral margins of the disk, the mesoderm separates into two discrete leaves of tissue, the somatic and splanchnic mesoderm. The somatic mesoderm layer is juxtaposed to the ectoderm while the splanchnic layer is juxtaposed to the endoderm. Mesoderm close to the axis on both sides of the embryo, the paraxial mesoderm, becomes organised as blocks of embryonic

Table 14.2 Fate of the mesoderm

Mesoderm zone	
Paraxial	Axial skeleton (vertebral column and ribs) dermis, muscles of body wall, limb muscles
Intermediate	Urogenital system, e.g. kidneys, ureters, gonads
Lateral plate:	
Somatic	Connective tissue of limbs; contributes to body wall, including parietal peritoneum
Splanchnic	Smooth musculature, connective tissue and vasculature of gut, visceral peritoneum

tissue called *somites*. Between these two zones lies the intermediate mesoderm.

The organisation of the paraxial mesoderm as tissue blocks represents preservation of an evolutionarily conserved process and leads to a segmented body structure. The somites represent the origins of much of the musculoskeletal system. Each somite corresponds to a spinal segment, and its derivatives are innervated by the spinal nerve emerging from the corresponding spinal cord segment. The fate of the various zones within the mesoderm are summarized in Table 14.2.

Embryonic Folding

At this point, the embryo is comprised of three layers stacked one on top of the other. With continued development of the neural tube and the somites, the embryonic disk undergoes a significant morphological change, resulting in a recognisable body form, with a cavity inside the embryo and ectoderm facing the external environment.

Thus the three-layered embryonic disk folds by rolling and tucking, to make a cylindrical body plan with inside and outside surfaces. The most significant consequence of this process, occurring in the fourth week of development, is that an anterior body wall is formed, along with the formation of an internal tube suspended in the first space inside the embryo, the intraembryonic coelom.

In order to conceptualise the process of embryonic folding, it is helpful to consider folding of the disk in two perpendicular planes. Firstly, in the longitudinal plane folds at the cranial and caudal extremities of the disk result in cephalocaudal folding (Fig. 14.4A).

Secondly, in the transverse plane, folding at the lateral margins completes the process of embryonic folding. By bringing together the lateral plate mesoderm from opposite sides of the disk, the spaces between the opposing somatic and splanchnic mesoderm layers join to become consolidated as a space now inside the embryonic body (Fig. 14.4B).

The amniotic sac is drawn around the embryonic body as it folds, with the result that the embryo is suspended within the amniotic sac. Much of the yolk sac is drawn into the developing body cavity from the primitive gut tube. The margins of the disk meet but do not quite close at the point at which the umbilical cord attaches at the ventral body wall, allowing for communication between the embryo and its supporting tissues (placenta) and consequently the uteroplacental circulation.

Teratogenesis

A large number of agents are capable of interfering with normal development leading to developmental defects. The nature of teratogenic agents varies widely and includes chemical and infectious agents as well as ionising radiation. Chemical agents include alcohol, a small molecule capable of free movement across the placenta, as well as certain classes of therapeutic drugs.

Whether or not exposure to a teratogenic agent will result in a developmental defect and the severity of any such defect caused is dependent on the time of exposure. In the pre-embryonic period, the first two weeks following fertilisation, the consequences of exposure to teratogenic agents at sufficient concentration, is likely to have lethal effects. This is a consequence of the basic cellular and developmental processes occurring during this period. The embryonic period from weeks 3–8 inclusive is the period of greatest sensitivity and carries the greatest risk of developmental defects. Furthermore, narrow windows of particular sensitivity exist for some systems of the body. Once the embryonic period has completed, the structural development of the systems of the body is complete and what remains to occur during the lengthy fetal period is continuing growth, and functional development and maturation of those systems and structures. The exception to this rule is, however, the central nervous system. Although it is the first system of the body to begin its development, its development continues throughout the fetal period and remains sensitive to teratogenic insult.

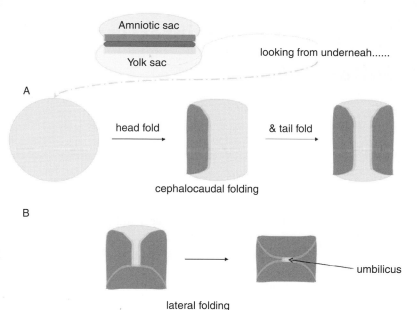

Figure 14.4 Schematic representation of folding of the embryo in the fourth week of development, showing [A] cephalocaudal folding; and lateral folding ; and [B] lateral folding resulting in the margins of the disk being drawn together to meet at the umbilicus.

References

Annona, G et al. 2015. *Evolution of the notochord. EvoDevo* **6**:30

Carlson, BM. 2014. *Human Embryology and Developmental Biology*, 5th edition. Elsevier

Fenwick, J et al. 2002. *Time from insemination to first cleavage predicts developmental competence of human preimplantation embryos in vitro. Human Reproduction* **17**, 407–12

Hill, MA. 2016. Embryology Neural System Development. Retrieved July 10, 2016, from https://embryology.med.unsw.edu.au/embryology/index.php/Neural_System_Development

Moore, KL et al. 2012. *The Developing Human: Clinically Oriented Embryology*, 9th edition. Elsevier

Sadler TW. 2015. *Langman's Medical Embryology*, 13th edition. Wolters Kluwer Health

Stemple, DL. 2005. Structure and function of the notochord: An essential organ for chordate development. *Development* **132**, 2503–12

Sutherland, AE. 2016. Tissue morphodynamics shaping the early mouse embryo. *Seminars in Cell and Developmental Biology*, **55**, 89–98

Chapter 15

Development of the Gastrointestinal and Urogenital Tracts

Laura C. Mongan

The Primitive Gut Tube and Its Divisions

The primitive gut tube arises as a consequence of folding of the embryo, a process which is complete by the end of the fourth week after fertilisation. The primitive gut tube is formed as an endoderm lined tube with blind diverticula at the cranial and caudal extremities. These blind-ending diverticula are bounded from the exterior by the buccopharyngeal and cloacal membranes at the cranial and caudal ends, respectively. At its formation, and critical to development of the gastrointestinal (GI) tract, the primitive gut tube maintains continuity with the yolk sac from which it is formed via the vitelline duct at the umbilicus.

The primitive gut tube is sub-divided into three divisions: the foregut, from the buccopharyngeal membrane to the liver bud; the midgut, from the liver bud to a point two-thirds of the length of the transverse colon; and the hindgut, from the last one-third of the transverse colon to the cloacal membrane.

These divisions of the embryonic primitive gut tube have important implications for arterial supply, venous and lymphatic drainage, and patterns of sensory processing.

The portion of the foregut cranial to the respiratory diverticulum, that is the portion that extends through the embryonic pharynx, is of particular significance for the development of the embryonic head and neck region. While this portion constitutes part of the foregut, detailed consideration of its development is beyond the scope of this chapter.

The primitive gut tube is suspended by a double fold of condensed mesoderm along its entire length dorsally and additionally ventrally in the region of the foregut only (Fig. 15.1). These membranes are the embryonic mesenteries that undergo considerable adaptation and morphological change as development and specialisation of the primitive gut tube proceeds.

Development of the gastrointestinal tract begins with the primitive gut tube as a simple linear tube,

Table 15.1 Summary of Key Points Relating to the Divisions of Primitive Gut Tube

Division	Derivative	Arterial supply	Visceral pain perceived
Foregut	Oesophagus Stomach Pancreas, liver and gall bladder Duodenum, proximal to the entrance of the bile duct	Coeliac trunk	Epigastrium
Midgut	Duodenum, duodenum, distal to the entrance of the bile duct Jejunum Ileum Caecum and appendix Ascending colon Proximal two-thirds of transverse colon	Superior mesenteric artery	Periumbilical region
Hindgut	Distal one-third of transverse colon Sigmoid colon Rectum Upper anal canal Internal lining of bladder and urethra	Inferior mesenteric artery	Suprapubic region

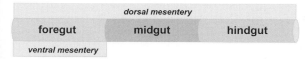

Figure 15.1 Embryonic mesenteries

which lengthens and undergoes considerable morphological and positional changes as the developmental programme progresses. These changes influence the disposition of the viscera and the morphology of the mesenteries that suspend the gut tube within the peritoneal cavity.

Morphological and Positional Changes of the Primitive Gut Tube during Embryonic Development

The developmental programme for the primitive gut tube involves positional changes of the foregut and midgut. It is helpful to consider these events as separate, discrete events. The stomach develops as a dilation within the foregut, a linear tube running cranial to caudal, and therefore a vertical relationship between the inlet and outlet of the stomach. As development proceeds, the stomach undergoes rotation in two distinct axes. Rotation around the longitudinal axis of the stomach results in positioning of the greater and lesser curvatures at first to the left and right sides, respectively. Concomitant rotation of the developing stomach around it anterio-posterior axis results in relative positioning of the cardia and pylorus toward the horizontal, and the greater curvature moves inferiorly.

These positional changes affecting the stomach inevitably result in changes to the shape of the mesenteries attaching the foregut to both dorsal and ventral body walls. As the stomach rotates, the mesenteries stretch and fold to accommodate the positional changes of the stomach.

As the stomach rotates around its longitudinal axis, the dorsal and ventral mesenteries attached to the dorsal and ventral borders of the developing stomach stretch and fold as shown in Fig. 15.2B. The ventral and dorsal borders of the stomach, the future lesser and greater curvatures, respectively, come to lie on the right and left sides.

Once rotation of the stomach around its antero-posterior axis is considered, there are further implications for the morphology of the mesenteries. Movement

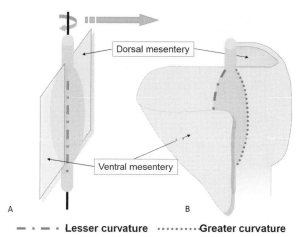

— — · — · **Lesser curvature** ·········**Greater curvature**

Figure 15.2 A & B Schematic representation of the consequences of rotation around the longitudinal axis of the stomach. Rotation around this axis, A, results in folding of the mesenteries, B.

of the greater curvature inferiorly, through rotation around the antero-posterior axis (Fig. 15.3B), draws with it the attached dorsal mesentery, creating the greater omentum, as shown in Fig. 15.3C.

The positional changes that the developing stomach undergoes impact the shape of the developing duodenum, which adopts its characteristic C-shape as a consequence of the shift in the position of the stomach. Furthermore, the pair of pancreatic buds that develop from duodenal endoderm within the leaves of each of the dorsal and ventral mesenteries are brought together to fuse as the duodenum adopts its mature shape.

The final consequence of the positional changes undertaken by the stomach during development is the final location of the lesser sac of the peritoneum. Prior to rotation of the stomach, the attachment of the foregut to both ventral and dorsal body walls results in separation of the intra-embryonic coelom into two spaces, right and left, in this region only (Fig. 15.4A). Of course, these two spaces are continuous with each other distal to the free edge of the ventral mesentery. With rotation of the stomach, the right sac moves posterior to the stomach (Fig. 15.4B). The liver bud appears within the leaves of the ventral mesentery which runs from the lesser curvature of the stomach to the ventral body wall. With continued growth of the liver, stomach and small bowel, the gut tube derivatives are packed ever more tightly within the peritoneal cavity. The result is that the duodenum,

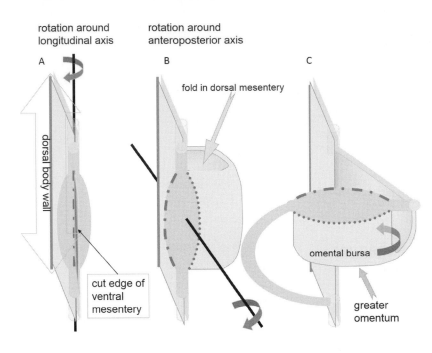

Figure15.3 A, B & C Schematic representation of the consequences of rotation around the antero-posterior axis of the stomach. Rotation around this axis, B, results in further folding of the mesenteries, C, and movement of the greater curvature inferiorly.

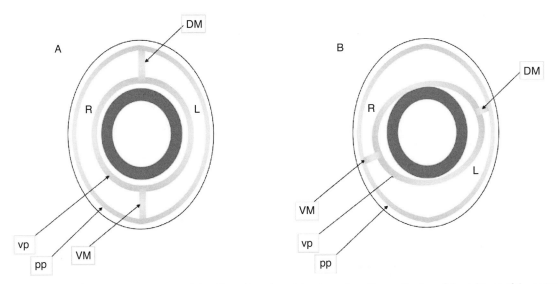

Figure 15.4 Schematic representation of the effect of rotation of the stomach on the positioning of the right sac of the peritoneum. DM: dorsal mesentery. VM: ventral mesentery. VP: visceral peritoneum. PP: parietal peritoneum. L: left sac. R: right sac.

other than the cap, and the pancreas become secondarily retro-peritoneal structures as the peritoneal membrane of overlying structures fuses. The once wide communication between right and left peritoneal sacs becomes narrowed, with the entrance to the lesser sac (the right sac derivative) at the epiploic foramen at the free edge of the lesser omentum once development is complete.

The midgut section of the primitive gut tube elongates and forms a loop as development proceeds. This loop, which has cranial and caudal limbs (Fig. 15.5A), forms around the superior mesenteric artery as its axis. This growth in length coupled with rapid growth of the liver results in physiological herniation of the midgut loop. The midgut is continuous with the yolk sac via the vitelline duct at the umbilicus. The midgut loop pushes out through the umbilicus into the proximal umbilical cord. As herniation begins, the midgut loop undergoes a 90° counterclockwise rotation (Fig. 15.5B). As herniation resolves, the loop undergoes a further 180° of rotation counter-clockwise (Fig. 15.5 C–E). The result is that the cranial limb (and consequently its derivatives) is positioned so that it returns to the adnominal cavity first, and consequently moves to the left side of the cavity. The transverse colon lies anterior to the duodenum, ensuring optimum arrangement of bowel loops and minimising the risk of volvulus and strangulation. Incomplete or reversed rotation, or malrotation, can give rise to significant complications (Lee, HC et al. 2012).

Once physiological herniation has resolved, the vitelline duct normally regresses; however, persistence of a vestigial remnant of the vitelline duct is not uncommon and results in a variety of structural abnormalities, most notably Meckel's diverticulum

Table 15.2 Derivatives of the limbs of the midgut loop

	Derivatives
Cranial limb	Duodenum (parts 2, 3 and 4), jejunum, proximal ileum
Caudal limb	Distal ileum, caecum and appendix, ascending colon, proximal 2/3 transverse colon

with a published prevalence of 0.2–3% (DiSantis DJ et al. 1991).

A number of defects are associated with the antero-lateral abdominal wall, notably umbilical hernia, omphalocoele and gastroschisis. An understanding of normal development affords the ability to discriminate among these conditions. The defect underlying umbilical hernia is weakness of the umbilical ring formed as the embryo folds, and the antero-lateral wall is formed as the edges of the embryonic disk are drawn together at the umbilicus. Umbilical hernia represents protrusion of a viscus through the defect in the anterior abdominal wall due to weakness of the umbilical ring. Omphalocoele may at first glance appear similar to umbilical hernia, as the viscera protrude through the umbilicus into the proximal part of the umbilical cord. However, the underlying defect in this case is persistence of physiological herniation. Consequently, in omphalocoele, the viscera are covered only by amnion, the membrane enclosing the umbilical cord, while all layers of the abdominal wall cover the viscus in umbilical hernia. Gastroschisis, a condition where bowel loops are found outside the abdominal cavity, is a result of a defect in closure of the antero-lateral body wall during its formation, and is seen lateral to the umbilicus.

Development of the Urogenital Tracts

The development of the reproductive and urinary tracts are closely linked, not only spatially, but also structurally. That is to say, structures at one time a constituent of one tract can be incorporated into the development of another. In addition, the development

Figure 15.5

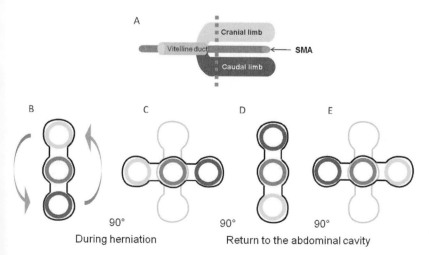

During herniation   Return to the abdominal cavity

of the urinary tract is interlinked with that of the developing gastrointestinal tract.

The kidney, gonad and duct systems appear within the intermediate mesoderm in a region known as the urogenital ridge. Mesonephric tubules capable of primitive renal function, together with a duct associated with this tubule system, the mesonephric duct, constitute an embryonic kidney. Developing in close proximity is the indifferent gonad. The indifferent gonad is comprised of tissue derived from two distinct cell types. Mesoderm-derived tissue constitutes the supporting tissue of the gonad. The primordial germ cells, from which gametogenesis will proceed, are extragonadal in origin. In fact, so critical is this population of cells – being the seed for the next generation – the precursors of primordial germ cells are specified prior to gastrulation from within the epiblast and moved to a site outside the developing embryo where they develop as primordial germ cells. From there they wait, ready to migrate back into the embryo from the yolk sac wall, to populate the indifferent gonad in the urogenital ridge (De Felici, M., 2013).

The indifferent gonad is organized into an outer cortex and an inner medulla. The developmental fate of the indifferent gonad is dependent on the karyotype of the primordial germ cells that populate it. If the primordial germ cells carry a Y chromosome, then as a consequence of expression of genes on the Y chromosome, the medulla continues to develop while there is no development of the cortex. In the event that the primordial germ cells do not carry a Y chromosome, the reverse is true and the cortex develops.

Therefore, if the karyotype of the primordial germ cells is XY, the indifferent gonad becomes committed to development as a testis, and consequently production of male sex steroid hormones. The primordial germ cells populate the developing medullary cords which go on to develop into the seminiferous tubules. If the karyotype of the primordial germ cells is XX, the indifferent gonad becomes committed to development as an ovary. Rather than being a default pathway, development of the ovary is driven by expression of ovary-specific genes which both ensure normal ovarian development and suppress testis development pathways (Dolci, S., et al, 2015).

Meanwhile, development of the urinary system proceeds; the mesonephric duct of the embryonic kidney makes contact with the cloaca of the distal hindgut. At its distal end, a new structure, the ureteric bud, sprouts from the mesonephric duct. The ureteric bud is essential for the development of the true, metanephric kidney. The ureteric bud acts on undifferentiated intermediate mesoderm in its vicinity to drive development of the metanephric blastema, which will ultimately become the true kidney. Once the mesonephric duct has completed this function, it is no longer required for the development of the urinary tract.

At this stage of development, the developing gastrointestinal, urinary and reproductive tracts end at a single structure – that is, the cloaca. The cloaca is the distal-most part of the endoderm-derived hindgut, which is bordered from the exterior by the cloacal membrane. The cloacal membrane lacks mesoderm, and is therefore avascular and consequently programmed to rupture, creating a caudal opening. The cloaca undergoes portioning to separate first the urinary and gastrointestinal tracts. The wedge of mesoderm grows caudally toward the cloacal membrane, dividing the cloaca into ventral and dorsal compartments. The ventral compartment is the urogenital sinus. The urogenital sinus proceeds to develop into the urinary bladder and urethra, and also makes a contribution to the development of the female internal genitalia (discussed later).

Development of the Duct Systems

As we have seen, a pair of mesonephric ducts develops to serve as the duct of the embryonic kidney. A further pair of ducts develops, in close proximity to the mesonephric ducts. These are termed *paramesonephric ducts*, or *Mullerian ducts*. The Mullerian ducts form as invaginations of the coelom and are open to the peritoneal cavity at their cranial end. The fate of these pairs of ducts is also dependant on the karyotype of the primordial germ cells and the consequent development of the indifferent gonad. Once the mesonephric duct has given rise to the ureteric bud, it will regress unless supported by testis-derived male sex steroid hormones. The converse is true of the paramesonephric ducts, which will proceed through their developmental programme unless actively suppressed by testis-derived Mullerian inhibiting hormone (MIH). Therefore, in the absence of a testis, the mesonephric ducts will regress and the paramesonephric ducts will not be subject to active suppression, so will develop into the uterus, fallopian tubes, cervix and part of the vagina. The mesonephric ducts are maintained in male embryos and are re-deployed as the duct system of the male reproductive tract.

Table 15.3 Derivative of the embryonic duct systems

	Male	Female
Mesonephric duct	Efferent ductules, epididymis, vas deferens, seminal vesicles, ejaculatory duct	Epoophoron, paroophoron in broad ligament Gartner cyst
Paramesonephric duct	Appendix testis	Fallopian tube, body and cervix of uterus, upper vagina

Table 15.4 Derivatives of the indifferent external genitalia

Male Derivative	Common Precursor	Female Derivative
Glans penis	Genital tubercle	Clitoris
Scrotum	Genital (labioscrotal) swellings	Labia majora
Ventral aspect of shaft of penis	Genital (urethral) folds	Labia minora

The pair of paramesonephric ducts, in the absence of MIH, develop by moving toward each other in the midline, ultimately fusing with each other to form the uterus, cervix and upper part of the vagina. They remain separate at their cranial ends, forming the fallopian tubes, the open ends of which lie close to the developing ovaries. The caudal tip of the fused paramesonephric ducts makes contact with the urogenital sinus, promoting development of the sinovaginal bulbs; these contribute an endoderm component to the vagina in its lower part.

External Genitalia

The external genitalia also proceed through an indifferent stage, being comprised of basic components, the genital tubercle, the genital folds and genital swellings.

If a testis develops, and the tissues are capable of responding to the male sex steroids it produces, then virilisation of the external genitalia will occur. In the male, the genital tubercle elongates, and there is fusion of the genital swellings and genital folds. In the female, there is no fusion, and consequently the urethra opens into the vestibule.

Descent of the Gonads

The gonads are tethered by their caudal pole to the developing genital swellings by a structure known as the *gubernaculum*. The gubernaculum passes through the inguinal canal, behind an evagination of the peritoneal cavity called the *processus vaginalis*. The gonad undergoes a caudal shift in position, due at least in part to the continued lengthening of the trunk of the embryo. In the male, the testis enters the inguinal canal via the deep inguinal ring and exits the abdomen via the superficial inguinal ring to pass into the developing scrotum, led by the gubernaculum. The spermatic cord, containing the vas deferens and vessels of the testis, consequently occupies the inguinal canal in males. In the female, the ovary undergoes a similar caudal shift in position, but is blocked from entry to the inguinal canal by the uterus. Consequently, the remnant of the gubernaculum, the round ligament of the uterus, is the only structure present in the inguinal canal in females.

References

Carlson, BM. 2014. *Human Embryology and Developmental Biology*, 5th edition. Elsevier

De Felici, M. 2013. Origin, migration, and proliferation of human primordial germ cells, in G. Coticchio et al. (eds.), *Oogenesis*. Springer-Verlag

Di Santis, DJ et al. 1991. Simplified approach to umbilical remnant abnormalities. Radiographics 11, 59–66.

Dolci, S et al. 2015. Gonadal development and germ cell tumors in mouse and humans. *Seminars in Cell and Developmental Biology*, **45**, 114–123

Lee, HC, et al. 2012. Intestinal malrotation and catastrophic volvulus in infancy. *Journal of Emergency Medicine*, **43**, e49–e51

Moore, KL et al. 2012. *The Developing Human: Clinically Oriented Embryology*, 9th edition. Elsevier

Sadler, TW. 2015. *Langman's Medical Embryology*, 13th edition. Wolters Kluwer Health

Problems in Early Pregnancy

Jemma Johns, Archana Vasireddy and Kugajeevan Vigneswaran

1 Normal Pregnancy

1.1 Hormonal Changes in Normal Pregnancy

1.1.1 The menstrual cycle: A detailed description of the menstrual cycle is not within the scope of this chapter. An understanding of dating early pregnancy from the last menstrual period (LMP) dates and adjusting this for cycle length is, however, essential in the management of early pregnancy problems. The first day of the LMP is the first day of bleeding and represents the shedding of the endometrium associated with the drop in ovarian hormone production in the absence of conception.

The follicular (proliferative) phase varies in length and corresponds to follicular stimulating hormone (FSH) driven follicle maturation (FSH). Each cycle starts with the recruitment of several primordial follicles one of which will become dominant causing regression of the others. The developing follicle releases increasing amounts of 17β-oestradiol inducing proliferative growth of the endometrium; eventual inhibition of FSH secretion (negative feedback) and triggers the luteinising hormone (LH) surge from the anterior pituitary (positive feedback). In a 28-day cycle, ovulation will occur on day 14 approximately 36 hours after the onset of the LH surge. After ovulation, the corpus luteum continues to produce oestrogen and progesterone, transforming the endometrium into its secretory phase in preparation for implantation if fertilisation occurs; supporting the conceptus until the early placenta takes over this role. If pregnancy does not occur, the corpus luteum begins to degenerate about four days prior to the onset of menstruation.

1.1.2 Hormonal changes in early pregnancy: As described above, the corpus luteum plays an important role in the hormonal maintenance of early pregnancy. It is initially maintained by the high LH level, but this role is taken over by β-hCG produced by the developing conceptus. The corpus luteum produces oestrogen and progesterone supporting the pregnancy until the developing placenta takes over this function. The production of hCG by the syncytiotrophoblast of the developing placenta but also by the extravillous trophoblast has both an endocrine and paracrine role in early pregnancy development and the β-subunit provides us with the first detectable and easily measurable sign of pregnancy. Most commercial pregnancy tests will detect β-hCG when it reaches a level of 25 IU/l or more, which coincides with a few days prior to the 'missed period'.

1.2 Development of the Feto-Maternal Circulation

At day 7, the blastocyst hatches and embeds into the decidualised endometrium. The surrounding trophoblast cells begin to invade the spiral arteries resulting in the necessary transformation from high resistance low capacity vessels to a high-flow, low-resistance circulation required for normal pregnancy. Traditionally it was thought that the fetomaternal circulation is established soon after implantation; however, there is good evidence to suggest that the extravillous trophoblast forms a trophoblastic 'shell' where the channels are plugged until the latter part of the first trimester when significant fetomaternal circulation becomes apparent.

1.3 Dating Normal Early Pregnancy

Before the development of transvaginal ultrasound (TVS), pregnancy was dated according to the LMP and cycle length. Today most pregnancies are formally dated at the first-trimester scan or 'nuchal scan'. In order to identify a deviation from normal, an understanding of how to date a pregnancy is essential in the management of women presenting with early pregnancy problems. The gestational age is calculated from the first day of the LMP and adjusted according to cycle length with the assumption that ovulation occurred on day 14 of a 28-day cycle. In a woman with a regular but longer or shorter cycle, the difference can be subtracted or added to the gestation, e.g. add 4 days for a 32-day cycle or subtract 2 days for a 26-day cycle. In women who have an irregular cycle, are breastfeeding, or have recently stopped hormonal contraception, it may not be possible to date pregnancy. Always enquire whether the LMP was a normal period for the patient. Frequently, particularly in cases of ectopic pregnancy, light bleeding relating to abnormal implantation is mistaken for a period and can lead to clinical error when interpreting ultrasound findings.

1.4 Landmarks and Ultrasound Features in Early Pregnancy

The landmarks for normal early pregnancy can be found in Fig. 16.1.

2 Early Pregnancy Problems

2.1 The Role of the Early Pregnancy Unit

The advent of high-resolution TVS revolutionised the care of women with early pregnancy problems allowing the development of dedicated early pregnancy units (EPUs). Prior to the introduction of the EPU, women with pain or bleeding in early pregnancy were admitted through the ED to await a scan in the ultrasound department. This often led to prolonged admissions while awaiting an ultrasound and also resulted in an unacceptable 'inconclusive scan' rate. The advantages of the EPU can be seen in Fig. 16.2.

The RCOG/NICE clinical guideline on the diagnosis and initial management of miscarriage and ectopic pregnancy recommended that an early pregnancy service should be available for women 7 days a week (1). They also recommended that this should be a dedicated service provided by healthcare professionals competent to diagnose and care for women with pain or bleeding in early pregnancy, offer ultrasound and hCG assays, and be staffed by clinicians trained in breaking bad news and sensitive communication.

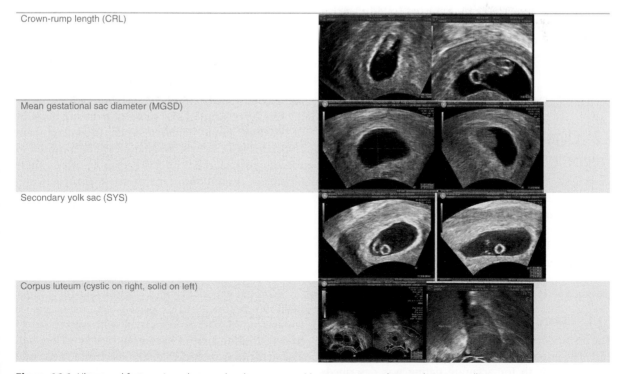

Crown-rump length (CRL)

Mean gestational sac diameter (MGSD)

Secondary yolk sac (SYS)

Corpus luteum (cystic on right, solid on left)

Figure 16.1 Ultrasound features in early normal early pregnancy. Measurements can be seen between callipers.

Table 16.1 Essential history relevant to early pregnancy problems

Age	
LMP	
Cycle length and regularity	Enquire whether this was a normal period
Recent contraceptive and pregnancy history	Including number of cycles since stopping contraception, recent births and pregnancy losses and lactation
Positive pregnancy test	When was the pregnancy test first positive
Was the pregnancy planned?	Ascertain in a sensitive manner whether the pregnancy was planned, unplanned, wanted, unwanted or undecided
Details of pain and bleeding	Amount and type of bleeding, amount and location of pain
Previous scans	Enquire about previous scans in the index pregnancy

Advantages of a dedicated Early Pregnancy Unit
- Open access, dedicated diagnostic facilities
- Quicker diagnosis, same day treatment
- Counselling & informed choice
- Improved management & patient satisfaction
- Less admissions
- Surgery performed in day with senior supervision (less out of hours)
- Teaching & research (new approaches)
- Structured training

Figure 16.2 Advantages of a dedicated Early Pregnancy Unit (EPU)

The potential disadvantages to EPU include increased emergency attendances with a lower threshold for referral, increased patient expectation and potential loss of training opportunities for junior gynaecology and ED staff. In addition, the evidence for their cost-effectiveness is not clear.

2.2 Clinical Features and Diagnosis in Early Pregnancy

In general, women experiencing a miscarriage, an ectopic or a molar pregnancy present with bleeding and/or lower abdominal pain. The role of the clinician is to establish the location of the pregnancy and its viability and to offer appropriate management.

The mainstay of assessment of women in the EPU is accurate and relevant history taking, clinical examination and high-quality ultrasound assessment.

2.2.1 History

The history that should be elicited is outlined in Table 16.1. The importance of accurately recording the LMP and cycle length for accurate dating was described

previously. Enquiring when the pregnancy test first became positive may be helpful when dates are uncertain or when diagnosing an early miscarriage.

Establishing in a sensitive manner whether the pregnancy is planned and wanted is paramount to the ongoing care of women in early pregnancy. Not only will it help you to deliver a diagnosis sensitively, but it will enable you to organise follow-up and referrals, giving you the opportunity to offer contraception if the pregnancy is not ongoing (see the discussion on the management of miscarriage and ectopic pregnancy, later in this chapter).

Additional history that should be elicited includes past gynaecological history, including a history of subfertility or pelvic inflammatory disease; past obstetric and medical history, surgical history (in particular, abdominal surgery or appendicectomy), allergies and medication.

The type, location and onset of pain and amount of bleeding should be documented. In general, pain associated with ectopic pregnancy will be localised to the iliac fossa and be colicky, becoming more generalised and continuous in the presence of rupture and intraperitoneal bleeding. Women will often also describe back pain or diarrhoea associated with blood causing irritation to the bowel. They will often also report irregular bleeding or that their last period was abnormal, associated with abnormal rises in hCG in the presence of an ectopic pregnancy.

Women experiencing a miscarriage are more likely to report central 'period-like' pain that is worsening in nature associated with moderate to heavy bleeding that is becoming heavier. They will also sometimes report that this reached a crescendo associated with very heavy bleeding followed by fairly

Box 1 Clinical Assessment of Women Presenting with Severe Pain or Heavy Bleeding to the ED

General	Pallor
	Mucous membranes
	BP, pulse, O_2 saturation
	Capillary return
	Conscious level
Abdomen	Guarding or rebound
Speculum (if bleeding moderate to severe)	Amount of bleeding
	Products of conception in cervical canal
Vaginal examination (rarely required; discussed later)	

quick resolution, which may represent a complete miscarriage. Women with delayed or missed miscarriages may be relatively asymptomatic with minor spotting or loss of pregnancy symptoms, and these are often detected for the first time during the first trimester routine screening scan at 11–14 weeks.

An understanding of the pathophysiology of early pregnancy loss is essential in order to interpret the history.

2.2.2 Examination

Women attending the EPU are examined as part of their ultrasound assessment, which should include an abdominal palpation during the scan. In general, women presenting to the EPU are well and do not require an assessment of their cardiovascular status. Women presenting either to the ED or EPU with heavy bleeding or severe pain should be assessed for signs of hypovolaemia and an acute abdomen (see Box 1).

2.2.3 Vaginal Examination

Traditional teaching has told us that part of the assessment of women with early pregnancy problems, includes a speculum and vaginal examination. In fact, in modern practice speculum examination is indicated when there is significant bleeding or hypotension, where a speculum examination will allow assessment of the amount and origin of bleeding but also allow visualisation and removal of products of conception in the cervical canal. It also enables the taking of swabs for microbiology if sepsis or infection is suspected. Digital vaginal examination is rarely required. It is painful and intrusive, and there is good evidence to suggest that it does not alter the differential diagnosis or course of subsequent management in women in early pregnancy and should be avoided (2).

2.2.4 Ultrasound Scan

In general, women who are stable with little or no pain or bleeding can be referred to the EPU for a scan within working hours to establish the location and viability of the pregnancy and to look for signs of intraperitoneal bleeding.

Haemodynamically unstable women or women who have heavy bleeding or severe pain with a positive pregnancy test should not be referred for a scan, which will only serve to delay definitive management; they should be managed clinically. The only exception to this may be in ED, where abdominal ultrasound performed similarly to the 'FAST' scan in trauma medicine may help exclude significant intraperitoneal bleeding. Caution should be exercised, however, and a clinician should never attempt this without sufficient training.

TVS has revolutionised the investigation of early pregnancy problems, and transabdominal scanning is rarely contributory in these circumstances. Situations in which TAS provides useful additional information can be found in Box 2.

There is no standardised way of reporting an early pregnancy ultrasound. The scan should be performed and reported in a systematic way including a description of pregnancy location (if visualised), mean gestational sac diameter (MGSD), crown-rump length (CRL), presence or absence of a fetal heartbeat (FHR) and the presence or absence of fluid in the POD. The presence of the secondary yolk sac and fetal heart rate are also frequently recorded (see Fig. 16.3). The ovaries are also examined and the presence of any ovarian cysts, including the corpus luteum, should also be recorded. Wherever possible, a definitive diagnosis should be made. The only exception would be in the case of a pregnancy of unknown location (PUL where the location of the pregnancy cannot be identified, as discussed

Box 2 Transabdominal Scanning May Be Useful in the Following Circumstances

Large fibroids	Pregnancy may be located high outside the true pelvis
High BMI	Possible less image distortion in some cases
Later gestations	
Suspected ovarian pathology	Where the history is suggestive of a non-pregnancy related pathology
Patient choice	It should be made clear to these women that a transabdominal scan may provide less diagnostic information which may delay diagnosis and management

Early Pregnancy Diagnoses in EPU

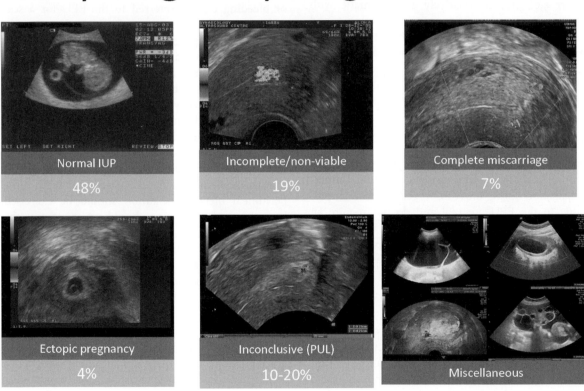

Figure 16.3 Early pregnancy diagnoses in EPU

later) and in pregnancies where the viability is uncertain (intrauterine pregnancies of uncertain viability IPUV).

It is important to interpret the scan according to the clinical picture and remember that the absence of landmarks does not necessarily imply a failing pregnancy. When there is a discrepancy between the history (e.g. size of the pregnancy and the LMP) and the ultrasound findings, it is always helpful to go back and ask further more specific questions. The potential differential diagnoses in the early pregnancy unit and their frequency can be found in Fig. 16.3.

Table 16.2 Definitions of miscarriage

Type of miscarriage	Description
Threatened miscarriage	Bleeding and or pain where there is a viable intrauterine pregnancy on ultrasound and a closed cervix
Incomplete miscarriage	Bleeding and or pain with residual pregnancy tissue in the uterine cavity on ultrasound. The cervix may be closed or open and may contain pregnancy tissue.
Inevitable miscarriage	Intact gestational sac within the cervical canal on ultrasound. The external os may be open or closed.
Complete miscarriage	Bleeding and or pain that has resolved where there is an empty uterine cavity on ultrasound *and* previous ultrasound evidence of an intrauterine pregnancy. The cervix is closed.
Missed miscarriage, Early embryonic demise, Delayed miscarriage	Intrauterine pregnancy on ultrasound with a CRL measuring >7mm or an empty sac >25mm in the absence of pain or bleeding. There is often a discrepancy between the LMP dates and the ultrasound findings (delayed miscarriage).
Septic miscarriage	An incomplete, inevitable or missed miscarriage in the presence of sepsis.
Recurrent miscarriage	More than three consecutive first trimester miscarriages.

2.2.5 Investigations

Women who are unstable or bleeding require urgent blood to be sent for group and save (or cross-match), full blood count and a clotting screen. Stable women who have experienced bleeding should have a blood group sent to check their rhesus status and given anti-D according to national guidelines (as discussed later). Serum β-hCG and progesterone measurements should only be performed after a scan assessment in order to guide ongoing management and are of little value (and a waste of money) and impossible to interpret without the benefit of an ultrasound assessment. The role of hCG and progesterone will be discussed later in the context of abnormal early pregnancy.

2.3 Miscarriage

2.3.1 Definitions and Epidemiology

Miscarriage is defined as the loss of an intrauterine pregnancy before 24 weeks gestation. It occurs in 20–25% of clinically recognised pregnancies, although the exact number is difficult to ascertain. This differs from the WHO definition as an expulsion of a fetus or embryo weighing 500 g or less and before 22 weeks of pregnancy. An early or first-trimester miscarriage is defined as less than 12 weeks, and a late or second-trimester miscarriage is defined as between 12 and 24 weeks. Approximately 4% of miscarriages occur in the second trimester (3). The different types of miscarriage have been defined by the NICE guidelines (1) and can be found in Table 16.2.

2.3.2 Risk Factors for Miscarriage

The cause of many miscarriages is unclear and likely to be multifactorial. There are, however, recognised maternal, paternal and fetal factors that are known to be associated with miscarriage (Table 16.3). Recurrent miscarriage affects 1–2% of couples and will be discussed later in this chapter.

Other factors associated with an increased risk of miscarriage can be found in Table 16.3.

2.3.3 Recurrent Miscarriage

Recurrent miscarriage affects 1–2% of fertile couples and in the UK is defined as three consecutive first trimester losses. The cause of recurrent miscarriage is often unclear and probably multifactorial (see Table 16.4). History taking is again essential in order to further investigate the cause of recurrent miscarriage.

Causes and Investigation of Recurrent Miscarriage

Uterine Anomalies – – Congenital uterine anomalies are associated with obstetric complications, including miscarriage. Women with recurrent miscarriage are more likely to have a uterine anomaly, although they are still rare with an incidence in the general population of 0.4–3.2%. Uterine septae are the only anomaly associated with an increased incidence of first-trimester miscarriage presumably related to implantation of the conceptus into a relatively avascular septum. Removal of the septum (septoplasty) has not been shown to improve reproductive outcome (in terms of live birth rate) in women with recurrent

Table 16.3 Factors associated with sporadic miscarriage

Association	Comments
Chromosomal	Single largest cause: approximately 50% Most common include autosomal trisomies (16, 21, 22)
Age	Significant acceleration in risk over 40 years Four-fold increase risk between 20 and 40 years Most likely to be related to increased chromosomal aneuploidy Increased paternal age (>45 years) also a factor
Obstetric history	Previous live birth reduces risk (up to 40% reduction) Increased risk with an increased number of miscarriages
Maternal medical conditions	Diabetes, thyroid disease, sickle cell disease, connective tissue disorders all associated More likely to be related to poorly controlled disease Well-controlled diabetes not associated with a significant increase Role of anti-thyroid antibodies and thyroxine currently under investigation (TABLET trial)
Other factors	Subfertility Assisted conception Low pre-pregnancy BMI (<18.5kg/m^2) Regular or heavy alcohol consumption Previous social termination of pregnancy Stress or anxiety Socio-demographic factors

Table 16.4 Causes of recurrent miscarriage

Main causes of recurrent miscarriage	Contribution (%couples with RM)	Investigation
Uterine anomalies	1.8–37.6%	3D transvaginal ultrasound scan
Antiphospholipid antibodies	15% (compared with 2% in background population)	Thrombophilia and cardiolipin antibody screen
Parental chromosomal rearrangements (balanced translocations)	4%	Karyotype of POC followed by parental karyotype if unbalanced translocation

miscarriage; however, it is associated with improvement in pregnancy rates in the subfertile population.

Antiphospholipid Syndrome (APLS) and the Thrombophilias –– APLS is the most investigated of the acquired thrombophilias associated with recurrent miscarriage and is diagnosed according to both clinical and laboratory criteria (Box 3). Women who fit the criteria for APLS are offered low molecular weight heparin and low-dose aspirin in subsequent pregnancies, as this has been shown to improve the live birth rate (RCOG Green Top 17).

The role of the other inherited or acquired thrombophilias in recurrent miscarriage is less clear; however, there is evidence for an association among factor V Leiden, prothrombin gene mutation and protein S deficiency with second-trimester miscarriage.

Parental Chromosomal Rearrangements –– The risk of miscarriage as a result of an abnormal fetal karyotype decreases with an increasing number of pregnancy losses. Parental balanced translocations have been found in 1.9% of couples with recurrent miscarriage, and products of conception should be routinely sent for karyotype in women who are experiencing their third pregnancy loss. If this shows an unbalanced translocation, then parental blood should be sent and referral to a clinical geneticist made if an abnormality is identified. The role of pre-implantation genetic diagnosis in these cases is unclear, as it requires couples to undergo IVF and their chance of a normal ongoing pregnancy may be higher with spontaneous conception in the longer term.

Other Causes of Recurrent Miscarriage –– There have been many other suggested causes of recurrent

Box 3 Diagnostic Criteria for Antiphospholipid Syndrome

Clinical criteria	• **Personal history of venous or arterial thromboembolism** • **Pregnancy-related morbidity: unexplained stillbirth, early-onset PET or** • **IUGR or three unexplained first trimester miscarriages**
Laboratory criteria	• Lupus anticoagulant: two or more occasions, 12 weeks apart or • Raised anticardiolipin IgM or IgG on two occasions 12 weeks apart or • Anti-β-2–glycoprotein IgM or IgG on two occasions 12 weeks apart

PET = pre-eclampsia
IUGR = intrauterine growth restriction

Box 4 Other Possible Associations with Recurrent Miscarriage

Cause	Comments
Natural killer cells	Association between uterine natural killer cells and reproductive failure
Endocrine factors	Progesterone has not been found to reduce the miscarriage rate in idiopathic RM (PROMISE). There is no evidence for a role for hCG
Insulin resistance and PCOS	No evidence that metformin reduces the miscarriage rate
Immune	There is currently no evidence for a beneficial effect of immunotherapy in recurrent miscarriage

miscarriage; however, the evidence for both a link and a treatment remains elusive (Box 4).

2.3.4 Ultrasound Diagnosis and Management of Miscarriage

In order to be confident to diagnose a miscarriage on ultrasound, it is essential to understand what is normal. Knowledge of the landmarks in early pregnancy and their relation to hCG is also essential, along with an understanding that these may not apply in an abnormal pregnancy (Box 5). The use of discriminatory zones in early pregnancy is often misleading and can even be dangerous without a methodical approach to history taking as described previously and also to the scan itself.

a. Missed Miscarriage or Early Embryonic Demise

The diagnosis of a missed miscarriage is often not possible on a single scan and is based on the finding of either a fetal pole with no cardiac pulsations or an empty sac. In order to minimise the risk of an erroneous diagnosis of miscarriage, various 'cut-offs' have been defined. The RCOG/NICE guidelines 2012 can

be seen in Table 16.2. In all cases, a second scan at least 7 days after the first should be recommended in order to confirm the diagnosis wherever possible, and a diagnosis of miscarriage should never be made if the CRL is less than 7 mm or there is an empty sac measuring less than 25 mm.

b. Incomplete Miscarriage

The ultrasound diagnosis of an incomplete miscarriage can also be difficult to make and is based on the finding of heterogeneous tissue distorting the midline with or without a vascular supply in the uterine cavity. The main concern when diagnosing an incomplete miscarriage is the chance that you may, in fact, miss an ectopic pregnancy. When a woman has had a previous scan confirming an intrauterine pregnancy, it is easier to be more confident of the diagnosis. There are no defined cut-offs for the diagnosis of an incomplete miscarriage, and history and symptomatology are often the most important indicators. If in any doubt, the diagnosis should be of a pregnancy of unknown location and the woman followed up until resolution of the pregnancy or a firm diagnosis can be made.

Box 5 Ultrasound Landmarks in Early Pregnancy

Early pregnancy landmarks

Gestational sac	Secondary yolk sac	Embryo, fetal heart beat
4.4–4.6 weeks	5–6 weeks	From ~6 weeks
2–4mm (TVS)	Diagnostic of IUP	6 Weeks (CRL ~4mm) / 7 Weeks (CRL ~10mm) / 8 Weeks (CRL ~16mm)
10mm (TAS		
Eccentric		

c. Complete Miscarriage

In women who have previous scan evidence of an intrauterine pregnancy, the diagnosis of a complete miscarriage on ultrasound is straightforward and the purpose of assessment is to exclude RPOC that require intervention. In women who have not had a previous ultrasound, the diagnosis is not so easy and the presence of an empty uterus on ultrasound is insufficient. History alone has been shown to miss ultrasonically detectable RPOC in up to 45% of women (4) – that is, just because the bleeding has stopped, this does not mean the pregnancy has miscarried completely. Of more concern is that 6% of women with a history suggestive of a complete miscarriage and an empty uterus on ultrasound will have an ectopic pregnancy (5). These women should be managed in the same was as a PUL until resolution of the pregnancy (negative hCG). If the hCG fails to fall or rises, a further assessment must be made. Caution should also be observed when POC apparently has been removed from the cervix. Confirmation of POC is difficult with the naked eye and is often confirmed to contain a blood clot only on the pathology report. Histopathology is the gold standard test for confirmation of RPOC, and clinicians should not be falsely reassured that removed tissue confirms the location of the pregnancy.

d. Threatened Miscarriage

Threatened miscarriage is defined as vaginal bleeding in the presence of an ongoing pregnancy and occurs in 16–25% of ongoing pregnancies. The risk of subsequent miscarriage in these pregnancies is difficult to ascertain but is thought to be about 2.6% above the background risk. There is no evidence that any single intervention (bed rest, progesterone, hCG, oestrogen) reduces the risk of miscarriage in these cases, although historically many women have been prescribed progestogens. The PRISM randomised controlled trial is currently attempting to answer the question of the role of progesterone supplementation in threatened miscarriage.

Management of Miscarriage — Incomplete and missed miscarriage has traditionally been managed with surgical evacuation under general anaesthetic (GA). Recently treatment has moved toward medical and expectant management. This move was partly driven by the success of the introduction of mifepristone and misoprostol for medical termination of pregnancy but also by research into patient outcomes and preferences and more recently by health economics.

In 2006 the MIST trial was published (6). This was a large randomised controlled trial comparing medical and expectant management with surgical evacuation. The main outcome measures the incidence of infection, and the need for unplanned admission and for surgical intervention. The study concluded that the overall risk of infection was low (2–3%), regardless of initial management. However, there were significantly more emergency admissions in the expectant and medical groups than after surgery.

a. Expectant

Expectant management is undoubtedly successful in selected cases; however, study outcomes differ widely in their success rates (25–91% for missed miscarriage and 71–96% for incomplete miscarriage). Women should ideally have access to 24-hour telephone advice and be warned that they may experience significant pain and bleeding at the time of the miscarriage. They should also be warned of the chance of emergency admission and surgical intervention (RR7.35) for heavy bleeding but also the chance of incomplete miscarriage (RR 3.98 at 2 weeks). They should be offered analgesia and advised about adequate sanitary protection.

b. Medical

Medical management of miscarriage with mifepristone and misoprostol has been used in some units for many years. More recent evidence suggests that, in fact, the mifepristone may not be required. Local protocols vary in the dose timing and route of administration of misoprostol, but in most units, women are discharged to miscarry at home. Again, they should be counselled about the risk of heavy bleeding requiring admission for emergency treatment and that the success rate overall is 85% at 3 weeks. Again women should be offered analgesia and advised about sanitary protection in case of very heavy or unexpected bleeding.

c. Surgical

Surgical management of miscarriage should be offered to all women as an option. Women who

should be advised to have surgical management include those with excessive bleeding or who are haemodynamically unstable, women in whom sepsis is suspected (with adequate antibiotic prophylaxis) or where molar pregnancy is suspected (see the discussion on gestational trophoblastic disease as follows).

Surgical evacuation can be performed under GA in theatres; however, many units now offer an outpatient procedure under local anaesthetic (LA) using the manual vacuum aspiration (MVA) technique. The decision whether to have the procedure performed awake lies entirely with the woman, and she should be informed of the pros and cons of either option.

The complications associated with surgical management must be discussed: as previously mentioned, the risk of infection appears to be equivocal; however, the surgical risks of perforation (estimated to be 1:1000) and Asherman's syndrome (rare and of uncertain significance) should be explained. Women should also be informed of the chance of retained tissue (3–5%), with a possible need for a repeat procedure.

The NICE guidelines in 2012 suggested that all women should be offered expectant management in the first instance, unless there were medical contraindications or the patient preferred medical or surgical intervention. In reality, effective counselling is what should be offered and women should be able to make an informed decision based on their personal preference, lifestyle and social factors such as employment and childcare.

2.4 Gestational Trophoblastic Disease

Gestational trophoblastic disease (GTD) is the collective term for a number of conditions, including hydatidiform mole (HM; complete and partial), invasive mole, choriocarcinoma and placental site trophoblastic tumour (PSTT). GTD is characterised by abnormal proliferation of the trophoblast layer of the placenta; if there is any evidence of persistent elevation of beta-human chorionic gonadotrophin (hCG), the condition is referred to as gestational trophoblastic neoplasia (GTN; Table 16.5) (7).

2.4.1 Epidemiology

The UK has a national register for HM pregnancies (the two registration centres are in Sheffield and Charing Cross Hospital). The reported incidence in the UK for complete hydatidiform mole (CHM) is 1 per 1000 pregnancies and 3 per 1000 for partial mole (PHM). Most other countries have less rigorous

Table 16.5 Clinical features and pathophysiology of GTN

Diagnosis	Clinical Features	Comments
Complete mole	Vaginal bleeding in 1st trimester No fetus, hydropic placental tissue	15% progress to GTN 46XX/XY 1:1000 pregnancies UK
Partial mole	Missed miscarriage Vaginal bleeding Abnormal/small fetus, hydropic placental tissue	0.5% progress to GTN 46XXX/XXY/XYY 3:1000 pregnancies UK
Invasive mole	Persistently elevated hCG following HM	Benign condition derived from myometrial invasion of HM 15% metastasise to lungs or vagina
Choriocarcinoma	Frequently presents with metastases	Malignant disease, occur following any pregnancy 50% post HM
Placental site trophoblastic tumour		Malignant disease Rare arising from placental implantation site (non-molar>molar pregnancies)

reporting systems but rates have historically been higher in Asian countries, with GTD occurring in 2 per 1000 pregnancies.

The incidence of HM increases with increasing maternal age. Women over the age of 40 years are 7.5 times more likely to develop HM. History of a previous molar pregnancy (partial or complete) carries a risk of recurrent molar pregnancy of 1–2% (8). This increases to 15–20% after two HMs, and the risk is not decreased by a change in partner (9).

2.4.2 Genetics

CHMs are diploid and the majority occur when a single spermatozoon fertilizes an empty oocyte and then duplicates. As the chromosomal material from the oocyte is missing, a 46XX karyotype is produced which is completely paternally derived. 20–25% of CHMs occur when two spermatozoa fertilise an empty oocyte, which leads to a 46XX or 46XY karyotype, again completely paternally derived. These then undergo mitosis to produce CHM. A 46YY fertilisation will not develop beyond an embryo of a few cells. CHMs contain no fetal tissue, only placental.

Rarely a CHM and twin pregnancy co-exist (approximately 1/20,000–100,000 pregnancies). They occur when two oocytes are fertilised: one abnormally (from an empty oocyte, as described previously), producing a CHM, and one normally, producing a normal pregnancy.

In patients with recurrent molar pregnancies studies have, in some cases, shown biparental CHM rather than solely paternally derived genetic material. In these patients, a gene mutation in NLRP7 has been

identified, which can occur sporadically or be autosomal recessively inherited.

Ninety percent of PHMs are triploid, containing two sets of paternal chromosomes derived from two separate spermatozoa and one set maternal chromosomes from the oocyte leading to a 69XXX, 69XXY or 69XYY karyotype. The other 10% of partial moles represent tetraploid or mosaic conceptions. PHMs have evidence of a fetus or fetal red blood cells.

2.4.3 Clinical Features and Diagnosis

Eighty to ninety percent of CHMs present with vaginal bleeding between 6 and 16 weeks gestation. There are also other classic signs and symptoms, such as uterine enlargement greater than expected for dates in 25%, hyperemesis in 10%, and pregnancy-related hypertension in the first or second trimester around 1%. There remain rarer presentations, such as hyperthyroidism, early-onset PET, abdominal distention due to theca lutein cysts, as well as acute respiratory failure or neurological symptoms such as seizures (secondary to metastatic disease), which would all warrant exclusion of HM. The later symptoms are incredibly rare, particularly in the UK due to early diagnosis.

PHMs tend to present later than CHMs but also present with vaginal bleeding (75%), or incomplete or missed miscarriage (90%). Other symptoms are rarer, which reflects the pathology of PHM compared to CHM. Focal trophoblastic hyperplasia rather than diffuse produces excessive uterine enlargement in only around 10% of cases; hCG is raised only marginally compared to normal pregnancies, rarely leading to hyperemesis, hyperthyroidism and theca lutein cysts.

2.4.4 Ultrasound Diagnosis of HMs

The US detection rate for HM has been shown to be between 44% and 56%. A UK study of more than 1000 cases at a regional referral centre found that 79% of complete moles and 29% of partial moles were suspected on ultrasound examination prior to histological diagnosis. In addition to this, 10% of cases that are thought to be molar on USS were diagnosed as non-molar hydropic abortions on histological review. The accuracy of USS is user-dependent, and operator experience contributes to detection rates. Therefore, although USS assists in the diagnosis of HMs, the products obtained from all medical or surgical miscarriages should undergo histological assessment to exclude trophoblastic neoplasia whenever possible. The typical US features of CHM are of an enlarged uterine cavity filled with heterogeneous material containing multiple cystic areas (the snowstorm appearance; Fig. 16.4), although this can be quite subtle in very early pregnancy. PHMs have less distinctive features on USS in both the first and second trimester compared to CHMs; however, USS remains helpful in facilitating their diagnosis. There is likely to be a gestational sac, but there may also be a thickened trophoblastic layer containing multiple avascular cystic spaces (Fig. 16.5). PHMs often present as an incomplete or missed miscarriage, and the findings on USS may be just this, with the diagnosis only becoming apparent at histopathological examination.

2.4.5 Management of HM

It is essential that when a non-viable pregnancy is diagnosed and molar pregnancy is suspected, surgical management is recommended and the products of conception are sent for histological analysis. This ensures that the correct diagnosis is established and the patient can be monitored for subsequent progression to GTN. It is widely accepted that surgical management should be performed via suction aspiration rather than sharp curettage to reduce the risk of perforation. Ultrasound examination throughout this procedure also aids in reducing the risk of perforation and ensuring that the uterine cavity is completely evacuated. In the UK, the average gestational age at evacuation is now less than 10 weeks. As previously mentioned, every attempt should be made to send POC for analysis after a miscarriage. POCs are not routinely sent after termination of pregnancy, and the risk of progression to GTN following induced abortion has been estimated to be 1:20000, although later diagnosis may lead to poorer prognosis. The RCOG recommends that women undergoing induced abortion are advised to perform a urinary pregnancy test 3–4 weeks post-abortion if they are still experiencing ongoing pregnancy symptoms, which should identify those women who have GTN.

The live birth rate for a CHM twin pregnancy has been found to be between 25% and 40%. The risk of GTN if the pregnancy continues is no higher. These pregnancies pose a management dilemma, and women should be counselled about the risks, including the increased risk of early fetal loss (40%), premature delivery (36%), and pre-eclampsia (4–20%).

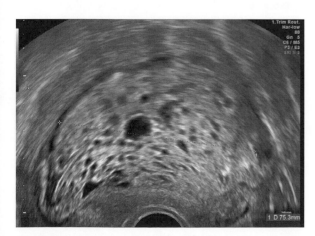

Figure 16.4 Typical US appearance of a CHM

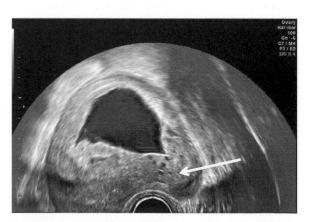

Figure 16.5 Typical US appearance of PHM where a missed miscarriage is diagnosed. Note the cystic appearance of the placental tissue (arrowed).

2.4.6 Follow-Up and Prognosis

All patients with identified HM are referred to one of the UK centres for histopathological review and placed on the national registry for hCG follow-up. This consists of serum and urine measurements every 2 weeks until the levels have normalised; following this, monthly hCG concentrations are measured. If the hCG returns to normal within 56 days of uterine evacuation, the patient has a reduced risk of developing GTN, and they are monitored for 6 months following evacuation. In patients where the hCG takes longer than 56 days to normalise, the risk of GTN is higher and the patients continue to be monitored for 6 months following the first normal hCG. Once the hCG has normalized, the risk of developing GTN is very low.

During the hCG follow-up period, women are advised to use reliable contraception. The RCOG Green-Top guidelines continue to recommend barrier methods; however, currently in the UK, the national centres advise that oral contraceptives after molar evacuation, before hCG returns to normal can be used safely. Studies have shown no increase in the development of invasive mole or choriocarcinoma in women taking oestrogen and or progestogens during this time. Intrauterine devices should be avoided due to the risk of uterine perforation.

Following a diagnosis of GTD, even when the hCG has normalised, if the patient becomes pregnant again, then she is once again at risk of developing GTN; therefore hCG levels should be checked at 6 weeks and 10 weeks after every pregnancy to ensure no reactivation of previous HM.

Gestational Trophoblastic Neoplasia

HMs are followed up closely due to the risk of development to GTN, which can be fatal if left untreated. The rate of development from CHM (Table 16.5) is around 15% and from PHM 0.5%. The diagnosis is made on the basis of an elevated hCG plateau or rising hCG titres over a period of several weeks. GTN is scored and staged using the International Federation of Gynaecology and Obstetrics (FIGO, 2000) scoring system for GTN. Approximately 95% of patients will have low risk, low resistance disease and will be treated with monotherapy chemotherapy (methotrexate or dactinomycin); if this fails, a second-line chemotherapy can be used. This group has an overall survival rate of nearly 100%.

High-risk disease occurs in only 5% of cases and usually presents with many metastases months or years after the causative pregnancy. Even in this high-risk group, there is a cure rate of around 84%.

2.5 Ectopic Pregnancy

2.5.1 Definitions and Epidemiology

An ectopic pregnancy is that which is implanted outside of the uterine cavity. The majority of ectopic pregnancies are located in the fallopian tube, 80% of which are ampullary (see Table 16.6).

More than 10,000 ectopic pregnancies are diagnosed annually in the UK with a rate of 11.3 per 1000 pregnancies and a mortality rate of 16.9 per 100,000 estimated ectopic pregnancies (CMACE, 2011). Non-tubal ectopic pregnancies are relatively uncommon, and their diagnosis and management are outside the scope of this chapter. The risk factors for ectopic pregnancy are outlined in Box 6, and in general, they are associated with tubal damage or infection.

Women undergoing IVF have an increased risk of ectopic and heterotopic pregnancy most likely because of the retrograde movement of the deposited embryo into a diseased tube. Current use of the IUCD/IUS and the progestogen-only pill have been associated with an increased risk of ectopic pregnancy, but it must be remembered that the overall pregnancy rate is lower and only if this method fails is the chance of ectopic pregnancy higher. Overall, a high proportion of tubal ectopic pregnancies are associated with tubal infection or surgery and cigarette smoking (possibly related to tubal function or altered immune function).

Table 16.6 Location and incidence of ectopic pregnancies

Location	Incidence
Ampullary portion of fallopian tube	80%
Isthmic portion of fallopian tube	12%
Fimbrial portion of fallopian tube	5%
Interstitial portion of fallopian tube	2%
Abdominal	1.4%
Ovarian	2%
Cervical	0.2%
Caesarean scar	<1%
Intramural	rare
Cornual (in rudimentary horn of abnormal uterus)	<1%

2.5.2 Clinical Features and Diagnosis of Tubal Ectopic Pregnancy (Fig. 16.6)

Diagnosis: Symptoms and Signs

The presentation of an ectopic pregnancy can be highly variable (Box 7). The majority of women will present with a history of amenorrhoea; however, the history can be variable, and on direct questioning, they will often report that their last 'period' was not normal (lighter or longer) and they are subsequently found to be more advanced in their pregnancy than expected on ultrasound, the bleed being associated with an abnormal rise in hCG associated with the abnormal pregnancy. Many women will be asymptomatic, the diagnosis being made on an early ultrasound scan prior to tubal rupture.

Clinical signs can also be variable and women can be relatively well with minimal tenderness. Women in whom there is significant blood loss will present with the clinical signs of haemorrhagic shock and an acute abdomen with hypotension, tachycardia, abdominal

Box 6 Risk Factors for Ectopic Pregnancy

High risk	Moderate risk	Low risk
Previous tubal surgery	Subfertility	Previous pelvic/abdominal surgery
Sterilisation	Previous PID	Ruptured appendix
Previous ectopic pregnancy	Multiple sexual partners	Cigarette smoking
Current IUCD use	Previous termination	Vaginal douching
Tubal pathology	Previous miscarriage	Age <18 years at first intercourse
DES exposure	Age >40 years	
Courtesy Emma Kirk 2011		

Adnexal mass

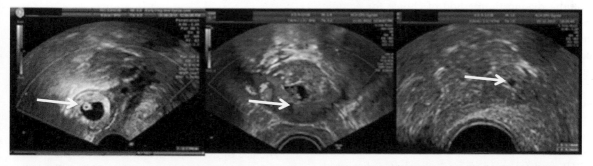

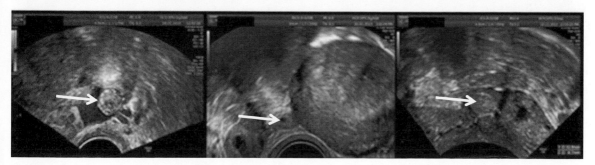

Figure 16.6 Ultrasound appearance of tubal ectopic pregnancies (arrows)

Box 7 Presenting Symptoms Associated with Ectopic Pregnancy

Symptom	Comment
Abdominal or pelvic pain	Often localised to iliac fossa More generalised in presence of haematoperitoneum Colicky in nature
Diarrhoea	Related to bowel and peritoneal irritation from haematoperitoneum Can be misleading if pregnancy not considered
Dizziness, fainting, shock	Related to hypovolaemia from haematoperitoneum
Shoulder tip pain	Blood irritating diaphragm
Urinary symptoms	Bladder irritation
Vaginal bleeding	Abnormal rise in hCG levels Can be heavy and erroneously lead to diagnosis of miscarriage
Asymptomatic	Diagnosis made on ultrasound in the absence of symptoms Associated with early scan

tenderness with guarding and rebound. All women presenting to the ED with an acute abdomen should have a urinary pregnancy test to exclude pregnancy. Vaginal and speculum examination rarely contributes to the assessment of women with suspected ectopic pregnancy and should only be undertaken if bleeding is heavy or cervical or vaginal swabs are clinically indicated.

Diagnosis: Ultrasound

TVS is the diagnostic method of choice for ectopic pregnancy carrying a sensitivity of 87–99%, with 91% of tubal ectopics being identified on the first scan in a specialist unit (10). The diagnosis of an ectopic pregnancy is usually made if there is an empty uterus and an adnexal mass with or without evidence of blood in the pelvis. Seventy percent of ectopic pregnancies occur on the ipsilateral side to the corpus luteum. If the scan is unable to identify an intra- or extra-uterine pregnancy, then this should be classified as a PUL and followed up accordingly (as discussed later).

The ultrasound appearance of an ectopic pregnancy varies ranging from an inhomogenous adnexal mass to an empty gestational sac surrounded by trophoblast to a live ectopic with a visible yolk sac, embryo and fetal heart pulsation (see Fig. 16.6). The presence of fluid between the endometrial layers of the uterine cavity (pseudosac) should not be mistaken for an intrauterine gestation, and the diagnostic criteria described previously should always be adhered to.

Diagnosis: Biochemistry

As discussed previously, the use of hCG and discriminatory zones is unhelpful in the diagnosis of ectopic pregnancy and can be misleading. The traditional use of hCG cut-offs (or discriminatory zones) over which the diagnosis of an ectopic can be made in the presence of a negative scan assumes that ectopic pregnancies with an hCG under this level do not exist and that after a spontaneous complete miscarriage the hCG is always below this level. It also assumes that all pregnancies look the same and that all scans are of the same quality. Cut-offs put women at risk of a negative laparoscopy which can carry significant operative complications and laparoscopy should be avoided if possible if the location of the pregnancy is undetermined. In contrast, women who present with signs of haemodynamic compromise should be managed clinically and promptly as a delay waiting for a scan could cause further compromise.

The use of hCG and progesterone for the prediction of outcome in women with a PUL will be discussed later in this chapter.

2.5.3   Management of Tubal Ectopic Pregnancy

Ectopic pregnancies have traditionally been managed surgically with a move to more conservative methods in more recent years.

Surgical

The indications for surgical management include the unstable patient with symptoms and signs suggestive of haemorrhage, moderate to severe pain or a live ectopic. Patient choice is also an indication following adequate counselling. The choice of surgical approach (laparotomy or laparoscopy) depends on the condition of the patient, the skills of the surgeon and the equipment available. The decision whether to perform a salpingectomy or salpingostomy should depend again on the condition of the contralateral tube. If it is healthy, then the chance of successful subsequent pregnancy is similar after both; however, the rate of persistent trophoblast and the repeat ectopic rates are higher after salpingostomy (11), and the RCOG guidelines (2004) suggest that salpingectomy should be performed in these circumstances.

Medical

Methotrexate for the treatment of ectopic pregnancy is commonly used in many units as a 'non-invasive alternative' to surgery, as it is relatively easy to organise and give and avoids surgical intervention. Methotrexate is a folate antagonist that inhibits synthesis of purines and pyrimidines, interfering with cell proliferation. Adverse effects are dose related and include conjunctivitis, stomatitis, liver dysfunction, bone marrow depression, photosensitivity and gastrointestinal upset, causing abdominal pain. In addition, women are advised against pregnancy for at least 3 months post-administration. While reported side effects after single use for ectopic pregnancy are low, it can be seen that its use is not entirely without risk, and careful counselling is required. The temptation to use methotrexate for 'persistent PUL' should be avoided, as the risk of teratogenicity is high in ongoing pregnancies.

The criteria for the use of methotrexate are a stable woman, with minimal or no pain; an hCG level that is rising and the baseline is below approximately 5000 IU/L. Ideally, the ectopic mass should be less than 3 cm with no fetal heart activity and there should be no contraindications to its use (renal impairment or dialysis). Again, patient choice after adequate counselling is essential; however, the patient must be able to commit to, often prolonged, follow-up and be able to head to the hospital quickly in the event of a change of symptoms. Most units in the UK use a single dose regimen as described in the RCOG guideline, with a repeat dose on day 7 if the fall in hCG is not sufficient. Follow-up should continue until the hCG reaches zero, and reassessment is essential if symptoms change. Reported success rates are variable and difficult to interpret due to the use of methotrexate in PUL (Table 16.7).

Expectant

Expectant management for ectopic pregnancy has been found to be safe and effective in selected cases. Again, the woman should be asymptomatic or have mild pain only, and she should be stable with a small ectopic with no visible fetal heart pulsations and a low initial hCG. As for methotrexate, she also needs to be able to attend for follow-up, which can be prolonged, and able to attend the hospital quickly if her symptoms persist. If the hCG is rising, then an alternative treatment should be considered, and each unit needs to establish protocols for expectant management based on their patient population and outcomes. Managed in this way, up to one-third of ectopic pregnancies can be managed conservatively, with good subsequent pregnancy rates and low repeat ectopic rates (Table 16.7) (11).

2.5.4   Follow-Up

The follow-up for women who have had medical or expectant management of their ectopic pregnancy and the prognosis for future pregnancy is described herein. Women who have had a salpingostomy should be followed up with serum hCG levels until they have returned to normal in view of the risk of persistent trophoblast tissue in these cases.

Table 16.7 Short- and long-term outcomes for the different management options in ectopic pregnancy

	Salpingotomy	Salpingectomy	Methotrexate	Expectant
Ongoing pregnancy	60.7%	56.2%	>80%	63–88%
Persistent trophoblast	7%	<1%	-	-
Repeat ectopic	8%	5%	13–24%	4–5%
Tubal patency rate			77–82%	93%

In the presence of healthy contralateral tube (Van Mello et al 2014)

Women who have had an ectopic pregnancy are advised to attend for an assessment at 6 weeks in subsequent pregnancies to confirm location. They should attend earlier if they are symptomatic; however, the chance of a diagnosis of a PUL and the subsequent follow-up inevitably will be higher.

2.6 Pregnancy of Unknown Location

A PUL refers to a case where there is a positive pregnancy test and no evidence of either an intra- or extrauterine pregnancy on TVS. The PUL rate between units can be highly variable, depending upon the service provided and the staffing of the unit. It can be a useful indicator of scan quality and is a useful audit tool to improve services with the ideal PUL rate suggested as <15%, with a good unit having a PUL rate of 10%. The PUL rate is also lower, the higher the gestation at which the first scan is performed, with the optimum gestational age having been suggested as 49 days (13; Bottomley 2009).

The possible diagnoses in the presence of a PUL will be that the assessment is too early (the pregnancy is too small to be seen), too late (the pregnancy has already miscarried/resolved) or that the pregnancy has not been identified due to scan quality. The quality of the scan as discussed before can depend on many factors, including the scan machine, the experience of the operator and the presence of factors such as adipose tissue, a full bladder or fibroids that may impair the view. Obviously, the biggest concern is that an ectopic pregnancy (Table 16.8) has been missed and a systematic approach to assessment will reduce this risk.

The approach to PUL should include a careful clinical assessment, expectant management unless there is evidence of bleeding or rupture, serum biochemistry and then follow up or treatment to complete resolution. The majority of PULs will resolve without intervention, the intervention rate has been variably described as being between 0.5% and 11%.

Neither hCG nor progesterone can identify the location of the pregnancy. hCG is an indicator of the amount of metabolically active trophoblast present doubling every 24–36 hours in normal early pregnancy; failing pregnancies will demonstrate a lower rise and plateau and in the case of a failed pregnancy will fall with a T ½ of 36 hours.

Progesterone is an indicator of pregnancy 'viability' but again are poor at predicting the location of the pregnancy. Low levels of progesterone <20 nmol/l have a high positive predictive value for a failing pregnancy. High levels >60 nmol/l are associated with viable pregnancies, and levels between 20 and 60 nmol/l are likely to predict viable pregnancies regardless of their location (RCOG, 2004).

The two most commonly used approaches to PUL management are the Single Visit Model, using a single progesterone and hCG level to plan ongoing follow-up, and various mathematical models using serial hCG levels with or without a progesterone measurement, all of which are designed to reduce risk while minimising unnecessary intervention.

2.7 Post-Pregnancy Contraception

It is generally and often erroneously assumed that all women attending with problems in early pregnancy have a planned and wanted pregnancy and therefore do not require ongoing contraception. Pregnancies are frequently unplanned and may or not be wanted, and a sensitive enquiry should be made regarding this and the desire for future pregnancies.

Women with planned pregnancies may also wish to use contraception in the short term to give them a break and a chance to recover both physically and psychologically, and clinicians should acquire training in contraception provision to enable them to offer appropriate contraception in a sensitive and appropriate fashion.

2.8 Anti-D Immunoglobulin

Table 16.9 outlines the recommended use of anti-D immunoprophylaxis in early pregnancy. The BCSH (British Committee for Standards in Haematology) guidelines published in 2014 recommend that a Kleihauer test for quantifying feto-maternal haemorrhage does not need to be performed in pregnancies prior to 12 weeks gestation. Individual units will have

Table 16.8 Final diagnosis of women presenting with a PUl

Final diagnosis	Percentage %
Ectopic pregnancy	6–20%
Intrauterine pregnancy	30–50%
Failing PUL	50–70%
Persistent PUL	<5%
Courtesy Kirk 2013	

Table 16.9 British Committee for Standards in Haematology (BCSH) Guideline on Anti-D Administration in Pregnancy, 2014: Recommendations for Use of Anti-D in Rhesus Negative Women

Should be offered anti-D	Do not require anti-D
Therapeutic management of miscarriage	Threatened miscarriage under 12 weeks
Vaginal bleeding or PSE over 12 weeks	Complete miscarriage under 12 weeks
Heavy vaginal bleeding with abdominal pain under 12 weeks	Pregnancy of unknown location
All ectopics and molar pregnancies	

PSE = potentially sensitising event, e.g. chorionic villus sampling or amniocentesis

local protocols based on these guidelines, which may also include different dosages of anti-D IgG, depending on their supplier.

References

1. Ectopic Pregnancy and Miscarriage: Diagnosis and Initial Management. NICE Guidelines. December 2012

2. Mol F et al. Should patients who are suspected of having an ectopic pregnancy undergo physical examination? *Fertil Steril* 1999 Jan; **71**(1): 155–7

3. French FE, Bierman JM. Probabilities of fetal mortality. *Public Health Rep.* 1962; **77**: 835–47

4. Alcazar JL, Baldonado C, Laparte C. The reliability of transvaginal ultrasonography to detect retained tissue after spontaneous first trimester abortion clinically thought to be complete. *Ultrasound Obstet Gynecol* 1995; **6**: 126–9

5. Condous G, Okaro E, Bourne T. Pregnancies of unknown location: Diagnostic dilemmas and management. *Curr Opin Obstet Gynecol* 2005 Dec; **17**(6): 568–73

6. Trinder J, Brocklehurst P, Porter R, Read M, Vyas S, Smith L. Management of miscarriage: Expectant, medical, or surgical? Results of randomised controlled trial (miscarriage treatment (MIST) trial). *BMJ* 2006 May 27; **332**(7552): 1235–40

7. Gestational Trophoblastic Disease. RCOG – Green-Top Guideline No. 38

8. Sebire NJ, Fisher RA, Foskett M, Rees H, Seckl MJ, Newlands ES. Risk of recurrent hydatidiform mole and subsequent pregnancy outcome following complete or partial hydatidiform molar pregnancy. *BJOG* 2003 Jan; **110**(1): 22–6

9. Seckl MJ, Sebire NJ, Berkowitz RS. Gestational trophoblastic disease. *Lancet.* 2010; **376**: 717–29

10. Kirk E, Papageorghiou AT, Condous G, Tan L, Bora S, Bourne T. The diagnostic effectiveness of an initial transvaginal scan in detecting ectopic pregnancy. *Hum Reprod* 2007 Nov; **22**(11): 2824–8

11. Mol F, van Mello NM et al. Salpingotomy versus salpingectomy in women with tubal pregnancy (ESEP study): An open-label, multicentre, randomised controlled trial. *Lancet* 2014 Apr 26; **383**(9927): 1483–9

12. Mavrelos D, Efficacy and safety of a clinical protocol for expectant management of selected women diagnosed with a tubal ectopic pregnancy. *Ultrasound in Obstetrics & Gynecology* 2013 July; **42**(1): 102–7

13. Bottomley C, Van Belle V, Mukri F, Kirk E, Van Huffel S, Timmerman D, Bourne T. The optimal timing of an ultrasound scan to assess the location and viability of an early pregnancy. *Hum Reprod* 2009; **24**: 1811–17

14. Qureshi H et al. BCSH guideline for the use of anti-D immunoglobulin for the prevention of haemolytic disease of the fetus and newborn. *Transfusion Medicine* 2014 February; **24**(1): 8–20

Single Best Answer Questions

1. What is the most common cause of a first-trimester miscarriage?

    a. Chromosomal

    b. Maternal disease

    c. Drugs

    d. Uterine anomalies

    e. Infection

2. What is the most common location for an ectopic pregnancy?

    a. Ampullary

    b. Isthmic

    c. Fimbrial

d. Interstitial

e. Cornual

3. What is the definition of a recurrent miscarriage?

a. Two or more non-recurrent miscarriages

b. Two or more recurrent miscarriages

c. Three or more non-recurrent miscarriages

d. Three or more recurrent miscarriages

e. Two second-trimester miscarriages

4. What is the frequent genetic composition of a complete hydatidiform molar pregnancy?

a. 46 XX

b. 46 XY

c. 47 XXX

d. 47 XYY

e. 45 XO

5. You are asked to review a 28-year-old woman in the EPU follow-up clinic. She underwent a surgical management of her miscarriage several weeks ago and has been asked to attend to discuss the results of the histology

Histology report: Multiple pieces of tan tissue. Microscopically, there is evidence of enlarged edematous villi and abnormal trophoblastic proliferation suggestive of a complete hydatidiform mole.

Once you have explained the findings to the patient, what is the appropriate next management step?

a. Refer to the nearest UK centre for histopathological review and placement on the national registry for hCG follow-up

b. Repeat serum and urine measurements of hCG in 2 weeks

c. Perform hCG in 56 days and yearly from then on

d. Recommend contraception in the form of an intrauterine device

e. Reassure the patient and discharge from the EPU

6. A woman with a first-trimester miscarriage opts for conservative management. How long is the recommended duration or conservative management?

a. 3–5 days

b. 5–7 days

c. 7–10 days

d. 7–14 days

e. 14–21 days

7. A woman presents with a short history of vaginal spotting and cramping abdominal pain after 7 weeks of amenorrhoea. A few days earlier, she had a positive result on a home pregnancy test. The cervix is closed on examination. A transvaginal ultrasound scan shows an intrauterine gestational sac measuring 23 mm, with no evidence of a fetal pole.

What is an appropriate management plan?

a. Explain the diagnosis of a missed miscarriage, and go through management options.

b. Ask the patient to repeat a urinary pregnancy test in a week and come back for a repeat scan if still positive.

c. Transvaginal scan in 5 days

d. Transvaginal scan in 7 days

e. Transvaginal scan in 2 weeks

8. In what early pregnancy clinical scenarios is anti-D not required for a patient who is Rhesus negative?

a. Molar pregnancies

b. Complete miscarriage under 12 weeks

c. Surgical management of miscarriage

d. Heavy vaginal bleeding with abdominal pain under 12 weeks

e. Surgical management of an ectopic pregnancies

Human Immunodeficiency Virus and Other Sexually Transmitted Infections

Taslima Rashid and Michael Rayment

Section 1: Introduction

1.1 Overview

The epidemiology of sexually transmitted infections (STIs) is unique and reflects societal, attitudinal, economic and technological changes.

The establishment of genito-urinary medicine (GUM) clinics, and latterly sexual health clinics, was designed to treat and deal with the complications of STIs and related genital conditions in a permissive and confidential environment. Confidentiality is paramount in sexual health, and clinical information is not routinely shared with other healthcare providers, unless it facilitates care, and then only with the express permission of the patient. Information is held separately from the general medical record and patients may register with partial or alternate demographic details. Services are delivered by a multidisciplinary team comprising doctors, nurses (often in advanced practitioner roles), health advisors, healthcare assistants and laboratory staff.

Partner notification is an important aspect of STI control and care. This is the process of gathering contact details and information about the recent sexual partners of a patient with a confirmed STI for the purposes of facilitating their assessment and treatment. Contacts of an infection may be offered 'epidemiological treatment' – the provision of therapy on the basis of exposure.

Taking a sexual history and discussing issues around sexual health are key aspects in a sexual health consultation. Table 17.1 outlines the key elements of a sexual health consultation. [1,2]

1.2 Female Examination

Symptomatic patients should have a clinical examination. In females, inspect the skin around the external

Table 17.1 Key components to be included in a sexual history [1,2]

Core sexual history components

- Reasons for attendance. Assess symptoms to guide examination and investigations required
- Exposure history to guide examination and investigations required. This will include:
  - Last sexual intercourse (LSI) and number of partners in preceding three months
  - Partner(s): gender, known or suspected infections, sites of exposure, condom use
- For women, assessment of contraceptive use and risk of pregnancy: last menstrual period (LMP), contraceptive use
- Previous STI history
- Assessment of other sexual health issues, including psychosexual problems
- HIV, hepatitis B and hepatitis C risk assessment for treatment and prevention purposes
  - Risk factors for blood-borne viruses (BBV) that should be assessed in the history include:
    1. Transfusions in lower/middle-income countries
    2. Sexual intercourse with a partner known to have a BBV, or partners from areas endemic for BBV infection
    3. Injecting drug use (themselves or by sexual partners)
    4. Men reporting sex with men (and their sexual partners)
    5. Sex with, or work as, a commercial sex worker
- Assessment of risk behaviour for purposes of health promotion (partner notification and sexual health promotion)
- Alcohol and recreational drug history
- Past medical and surgical history (including cervical cytology history in women), medication and drug allergies
- Establish Fraser competency/child protection concerns if aged under 16 years
- Be aware of vulnerable adults, intimate-partner violence and gender-based violence

Table 17.2 Summary of diagnostics used in the detection of STIs and related genital conditions

	Nucleic acid amplification test (NAATs)	Culture	Microscopy	Serology	Sites and samples
Chlamydia	✔	✔			Vulvo-vaginal swab (VVS) (Culture not widely available)
Gonorrhoea	✔	✔	✔		Endo-cervical swab for culture Vulvo-vaginal swab (NAATs)
Bacterial vaginosis			✔		Vaginal wall swab (Gram stain microscopy: Hay/Ison criteria)
Trichomonas vaginalis	+/-	✔	✔		Posterior fornix swab (Wet-mount microscopy) NAATs increasingly available
Herpes simplex					Swab of lesion (PCR)
Candidiasis		✔	✔		Vaginal wall swab (Gram stain microscopy)
HIV				✔	Point-of-care tests widely available
Hepatitis B				✔	
Hepatitis C				✔	
Syphilis		✔		✔	Dark ground microscopy of ulcer material

genitalia and pubic area and palpate for inguinal lymphadenopathy. A speculum examination is performed to visualise the vagina, posterior fornices and cervix for lesions, inflammation and discharge, and to take samples for near-patient and laboratory investigations. [3]

A bimanual examination should be performed in all women who attend with pelvic or lower abdominal pain or deep dyspareunia.

Urine samples may be required to test for pregnancy and urinary tract infection.

1.3 Investigations

Many near-patient tests (such as Gram staining, wet-mount and dark-field microscopy, and HIV point-of-care testing) are undertaken in sexual health clinics. These investigations may facilitate same-day diagnosis and treatment.

Further details on specific investigations are presented in the topic sections, but a general summary of testing for specific STIs is given in Table 17.2.

1.4 General Management Considerations

Standard management considerations applying to all individuals diagnosed with an STI include:

- The provision of written and verbal information regarding the diagnosis
- Safer sex and risk reduction advice (including discussions around drug and alcohol use)
- Advising on sexual abstinence immediately after treatment. Patients should ordinarily abstain from sexual intercourse (including oral sex) for seven-fourteen days and until after ongoing partners have completed their treatment
- Screening for other sexually transmitted infections
- Discussions relating to the notification and treatment of exposed partners (partner notification)

Section 2: Vaginal Discharge

2 Altered Vaginal Discharge

Altered vaginal discharge within the sexual health setting is one of the commonest presentations in women encountered. The combination of a detailed and directed sexual health history in conjunction with appropriate clinical examination, specimen collection and near-patient and laboratory testing can yield a diagnosis in a timely fashion.

Table 17.3 Comparison between Amsel's and Hay/Ison criteria for BV

Amsel's criteria	Hay/Ison criteria or the Nugent criteria
Thin, white, homogenous discharge	**Grade 1:** Lactobacilli predominantly (normal)
Clue cells on microscopy	**Grade 2:** Mixed flora with some lactobacilli. Gardnerella and Mobiluncus morphotypes present (intermediate)
pH of vaginal fluid is more than 4.5	**Grade 3:** Gardnerella and mobiluncus morphotypes predominate. Few or absent lactobacilli (BV) – see Fig. 17.1
Release of a fishy odour on adding alkali (10% potassium hydroxide)	

2.1 Bacterial Vaginosis

2.1.1 Aetiology

Bacterial vaginosis (BV) is characterised by an imbalance of the normal vaginal microbiome, with dominance of anaerobic and facultative anaerobic bacteria. This causes a rise in the vaginal pH from its norm of 4.5 to 6.0.

The vaginal flora is made up mainly of hydrogen peroxide producing Lactobacilli. In bacterial vaginosis, bacteria such as *Gardnerella vaginalis*, *Prevotella spp.*, *Mycoplasma hominis* and *Mobiluncus spp.* are the most commonly found using conventional culture techniques.

Please refer to Table 17.5 for risk factors, clinical features, diagnosis and treatment.

2.1.2 Diagnosis

There are two sets of clinical and microbiological criteria that can be used to diagnose BV (see Table 17.3):

1. Amsel's criteria in which the diagnosis can be made if three of the four factors are present
2. The Hay/Ison Criteria or the Nugent Criteria, based on the microscopic appearance of a Gram-stained vaginal wall smear

The British Association for Sexual Health and HIV (BASHH) recommends the Hay/Ison criteria as the gold standard for diagnosis of BV. [4]

2.1.3 Management

– General advice regarding avoidance of practices such as vaginal douching and use of soaps and shampoos in the bath, which may precipitate or perpetuate BV through reducing numbers of lactobacilli
– Antimicrobial treatment (oral or topical) – refer to Table 17.5

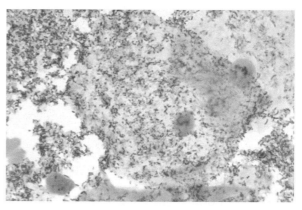

Figure 17.1 Gram-stained smear of vaginal wall sample demonstrating Grade 3 Hay/Ison – a complete absence of lactobacilli is noted, with a preponderance of gram-variable cocci and bacilli. The epithelial cell 'coated' with bacteria is known as a 'clue cell'.

Patients should avoid alcohol with metronidazole oral treatment, as it may cause a disulfiram-like reaction.

2.1.4 Pregnancy

See Table 17.6 for a summary of treatment considerations of women with vaginal discharge in pregnancy.

2.2 Vulvo-Vaginal Candidiasis

2.2.1 Aetiology

Vulvo-vaginal candidiasis, also referred to as candidosis or thrush, is considered to be due to pathogenic activity of commensal yeasts associated with dermatitis of the vulva and non-offensive vaginal discharge (see Fig. 17.2).

Candida albicans is responsible for 80–89% cases, and *C. glabrata* for 3–15% of cases of acute candidiasis. Other yeasts are rarely implicated: these include *C. crusei*, *C. tropicalis* and *C. parapsilosis*.

Refer to Table 17.5 for risk-factors, clinical features, diagnosis and treatment.

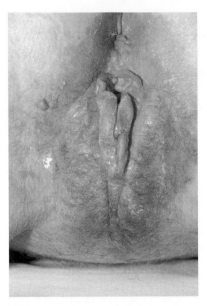

Figure 17.2 Acute candidiasis: Note the vulvovaginitis, with erythema and swelling, with white vaginal discharge

2.2.2 Diagnosis

- Clinical history (signs and symptoms)
- Direct microscopy: Gram stain of vaginal discharge collected from the anterior fornix or lateral vaginal walls looking for spores and hyphae (Fig. 17.3).
- Laboratory culture: Samples are taken from the lateral vaginal walls and sent in a transport medium (Amies, Feinburg-Whittington), and cultured on a growth medium (Sabouraud). Cultures are helpful when microscopy is inconclusive, and in cases of recurrent candidiasis where speciation may change management

Note: As yeasts are commensals, the visualization or isolation of treatment of *Candida sp.* does not merit treatment in the absence of signs or symptoms.

2.2.3 Management

- General advice:
  - Avoidance of local irritants such as perfumed products, shower gels, deodorants
  - Avoidance of wearing tight-fitting, synthetic clothing
  - Anti-fungal treatment (topical or systemic)
- Topical treatments (Table 17.4a)
- Oral treatments (Table 17.4b)

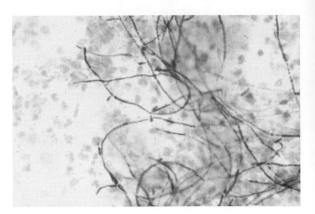

Figure 17.3 Gram stain of vaginal wall smear, showing spores and hyphae in a female with acute candidiasis

2.2.4 Recurrent Candidiasis

Recurrent candidiasis is defined as more than four confirmed episodes of thrush a year. Approximately 5% of women of reproductive age will develop recurrent candidiasis. Host factors are more likely to drive recurrence and these include (uncontrolled) diabetes, immunocompromise, high levels of oestrogen (HRT or COCP), vaginal microbiome imbalance due to, for example, broad-spectrum antibiotic use, and a possible link to atopy. Women with recurrent thrush should have a comprehensive assessment, and risk factors should be addressed. Hygiene and lifestyle practices should be discussed (e.g. encouraging the use of emollients for washing, and advising the avoidance of douching, perfumed products, and synthetic underwear and sanitary products). Non-typical *Candida* species (such as *C. glabrata*) are more likely to isolated in women with recurrent candidiasis, and speciation and anti-fungal susceptibility testing should be performed, as non-*albicans* species may have lower susceptibility to imidazole anti-fungals. A variety of induction-maintenance regimens of oral and topical anti-fungals have been used with success, with regimens lasting weeks to months, although relapse and recurrence is common. [5]

2.3 Trichomonas Vaginalis

2.3.1 Aetiology

Trichomonas vaginalis (TV) is a flagellated protozoan infecting the vagina, urethra and para-urethral glands. Infection can only follow intravaginal or intraurethral inoculation. Due to this site specificity, TV is therefore almost exclusively transmitted through sexual contact.

Table 17.4a BASHH topical treatments for vulvovaginal candidiasis [5]

Drug	Formulation	Dosage regimen
Clotrimazole*	Pessary	500 mg stat
Clotrimazole*	Pessary	200 mg × 3 nights
Clotrimazole*	Pessary	100 mg × 6 nights
Clotrimazole*	Vaginal cream (10%)	5 g stat
Econozole	Pessary	150mg stat OR 150mg × 3 nights
Fenticonazole	Intravaginal capsule	600mg stat OR 200mg × 3 nights
Miconazole	Intravaginal capsule	1200mg stat OR 400mg × 3 nights
Miconazole	Intravaginal cream (2%)	5g × 7 nights

NB * Effect on latex condoms and diaphragms not known

Table 17.4b BASHH oral treatments for vulvovaginal candidiasis [5]

Drug	Formulation	Dosage regimen
Fluconazole	Capsule	150 mg stat
Itraconazole	Capsule	200 mg bd × 1d

NB Avoid in pregnancy/risk of pregnancy and breastfeeding

Refer to Table 17.5 for risk-factors, clinical features, diagnosis and treatment.

2.3.2 Diagnosis

1. **Direct microscopy** – Vaginal discharge from swabs taken from the posterior fornix are examined as a suspension in isotonic saline by light-field microscopy. Motile protozoa being propelled by flagella are seen

2. **Culture** – Culture has a higher sensitivity compared with microscopy and can be used to diagnose TV in men. Samples are spun down by centrifugation and placed in culture medium (e.g. Feinburg-Whittington) or dispatched initially in transport medium (e.g. Amies). Culture was considered the 'gold standard' until molecular testing revealed higher sensitivity

3. **Polymerase chain reaction (PCR)** – Nucleic acid amplification tests (NAATs) for TV are available, but not yet widely so. NAATs have been shown to have sensitivities of 88–97% and specificities of 98–99%, depending on the specimen and the reference standard

2.3.3 Management

Treatment – See Table 17.5. Treatment should be systemic and not topical in view of high urethral and peri-urethral gland involvement. Spontaneous clearance can occur in 20–25% of cases.

Note Regarding Pregnancy and Treatment

It is not known whether metronidazole affects pregnancy outcomes but meta-analyses have shown that it does not affect pregnancy in terms of teratogenicity in the first trimester. High-dose metronidazole is not recommended by the British National Formulary (BNF) in pregnancy. Metronidazole does enter breast milk. The safety of tinidazole in pregnancy has not been fully evaluated and manufacturers advise against use in the first trimester. [6]

Section 3: Cervicitis and Pelvic Inflammatory Disease

3 Cervicitis

3.1 Chlamydia

Genital chlamydia infection is the most common curable bacterial sexually transmitted infection (STI) in Britain, with a prevalence of 5–10% in women less than 24 years of age. Most individuals are asymptomatic. *Chlamydia trachomatis* is an obligate intracellular bacterium infecting endothelial cells. It derives its energy from host cell adenosine triphosphate. Serovars D-K are implicated in urogenital infection. In females, the cervix is the most common site of infection, and the infection may be carried asymptomatically or cause mucopurulent cervicitis (manifest as intermenstrual and post-coital bleeding – Fig. 17.4).

Table 17.5 Summary of conditions of altered vaginal discharge

Condition	Risk factors	Symptoms and signs	Investigations	Treatment	Complications
Bacterial vaginosis	Black ethnicity Vaginal douching Recent change in sexual partner Cigarette smoking Presence of an STI Receptive cunnilingus	Fishy smelling discharge Asymptomatic approx. 50% No vulvo-vaginal irritation	Amsel's criteria Hay/Ison criteria	Metronidazole 400 mg PO BD 5–7 day Metronidazole 2 g PO STAT Metronidazole gel 0.5% PV TOP OD 5–7 days Clindamycin gel 2% PV TOP OD 7 days	Post termination of pregnancy (TOP) endometritis Increased risk of HIV acquisition
Vulvo-vaginal candidiasis	Inflammation Diabetes mellitus Broad spectrum antibiotic use Impaired immunity	Vulvovaginal itch Lumpy/abnormal discharge	Gram stain microscopy Culture	Clotrimazole 500 mg STAT pessary Clotrimazole 200 mg ON 3/7 pessary Clotrimazole 1% topical cream BD 5–7 days Fluconazole 150 mg PO STAT Itraconazole 200 mg BD (1/7)	Recurrent candidiasis
Trichomonas vaginalis	Sexually active women Presence of other STIs	Discharge Dysuria Offensive smelling urine Vulvitis/vaginitis 'Strawberry' cervix	Wet preparation microscopy Culture NAAT	Metronidazole 2 g PO STAT Metronidazole 400 mg BD 5–7 days	Enhanced HIV acquisition

Table 17.6 Summary of Pregnancy complications with BV, candidiasis and TV

	Pregnancy
Bacterial vaginosis	Late miscarriage Preterm birth Premature rupture of membranes (ROM) Post-partum endometritis
Vulvovaginal candidiasis	Asymptomatic colonization 30–40% More symptomatic infections also Oral therapy is contraindicated Topical imidazoles may be used but pregnant women require longer treatment courses
Trichomonas vaginalis	Preterm delivery Low birth weight High dose single treatment for TV should be avoided in pregnancy Metronidazole is relatively contraindicated in the first trimester

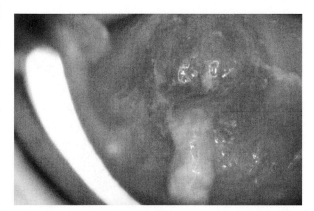

Figure 17.4 Appearances of muco-purulent cervicitis. Such an appearance may result from cervical infection with either *Chlamydia trachomatis, Mycoplasma genitalium or Neisseria gonorrhoeae.*

3.1.1 Risk Factors

- New sexual partner
- >1 sexual partner in the past year
- Lack of condom use

Chlamydia has a high frequency of transmission with concordance rates of up to 75%. Infection in women is known to cause complications such as tubal infertility, ectopic pregnancy and pelvic inflammatory disease (PID). In view of its high prevalence and the risk of significant long and short-term morbidity, the National Chlamydia Screening Programme was set up in the UK in 2003 targeted at young men and women under the age of 25. Large numbers of tests are now performed outside of sexual health settings, and the prevalence of chlamydia has been seen to decline in recent years.

3.1.2 Extra-genital Infection

Rectal and pharyngeal infections are usually asymptomatic, although rectal infections can cause discharge and discomfort. Extra-genital carriage rates in heterosexual women vary in studies and may not relate clearly to self-reported sexual behaviour. Extra-genital carriage is almost certainly an important factor in ongoing transmission. Conjunctival chlamydial infection in adults is usually sexually acquired and presents with unilateral, mild conjunctivitis, though bilateral infection can occur.

Please refer to Table17.8 for risk-factors, clinical features, diagnosis and treatment.

3.1.3 Samples for Diagnosis

For women, vulvo-vaginal swabs (self-taken or clinician collected) are the recommended samples for NAATs. For men, first catch urine is recommended and patients should hold their urine for an hour before passing urine for the specimen. Extra-genital swabs include rectal and pharyngeal swabs.

3.1.4 Sexually Acquired Reactive Arthritis (SARA) (Table 17.7)

This is a complication of chlamydial infection with preponderance to Caucasian ethnicity and HLA B27 carriers (approximately 75%). It is a seronegative spondyloarthropathy, presenting with clinical features of low back pain, oligo-arthritis, and extra-articular manifestations. Reiter's triad consists of conjunctivitis, urethritis and arthritis.

3.1.4 Lymphogranuloma Venereum (LGV)

LGV is caused by *Chlamydia trachomatis* serovars L1–L3. It was previously rare in Western Europe and

Table 17.7 Features of Sexually Acquired Reactive Arthritis

Sub-categories
Post gastrointestinal infection
  Post urogenital infection
Time frame
From 1 week to max 3–6 weeks post infection
Articular manifestation
Low back pain
    Oligo-arthritis – asymmetrical, lower extremities
Extra-articular manifestations
Acute onset fever, malaise
    Achilles tendonitis
    Eyes – uveitis, episcleritis, keratitis, corneal ulceration
    Skin – circinate balanitis, erythema nodosum
    Mucous membranes – ulcers
    Nails – dystrophic changes
    Gastrointestinal – diarrhoea, abdominal pain, colonic features of colitis/inflammation
    Cardiovascular – aortitis, conduction defects

the US but has increased since 2003 and is now hyper-endemic in the UK, mainly affecting men who have sex with men (especially those living with HIV infection). Heterosexual cases have been reported in women with partners who are bisexual or from endemic regions (South Africa, West Africa, Madagascar, South East Asia).

Symptoms consist of anorectal discharge (can be bloody) and pain, diarrhoea and tenesmus. Women may present with tender and/or suppurative inguinal lymphadenopathy. LGV is diagnosed on PCR from swabs taken from affected sites. Treatment is with doxycycline 100 mg BD PO for 3 weeks. [7]

3.2 Gonorrhoea

Neisseria gonorrhoea is an intracellular gram-negative diplococcus that infects mucous membranes of the endocervix, urethra, rectum, oropharynx and conjunctiva.

It can also extend to the epididymis and prostate in men and the endometrium and pelvic organs in women, and (rarely) haematogenously.

3.2.1 Disseminated Gonococcal Infection (DGI)

Caused by bacteraemic spread of *Neisseria gonorrhoea*, leading to a variety of clinical features, including:

– Tenosynovitis

– Dermatitis
– Skin lesions
– Arthralgia/arthritis

Refer to Table 17.8 for risk factors, clinical features, diagnosis and treatment.

Surveillance data has shown significant resistance to penicillin, tetracyclines and ciprofloxacin and other quinolones.

3.2.2 Diagnosis

NAATs and culture are both used for the diagnosis of gonorrhoea. In symptomatic patients, a Gram-stained smear from an infected site may identify gram-negative intracellular diplococci and a presumptive diagnosis may be made (the sensitivity varies from >95% in the male urethra to <50% at the cervix – Fig. 17.5). NAATs are very sensitive but lack specificity in extra-genital sites. All extra-genital NAATs should be tested against two gene targets to increases specificity. Culture offers confirmatory diagnosis but also antimicrobial sensitivity/susceptibility testing, but may lack sensitivity

3.2.3 Indications for Treatment:

1. Epidemiological treatment if contact with a recent sexual partner who has a confirmed diagnosis

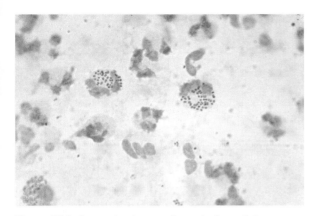

Figure 17.5 Gram-stained smear of a urethral sample in a symptomatic male. Note the intracellular Gram-negative diplococcic infecting polymorphonuclear cells.

2. Epidemiological treatment should be considered in sexual assault cases

3. Diagnosis on direct microscopy, NAATs or culture

3.2.3 Management

General:

– A test of cure (TOC) is now recommended in all infected patients following treatment. This is to identify emerging antimicrobial resistance. The timings as recommended by BASHH are more than 72 hours after completion of treatment in symptomatic patients and two weeks after completion of treatment in those who are not.

All clinically suspicious cases, or those with microscopy positive or NAAT positive gonorrhoea, should have cultures taken from all susceptible sites (e.g. vaginal, urethral, rectal, pharyngeal) prior to antibiotic therapy, if possible.

Treatments

See Table 17.8. [8]

Alternative Regimens for Gonorrhoea in Patients Allergic to Penicillins

Spectinomycin 2 g IM STAT + Azithromycin
2 g PO STAT
OR
Azithromycin 2 g PO STAT
OR
Ciprofloxacin 500 mg PO STAT

Treatment of Complicated Gonococcal infection

1. PID – Ceftriaxone 500 mg IM STAT + Doxycycline 100 mg BD 14/7 + Metronidazole 400 mg BD 5–14/7

2. Gonococcal conjunctivitis – ceftriaxone 1000 mg IM STAT

3. Disseminated gonococcal infection (DGI) – ceftriaxone 1 g IM or IV OD 7/7 or Cefotaxime 1 g IV TDS 7/7 or Ciprofloxacin 500 mg IV BD 7/7 or Spectinomycin 2 g IM BD 7/7 (These can be switched to oral preparations after 24–48 hrs if there is clinical improvement.)

Pregnancy and Breastfeeding

Patients who are pregnant or breastfeeding should not be treated with quinolones or tetracyclines; therefore recommended regimens are:

Ceftriaxone 1000 mg IM STAT
or
Spectinomycin 2 g IM + Azithromycin 2 g PO STAT

3.3 Mycoplasma genitalium

Mycoplasma genitalium was first isolated in 1981, having been cultured from urethral specimens of two men presenting with non-gonococcal urethritis (NGU). M. genitalium belongs to the Mollicutes class, and with a genome of only 580 kilobases in size, is the smallest known self-replicating bacterium. The specialised tip-like structure of M. genitalium enables it to adhere to and invade epithelial cells. Infection may persist for months or years.

Evidence suggests that the majority of people infected with M. genitalium in the genital tract do not develop disease. M. genitalium infection is unequivocally and strongly associated with non-gonococcal urethritis in men. Several studies support an association of M. genitalium infection in cisgender women with post coital bleeding and cervicitis, endometritis and pelvic inflammatory disease (PID).

Antimicrobial therapy for Mycoplasma genitalium has been complicated by the emergence of high levels of resistance to macrolide antibiotics. Because of this, more widespread testing for Mycoplasma genitalium is now advocated. Genotypic resistance tests for macrolide resistance are becoming available.

Table 17.8 Clinical features, investigations and treatment of *Chlamydia trachomatis* and *Neisseria gonorrhoea*

Condition	Symptoms and signs	Infections sites	Investigations	Treatment	Complications	Pregnancy
Chlamydia	Post-coital or intermenstrual bleeding Lower abdominal pain Dysuria Vaginal discharge (rare) Mucopurulent cervicitis (see Fig. 17.4) Cervical motion excitation or adnexal tenderness	Vagina Urethra Rectum Pharynx Ocular	Nucleic acid amplification tests (NAATs) from a vulvovaginal, rectal, pharyngeal, or conjunctival swab	Doxycycline 100 mg BD PO 7 days OR Azithromycin 1 g PO STAT followed by 500mg PO once daily for 2 days Rectal Chlamydia: Doxycycline 100 mg BD PO 7 days	PID, salpingitis, endometritis Tubal infertility Ectopic pregnancy Sexually acquired reactive arthritis (SARA) Perihepatitis	Doxycycline and ofloxacin are contra-indicated All pregnant women should be offered TOC >3weeks after completing treatment
Gonorrhoea	Asymptomatic in up to 50% Lower abdominal pain Dysuria Intermenstrual bleeding Vaginal discharge Contact bleeding of the cervix (see Fig. 17.4)	Urethra Endocervix Rectum Pharynx Conjunctiva	Direct microscopy NAATs Culture	Ceftriaxone 1000 mg IM STAT +	PID Gonococcal arthritis Disseminated Gonococcal infection (DGI)	Quinolones and tetracyclines contra-indicated

Table 17.9 Summary of pelvic inflammatory disease

Clinical features	**Symptoms** – Lower abdominal pain, deep dyspareunia, abnormal vaginal discharge, abnormal vaginal bleeding **Signs –** Cervical motion tenderness on bimanual examination, adnexal tenderness on bimanual examination, fever, abdominal tenderness
Diagnosis	Clinical examination and history. The presence of vaginal and endo-cervical pus cells (polymorphonuclear cells [neutrophils]) on microscopy is a non-specific sign but the absence of pus cells has an excellent negative predictive value (95%). NAATs for chlamydia, gonorrhoea and *Mycoplasma genitalium*; inflammatory markers (ESR/CRP); ultrasound +/- endometrial biopsy; diagnostic laparoscopy
Treatment	OUTPATIENT: IM Ceftriaxone 1000 mq STAT **PLUS either** Doxycycline 100 mg BD **+** Metronidazole 400 mg PO 14 days **OR** Ofloxacin 400 mg BD **+** Metronidazole 400 mg BD 14 days (avoid in gonococcal PID) If *Mycoplasma genitalium* is detected: Moxifloxacin 400mg OD 14 days
Complications	Fitz-Hugh-Curtis syndrome occurs in approximately 10–20% of patients with PID. HIV positive women tend to get more severe disease There is inconclusive evidence to recommend removal of IUDs/IUSs in PID. The balance must be made with the possibility of better short term clinical outcomes with the risk of pregnancy in women who have had unprotected sex in the last seven days Tubo-ovarian abscess should be suspected in patients who are systemically unwell +/- severe abdominal pain, and should be considered for inpatient admission for parenteral antimicrobial therapy and further imaging investigations.
Inpatient vs outpatient	PID should be assessed in terms of clinical severity in order to triage those that need inpatient care and those that can be treated on an outpatient basis. **General severe clinical indicators**: haemodynamic instability, signs of tubo-ovarian abscess and signs of peritonitis. **Specific indicators:** a surgical emergency cannot be safely excluded, lack of response to oral therapy, Intolerance to oral therapy, pregnancy

All women with PID should be tested for infection with Mycoplasma genitalium with a nucleic acid amplification test, and testing may be considered in women with muco-purulent cervicitis. There are no data to support screening asymptomatic people for infection.

Recommended treatments for urethritis and cervicitis include:

- Doxycycline 100mg bd for seven days followed by azithromycin 1g orally as a single dose then 500mg orally once daily for 2 days where organism is known to be macrolide-sensitive or where resistance status is unknown (1D)
- Moxifloxacin 400mg orally once daily for 10 days if organism known to be macrolide-resistant or where treatment with azithromycin has failed (1B)

Women with PID in whom Mycoplasma genitalium is detected should receive moxifloxacin 400mg orally once daily for 14 days.

Women should abstain from sex for the duration of treatment, and their current sexual partners should be tested and offered treatment (to reduce the risk of re-infection in the symptomatic partner).

3.4 Pelvic Inflammatory Disease

3.4.1 Aetiology

Pelvic inflammatory disease (PID) is an ascending genital tract infection leading to symptoms of lower abdominal pain, deep dyspareunia and systemic upset. It is a significant health concern that needs prompt diagnosis and treatment. PID can lead to endometritis, parametritis, salpingitis, oopheritis, tubo-ovarian abscess and pelvic peritonitis. Long-term sequelae include tubal factor infertility, pelvic adhesions, and chronic pelvic pain. PID is aetiologically associated with ectopic pregnancy.

Organisms implicated in PID include *Neisseria gonorrhoea* (5%), *Chlamydia trachomatis* (20–40%), *Mycoplasma genitalium* (10–15%) and *Gardnerella vaginalis,* although most commonly no single organism is implicated.

3.4.2 Clinical Features and Management

Refer to Table 17.9 for clinical features, diagnosis, treatment and complications. The clinical features of PID are relatively non-specific, and it must be remembered that other conditions present with similar features. These must be excluded:

Table 17.10 Summary table of HSV-1 and HSV-2

	Clinical features	Diagnosis	Treatment	Complications
HSV-1/HSV-2	– Painful ulceration – Dysuria – Discharge – Systemic unwell – Local lymphadenitis	– HSV PCR swab of infected fluid with typing – Serology *	**GENERAL:** – Saline bathing – Analgesia – Topical anaesthetics **SPECIFIC:** – Aciclovir 400 mg PO TDS 5/7 – Valaciclovir 500 mg BD 5/7	– Superadded infection with Candida or Streptococcus species – Autonomic neuropathy -> urinary retention – Autoinoculation – Aseptic meningitis – Herpes proctitis – Disseminated herpes infection (hepatitis, disseminated skin lesions, encephalitis)

1. Ectopic pregnancy – this must always be ruled out in patients being investigated for PID
2. Acute appendicitis – up to 25% of women with appendicitis have cervical motion tenderness
3. Endometriosis – a menstrual cycle history is helpful to assess the likelihood of endometriosis being the cause
4. Ovarian cyst complications – can be sudden onset
5. Functional pain – often longstanding

Practice point: If PID is in the differential and other conditions are excluded, treat empirically for PID to reduce the risk of short and long-term complications. A full STI screen should be performed and PN pursued. (Even in STI-negative cases, treating partners epidemiologically improves outcomes.)

Section 4: Genital Ulceration

4.1 Genital Ulceration – Herpes Simplex

4.1.1 Aetiology

Anogenital herpes is caused by herpes simplex virus (HSV) types 1 and 2. HSV-1 (the cause of orolabial herpes) is now the most common cause of genital herpes in the UK (>50%). HSV-2 tends to cause more recurrent episodes, with recurrences occurring four times more often than HSV-1. Acquisition is sexual, and the incubation period is between two days and two weeks. However, only one-third of patients develop symptoms at time of acquisition, although most will go on to develop symptoms at some point. The clinical presentation and natural history is hugely variable between patients.

Following infection, the virus migrates along cutaneous nerves to local sensory ganglia and establishes persistent infection. The virus periodically re-activates and may cause a symptomatic episode or shedding of infectious viral material asymptomatically (an important cause of transmission). Newer data suggest that the natural history is far more dynamic, with viral replication occurring very frequently, controlled by T-cell mediated cutaneous immunity.

4.1.2 Management

Management is similar in primary infection and recurrent episodes. Primary infection is commonly more symptomatic and tends to have a longer symptomatic period (can last for up to three weeks). Patients with primary infection can become systemically unwell and appropriate clinical assessment is needed to assess whether patients need management as an inpatient or outpatient.

Refer to Table 17.10 for a summary of clinical features, investigations, treatment and complications.

*Serology – this may be useful in the context of:
– Patients with genital ulceration who do not have an established diagnosis
– Pregnant women
– Women planning to get pregnant who have HSV-1/2 positive partners.
– Asymptomatic partners of HSV-1/2 positive partners

Recurrences are usually self-limiting and can be treated supportively, with episodic antiviral treatment or with suppressive antiviral treatment. Episodic treatment regimens may be the same as treatment for an initial infection and should be initiated within 24–72 hours of onset of symptoms, and may reduce the duration and severity of the attack. Shorter treatment regimens may also be effective (aciclovir 800 mg TDS 2/7, for example). Patients with frequent recurrences (>6/annum) may be offered continuous daily therapy – 'suppressive treatment'. Regimens include:

Aciclovir 400 mg BD

Aciclovir 200 mg QDS

Famciclovir 250 mg BD

Valaciclovir 500 mg OD

Suppression should reduce recurrences by 95% for the duration of therapy. Treatment does not affect the natural history of the infection, but may improve quality of life until host and viral factors reduce recurrences naturally. Recurrence frequency should be assessed after suppression is discontinued. Suppressive treatment should be for 6 to 12 months in the first instance, and may be restarted as required.

Counselling is essential. The disease remains stigmatised, and misinformation is common. Patient advocacy organisations (such as the Herpes Viruses Association) are helpful resources. Key points to include in a conversation with patients newly diagnosed should include:

1. Refraining from sexual intercourse during a symptomatic episode when lesions are present
2. The role of asymptomatic viral shedding as a factor for transmission
3. Disclosure is advised to sexual partners
4. Male condoms can reduce the risk of transmission
5. Suppressive treatment can reduce the risk of transmission in sero-discordant couples

4.1.3 HSV in Pregnancy

Neonatal herpes is rare in the UK. Both HSV-1 and -2 are implicated in infection, causing approximately 50% of neonatal infection each. Transmission is most commonly through direct contact of infected maternal secretions. There are three phenotypes in the neonate:

1. Localised infection on the skin, eyes and/or mouth. This is the mildest form.
2. Localised central nervous system (CNS) disease (encephalitis) with neurological morbidity of up to 70%
3. Disseminated multi-organ involvement. This is the most severe and has a mortality rate of approximately 30%. This is most often associated with primary HSV infection

Factors related to transmission include:

– Maternal infection – whether it is a primary or recurrent episode (the former is high risk; the latter is very low risk)
– Presence of trans-placental maternal neutralising antibodies
– Duration of rupture of membranes (ROM) prior to delivery
– The use of fetal scalp electrodes
– Mode of delivery

The risk for the neonate is greatest if the mother has acquired primary infection in her third trimester (particularly if the infection was acquired within 6 weeks of delivery). This is due to high levels of viral shedding and the fact that the timeframe is likely to be too short for the formation of protective trans-placental passage of antibodies before delivery.

The management of herpes in pregnancy is summarised in Table 17.11.

Disseminated infection is associated with primary infection. Importantly, recurrent episodes in the third trimester can cause the more localised forms of disease, as recurrent episodes are often asymptomatic or unrecognized. [9]

4.2 Genital Ulceration – Syphilis

4.2.1 Aetiology

The spirochete bacterium *Treponema pallidum* is the aetiological agent of venereal syphilis. Rare at the end of the twentieth century, cases in the UK have risen >600% since 2000, mainly among men who have sex with men. Transmission occurs through direct contact of infected lesions (acquired) or vertically (congenital).

4.2.2 Staging and Clinical Features

Acquired syphilis is categorised as symptomatic or latent, and as early or late. Early disease is diagnosed within two years of acquisition, late disease after two years. Latent disease exists in both stages, and neuro-syphilis may occur early (typically meningo-vascular syphilis or mononeuritis, especially of the cranial nerves) or late (tabes dorsalis and general paresis).

Staging and clinical features are as per Fig. 17.6.

Figure 17.7 shows the features of the chancre, the site of initial inoculation. These are anaesthetic, indurated papules that occur most commonly on genital

Table 17.11 Summary of management points for primary and recurrent anogenital herpes infection in pregnancy

	First and second trimester	Third trimester	Labour
First episode	– Diagnosis with swab PCR at GU clinic – Treatment with Aciclovir 400 mg TDS for 5 days – Inform obstetrician or refer if under midwife – Continue pregnancy plan/birth plan as previous – Aciclovir suppression therapy 400 mg TDS daily from 36 weeks till delivery	– Some evidence of preterm labour, low birthweight, stillbirth – Treatment with Aciclovir 400 mg TDS for 5 days – This should then be continued as suppression at the same dose until delivery – Caesarean section (CS) is recommended (risk of transmission is 41%) – Differentiate primary and recurrent episode with a type-specific IgG, especially if <6 weeks till delivery	General management points: – all pregnant women with lesions at delivery should be referred to the neonatology team – swabs should be taken (although they will not be available in time) Primary: – All women should be offered Caesarean sections (CS) – Intravenous aciclovir intrapartum to the mother (5 mg/kg TDS) and then to the child (20 mg/kg) in those not having a CS (the risk of transmission untreated is 41%) – Avoid instrumentation in vaginal deliveries Recurrent: – The risk of transmission is low (0–3%) – Vaginal delivery should be offered to all women – Invasive procedures may be used if required – Spontaneous ROM – no evidence to guide management here but some would advocate expediting delivery
Recurrent episode	– Risk of transmission is low (0–3%) – Does not necessarily have to be treated with antivirals, it can be managed supportively – Consider suppression at 36 weeks – insufficient evidence to suggest a reduction in neonatal transmission but does reduce viral shedding and recurrence and therefore the need for CS		

sites, but may occur anywhere. Congenital syphilis is also categorised as early and late, with a two-year cutoff. In early congenital syphilis (age less than two years at diagnosis), signs include rash, haemorrhagic rhinitis ('bloody sniffles'), lymphadenopathy, hepatosplenomegaly and skeletal abnormalities. Syphilis diagnosed over the age of two years tends to cause chronic inflammatory changes with manifestations similar to those of gummatous disease in adults.

The less common manifestations of congenital syphilis are shown in Table 17.12.

4.2.3 Diagnosis

1. Dark ground microscopy from infectious lesions
2. Polymerase chain reaction (PCR) from infectious lesions
3. Clinical features – e.g. the rash of secondary syphilis, condylomata lata
4. Serology – can be classified as specific or non-specific. Of note, the serological investigations

cannot differentiate between syphilis and endemic treponematoses such as yaws or pinta. Therefore, clinical judgment and a thorough sexual history are needed.

Non-specific Serological Tests

1. Venereal Diseases Research Laboratory (VDRL)
2. Rapid Plasma Reagin (RPR)

Specific Tests

1. ELISA Immune Assay (EIA)
2. Treponema Pallidum Haemagglutination Assay (TPHA)
3. Treponema Pallidum Particle Agglutination (TPPA)

Positive specific serological tests should be confirmed with another specific test and a non-specific test. Positive non-specific tests are expressed as a dilutional titre (e.g. 1:16), with higher dilutions representing greater anti-treponemal immune

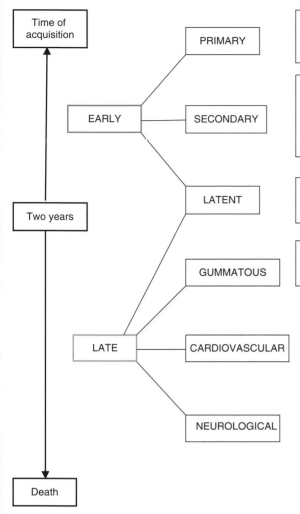

Time of acquisition	PRIMARY	A single papule with regional lymphadenopathy. This develops into an indurated, anaesthetic ulcer with a clean base that discharges clear serum –the chancre. Incubation is approximately three weeks (classically 9–90 days).

EARLY

SECONDARY

Approximately 4–10 weeks after the chancre, 25% of those will develop secondary syphilis. This is a multisystem insult with:
- Rash (maculopapular / macular / papular)
- Lymphadenopathy
- Mucous patches
- Condylomata lata (highly infectious warty lesions)

LATENT

Latent syphilis is a quiescent stage of the disease that can occur both with the early stage (<2 years) or the in the late stage (>2 years)

Two years

GUMMATOUS

Inflammatory, granulomatous, destructive lesions that mainly affect skin and bone. Affects approximately 15% of late syphilis patients.

LATE

CARDIOVASCULAR

10% of late syphilis patients will get cardiovascular problems:
- Aortitis (+/-aneurysm formation)
- Aortic regurgitation
- Heart failure
- Angina

NEUROLOGICAL

7% of late syphilis patients will get neurosyphilis:
- Asymptomatic
- Meningo-vascular
- General paresis; memory impairment, personality change, emotionally labile, dementia, psychosis
- Tabes dorsalis; areflexia, shooting pains, Charcot Joints, sensory ataxia, Argyll-Robertson pupil

Death

Figure 17.6 Clinical features and stages of venereal syphilis

Table 17.12 Comparison between early and late congenital syphilis

Congenital early syphilis	Congenital late syphilis
– Condylamata lata	– Hutchinson's incisors
– Mucous patches	– Clutton's joints
– Perioral fissures	– Mulberry molars
– Glomerulonephritis	– High palatal arch
– Haemolysis	– Sensorineural deafness
– Thrombocytopenia	– Frontal bossing
– Periostitis	– Mandibular protrusion
– Neurological	– Saddle nose deformity
	– Intellectual disability
	– Cranial nerve palsies

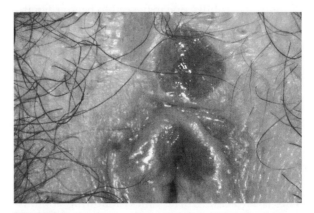

Figure17.7 The chancre of primary syphilis. This patient has two chancres in close proximity.

Table 17.13 Examples of serological results and corresponding clinical interpretation

Syphilis EIA	TPPA	Current RPR level	Last previous RPR level	Possible diagnoses
Positive	Positive	1:128	Negative	Active (likely acute) infection
Negative	Negative	Negative	Nil previous	Never been exposed
Positive	Positive	Negative	1:32 (12 months ago)	Previous treated infection
Positive	Positive	1:2	1:2 (3 months ago)	Possible latent infection Possible serofast result Possible untreated infection Possible inadequately treated infection
Positive	Negative	Negative	Nil previous	Likely biological false positive

activity. Higher titres are typically seen in early and symptomatic disease. Titres are used to detect response to treatment. When positive, titres should have fallen at least four-fold six months after treatment (e.g. 1:32 to 1:8 or less). Failure to achieve 'serological cure' may be due to treatment failure (from non-compliance, re-infection or CNS disease). A small proportion of patients fail to achieve low-level titres or negative results. Provided treatment has been given and relapse or re-infection excluded, this state is termed 'sero-fast'.

Examples of serological patterns, and their interpretation, are given in Table 17.13.

Patients should be fully examined, including examination of the mucous membranes, skin, genitals, eyes, and central and peripheral nervous system.

4.2.4 Management

General:

1. Partner notification; in early disease, a look back period of three months is sufficient. In secondary and late syphilis, one may need to back as far as two years ago. All contacts within those look back periods should be offered epidemiological treatment.
2. Abstain from sexual intercourse until after the lesions have healed (in primary) and two weeks after treatment has been completed.

4.2.5 Treatment

See Figure 17.8.

4.2.6 Jarisch-Herxheimer Reaction

This is an acute febrile illness following administration of an antimicrobial that can cause myalgia,

headache, and chills but usually resolves within 24 hours of onset. It occurs as a result of lysis of spirochaetes. Patients must be counselled on the possibility of this reaction occurring with the use of penicillins, and can be reassured and advised to use simple analgesia and anti-pyretics.

4.2.7 Syphilis in Pregnancy

Syphilis is easily transmissible via placental passage in vertical transmission, where the risk of transmission is greatest in early disease. It is recommended that a full obstetric history should be taken to identify any risk of congenital disease in previous live births and any adverse outcomes in pregnancies that may indicate previous/current infection. Management of women being treated should be jointly undertaken with fetal medicine and paediatrics. Good communication between all is key to successful management.

Infection in early pregnancy may result in polyhydramnios, miscarriage, pre-term labour, stillbirth and hydrops and placental oedema.

Specific Considerations in Pregnancy

- All pregnant women should have a full sexual health screen during antenatal screening
- If risk is recognised, repeat screening should be done later in the pregnancy
- If women have been cured prior to pregnancy, and are not at risk of re-infection, the neonate does not require testing
- Re-treatment is indicated where there is uncertainty of treatment *or* the serological cure is in doubt
- Treatment for early syphilis in the third trimester should be benzathine penicillin followed by a second dose one week later

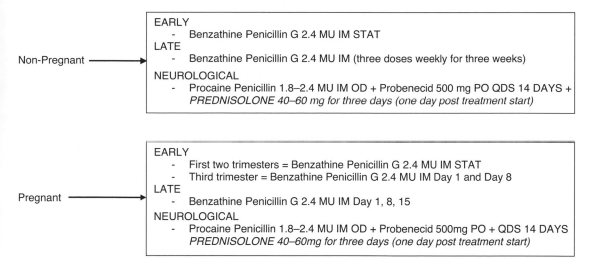

Non-Pregnant

EARLY
- Benzathine Penicillin G 2.4 MU IM STAT
LATE
- Benzathine Penicillin G 2.4 MU IM (three doses weekly for three weeks)
NEUROLOGICAL
- Procaine Penicillin 1.8–2.4 MU IM OD + Probenecid 500 mg PO QDS 14 DAYS +
  PREDNISOLONE 40–60 mg for three days (one day post treatment start)

Pregnant

EARLY
- First two trimesters = Benzathine Penicillin G 2.4 MU IM STAT
- Third trimester = Benzathine Penicillin G 2.4 MU IM Day 1 and Day 8
LATE
- Benzathine Penicillin G 2.4 MU IM Day 1, 8, 15
NEUROLOGICAL
- Procaine Penicillin 1.8–2.4 MU IM OD + Probenecid 500mg PO + QDS 14 DAYS
  PREDNISOLONE 40–60mg for three days (one day post treatment start)

NB – All late syphilis with cardiovascular involvement should have prednisolone 40–60mg for three days (one day post treatment start) included in the treatment, as with late syphilis with neurological involvement.

Figure 17.8 Treatment of syphilis

– A template birth plan can be found in the 2015 BASHH guidelines on syphilis

4.2.8 Congenital Syphilis: Diagnosis and Treatment

Assessment of the neonate should take place in all cases where the mother was treated or re-treated for syphilis during the pregnancy. Serological examination of neonatal blood (not cord blood) should comprise EIA IgM and VRDL/RPR. A positive IgM or a high or rising VDRL/RPR is suggestive of congenital infection. In children, intravenous penicillin therapy is preferable due to the pain caused by intramuscular injections. Thus:

1st line treatment: Benzyl penicillin sodium 60–90 mg/kg daily IV (in divided doses given as - 30 mg/kg 12 hourly) in the first seven days of life and 8 hourly thereafter for a further 3 days for a total of 10 days

4.2.9 Follow-Up

The recommended follow-up must involve assessment serologically and clinically. The recommendation is for 3-, 6- and 12-month follow-up from treatment and six monthly thereafter until the VDRL/RPR is negative or sero-fast.

Section 5: Genital Lumps and Infestations

5.1 Genital Lumps – Anogenital Warts

5.1.1 Aetiology

There are more than 100 human papilloma virus (HPV) genotypes. Ninety percent of anogenital warts are caused by HPV types 6 and 11. They are one of the commonest conditions treated in the sexual health setting, with more than 130,000 cases treated in the UK per annum. The bivalent HPV vaccine was introduced in the UK in 2008 for girls and 2018 for boys aged 12–13. This was intended to provide protection against oncogenic virus strains 16 and 18 before sexual debut. The bivalent vaccine was upgraded to quadrivalent to include genotypes 6 and 11 in 2012. Both vaccines are highly efficacious, and many countries (including the UK) are seeing reductions in first presentations of anogenital warts in young heterosexual women and men, and in cervical dysplasia. No reductions have been seen in men having sex with men, although vaccination has been offered to this group since 2017 via sexual health clinics in men up to 45 years of age.

Warts are benign epithelial skin tumours. They can be mulitmorphic in appearance, ranging from soft and fleshy growths to hard, keratinized warts. They tend to occur at sites of microtrauma secondary to penetrative sexual intercourse. HPV DNA is found in approximately 10–20% of 15–49-year-olds, and the majority will have no symptoms. Most clear the infection within two years, but remain at risk of infection of other genotypes. The risk of symptomatic and persistent infection is increased five-fold in smokers.

Sites and locations of lesions can include the vagina, the cervix, urethral meatus and anal canal. The incubation period for HPV is between three weeks and eight months. Rarely, warts can grow rapidly causing local invasion and destruction; these lesions are known as Buschke Lowenstein lesions.

5.1.2 Diagnosis

This is a clinical diagnosis although more detailed visualisation may be required when seen on the cervix with colposcopy. Consider malignant change in atypical presentations (e.g. hyper/hypopigmentation, contact bleeding, pruritus, immunodeficiency or previous history of intraepithelial neoplasia).

5.1.3 Assessment

Mapping is required to aid follow up and comparison. Information recorded should include site, size, shape morphology number and distribution. A speculum exam should be undertaken in women as part of their initial assessment.

5.1.4 Management:

General

- Smoking cessation

Specific Regimens (Table 17.14)

All treatments should have an end of treatment review. This should include assessments on:
- Response to treatment
- Need for further treatment
- Change in treatment –> not tolerating current regimen, <50% response at week 4–5

5.1.5 Pregnancy

Vertical transmission of HPV is rare, and the only serious condition in the neonate is respiratory papillomatosis. Changes in humoral immunity may mean warts appear for the first time or worsen in pregnancy, especially in the third trimester. Treatment is usually delayed until after delivery, and caesarean sections are not indicated for women with anogenital warts. Conservative management is often appropriate. Reassure the patient that typically 95% of cases resolve spontaneously by six weeks post-partum.

However, if the warts are numerous, treatment may reduce the risk of transmission at vaginal delivery, in which case cryotherapy, ablative therapy and excision are deemed appropriate treatments to use during pregnancy.

Caesarean section is indicated only if there is obstruction of the vaginal outlet from large warts or large cervical warts. Podophyllotoxin and 5FU are teratogenic in pregnancy and are therefore contraindicated in pregnancy.

5.1.6 Special Situations (Table 15.15)

5.2 Genital Lumps – Molluscum Contagiosum

5.2.1 Aetiology

Molluscum is a self-limiting infection by the DNA pox virus molluscum contagiosum. Most infections are probably asymptomatic. It causes an eruption of smooth, round papules with a central punctum (Fig. 17.9). Genital infection by molluscum can occur in the pubic region, the genitals, the buttock and the abdomen. Increased rates and more severe disease tend to occur in immunocompromised individuals – in particular, those with late-stage HIV.

Lesions can occur in crops of up to 30. They can cause itch, discomfort or have superadded bacterial infection, though in the majority of cases, they are painless. The differential diagnoses include warts, cysts, sebaceous glands and basal cell carcinoma.

In immunocompromised patients, it is important to rule out disseminated fungal infections such as cryptococcosis, histoplasmosis, and aspergillosis.

5.2.2 Management

The mainstay of treatment is expectant. The condition is self-limiting, but the time to spontaneous clearance is highly variable. If patients attend because of cosmetic reasons, stigma or symptoms (itch, bacterial infection, discomfort), then treatment with podophyllotoxin, imiquimod or liquid nitrogen therapy can be used, although all are off-license, and there are limited data to support one treatment over another.

Table 17.14 Summary of treatments of anogenital warts

	Topical				Ablative		
podophyllotoxin	**Imiquimod**	**Catephen 10%**	**TCA (trichloroacetic acid)**	**Cryotherapy**	**Excision**	**Laser**
– Self-applied – Three consecutive days BD treatment with a 4-day break – Review after 4–5 weeks – Can cause soreness and ulcerations – Avoid unprotected sexual intercourse – Avoid in pregnancy	– Self-applied – Stimulates innate and acquired immune response – Apply three times a week for 6–10 hours and then wash off – Can be used for up to 16 weeks – Avoid unprotected sex – Can cause skin irritation – Review if no response in 12–16 weeks – Caution in use in patients who have autoimmune conditions or inflammatory skin conditions – Not approved in pregnancy	– Self-applied – Green tea extract – Apply three times a week for up to 16 weeks	– Caustic agent that causes chemical coagulation and necrosis – Used weekly in specialist setting – Use is limited due to significant side effects (dermal ulceration) – Intense burning occurs for 5–10 minutes after application – Petroleum jelly should be used on surrounding skin	– The use of liquid nitrogen spray to cause cytolysis at the dermal-epidermal junction – Applied directly to the wart with a surrounding margin ('halo') which blisters and causes local necrosis – Healing takes 7–10 days – Repeat weekly – Review in 4 weeks and consider alternatives if no response at 4 weeks	– Should be considered for large or pedunculated warts	– Vaporisation of warts – Good for large volume warts – Note – masks should be worn to avoid respiratory HPV transmission from plumes produced in laser and electro surgery

Table 17.15 Treatment of specific situations in the treatment of anogenital warts

Intra-vaginal	Cervical	Intra-meatal	Intra-anal
Cryotherapy, electrosurgery and TCA can be used but usually no treatment is advised	Routine colposcopy is not recommended for cervical warts. Cryotherapy, TCA, laser, and excision can be used but repeat examination should be performed to assess treatment efficacy	Cryotherapy, laser, podophyllotoxin, imiquimod can be used, but if lesions are deeper, referral to urology for surgical ablation is required	Cryotherapy, imiquimod (although not licensed), laser, electrosurgery and TCA can be used

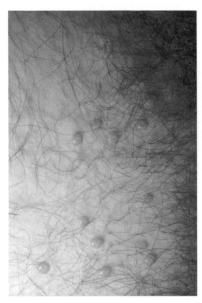

Figure 17.9 Smooth, umbilicated papules typical of molluscum contagiosum infection

Provide verbal and written information. Basic advice includes avoiding waxing, not sharing bed linen/towels, risk of autoinoculation and to avoid squeezing (can cause added bacterial infection and worsen spread). Always offer a full sexual health screen. Partner notification is not necessary.

5.2.3 Pregnancy and Breastfeeding
Cryotherapy is safe in pregnancy and breastfeeding. Podophyllotoxin and imiquimod should be avoided.

5.3 Infestations – Scabies

5.3.1 Aetiology
Sarcoptes scabei is a parasitic mite that burrows under the skin and lays eggs during its lifespan of approximately four to six weeks. Any part of the body of the host may be affected and transmission is through skin to skin contact.

Primary infection may be asymptomatic and symptoms can take up to four to six weeks to develop. Pruritus is the most common symptom and can be severe.

5.3.2 Signs
- Silvery lines may be visible indicating burrows along the interdigital folds, wrists, nipples and elbows.
- Papules or nodules may be seen around the genital area
- Superadded bacterial infection from excoriation and itching may occur

5.3.3 Diagnosis
The diagnosis is usually clinical, but mites may be visualised by taking skin scrapings from burrows and observing mites under light microscopy.

5.3.4 Management
General
- Avoid close contact with others while being treated
- Contaminated bedding and clothes should be washed at high temperatures (>50 degrees)
- Advise that the itch may persist for up to four to six weeks

Specific Treatment
- Permethrin 5% cream applied in all areas neck down, taking care around mucous membranes
- Malathion 0.5% aqueous lotion

Both are usually applied overnight for approximately 12 hours and then washed off. Application may be repeated in one week.

5.4 Infestations – Pediculosis
Pubic lice are seen with less frequency in sexual health clinics than previously. The condition is associated

with crowded living, and poor personal hygiene in young, sexually active people and it is associated with other sexually acquired infections. Transmission is via skin to skin contact.

5.4.1 Clinical Features

- Intense itching/irritation due to hypersensitivity
- Erythema around area of itch

5.4.2 Diagnosis

Lice can be visualised on the skin by the naked eye, and crabs, lice or eggs may be seen.

5.4.3 Management

General

- Partner notification should be carried out with a lookback period of three months

Specific Treatment

- Malathion 5% apply and leave on the skin for 12 hours and then wash off
- Permethrin 1% cream rinse (safe in pregnancy and breastfeeding)
- Eyelashes – Permethrin lotion can be applied on the lashes for 10 minutes ensuring *eyes are shut throughout* OR soft paraffin twice a day to the eyelashes for 8–10 days. This suffocates the lice.

Section 6 – Blood-Borne Viruses

6.1 Human Immunodeficiency Virus (HIV)

UNAIDS states that the number of individuals living with HIV globally exceeds 36 million. The most common mechanism of transmission is sexual transmission, but the virus may be transmitted vertically, and from unscreened blood products and shared injecting drug equipment.

In the UK in 2019, 105,200 people were thought to be living with HIV infection, 6% of whom did not know their HIV-positive status. 42% of adults were diagnosed late, with a CD4 count at diagnosis of <350 cells/mcl. Late diagnosis incurs significant health costs, and undiagnosed HIV contributes to on-going transmission.

However, the advent of highly active antiretroviral therapy (ART) means people living with HIV can live healthy lives with normal to near-normal life expectancies if diagnosed at early stages of the infection.

Understanding the pathogenesis of HIV-1 infection is important in the management of patients but also the development of new drug therapies and novel preventative/prophylactic strategies such as a vaccination.

6.1.1 Aetiology

HIV is a retrovirus from the lentivirus family; there are two known types HIV-1 and HIV-2. Both types, as with other lentiviruses, have a chronic disease course with a period of latency and persistent viral replication. Both infect and replicate within cluster of differentiation 4 (CD4) immune cells, most notably T-helper cells.

The structure of the HIV particle contains a lipoprotein membrane, the capsid (containing p24 proteins), and two copies of the HIV-1 RNA genome. Within this structure are enzymes necessary for viral replication – reverse transcriptase, integrase and protease.

CD4 is a glycoprotein that binds T cell receptors. The gp120 protein exposed on the surface of HIV binds CD4 and through this step gains viral entry. Membrane fusion allows the capsid to be introduced into the target cell cytoplasm where reverse transcriptase creates non-integrated HIV DNA. Integration (using viral integrase) into the host cell genome occurs after the transportation of the complex into the host cell nucleus. Synthesis of new virions can then be achieved (Fig. 17.10).

6.1.2 Natural History of HIV Infection

Without effective antiretroviral treatment, HIV replication continues unopposed with progressive loss of immune function leading to the development of opportunistic infections and malignancies. The mean time between initial infection and development of an Acquired Immunodeficiency Syndrome (AIDS) defining illness is approximately 10 years. The time between infection and death can be categorised into primary infection, early, middle (chronic phase) and advanced infection (leading to AIDS – Fig. 17.11).

Acute infection or seroconversion illness occurs within a few weeks of initial infection and is categorised by fever, lymphadenopathy, maculopapular rash and myalgia. Up to 90% of patient experience seroconversion illness, but the spectrum of severity is broad, and the symptoms are non-specific. The syndrome can last for up to four weeks. Clinically asymptomatic infection occurs after this and can continue

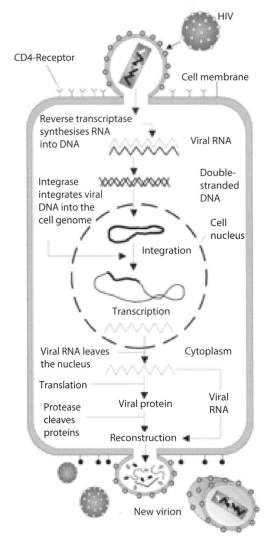

Figure 17.10 Life-cycle of human immunodeficiency virus

for several years. Abnormal immune function can manifest after this period, although this may not include AIDS-defining illnesses. Non-AIDS-defining conditions include herpes zoster infection, cervical intra-epithelial neoplasia, oral candidiasis and chronic vulvovaginal candidiasis. These conditions should prompt HIV testing. See Table 17.16 for the classification of HIV disease as defined by the World Health Organisation (WHO).

6.1.3 Modern Management of HIV

People living with HIV (PLWH) can expect a favourable prognosis in the era of effective antiretroviral therapy. HIV infection is now widely recognised

as a chronic, manageable, albeit lifelong condition. A full and normal life expectancy is anticipated with treatment. This has been made possible with the advent of newer, safer and more effective drug regimens, of which nine are single tablet preparations.

Antiretroviral therapies fall under five broad categories by mode of action:

1. Nucleoside reverse transcriptase inhibitors (NRTIs)
2. Non-nucleoside reverse transcriptase inhibitors (NNRTIs)
3. Protease inhibitors (PIs)
4. Integrase inhibitors (INIs)
5. Entry inhibitors

The British HIV Association (BHIVA) recommends that all therapy-naïve patients should be started on ART containing two NRTIs and one of the following:
– A ritonavir- or cobicistat-boosted PI
– NNRTI
– INI

The consultations around starting treatment should encourage patient involvement, support, adherence counselling and a full drug history to avoid and manage drug-drug interactions. The aim of treatment is to arrest viral replication and facilitate and preserve immune recovery. Patients on successful treatment have undetectable levels of HIV RNA in blood. An undetectable viral load eliminates the risk of transmission to others (including mother to child in pregnancy). This concept of undetectable = untransmittable (U=U) is scientifically justified, and means HIV treatment is an important HIV prevention tool

Indications for starting antiretroviral therapy:

All patients living with HIV should be offered antiretroviral therapy, and they should start as soon as they are ready.

6.1.4 HIV Transmission Routes

The main routes of transmission are:
– Unprotected sexual intercourse with an HIV positive partner
– Sharing injecting paraphernalia with an HIV infected individual
– Vertical transmission

Table 17.16 WHO clinical staging of HIV/AIDS for adults and adolescents

Clinical stage	Clinical conditions or symptoms
Primary HIV Infection	Asymptomatic Acute retroviral syndrome
Clinical Stage 1	Asymptomatic Persistent generalized lymphadenopathy
Clinical Stage 2	Moderate unexplained weight loss (<10% of presumed or measured body weight) Recurrent respiratory infections (sinusitis, tonsillitis, otitis media, and pharyngitis) Herpes zoster Angular cheilitis Recurrent oral ulceration Papular pruritic eruptions Seborrheic dermatitis Fungal nail infections
Clinical Stage 3	Unexplained severe weight loss (>10% of presumed or measured body weight) Unexplained chronic diarrhoea for >1 month Unexplained persistent fever for >1 month (>37.6°C, intermittent or constant) Persistent oral candidiasis (thrush) Oral hairy leukoplakia Pulmonary tuberculosis (current) Severe presumed bacterial infections (e.g. pneumonia, empyema, pyomyositis, bone or joint infection, meningitis, bacteraemia) Acute necrotizing ulcerative stomatitis, gingivitis, or periodontitis Unexplained anaemia (haemoglobin <8 g/dL) Neutropenia (neutrophils <500 cells/μL) Chronic thrombocytopenia (platelets <50,000 cells/μL)
Clinical Stage 4	HIV wasting syndrome, as defined by the CDC as wasting caused by HIV (involuntary weight loss >10% of baseline body weight) associated with either chronic diarrhoea (two or more loose stools per day for ≥1 month) or chronic weakness and documented fever for ≥1 month *Pneumocystis* pneumonia Recurrent severe bacterial pneumonia Chronic herpes simplex infection (orolabial, genital or anorectal site for >1 month or visceral herpes at any site) Oesophageal candidiasis (or candidiasis of trachea, bronchi, or lungs) Extrapulmonary tuberculosis Kaposi sarcoma Cytomegalovirus infection (retinitis or infection of other organs) Central nervous system toxoplasmosis HIV encephalopathy Cryptococcosis, extrapulmonary (including meningitis) Disseminated nontuberculosis mycobacteria infection Progressive multifocal leukoencephalopathy Candida of the trachea, bronchi, or lungs Chronic cryptosporidiosis (with diarrhoea) Chronic isosporiasis Disseminated mycosis (e.g. histoplasmosis, coccidioidomycosis, penicilliosis) Recurrent nontyphoidal *Salmonella* bacteraemia Lymphoma (cerebral or B-cell non-Hodgkin) Invasive cervical carcinoma Atypical disseminated leishmaniasis Symptomatic HIV-associated nephropathy Symptomatic HIV-associated cardiomyopathy Reactivation of American trypanosomiasis (meningoencephalitis or myocarditis)

Rare routes of transmission include transmission via infected blood products, although this is less relevant since the introduction of screening of blood-borne viruses in blood products in the UK in the early 1980s.

6.1.5 A Note on Pre-test HIV Testing Discussions

All medical professionals should be able to take informed consent from a patient for an HIV test. Current practice aims to normalise the process and

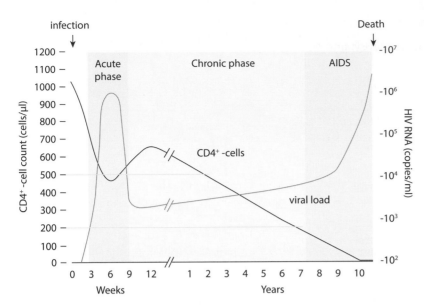

Figure 17.11 Natural history of HIV infection

avoid lengthy conversations around testing. Testing should be offered universally at:

– Genito-urinary clinics
– Antenatal clinics
– Termination of pregnancy clinics
– Drug dependence programmes
– Blood-borne viruses / TB / lymphoma services

Testing should routinely be performed in:

– Blood donors
– Dialysis patients
– Organ donors and recipients

The outline of the pre-test discussion should be two-fold:

1. Benefits of testing
2. How the results will be given

Laboratory tests are usually performed on serum. Point-of-care tests may use capillary blood (a finger-prick test) or oral fluid (saliva), collected by swab.

The recommended blood test should be a test that detects the presence of HIV antibodies and p24 antigen (a virally derived antigen detectable in early infection). These are known as fourth-generation assays and are able to reduce the period between infection and reliable diagnosis to six weeks. All positive results should be followed up with a second confirmatory test. Antibody-only tests have a 'window period' of 6–12 weeks.

6.1.6   HIV and Pregnancy

The mother-to-child transmission (MTCT) rate without treatment, and including breastfeeding, is approximately 40%. The most important element in vertical transmission is viral load at the time of delivery. With appropriate management in pre-and post-pregnancy, rates of transmission are very low in the UK (overall rate of 0.57%). The risk factors and protective factors against MTCT are listed in Table 17.17.

Guidance from BHIVA [10] suggests that:

– All pregnant women with a new diagnosis of HIV should be offered a full sexual health screen for other STIs
– For monitoring purposes, women already known to be HIV-positive and stable on treatment should have CD4 count monitoring at baseline and at delivery
– All women should commence anti-retroviral therapy by week 24, but should be started as soon as possible to ensure an undetectable viral load is achieved by week 36
– Any woman in rupture of membranes (ROM), labour or requiring emergency delivery without a documented HIV test should have a point of care test
– New starters on ART should have viral load monitoring at baseline, at 2–4 weeks after starting therapy, each trimester, at week 36 and at delivery, with liver function test monitoring with each visit

Table 17.17 The risk factors and protective factors against mother-to-child transmission

Protective factors against MTCT	Risk factors for MTCT
Elective caesarean section	High maternal viral load
Mother on combined antiretroviral therapy	Low CD4 T cell count, AIDS-defining illness of the mother
Prophylactic antiretroviral therapy for baby	Vaginal delivery with viral load >50 copies without ART
No breastfeeding	Premature rupture of membranes of >4 h, preterm infants (<37 weeks of gestation)
	Breastfeeding

– No routine dose adjustments of antiretrovirals are required in pregnancy
– Women starting therapy during pregnancy should usually be started on a combination containing efavirenz + 2 NRTIs, or atazanavir/ritonavir + 2 NRTIs
– Women already on ART at conception should usually continue their existing regimen, with the exception of regimens that have been demonstrated to show lower pharmacokinetics in pregnancy such as darunavir/cobicistat and elvitegravir/cobicistat, or where there is an absence of pharmacokinetic data such as for raltegravir 1200 mg once daily. A woman conceiving on dolutegravir should see her physician as soon as possible to discuss current evidence on neural tube defects

Most modern antiretrovirals are believed to be safe in pregnancy. Data are held in a national register of use in pregnancy.

In all women who have not achieved an undetectable viral load at week 36, recommendations are:

– A full review of adherence and co-medications review should be undertaken
– A viral resistance test should be undertaken
– Therapeutic drug monitoring should be considered
– Optimise ART under specialist review
– Consider intensification of ART

Table 17.18 summarizes the obstetric management of women living with HIV infection.

6.2 Viral Hepatitis

6.2.1 Hepatitis A

Hepatitis A is a highly infectious viral infection primary transmitted faeco-orally. It mainly affects children in developing countries but can also affect men who have sex with men and injecting drug users. The incubation period is between 2–6 weeks.

Fifty percent of patients are asymptomatic, and those that do have symptoms may have a prodromal illness with lethargy and malaise. Jaundice and right upper quadrant pain can occur, and this illness may last for up to three weeks.

Vaccinations should be offered to travellers going to endemic regions, injecting drug users, HIV positive patients, and patients with chronic hepatitis B and C. Vaccination may be offered to men who have sex with men, but it is not routinely recommended.

See the following discussion on treatment, complications, vaccination and pregnancy/breastfeeding.

6.2.2 Hepatitis B

The clinical features of acute hepatitis B are similar to those of acute hepatitis A, although 10–50% will have no symptoms of acute infection. Eighty percent of children with acute hepatitis B, and 20% of adults, will go on to develop chronic infection as a failure of immune clearance. Chronic hepatitis B (defined as the presence of hepatitis B surface antigen in blood) can progress to chronic liver disease, cirrhosis and hepatocellular carcinoma. Higher levels of hepatitis B DNA predict risks of complications. People at risk of chronic progression include HIV positive patients, chronic kidney disease, immunosuppression and children infected by vertical transmission.

Those that should be offered screening include:

– Injecting drug users (other parenteral routes – acupuncture, tattoos)
– Men who have sex with men
– Commercial sex workers
– Sexual contacts of
– Sexual assault victims
– Those from endemic regions

Patients at risk of hepatitis B infection (the groups listed here) should be offered vaccination if they are

Table 17.18 Summary of obstetric management in HIV

Antenatal care	Delivery	Intrapartum zidovudine	Neonatal management	Neonatal testing	Rupture of membranes
Ultrasound imaging as per national guidance	Women with VL<50 and on combined antiretrovirals at week 36 should be offered vaginal delivery	Recommended in mothers with VL>1000 copies/ml in labour, ROM, PLCS	All infant PEP should be started within four hours of birth	First test should be done in the first 48 hours (non-breastfeeding)	Mothers with VL<50 RNA copies/ml should have immediate induction of labour
Invasive fetal sampling; avoided until an up to date viral load is known. Can be undertaken in women with VL<50 RNA copies/ml. If not on ART and the invasive diagnostic test procedure cannot be delayed it is recommended that women should commence ART to include raltegravir and be given a single dose of nevirapine 2–4 hours prior to the procedure	Mothers with a VL between 50 and 399 RNA copies/ml at 36 weeks should be considered for PLCS, taking into account length of ART use, adherence issues, obstetric factors and the mother's views	Recommended in women who are untreated with unknown VL	Zidovudine monotherapy should be started in infants with mothers who have undetectable viral loads. Two weeks therapy if: • The woman has been on ART for longer than 10 weeks AND • Two documented maternal HIV viral loads <50 HIV RNA copies/ml during pregnancy at least 4 weeks apart AND • Maternal HIV viral load <50 HIV RNA copies/ml at or after 36 weeks Extend to FOUR weeks if the criteria above are not met OR the infant is born prematurely (<34 weeks) but most recent maternal HIV viral load is <50 HIV RNA copies/ml	Then two weeks post PEP (at six weeks of age) (non-breastfeeding)	Mothers with VL 50–399 RNA copies/ml; immediate CS should be considered
Combined trisomy testing is recommended in HIV positive women	Mothers with VL>400 RNA copies/ml at 36 weeks should have PLCS recommended	The use of intrapartum intravenous zidovudine infusion can be considered in women on ART with a plasma HIV viral load between 50 and 1000 HIV RNA copies/ml	Three drug combination therapy is indicated in all infants born to mothers with detectable viral loads at 36 weeks	Then at two months post PEP (age three months) (non-breastfeeding)	Mothers with VL>400 RNA copies/ml; immediate CS is recommended

External cephalic version can be offered to women with plasma viral load >50 HIV RNA copies/ml	Vaginal delivery after Caesarean (VBAC) should be offered to all women with VL<50 RNA copies/ml on antiretrovirals	Routine immunisation should be carried out in all infants as per national guidance	PROM>34 weeks should be treated as term ROM but with the addition of Group B streptococcus prophylaxis for women >34 but <37 weeks
	Breastfeeding mothers should have additional monthly testing of both mother and baby	HIV antibody testing for seroconversion should be done at 18 months of age (non-breastfeeding)	PROM<34 weeks: IM steroids Virological control optimisation MDT approach to timing and mode of delivery

Note: PROM = premature rupture of membranes, VL = viral load, PLCS = pre-labour Caesarean section

Table 17.19 Summary table for viral hepatitis A, B and C

	Incubation period	Diagnosis	Treatment	Complications	Vaccination schedule	Pregnancy/breastfeeding
Hepatitis A	2–6 weeks	IgM IgG	Information Notifiable Supportive	Fulminant hepatitis (0.4%) Admission for supportive treatment	0, 6–12 months	Premature labour Miscarriage Uncertain breastfeeding risk – avoid
Hepatitis B	6 weeks–6 months	SEE TABLE	**Acute:** Information PN/notifiable Avoid sex Avoid alcohol Assess for need for admission **Chronic:** Information Referral to hepatology Vaccination against hepatitis A Contact tracing Disclosure to future sexual partners	Chronic carriage (5–10%) Chronic liver disease (cirrhosis, hepatocellular carcinoma) Acute liver failure <1%	**Ultra-rapid:** 0, 1, 3 weeks and 12-month booster **Rapid:** 0, 1, 2 months and 12-month booster **Standard:** 0, 1, 6 months	Premature labour Miscarriage 90% vertical transmission with no intervention (90% of those infants will become chronic carriers) All infants must be vaccinated at birth Hep B specific immunoglobulin (200 I.U. IM) given to infants with highly infectious mothers (e antigen positive) Vaccination +/- immunoglobulin reduces vertical transmission rates by >90% Tenofovir monotherapy may be considered in third trimester in women with high viral loads
Hepatitis C	4–20 weeks	RNA	As above in HBV Specific: Liver staging with elastography Ultrasound liver Vaccination for hepatitis A + B Pegulated interferon and ribavirin are no longer recommended Direct Acting Antivirals (DAAs) are increasingly available	Chronic infection Chronic liver disease (cirrhosis, hepatocellular carcinoma)	None available	Low rates of vertical transmission: 5% Higher rates in HIV+ (7%) No clearly demonstrated intervention to reduced transmission Ribavirin is teratogenic DAAs may be used to clear the virus before attempting conception Treatment is not currently indicated in pregnancy but trials are ongoing

Table 17.20 Summary for serological investigations for hepatitis B

	HBV core Ab	HBV surface Ag	HBV DNA	HBV surface Ab
Acute hepatitis N infection	+	+	+	–
Chronic hepatitis B infection	+	+	+/–	–
Previously cleared infection ('natural immunity')	+	–	–	–
Previous vaccination	–	–	–	+

not chronically infected or previously exposed. General advice for patients with hepatitis B includes the avoidance of unprotected sexual intercourse, and screening +/– vaccination of household and sexual partners. As with all the viral hepatitides, hepatitis B is a notifiable illness. Patients with chronic hepatitis should be referred to specialist services for consideration of treatment – namely, pegylated interferon-alpha (used rarely) or oral treatments such as nucleoside analogues (entecavir and tenofovir).

The screening tests of choice for blood tests are hepatitis B core antibody and hepatitis B surface antigen. Refer to Table 17.19 for advice on management in pregnancy. Refer to Table 17.20 for information on interpreting hepatitis B serology.

6.2.3 Hepatitis C

There are six genotypes of hepatitis C, and G1 is the most common in the UK. The clinical signs and symptoms again are similar to hepatitis A and B in the acute phase and hepatitis B in the chronic. Fulminant hepatitis is more likely to occur with hepatitis A co-infection. The acquisition of hepatitis C through sex in heterosexual couples is very rare, but there has been a recent increase in incidence in men who have sex with men, with higher rates seen in those living with HIV.

Risk factors for hepatitis C transmission include:

– Renal dialysis
– IVDU/needlestick injuries
– Sharing razors
– Sharing equipment for snorting cocaine
– Sexual activity

Self-clearance is defined as loss of hepatitis RNA within 6 months of infection. However, 50–85% of patients will progress to chronic infection, and these patients remain at risk of chronic liver disease, cirrhosis and hepatocellular carcinoma. Treatment of hepatitis C has previously involved the use of pegylated interferon-alpha, with ribavirin. This can lead to cure in 40–70% of patients but carries significant side effects, and these regimens are no longer recommended. Newer oral agents that act directly on the virus (directly acting antivirals, DAAs, such as sofosbuvir and grazoprevir) are now widely available. These agents achieve cure in >95% of patients.

Pregnancy

Treatment of HCV in pregnancy with pegylated interferon and ribavirin is not currently recommended, as ribavirin is teratogenic. Conception should be avoided for up to six months after the use of ribavirin in women of reproductive age. DAAs may be offered to women to clear the virus before conception, but there are limited data regarding their safety in pregnancy at present, but trials are ongoing. No obstetric interventions have been found to reduce/prevent mother to child transmission. The risk of transmission in pregnancy is approximately 5% (7% in HIV co-infected women), and there is no robust evidence to advise regarding additional risk of transmission through breastfeeding.

References

1. Rayment, Michael and Jones, Rachael. Let's Talk about Sex. *Student BMJ*. 14 June 2012. http://student.bmj.com/student/view-article.html?id=sbmj.e3466.

2. Brooks, Gary, et al. UK National Guidelines for Consultations Requiring Sexual History Taking. *British Association of Sexual Health and HIV*. 2013. www.bashh.org/documents/Sexual%20History%20Guidelines%202013%20final.pdf.

3. Pattman, Richard, et al. *Oxford Handbook of Genitourinary Medicine, HIV, and Sexual Health 2/e*. Oxford: Oxford University Press, 2010.

4. Hay, Phillip, Patel, Sheel and Daniels, David. UK National Guideline for the Management of Bacterial

Vaginosis. *British Association for Sexual Health and HIV*. 2012. www.bashh.org/documents/4413.pdf.

5. White, David and Robertson, Claire. The United Kingdom National Guideline on the Management of Vulvovaginal Candidiasis. *British Association of Sexual Health and HIV*. 2007. www.bashh.org/documents/50/50.pdf.

6. Sherrard, Jackie, et al. United Kingdom National Guideline on the Management of Trichomonas Vaginalis. *British Association of Sexual Health and HIV*. 2014. www.bashh.org/documents/UK%20national%20guideline%20on%20the%20management%20of%20TV%20%202014.pdf.

7. Nwokolo, N. et al. 2015 UK National Guideline for the Management of Genital Tract Infection with Chlamydia Trachomatis. *British Association of Sexual*

Health and HIV. 2015. www.bashhguidelines.org/media/1192/ct-2015.pdf.

8. Fifer, H et al. UK National Guideline for the Management of Gonorrhoea in Adults, 2019. *British Association of Sexual Health and HIV*. 2019. www.bashhguidelines.org/media/1208/gc-2019.pdf

9. Foley, E, et al. Management of Genital Herpes in Pregnancy. *Royal College of Obstetricians and Gynaecologists*. October 2015. www.rcog.org.uk/globalassets/documents/guidelines/management-genital-herpes.pdf.

10. Gilleece, Y et al. British HIV Association Guidelines for the Management of HIV Infection in Pregnant Women 2018. *British HIV Association*. 2018. www.bhiva.org/file/5bfd30be95deb/BHIVA-guidelines-for-the-management-of-HIV-in-pregnancy.pdf

Pharmacokinetics, Pharmacodynamics and Teratogenesis

Kevin Hayes

Pharmacokinetics (Pk)

Describe what the body does to the drug and encompasses:

- Drug absorption (from the GI tract)
- Drug distribution (bioavailability + volume of distribution)
- Drug elimination (drug clearance is largely renal and hepatic)

Drug Absorption

- Lipid soluble drugs cross membranes and are easily absorbed from the stomach and duodenum
- Water-soluble drugs do *not* cross membranes; they need to be moved by facilitated diffusion or actively by carriers, e.g. ion channels
- Most drugs are given orally unless:
  - Oral intake is not possible, e.g. an unconscious patient
  - The drug is not absorbed, altered or digested, e.g. insulin

Drug Distribution (This Describes Where the Drug Goes throughout the Body)

Most drugs are designed to reach the systemic circulation, but others are deliberately intended to reach other tissues, depending upon the desired drug effect (e.g. across the blood-brain barrier for meningitis or into the urinary tract for the treatment of UTIs).

- *Bioavailability* is the amount of drug that reaches the systemic circulation unchanged; IV drugs therefore have 100% bioavailability. Oral drugs will lose considerable amounts of bioavailability due to first-pass hepatic metabolism; their dosing schedules will reflect this for them to be effective.
- *Volume of distribution (VD)* is the theoretical volume of water in which the amount of drug would need to be uniformly distributed to produce an observed blood concentration. Fat-soluble drugs may have an enormous VD and they may have prolonged duration of action, as they can have a reservoir in fat tissue.

While the provided two measures are principally theoretical concepts, they have a practical application as pharmacologists use them to help calculate doses and timings of drug administration.

Drug Elimination

Hepatic metabolism generally changes the original drug and then makes them more water soluble to aid elimination

- *Phase I* – Metabolism is by reduction/oxidation/hydrolysis principally due to the cytochrome p450 enzyme complex. After metabolism drugs can become:
  - *Inactive* – The vast majority of drugs are initially turned into inert biologically non-active chemicals following enzymatic change.
  - *Active* – Some compounds do not store well or are best delivered in an alternative chemical format. The cytochrome p450 complex is used to convert the inert form into the desired active chemical, e.g. enalapril and diazepam.
  - *Toxic* – Occasionally the initial drug is converted to a chemical that can cause harm. This is rare under normal pharmacological conditions, but in overdose the drug can be sent down an alternative red-ox pathway, e.g. paracetamol overdose.

- *Phase II* – Once converted to an alternative chemical, the drugs are made more soluble by *conjugation* with another compound. These tend to be:
  - *Glucuronate (for basic drugs)* – e.g. paracetamol, morphine
  - *Acetate (for acidic drugs)* – e.g. hydralazine, procainamide, isoniazid
  - *Sulphate* – e.g. oral contraceptives

Once soluble, they are excreted into:

- Urine via filtration from afferent renal blood flow from the liver OR
- Bile if the molecular weight (MW) is greater than 300 Da – the drug is then excreted in the faeces. Some drugs (e.g. combined oral contraceptive) have a recycling via breakdown by colonic bacteria so that some of the chemical is reabsorbed from the lower GI tract before excretion (the entero-hepatic circulation).

Renal elimination depends principally upon glomerular filtration rate and renal function:

- Drugs with MW less than 500 Da are filtered, so very large drugs (e.g. heparin) are not renally excreted.
- Filtration is reduced in highly protein-bound drugs (e.g. warfarin), as the protein carriers are negatively charged and are repelled from the glomerular basement membrane (GBM). Only 'free' non-bound drugs will be filtered.
- Excretion can be active in the proximal convoluted tubule (PCT) or by passive diffusion in the descending limb of the Loop of Henle due to drug concentration gradients between the tubule and the peri-tubular capillaries. It is a dynamic process and, depending upon concentration gradients inside or outside the tubule, the drug will diffuse in or out, particularly if lipid soluble.

- Active transport depends upon the acid-base status of a given drug:
  - Anion transporters are required for acidic drugs, e.g. penicillins, cephalosporins, salicylates, frusemide.
  - Cation transporters are required for basic drugs, e.g. morphine, pethidine, amiloride, quinine.
- Once a drug reaches the ascending limb of the loop of Henle, it will invariably be excreted in the urine

Therapeutic Window

All drugs have a dose at which they will be ineffective and a higher dose at which they may become toxic or cause significant side-effects. The area between these doses is the therapeutic window. Most drugs have a wide therapeutic window. Some drugs, however, have a narrower therapeutic window, e.g. gentamicin, cyclosporin (Fig. 18.1).

Drug Monitoring

The vast majority of drugs do not need close monitoring, as long as recommended doses and timings are adhered to. Certain drugs do, however, need close-level monitoring. Their dosing is often related to individual patient weight and or height (e.g. methotrexate). The need for monitoring will be dependent upon the following factors:

- Narrow therapeutic window – the narrower the window the greater the risk of either being ineffective (e.g. increased fit frequency in anti-epileptic drugs (AEDs)) or toxic causing significant side effects (AEDs again).

Figure 18.1 The difference between a wide and narrow therapeutic window

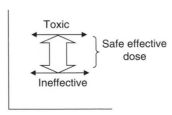

Wide therapeutic window

Narrow therapeutic window

- Intrinsic toxicity of the drug / how serious its side effects are, e.g. gentamicin causing renal impairment and/or oto-toxicity (vestibular component of VIIIth nerve). Minor side effects are clearly less important.
- Impaired renal or hepatic function – These will invariably reduce clearance and increase the risk of toxicity.
- Certain special circumstances affecting Pk or where other harm is possible e.g. pregnancy, breastfeeding, extremes of age – Paediatric and very elderly patients handle drugs differently and care is required in dosing.

Pregnancy and Pharmacokinetics

Due to the very large physiological changes associated with pregnancy, it is mainly drug handling that is affected rather than intrinsic drug actions.

The most relevant factors include:

- Large increase in circulating volume (40–50%)
- Concomitant large increased in renal blood flow and consequent GFR
- Increased third space availability (amniotic fluid and peripheral oedema)
- Relatively increased fat content due to laying down of maternal fat reserves
- Reduced albumin and other binding proteins due to the overall plasma dilution effect
- Progressive insulin resistance affecting medication for diabetes

This results in:

- Increased clearance of most drugs reducing serum concentrations and sometimes efficacy. There are certain clinical conditions in pregnancy where this may require close drug monitoring and usually increases in drug doses over the course of pregnancy:
  - Anticonvulsants such as carbamazepine, phenytoin, valproate, lamotrigine and gabapentin, especially where fit frequency is closely related to serum levels.
  - Mood stabilizers such as lithium where stable mood is vital and toxicity is particularly significant.
  - Common endocrine disorders in young women such as hypothyroidism – Thyroxine inevitably needs to be increased to keep thyroid function normal.

- Pregnancy is characterised by progressive insulin resistance – Women with pre-existing diabetes invariably need large increases in diabetic medication, especially insulin, as pregnancy advances.
- While most drugs have reduced levels due to altered Pk, the effect may be less marked for:
  - Highly protein-bound drugs, as the free, active concentration is less affected due to the reduction in albumin levels, e.g. warfarin
  - Fat-soluble drugs due to the increased fat reservoir, e.g. chloroquine. The drug can be stored in fat reservoirs, increasing the time scale of the available drug.

Pharmacodynamics

Describe what the drug does to the body i.e. the drug effect. There are generally four major drug effects:

- Receptors – tend to be metabotropic or ionotropic
  - Ionotropic receptors directly open or close an ion-pore in a membrane
  - Metabotropic receptors are indirectly linked to ion channels in plasma membranes via signal transduction by secondary messengers, usually G-coupled proteins.

Drugs can be *agonists, antagonists* or occasionally have a *mixed* effect on receptors (Fig. 18.2).

- Agonists (Table 18.1)
- Antagonists (Table 18.2)
  - Enzyme interaction – The majority of licensed drugs that influence enzymatic reactions tend to inhibit them (Fig. 18.3; Table 18.3).
  - Membrane ion channels – Most licensed drugs are generally designed to block ion channels (Fig. 18.4; Table 18.4).
  - Metabolic processes, e.g. antibiotics and ribosome / DNA synthesis (Fig. 18.5; Table 18.5)

Drug Interactions

These occur when one drug has an effect on the pharmacokinetics +/or dynamics of another used at the same time. The more drugs a person takes the more likely there is to be an interaction. These can occur by:

Table 18.1 Agonists and their receptors

Drug name	Receptor
Salbutamol	β1 and β2 adrenergic
Methyldopa	α2 adrenergic
Phenylephrine	α1 adrenergic
Pilocarpine	Muscarinic
Diazepam	GABA
Morphine	μ-opioid
Cabergoline	Dopamine

Table 18.2 Antagonists and their receptors

Drug name	Receptor
Atenolol	β1 adrenergic
Labetolol	α1, β1 adrenergic
Doxazocin	α1 adrenergic
Tolterodine	Muscarinic
Ranitidine	Histamine (H2)
Cyproterone acetate	Testosterone
Metoclopramide	Dopamine

Table 18.3 Enzyme interactions with drugs

Drug name	Enzyme
Diclofenac	Cyclo-oxygenase (COX) inhibition
Ramipril	Angiotensin-converting enzyme (ACE) inhibition
Neostigmine	Anti-cholinesterase inhibition
Zidovudine	Reverse transcriptase inhibition
Acyclovir	HSV-specific thymidine kinase inhibition
Warfarin	Vitamin K epoxide reductase inhibition
Methotrexate	Dihydrofolate reductase inhibition

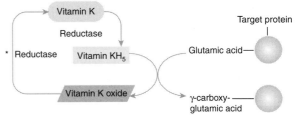

*= step blocked by warfarin

Figure 18.3 The enzyme block due to warfarin

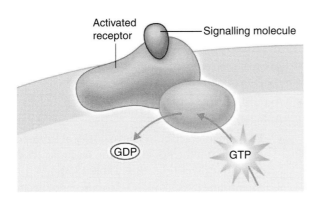

The signalling molecule acts via a G-protein-coupled receptor to influence intracellular events. An antagonist will block the receptor and hence the signalling molecule's action.
I GDP = Guanosine diphosphate I
GTP = Guanosine-5'-triphosphate

Figure 18.2 Muscarinic receptors as a signalling molecule act via G-protein coupled receptors to influence intracellular events. An antagonist will block the receptor and hence its action.

- *Enzyme induction* – Phenytoin is a potent inducer of cytochrome p450 enzyme complex activity and leads to reduced levels of many drugs metabolised in the liver and indeed reduced efficacy, e.g. COCP, warfarin. Other examples of enzyme inducers are rifampicin, griseofulvin and spironolactone.
- *Enzyme inhibition* – Sulphonamides inhibit hepatic metabolism and therefore increase plasma levels increasing the risk of toxicity and side effects, e.g. phenytoin.
- *Individual effects* – Ampicillin alters the bacterial gut flora and thus leads to a reduced entero-hepatic re-circulation of oestrogens, thus potentially impairing the efficacy of the COCP.

These effects may be potentiated in the very young and very old and where there is altered renal and hepatic function

Drugs in Relation to Pregnancy

General principles to consider:

- Remember all women of reproductive age might be pregnant
- Always question the need for drug therapy
- Avoid drugs in the first trimester if possible
- The benefits to the mother should outweigh the risks to the fetus (fetal therapy is sometimes a notable exception here)

Table 18.4 Drugs that block ion channels

Drug name	Ion channel
Nifedipine	Calcium blocker
Diltiazem	Calcium blocker
Verapamil	Calcium blocker
Lignocaine	Sodium blocker
Amiloride	Sodium blocker

Table 18.5 Drugs that affect metabolic processes

Drug name	Process
Gentamicin	Inhibition of ribosome synthesis
Erythromycin	Inhibition of protein translocation
Doxycycline	Inhibition of protein translation
Carboplatin	DNA alkylating agent
Paclitaxel	Cellular microtubule function
Vincristine	Spindle poison

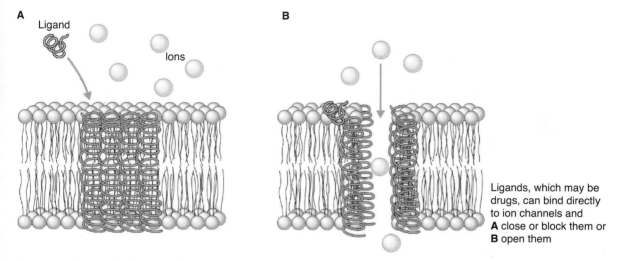

A Ligand Ions

B

Ligands, which may be drugs, can bind directly to ion channels and
A close or block them or
B open them

Figure 18.4 Ligands which may be drugs can bind directly to ion channels and open or close them. Nifedipine blocks the calcium influx seen here.

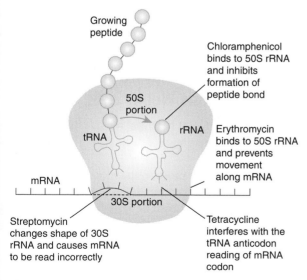

Growing peptide

Chloramphenicol binds to 50S rRNA and inhibits formation of peptide bond

50S portion

tRNA

rRNA

Erythromycin binds to 50S rRNA and prevents movement along mRNA

mRNA

30S portion

Streptomycin changes shape of 30S rRNA and causes mRNA to be read incorrectly

Tetracycline interferes with the tRNA anticodon reading of mRNA codon

Figure 18.5 Various actions of antibiotics on metabolic processes

- Do not stop a useful drug without careful risk-benefit analysis – drugs for epilepsy, asthma and thrombo-embolic disease are good examples
- Most drugs cross the placenta; few have been shown to be teratogenic
- Pre-pregnancy counselling for chronic medical conditions is the gold standard to optimise, alter or stop treatment to reduce the risk of harm
- Consider screening if exposure has occurred

When you need to prescribe:

- Use the smallest effective dose for the shortest possible time
- Choose a drug of which there is extensive experience in human pregnancy wherever possible
- Avoid poly-pharmacy where possible – the risk of teratogenesis with anti-epileptics increases each time another agent is introduced

Teratogenesis

Teratogenesis due to prescribed drugs would not exist if pregnant women never took medication. So, can we avoid drugs in pregnancy? Facts to consider:

- 35% of women take prescribed drug therapy at least once in pregnancy
- This is increasing as ever more women with medical problems becoming pregnant
- 6% of women take prescribed drug therapy in the first trimester (excluding iron and folic acid)
- 90% of women take something!

The reality is that prescribing is common in pregnancy as many medical problems arise (e.g. hyperemesis gravidarum) or pre-exist and can be exacerbated by pregnancy (e.g. heart disease). There are also times when it is considered safer to prescribe known teratogens, or drugs where safety is unknown, as the risk to the mother outweighs the risk of teratogenesis. Two good examples of this are for potentially life-threatening conditions where pregnancy has a big effect on disease occurrence and potentially prognosis: epilepsy and malaria. Withholding or withdrawing treatment because of fetal concerns puts the mother at unacceptable risk.

The background incidence of congenital abnormalities is approximately 2–3%. So, what proportion of these is likely to be caused by drugs? It is calculated that up to 1% may be due to prescription drugs. However, a recent UK review looking at two of the most commonly studied drugs in pregnancy, anti-epileptic drugs (AEDs) and anti-depressants (especially SSRIs), was clear that the true risks to the fetus remain unknown [1].

There are lots of problems with known data:

- Pregnant women are excluded from drug trials – teratogenic risk is therefore not assessed
- Retrospective cohort studies comparing exposed with non-exposed women are difficult to interpret because:
  - Congenital abnormalities are relatively common (2–3%)
  - Detection of a significant drug effect is therefore very difficult as it would need to be a large effect
  - Retrospective data is highly prone to recall bias – Pregnancies affected by congenital anomaly are much more likely to remember taking a drug if asked
- Most drugs do reach the fetus to some extent, but teratogenesis remains difficult to predict, e.g. warfarin, as a known teratogen has an exposure risk estimated at around 5%; therefore 95% of exposed pregnancies are unaffected
- Animal studies are idiosyncratic; many risks are likely to be dose and/or species specific
- Negative animal study results therefore provide information but do not guarantee that a drug is safe

Drugs that do *not* cross the placenta:

- Heparin (unfractionated or LMWH)
- Tubocurarine
- Insulin

Teratogenic Categorisation

The US Food and Drug Administration (FDA) has a categorisation of drugs as per Fig. 18.6 (other categorisation systems exist in Germany and Australia, with slight variation but essentially the same message).

When and Where Do Drugs Have an Effect?

- *Pre-embryonic up to day 17* – As the conceptus consists of totipotent cells, there is an 'all or nothing effect', i.e. death and resorption or survival. Therefore, if there is drug exposure at this specific time and the pregnancy continues, then a woman can be reassured.
- *Caution*: As well as drugs taken during this time, caution is required with certain drugs taken previously, e.g. retinoids can be present for up to two years, methotrexate for up to three months.

Embryonic from Day 18 to 55 (Organogenesis Weeks 2–8)

- Here is the biggest potential for structural damage and major anatomical defects due to irreparable tissue damage
- The earlier the exposure, the more marked the effect is likely to be
- Every individual organ or system has a period of maximum sensitivity
- Some systems (e.g. external genital tract) are not complete till well after the embryonic period and are therefore at risk much later, e.g. cyproterone acetate having an anti-androgenic effect on male genitalia
- Table 18.6 shows some examples of timings for some of the more common defects

FIG. 18.6 Pregnancy Categories

Pregnancy category	Description
A	**No risk in controlled human studies:** Adequate and well-controlled human studies have failed to demonstrate a risk to the fetus in the first trimester of pregnancy (and there is no evidence of risk in later trimesters).
B	**No risk in other studies:** Animal reproduction studies have failed to demonstrate a risk to the fetus and there are no adequate and well-controlled studies in pregnant women OR animal studies have shown an adverse effect, but adequate and well-controlled studies in pregnant women have failed to demonstrate a risk to the fetus in any trimester.
C	**Risk not ruled out:** Animal reproduction studies have shown an adverse effect on the fetus and there are no adequate and well-controlled studies in humans, but potential benefits may warrant use of the drug in pregnant women despite potential risks.
D	**Positive evidence of risk:** There is positive evidence of human fetal risk based on adverse reaction data from investigational or marketing experience or studies in humans, but potential benefits may warrant use of the drug in pregnant women despite potential risks.
X	**Contraindicated in pregnancy:** Studies in animals or humans have demonstrated fetal abnormalities and/or there is positive evidence of human fetal risk based on adverse reaction data from investigational or marketing experience, and the risks involved in use of the drug in pregnant women clearly outweigh potential benefits.
N	FDA has not yet classified the drug into a specified pregnancy category.

- Post-embryonic from eight weeks to term – The effects may be:
  - On fetal growth and development leading to intra-uterine growth restriction (IUGR), e.g. β-blockers
  - Continued differentiation and maturation in organs such as the brain and kidney, e.g. ACE inhibitors reducing fetal renal function
  - Shortly before term and labour, e.g. pethidine immediately before delivery leading to neonatal respiratory depression
  - Potential late effects such as sub-fertility and/or carcinogenesis, e.g. chemotherapy exposure in utero

Table 18.6 Examples of timing for some common embryological defects

Days	Defect
12–40	Limb reduction defects
24	Anencephaly
34	Transposition of great vessels
36	Cleft lip
42	VSD Syndactyly
84	Hypospadias

Further sources of information available:

- Appendix 4 of the BNF in pre-version 70. In versions 70 onwards, the risks are with each drug
- National Teratology Information service: 0191 232 1525
- www.nyrdtc.nhs.uk/Services/teratology/teratology .html

Known Teratogens

Particular teratogenic drugs to consider – Remember: *All the A's*

- Anticonvulsants
- Antibiotics
- Anticoagulants
- Antimetabolites
- Antipsychotics
- Androgens
- Acne drugs ('A-Vitamin')
- Alcohol

Certain drugs that may result in miscarriage

- Ergotamine
- Misoprostol
- Mifepristone
- Thrombolytics

The following highlight some of the issues with the more commonly known teratogens in pregnancy:

Anticonvulsants

- 90% of women with epilepsy have a normal pregnancy
- The risk is slightly increased regardless of anti-epileptic therapy (2.4% no therapy, 3–4% single-agent carbamazepine or phenytoin, 6% valproate, 3% lamotrigine [2])
- The risk increases with polypharmacy

- Valproate repeatedly been shown to have the highest risks
- Valproate also appears to have a dose-related effect on verbal IQ [3]
- Current data on lamotrigine suggests no extra risk above baseline
- Topiramate, gabapentin, levetiracetam currently have no firm information in pregnancy to guide risk assessment

Phenytoin is associated with malformations mainly due to alterations in folate metabolism. The fetal anticonvulsant syndrome is:

- Cleft lip/palate
- Microcephaly
- Cardiac abnormalities
- Mental retardation

Carbamazepine

- Similar effects to phenytoin
- Plus neural tube defects

Valproate

- Neural tube defects also

Risk reduction appears to be possible if:

- Pre-conceptual folic acid 5 mg once daily is taken for at least three months
- Polypharmacy is avoided wherever possible
- The lowest dose required for fit control is used (this may require level monitoring)
- Vitamin K is routinely given to mothers from 36 weeks and IM to babies to reduce the risk of post-partum haemorrhage and neonatal haemorrhage (evidence for a significant effect is, however, lacking)

Antibiotics

Antibiotics are one of the commonest classes of drugs prescribed in pregnancy as infective morbidity is relatively common.

Antibiotics to avoid are:

- Tetracyclines
  - Animal and human teratogenicity has been demonstrated
  - They cause permanent discolouration of teeth and impaired bone growth in utero and up to age seven as they chelate calcium
- Sulphonamides
  - They inhibit folate metabolism – benzoic acid to folate (sulphonamides) and folate to tetrahydrofolate (trimethoprim)
  - Sulphonamides displace bilirubin from protein and may cause kernicterus in the neonate
  - Sulphasalazine, used for inflammatory bowel disease, is probably safe

Caution is required and safer alternatives are preferred if possible with the following:

- Aminoglycosides (usually used for uro-sepsis and/or severe general sepsis):
  - They are nephrotoxic causing tubular destruction
  - They cause VIIIth nerve damage (the vestibular component)
  - Use only if essential and levels need to be monitored
- Quinolones
  - There appears to be a risk of permanent arthropathy in animals – data too limited in humans
  - Better alternatives are usually available
- Nitrofurantoin
  - Has been associated with neonatal haemolysis
- Chloramphenicol
  - May cause cardiovascular collapse (Grey baby syndrome) if given close to term. Local eye treatment with chloramphenicol eye drops is safe, as the systemic absorption is minimal.

The following antibiotics have the most experience in their use in pregnancy and appear to be safe:

- Penicillins
  - 70% of maternal serum levels are present in the fetus so can also treat fetal infection, e.g. syphilis
  - There is a theoretical risk of allergic sensitisation of the fetus, though this appears to be very rare
- Cephalosporins appear safe and are often first line
- Macrolides e.g. erythromycin appear safe
  - There is a small risk of neonatal cholestatic jaundice

Anticoagulants

- Heparin
  - Both unfractionated + LMW heparins are very large and do not cross the placenta – they are extensively used in pregnancy for prophylaxis and

treatment of thrombo-embolic disease. They have no teratogenic risks but like all drugs have some maternal side effects:

- Haemorrhage
- Heparin-induced thrombocytopaenia
- Local skin reaction and bruising

■ Warfarin is contraindicated between 6 and 12 weeks gestation as a recognised teratogen unless the thrombo-embolic risk is so high that it needs to be continued, e.g. metallic heart valves. They are not teratogenic after 12 weeks and may be used between 12 and 36 weeks if absolutely necessary, but as they cross the placenta, they cause anti-coagulation in the fetus. There is no relationship between maternal INR measurements and fetal ones, and as such, there is a risk of fetal intracranial haemorrhage, especially if taken close to delivery.

- They are teratogenic between 6–12 weeks gestation – Risk appears to be around 5% if exposed
- They are causally associated with multiple cranio-facial and skeletal abnormalities (Conradi-Hunnerman syndrome)

Antimetabolites

■ Most anti-neoplastics have been shown to be teratogenic at some stage

- However, information is based on mainly animal studies (relatively small numbers of humans); most fetuses have multi-agent exposure and the longer-term effects are not yet known
- They are contraindicated in the first trimester and breastfeeding
- They should be avoided within 2–3 weeks of delivery to allow marrow suppression to recover in the mother
- Most agents have actually been safely used in the second and third trimester [4]

Drugs in Relation to Lactation

■ Most drugs enter breast milk – therefore all the principles of prescribing in pregnancy are equally applicable to lactation
■ Drugs in breast milk may:

- Be harmful e.g. lithium
- Have no effect, e.g. digoxin

- Potentially cause hypersensitivity in the neonate, e.g. penicillin
- Suppress lactation, e.g. bromocriptine and cabergoline
- Reduce suckling due to neonatal sedation, e.g. phenobarbitone

■ The likelihood of a problem in the neonate is determined by a number of factors:

- The concentration of drug in the milk
- The transfer of drugs depends on molecule size and lipid solubility – The smaller and more lipid soluble they are, the more likely they are to cross into breast milk
- The volume of milk taken (hind-milk has a higher fat concentration than fore-milk so longer, deeper suckling will contain more drug if it is lipid soluble)
- The Pk of the drug in the infant – The ability of the infant to absorb and then clear any given drug will determine its serum concentration
- The inherent toxicity of the drug – Some drugs matter and some do not!

■ If a drug is deemed necessary post-natally and known to be harmful to the neonate, then invariably the best advice is to bottle feed
■ Below are drugs which are contraindicated in breastfeeding mothers:

- Cytotoxics
- Mood stabilizers – Lithium
- Sedatives – Benzodiazepines, barbiturates
- Amiodarone
- Antibiotics – Tetracyclines, metronidazole, chloramphenicol
- COCP (reduced milk)
- Theophylline (irritability)
- Aspirin (Reyes syndrome)

Further Sources of Information Available

Appendix 5 of the BNF in pre-version 70. In versions 70 onwards, the risks are with each drug.

Fetal pharmaco-therapy

Drugs that cross the placenta are deliberately administered via the mother to treat fetal conditions. They have the potential for maternal harm due to side effects and can present a clinical and ethical dilemma. Examples in use are:

- Betamethasone – Proven to reduce RDS and IVH between 26–32 weeks
- Corticosteroids to prevent masculinisation of female fetuses in CAH
- Flecainide for fetal tachycardia
- Amiodarone for resistant fetal tachycardia
- Salbutamol for hydrops fetalis due to congenital heart block
- Penicillin for the treatment of congenital syphilis

References

1. Chan M, Wong ICK, Sutcliffe AG. Prescription drug use in pregnancy: More evidence of safety is needed. *The Obstetrician & Gynaecologist* 2012;**14**:87–92.
2. Tomson T, Hiilesmaa V. Epilepsy in pregnancy. *BMJ* 2007;**335**:769–73.
3. Adab N, Kini U, Vinten J, Ayres J, Baker G, Clayton-Smith J, Coyle H et al. The longer term outcome of children born to mothers with epilepsy. *J Neurol Neurosurg Psychiatry* 2004;**75**:1575–83.
4. Cardonick E, Iacobucci A. Use of chemotherapy during human pregnancy. *Lancet Oncol.* 2004 May;**5**(5):283–91.

Single Best Answer Questions

1. Chloroquine for malarial prophylaxis has a very large volume of distribution of approximately 15,000 litres.
   What is the most important factor influencing such a large volume of distribution?
   a. High bioavailability
   b. High degree of renal excretion
   c. High first-pass metabolism
   d. High lipid solubility
   e. High therapeutic dosing

2. Gentamicin has a narrow therapeutic window necessitating level monitoring.
   What is the definition of the therapeutic window?
   a. The average time taken for a drug to reach therapeutic levels
   b. The bioavailable level once steady state has been reached
   c. The difference between minimal effective dose and toxic levels
   d. The level at which the drug causes side effects
   e. The trough level used for monitoring clearance

3. Pregnant women handle drugs differently when they are not pregnant.
   What is the single biggest factor that accounts for this in pregnancy?
   a. Increased availability of the amniotic fluid as a new third space
   b. Increased cardiac output presenting drugs to target areas more efficiently
   c. Increased clearance reducing serum levels
   d. Increased intrinsic hepatic activity
   e. Increased maternal fat stores altering volumes of distribution

4. Polypharmacy can result in drug interactions. Phenytoin is a good example of a drug that can have a significant effect on other drugs.
   What is the principal reason phenytoin can cause drug interactions?
   a. Cytochrome p450 inhibition
   b. Folate reduction leading to reduced cellular metabolic activity
   c. Hepatic enzyme induction
   d. It drives down albumin production leading to increased free drug availability
   e. It out-competes other drugs and is selectively reabsorbed in the kidney

5. Warfarin is a known teratogen.
   What is/are the most common abnormalities seen with affected pregnancies?
   a. Anencephaly
   b. Cranio-facial and skeletal
   c. Holoprosencephaly
   d. Ompholocoele
   e. Tetralogy of Fallot

6. Most anti-convulsants are known teratogens.
   Which anti-convulsant is known to have the single highest individual risk?
   a. Carbamazepine
   b. Gabapentin
   c. Lamotrigine
   d. Phenytoin
   e. Sodium valproate

Chapter 19

Non-hormonal Therapy in Obstetrics and Gynaecology

Kevin Hayes

Drugs in Common Use in Pregnancy

Anti-hypertensives

Hypertension and pre-eclampsia (PET) affect approximately 10% and 3% of all pregnancies, respectively, and are one of the commonest medical problems in pregnancy. While the benefits of treatment are clear for a minority with severe hypertension, much controversy exists over the benefit of treatment in women with mild and moderate hypertension. The purpose of treatment is to reduce the risk of acute intra-cerebral events in the mother.

The only clear indications for treatment are:

Persistent blood pressure (BP) ≥ 160/100

Acute severe hypertension

Fulminating PET

Eclampsia

The merit of treatment when BP is between 140/90 and 160/110 is debatable, but most obstetricians pragmatically medicate from 150/100 upwards.

- The β-blocker labetalol is considered safe and has been used extensively in human pregnancy – it is generally considered as first-line treatment
  - It has non-specific α + β blockade actions
  - It may be also be used for acute hypertension as a first-line intravenous (IV) infusion

Side effects:

  - It may cause fetal growth restriction (FGR) (even after controlling for BP) with prolonged use
  - Neonatal hypoglycaemia or bradycardia have rarely been reported

The safety of other β-blockers, atenolol in particular, in the early and late stages of pregnancy is unresolved; their use is therefore generally contraindicated according to several guidelines [1].

- α -Methyldopa is considered safe and has been used extensively in human pregnancy – it is now generally considered as second-line treatment in addition to labetalol but may be used as first-line instead
  - It is centrally acting and is metabolised to α-methylnoradrenaline (its active component)
  - It works as a post-synaptic α2 agonist, reducing central sympathetic outflow

Side effects include:
  - Rebound hypertension
  - Depressed mood (with long-term use)
  - Reduced cardiotocograph (CTG) variability
  - Autoimmune haemolytic anaemia (rare)
  - Raised prolactin (outside of pregnancy)
  - Hepatitis

- Nifedipine – nifedipine is not licensed for use in pregnancy but is a commonly used second-line treatment; a modified release (MR) preparation is recommended due to the potential acute hypotensive effect it can have [2].
  - It is a member of the dihydropyridine group and blocks inward flux of calcium through voltage-gated calcium channels
  - It has a preferential effect on vessels (as a vasodilator) rather than on the myocardium
  - It can also be used to treat acute hypertension
  - It has no anti-arrhythmic activity
  - It also has a known effect on the myometrium – it may inhibit premature labour (unlicensed use) and has been used as a tocolytic agent

Side effects include:
  - Acute hypotension if given sub-lingually
  - Peripheral oedema
  - Headache and flushing

- Hydralazine IV is used for acute hypertension
  - It needs to be given slowly over a minimum of 5 minutes IV
  - It can be repeated IV every 15 minutes if needed
  - It is a potent vasodilator with a poorly understood mechanism of action
  - It is metabolised by acetylation in the liver (fast and slow acetylators are genetically determined)

  Side effects include:
  - Acute hypotension if given too fast or too often
  - There is a recognised rare idiosyncratic adverse event (AE) of a lupus-like syndrome in slow acetylators
- $MgSO_4$ is proven to be the best prevention and best treatment of seizures in severe PET / eclampsia. The landmark MAGPIE trial showed that it halved the risk of eclampsia and probably reduced the risk of maternal death. There did not appear to be any substantive harmful effects to mother or baby in the short-term [3]. Its mechanism of action:
  - It acts as a membrane stabiliser
  - It has a rapid onset of action – maintained for 24 hours post delivery / seizure
  - It usually requires Mg level monitoring only if the patient is oliguric

  Side effects in toxicity:
  - Hyporeflexia presents in advance of more serious effects
  - Respiratory depression
  - Cardio-respiratory arrest

Drugs to Avoid for Hypertension

- ACE-Inhibitors are contraindicated in pregnancy. They are associated with:
  - Congenital malformations – especially CVS
  - Skull defects
  - Oligohydramnios and impaired fetal renal function
  - Sudden intra-uterine fetal death
- Thiazide diuretics – diuretic-associated harmful effects on maternal and fetal outcomes are controversial: their use is discouraged in pregnancy.

- Neonatal thrombocytopenia has been reported with bendromethafluazide

Tocolytic Agents

Tocolytic agents are used to abolish unwanted uterine activity, most commonly for preterm labour (PTL), but also for acute hyperstimulation and external cephalic version (ECV).

Preterm Labour

There is little evidence of benefit to overall outcome for the fetus with blanket tocolysis for PTL, and not using it is reasonable. Currently, the two clinical uses are:

- To achieve 24-hour steroid latency < 34 weeks
- When in utero transfer is necessary for appropriate level neonatal care

The following drugs have been and are used. The recent NICE guidelines [4] recommend nifedipine as first-line if used, reserving Atosiban for when there is a contraindication to nifedipine:

- Nifedipine (unlicensed use) – Its effectiveness is at least comparable with the agents described below and appears to have a better side-effect profile
- Atosiban (oxytocin antagonist) – Has fewer side effects than most other tocolytics but the Cochrane review suggests no overall benefit. Side effects: nausea, tachycardia, hypotension. Appears to cause no fetal/neonatal harm
- Beta-sympathomimetics (salbutamol, ritodrine, terbutaline). These are historically the most used tocolytic agents. However, their use is limited by significant side effects: tachycardia, hypotension, pulmonary oedema, hypokalaemia, hyperglycaemia. Current NICE guidelines advise avoiding their use
- Mg SO_4 – More commonly used in the United States. This is now recommended for fetal neuroprotection from 24–30 weeks gestation and possibly from 30–34 weeks
- Glyceryl trinitrate (GTN) patches – No evidence of benefit over ritodrine, but side effects are relatively less. Side effects: headache, rarely hypotension
- NSAIDS have been used historically but are currently not recommended

External Cephalic Version

Terbutaline given subcutaneously (s/c) prior to ECV has some evidence of increased procedural success in primigravidae and should be used only for this group. It is given as a one-off dose so the only common side effect is usually a transient maternal tachycardia and tremor.

Emergency Tocolysis

Terbutaline IV has been shown to improve fetal heart rate patterns and fetal pH in the presence of hyperstimulation (usually due to oxytocin) and possibly even without hyperstimulation. Side effects are as listed previously for beta-sympathomimetics.

Analgesia

Analgesics are arguably the most commonly prescribed drugs in pregnancy and gynaecological care.

Paracetamol

Paracetamol has both analgesic and anti-pyretic effects. It is considered safe in pregnancy for simple analgesia and is thus the first-line analgesic recommended. It has very few side effects in recommended doses but in excess can cause irreparable liver damage (usually seen with deliberate overdose).

Non-steroidal Anti-inflammatory Drugs (NSAIDs)

Aspirin has been studied extensively in low doses (75 mg), principally as a method of preventing PET and FGR. It should not be used liberally in low-risk women. Current advice is that women at high risk of PET should take 75 mg of aspirin daily from 12 weeks until 36 weeks gestation. Women at high risk are those with any of the following [2]:

- hypertensive disease during a previous pregnancy
- chronic kidney disease
- autoimmune disease, such as systemic lupus erythematosus (SLE) or antiphospholipid syndrome
- type 1 or type 2 diabetes
- chronic hypertension

Aspirin in low doses appears to have few adverse effects, although common practice seems to be stopping 2–3 weeks before delivery due to the theoretical risks of neonatal haemorrhage at delivery due to its anti-platelet effect.

Other NSAIDs have been used for the prevention and treatment of pre-term labour, as noted previously, as well as for their analgesic properties. Their use is controversial but current evidence suggests that they are associated with:

- A possible increase in the risk of miscarriage [5]
- Fetal renal impairment and oligohydramnios
- Increased risks of premature closure of the ductus arteriosus – the evidence for this is actually poor
- A potential small increased risk in necrotising enterocolitis (NEC)
- They can also cause maternal upper GI symptoms and, over prolonged periods, renal impairment

As analgesics, they are essentially contraindicated in pregnancy, and alternative drugs should be used in pregnant patients.

Opioids

Codeine phosphate and dihydrocodeine are commonly used for the relief of moderate pain and belong to the opioid family. They work by activating μ-opioid receptors, reducing cerebral appreciation of pain. They are also often given with paracetamol in the combined proprietary compounds Co-codamol® and Co-dydramol®.

Dextropropoxyphene is a more potent oral opioid reserved for more severe pain; it is therefore used more sparingly.

They are considered safe in pregnancy in recommended doses, and there is a large experience of human pregnancy exposure.

Side effects include:

- Sedation
- Nausea and vomiting
- Constipation
- In large quantities (invariably as drugs of abuse), they may cause a neonatal withdrawal syndrome

Drugs Used for Pain Relief in Labour

- Entonox – 50/50 nitrous oxide / O_2 mix. This is safe, stable and has a very rapid onset and offset. It is widely used and highly effective for many. Side effects: nausea, 'feeling drunk'
- Pethidine IM is widely used despite little evidence of effective pain relief. It has a rapid onset and

short half-life. Side effects: nausea and vomiting, narcosis, respiratory depression in the neonate if within 2 hours before delivery

- Morphine, though less widely used, appears to be more effective than and as safe as pethidine. Both pethidine and morphine are μ–opioid receptor agonists
- Combinations of bupivacaine (local anaesthetic) and fentanyl (opiate) in epidural administration provide highly effective pain relief.

  Side effects: hypotension, loss of mobility, increased chance of assisted delivery and, rarely, complications associated with insertion (dural tap, haematoma, high blockade).

Drugs Used in the Third Stage of Labour

Active management of the third stage has been shown to reduce the rate of postpartum haemorrhage (PPH) by around 50%. Most women receive drugs for their third stage as recommended routine practice. Drugs commonly used are:

- Syntometrine® (Ergometrine 500mcg / Sytocinon 5IU) IM. Ergometrine causes prolonged vasoconstriction. Side effects: nausea and vomiting, hypertension.

  It is contraindicated in hypertensive women. Syntocinon is synthetic oxytocin and causes short-term uterine contraction.

- Oxytocin (infusion of 40IU in saline) and ergometrine can also be used singly for the treatment of PPH
- Misoprostol 800mcg (PGE_1 analogue) taken orally/vaginally/rectally is effective in preventing and treating PPH. Stable and cheap and does not need refrigeration. Side effects: commonly diarrhoea and nausea/vomiting
- Carboprost ($PGF_{2\alpha}$ analogue) is an effective IM or intra-myometrial as a second-line treatment of PPH. Caution is required in hypertension, and this should be avoided in women with asthma.

Anti-emetics

Nausea and vomiting are common, particularly in the first trimester. Hyperemesis gravidarum affects up to 1–2% of pregnancies throughout the first trimester

and can be highly debilitating necessitating hospital admission, often on multiple occasions. As well as hydration, anti-emetics are used liberally to try to reduce nausea and vomiting. The evidence for their efficacy is relatively weak.

Commonly Used Agents

Promethazine (from the phenothiazine family) is the current first-line recommended drug, as a long-established anti-emetic with extensive experience in human pregnancy. It works principally by its antagonist action on H1 (histamine) receptors but does have a weaker anti-muscarinic effect. Side effects include sedation and, more rarely, extra-pyramidal neurological effects such as tardive dyskinesia.

Second-Line Agents

Metoclopramide is another drug with no recognized fetal harm. It is a dopamine (D2) antagonist and a 5-HT3 antagonist and has its anti-emetic effect centrally, as well as increasing gastric emptying. Side effects include akathisia (restlessness) and tardive dyskinesia.

Prochlorperazine (also from the phenothiazine family) is another potent D2 antagonist used extensively in pregnancy without demonstrable harm. Side effects are as per promethazine.

Third-Line Agents

Ondansetron and related compounds are potent 5-HT3 antagonists. They are not licensed for use in pregnancy and are used only when the above first- and second-line agents have failed. They appear to be safe in pregnancy. Side effects include headache, diarrhoea and sedation.

Fourth-Line Agents

Corticosteroids (either methylprednisolone or hydrocortisone) are used in resistant cases once the drugs listed above have been tried without success. They have some evidence of efficacy, though large trials have not been performed [6]. They have not been shown to be teratogenic, though most women are at the post-embryonic stage at commencement, and treatment is usually of short duration.

Antacids

Reflux and 'heartburn' are very common in pregnancy due to the reduced lower oesophageal sphincter tone induced by progesterone and increased gastric acidity.

Most pregnant women will experience this to some degree. These agents are basic and work by neutralising gastric acid; they do not affect its production. The commonest used in the UK is Gaviscon®, which contains sodium alginate, calcium carbonate and sodium bicarbonate. Maalox® is an aluminium and magnesium hydroxide–containing alternative. They appear safe in pregnancy and are widely used.

Drugs Commonly Used in Gynaecological Practice

Drugs Used for Menorrhagia

Mefenamic acid is an NSAID widely used for the treatment of dysmenorrhoea and menorrhagia. As an inhibitor of prostaglandin production, it is highly effective for menstrual pain when taken at the time of menstruation. It has also been shown to reduce average menstrual blood loss by up to 30% in dysfunctional uterine bleeding and is therefore effective for managing menorrhagia. Side effects are as for other NSAIDs used for analgesia.

Tranexamic acid is an anti-fibrinolytic drug which works by blocking the conversion of plasminogen to plasmin and reducing fibrinolysis. It has been shown to be a highly effective treatment for menorrhagia, reducing mean blood loss by 40–50%.

Side effects include mild GI upset, and caution is needed in women with pre-existing heart disease.

Urogynaecological Agents

Urge incontinence is commonly treated by drugs with anti-muscarinic properties.

Tolterodine and oxybutynin are both muscarinic antagonists (particularly the M3 receptor; there are 5 subtypes of muscarinic receptor M1–M5; oxybutynin is somewhat less selective). Both are effective in reducing symptoms of detrusor over-activity. Improvements in incontinence and irritative symptoms such as urgency and frequency are seen in up to 60–70%. The side effects are predictable, given their anti-muscarinic action: dry mouth, dry eyes, constipation and dizziness. These unwanted effects can limit their use but usually habituate over time. The use of modified-release products also seems to reduce side effects.

- Imipramine is often used as second-line but may be effective due to its anti-muscarinic effect
- Trospium chloride, propiverine and desmopressin also prove effective for some women

Stress Urinary Incontinence

Duloxetine is a balanced serotonin and noradrenaline reuptake inhibitor (SNRI). It increases urinary sphincter tone and has been shown to reduce (but not cure) stress incontinence by about 50%, with improvements in quality of life.

Side effects: nausea, dizziness, insomnia occur in 10–20% of patients.

Chemotherapeutic Drugs Used in Gynaecological Oncology

Chemotherapeutic agents (usually given as an out-patient) interfere with cell division by acting on a specific phase of the cell cycle (e.g. taxanes are active against cells in the G2/M phases) or non-specifically (e.g. alkylating agents which exert their effects throughout the cell cycle). As chemotherapy has a propensity for actively proliferating cells, cancer cells are more vulnerable than normal cells. However, chemotherapeutic agents also act on normal cells, so side effects are common. Chemotherapy has a narrow therapeutic index, and close monitoring under oncological guidance is essential while on treatment.

Some classes of cytotoxic agents:

- Antimetabolites – interfere with DNA and RNA synthesis, e.g. 5-FU, methotrexate (folate antagonist)

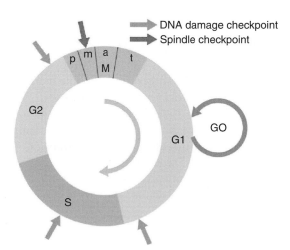

a= anaphase I Go = quiescent phase I G1 = gap 1 I
G2 = gap 2 I m = metaphase I M-mitosis I p = prophase I
S = synthesis phase I t = telophase

Figure 19.1 The cell cycle

- Alkylating agents – form covalent bonds with DNA bases, e.g. cyclophosphamide, ifosfamide
- Intercalating agents – bind to DNA, thus inhibiting its replication, e.g. cisplatin, carboplatin
- Anti-tumour antibiotics – complex mechanisms leading to inhibition of DNA synthesis, e.g. bleomycin, doxorubicin, etoposide
- Drugs directed against spindle microtubules inhibiting mitosis, e.g. paclitaxel, vincristine

Common Regimens

- Ovarian cancer – These are usually sensitive to platinum-based regimens. Response rates around 70% are seen in clinical practice. Carboplatin +/– paclitaxel may be used neoadjuvantly, adjuvantly or palliatively. More than 50% of patients will relapse and require further treatment, usually due to advanced stage of disease at diagnosis. If more than six months have elapsed since initial chemotherapy, the tumour is more likely to be sensitive to carboplatin and it is often given again.
- Endometrial cancer – Chemotherapy has a more limited role and is usually reserved for recurrent or metastatic disease; carboplatin +/– paclitaxel or doxorubicin and cisplatin are the most commonly used combinations.
- Cervical cancer – Cisplatin combined with radiotherapy has been shown to reduce the risk of recurrence for those undergoing radiotherapy after surgery. Cisplatin and methotrexate may be used for metastatic disease although the reported response rate is low.
- Vulval cancer – 5-FluUracil (5-FU) +/– cisplatin is used in combination with radiotherapy for patients unfit for surgery or as the sole therapy for symptom control in metastatic disease.
- Trophoblastic disease – Chemotherapy alone is highly curative. Methotrexate is used for simple trophoblastic disease. EMA-CO (Etoposide, Methotrexate, Dactinomycin, Cyclophosphamide, Vincristine) is used for high-risk trophoblastic disease. Both have cure rates of around 99%.

Side Effects of Chemotherapy

- Haematological – Bone marrow suppression which eventually recovers. Cellular nadir is at around 7–14 days, resulting in neutropenia, anaemia and thrombocytopenia
- Gastrointestinal – Side effects are due to loss of epithelial cells:
  - Nausea and vomiting are very common with most agents and are actively prevented with anti-emetics
  - Mucositis (especially methotrexate), resulting in ulcers in mucous membranes, particularly oral – these usually resolve spontaneously
  - Diarrhoea is less common and usually transient
- Alopecia – Taxanes (e.g. paclitaxel), doxorubicin and etoposide commonly cause temporary hair loss. This is seen less commonly with carboplatin and cisplatin.
- Neurological – Usually dose-related and improve on dose reduction or stopping:
  - Peripheral neuropathy is commonly seen with paclitaxel and cisplatin
  - Tinnitus is associated with cisplatin
- Constitutional – Tend to have cumulative effects but resolve on cessation:
  - Lethargy
  - Anorexia

References

1. Al Khaja KA, Sequeira RP, Alkhaja AK, et al. Drug treatment of hypertension in pregnancy: a critical review of adult guideline recommendations. *J Hypertens.* 2014;**32**(3):454–63.

2. Hypertension in Pregnancy. NICE Guideline 2015.

3. Altman D, Carroli G, Duley L, et al. Do women with pre-eclampsia, and their babies, benefit from magnesium sulphate? The Magpie Trial: A randomised placebo-controlled trial. *Lancet.* 2002 Jun 1;**359**(9321):1877–90.

4. Pre-term Labour and Birth. NICE guideline 2015.

5. Nakhai-Pour H, Broy P, Sheehy O, et al. Use of non-aspirin nonsteroidal anti-inflammatory drugs during pregnancy and the risk of spontaneous abortion. *CMAJ* 2011: DOI: 10.1503/cmaj.110454.

6. Wegrzyniak L, Repke J, Ural S. Treatment of hyperemesis gravidarum. *Rev Obstet Gynecol.* 2012;**5**(2):78–84.

7. Philadelphia College of Osteopathic Medicine, Philadelphia, PA.

8. The Pennsylvania State University College of Medicine, Department of Obstetrics and Gynecology, Hershey, PA.

Single Best Answer Questions

1. According to current national UK guidelines, what is the first-line drug of choice for the treatment of hypertension in pregnancy?

    a. Atenolol
    b. Bendromethafluazide
    c. Enalapril
    d. Labetalol
    e. Methyldopa

2. What is the mechanism of action of methyldopa?

    a. α1 agonist
    b. α1 antagonist
    c. α2 antagonist
    d. α2 agonist
    e. Balanced α1/ α2 antagonist

3. Magnesium sulphate ($MgSO_4$) is the international first choice for seizure prophylaxis in pre-eclampsia. By what proportion did $MgSO_4$ reduce the rate of seizures in the MAGPIE trial?

    a. 10%
    b. 20%
    c. 30%
    d. 40%
    e. 50%

4. What is the first-line tocolytic agent recommended by the 2015 NICE guidance for the management of preterm labour in the absence of contraindications?

    a. Atosiban
    b. $MgSO_4$
    c. Nifedipine
    d. Salbutamol
    e. Terbutaline

5. Promethazine is used as first-line treatment for hyperemesis gravidarum.
   Which receptor is the site of its principal mechanism of action?

    a. 5-HT3
    b. Dopamine D2
    c. Dopamine D3
    d. Histamine H1
    e. Muscarinic

6. Gaviscon®, which contains sodium alginate, calcium carbonate and sodium bicarbonate, is commonly used to treat heartburn in pregnant women.
   What is its mechanism of action?

    a. Direct competition for Substance P receptors, reducing the drive to gastric acid production
    b. Increasing lower oesophageal sphincter tone, thereby preventing gastric acid retrograde escape
    c. Increasing gastric emptying, thereby sending gastric acid antegrade
    d. Neutralisation of gastric acid
    e. Reduction in gastric acid production by histamine blockade

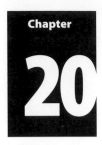

Drugs in Gynaecology and Contraception

Alastair Graham

Hormone Replacement Therapy (HRT)

Oestrogens (Table 20.1)

In low dose, oestrogen (together with a progestogen in women with a uterus) can reduce menopausal symptoms such as **vasomotor instability** or **vaginal atrophy**.

The natural oestrogens, *estradiol* and *estriol* are used for HRT as they have a better therapeutic profile as compared with synthetic *ethinylestradiol*. When given systemically in the perimenopausal and postmenopausal period, they, also diminish **postmenopausal osteoporosis**.

Since they are at high risk of osteoporosis, women with **early natural** or **surgical menopause**, can be given HRT until they have reached an age at which their menopause should have normally started – although, if osteoporosis is the main concern alternatives to HRT should be considered.

At least 20 different oestrogen plus progesterone HRT preparations are available; mostly as tablets or patches. As is the case with all other systemic HRT the vast majority contain *estradiol*. Premarin® uses *conjugated oestrogens*, sourced from **pregnant mare urine**. Both drugs are formulated either separately or in combination. *Cyclical HRT* (also know as *Sequential HRT*) is where a progestogen is taken for 12–14 days of each 28-day oestrogen treatment cycle. It is used when periods are still regular and usually results in regular withdrawal bleeding towards the end of the progestogen phase. The progestogen is usually formulated with the oestrogen in a combined tablet/patch. Each monthly pack also contains 12–14 days of an oestrogen only preparation. Many have 'sequi' in their brand name. When periods are irregular an option is Tridestra®: od oestrogen plus every 3 months a progestogen for 14 days, followed by 7 days of placebo. *Continuous Combined HRT* (where a combination of oestrogen and progestogen is taken, usually as a single tablet/patch) is to avoid bleeding – but irregular

bleeding may occur during the early treatment stages. If it continues, endometrial abnormality should be excluded and consideration given to *Cyclical HRT*.

There are at least 14 different *Oestrogen Only HRT* formulations – most are patches, some are tablets or gels. They are used continuously and are only suitable for women without a uterus. However, in endometriosis endometrial foci may remain despite hysterectomy and the addition of a progestogen should be considered.

Tibolone (Table 20.2)

Combines ***oestrogenic and progestogenic activity with weak androgenic activity***. Licensed for short-term treatment of **symptoms of oestrogen deficiency** (including women being treated with gonadotropin-releasing hormone analogues) and **osteoporosis prophylaxis** in women at high risk of fractures when other prophylaxis is contraindicated or not tolerated. Radiological detection of breast cancer can be more difficult as mammographic density may be increased with HRT – tibolone's effect is apparently limited.

Like Continuous Combined HRT preparations, *tibolone* is not suitable for use in the perimenopause or within 12 months of the last menstrual period.

Risks Associated with HRT

For the treatment of menopausal symptoms, that **adversely** affect quality of life, the benefits of short-term HRT outweigh the risks in the majority of women – especially in those aged < 60 yrs.

It increases the risk of *VTE, stroke, breast cancer, endometrial cancer*, (latter reduced by a progestogen), and to a small extent *ovarian cancer*. There is an increased risk of *coronary heart disease (CHD)* in women who start *Continuous Combined HRT* > 10 years after the menopause. The risk of *breast cancer* is increased with all forms of systemic HRT, used for > 1 year. It increases **further** with duration, use of *Continuous Combined HRT* (*Cyclical HRT* is less

Table 20.1 Oestrogen only HRT: For combined preparations – see each preparation's Summary of Product Characteristics at www.med icines.org.uk

Cautions	Contraindications	Side effects
Acute porphyrias*; diabetes[T] (risk of heart disease); endometrosis history (Hx) of breast nodules/endometrial hyperplasia/fibrocystic disease[T]; hypophyseal tumours; **migraine**[I]; **positive antiphospholipid antibodies[T 2]**; risk factors for oestrogen-dependent tumours (e.g. breast cancer in first-degree relative)[T]; risk of gall-bladder disease; **risk factors for thromboembolism**[T] (TE); uterine fibroid size may increase. For *ethinylestradiol* exclude* but add; cardiovascular disease (risk of fluid retention) and personal or family history of hypertriglyceridaemia (increased risk of pancreatitis)^[T] Key:[T] also a caution for *tibolone*. also a caution with **POPs** (Progestogen Only Pills) or **POPs and COCs** (Combined Oral Contraceptives). ^also a caution for COCs (and *tibolone*).	Active arterial TE disease (e.g. angina or myocardial infarction (MI)); abnormal liver function tests (LFTs); *Hx of breast cancer* (BC)[a]; **Hx of VTE**; oestrogen-dependent cancer; thrombophilic disorder; untreated endometrial hyperplasia; **undiagnosed vaginal bleeding** (UVB). Key: also a contraindication with **all progestogens (except levonorgesterol)**; all progestogens (except conjugated oestrogens, dienogest and estradiol) and all *COCs*. *Breastfeeding*: adversely affects lactation **Significant interactions:** ospemifene, raloxifene, pomalidomide, thalidomide.	Nausea & vomiting (N&V), abdominal cramps and bloating, weight changes, breast enlargement and tenderness, Premenstrual syndrome (PMS) sodium and fluid retention, cholestatic jaundice, glucose intolerance, altered blood lipids – may lead to pancreatitis, rashes and chloasma, changes in libido, depression, mood changes, headache, migraine, dizziness, leg cramps (rule out VTE), vaginal candidiasis, contact lenses may irritate; patches may cause severe hypersensitivity reaction, headache on vigorous exercise.

risky) and persists for > 10 years after stopping – see Table 20.3. In Sept. 2019, the MHRA advised that these updated risks are discussed with women who use or are considering starting HRT. It also encourages current and past users to

- look out for signs of *breast cancer*,
- attend routine breast screening
- stop HRT gradually (so as to minimise recurrence of symptoms),
- to always use the minimum effective dose.

Tibolone increases the risk of stroke about 2.2 times from the first year of treatment and is age-dependent. It also increases the risk of BC but to a lesser extent than with *Continuous Combined HRT*, while for endometrial cancer 1 licensing study reported an increased case rate of 0.8 per 1000 per 1 year. Limited data do not suggest an increased risk of thromboembolism and there is insufficient data to draw any conclusions regarding the risk of CHD.

HRT does not provide contraception. Women < 50 years and free of all risk factors for venous and arterial disease can use a low-oestrogen COC pill for relief of menopausal symptoms and contraception.

Menopausal Atrophic Vaginitis

Options are *moisturisers* (such as ReplensMD® or Sylk®) or intravaginal cream (*estriol* 0.01% or 0.1%) or vaginal tablets (*estradiol* 10 micrograms).

Dosing: Insert daily for 3–4 weeks (cream) and 2 weeks (tablet), preferably in the evening, then reduce to twice a week. Attempt to discontinue every 3–6 months with re-examination. Endometrial safety of long-term or repeated use is uncertain.

Table 20.2 Tibolone

Cautions	Contraindications	Side effects	Prescribing
See Oestrogen Only HRT; also, vaginal bleeding (investigate for endometrial cancer if bleeding > 6 months or after stopping treatment); Hx liver disease, epilepsy, migraine, diabetes, hypertriglyceridaemia; withdraw if signs of TE, abnormal LFTs or cholestatic jaundice	See oestrogen for HRT; also, Hx cardiovascular or cerebrovascular disease (e.g. thrombophlebitis, TE UVB; acute porphyria Avoid in acute liver disease or abnormal LFTs; untreated endometrial hyperplasia; pregnancy	Abdominal pain, weight changes, vaginal bleeding, leucorrhoea, facial hair, and *rarely* amnesia; gastrointestinal disturbance (GI dist.), oedema, dizziness, headache, migraine, depression, arthralgia, myalgia, visual disturbance, seborrhoeic dermatitis, rash and pruritus also reported	2.5 mg od. Unsuitable in the premenopause (unless being treated with GnRH analogue) and as or with an oral contraceptive; also unsuitable < 1yr. of last period (may cause irregular bleeding). If transferring from *Cyclical HRT*, start at end of regimen; if from *Continuous-combined HRT*, start at any time. **Possible interactions** with drugs that increase risk of TE.

Table 20.3 Oestrogen only and Combined HRT Risks for Women aged 50–59 (for CHD 70–79†)

	Background incidence per 1000 women in Europe not using HRT		Additional cases per 1000 women using Oestrogen only HRT (estimated)		Additional cases per 1000 women using a Combined HRT preparation (estimated)*	
	Age		Years Used		Years Used	
	50–54	50–59	5	10	5	10
Breast Cancer	13	27	3	7	8	20
Endometrial Cancer	2	4	4	32	NS	NS
Ovarian Cancer	2	4	<1	1	<1	1
VTE	5	10	2	3	7	13
Stroke	4	8	1	2	1	2
CHD†	29–44	ND	NS	ND	15	ND

NS = a non-significant difference. ND = no data. *combined figures for cyclical and continuous HRT. Further details - HRT Risk tables, BNF Chapter 6.8 or https://assets.publishing.service.gov.uk/media/5d680409e5274a1711fbe65a/Table1.pdf

Prasterone

This daily pessary is a relatively new treatment (2018) for **vulvar** and **vaginal atrophy**. It is biochemically and biologically *identical to endogenous dehydroepiandrosterone* (DHEA). Compared to oestrogens the *cautions* of hypophyseal tumours, positive antiphospholipid antibodies and risk of gall-bladder disease are not listed. Cholelithiasis and liver disorders are extra and it shares hypertriglyceridaemia with *ethinylestradiol* and *tibolone*. *Contraindications* are the same as oestrogens. Reassess need 6 monthly.

Common *side effects* are cervical abnormalities and weight change; others are benign breast neoplasm and uterine polyps. *No interactions*.

Ospemifene

A *selective oestrogen receptor modulator*. This daily tablet was licensed in 2015 for **moderate to severe symptomatic vulvar and vaginal atrophy where vaginal oestrogen therapy is not suitable**. It has the same *contraindications* as oestrogens except for abnormal LFTs, acute porphyrias, arterial TE disease and thrombophilic disorders; while its only *cautions* are risk factors for stroke and VTE.

Common *side effects* are genital/vaginal discharge, hot flushes, muscle spasm and skin reactions; others are endometrial thickening and tongue swelling. Only *interacts* with HRT and Combined Oral Contraceptives (COCs).

Raloxifene (Table 20.4)

This is another **selective oestrogen receptor modulator**. Licensed for the treatment and prevention (NICE recommended only for *secondary* prevention) of **post-menopausal osteoporosis**, but it does not reduce vaso-motor symptoms. Only licensed for chemoprotection of BC in USA.

Menopausal Symptoms in Breast Cancer

Treatments, such as *tamoxifen* or ovarian function suppression may lead to menopausal symptoms or early menopause. Women should be counselled about these potential side effects. HRT can cause tumour stimulation and interfere with adjuvant endocrine therapy of BC and so should be discontinued. History of BC is a *contraindication*, but in exceptional circum-stances HRT can be offered after a risk/benefit discus-sion with the patient. Other options are as follows.

Fluoxetine and Paroxetine

These are Selective Serotonin Re-uptake Inhibitors (SSRIs). Both are licensed but **decrease** tamoxifen levels. Only *contraindicated* in poorly controlled epi-

lepsy and manic patients. *Cautions* are cardiac disease, electroconvulsive therapy, diabetes mellitus, epilepsy, history of bleeding disorders or mania and suscepti-bility to angle-closure glaucoma. For *side effects* see p.200. *Significant interactions* are with anticoagulants, tricyclic antidepressants and tramadol – as well as some other uncommon drugs.

Other Menopausal Treatments

Clonidine (Table 20.5)

May be used in those who cannot take oestrogen, but can cause unacceptable side effects. It is an antihyper-tensive which **acts centrally by stimulating alpha$_2$-adrenergic receptors**. The resulting fall in blood pressure and heart rate helps prevent **menopausal flushing**. The usual starting dose is 50mcg bd for 2 weeks and then 75mcg bd if necessary. Other, but <u>unlicensed</u>, options are *Gabapentin* and *Venlafaxine*.

Progestogens and Progesterone Receptor Modulators

There are 2 main groups of progestogens: **progesterone and its analogues** (*dydrogesterone**

Table 20.4 Raloxifene

Cautions	Contraindications	Side Effects
Risk factors for VTE (discontinue if prolonged immobilisation); risk factors for stroke; BC; Hx of oestrogen-induced hypertriglyceridaemia	Hx of VTE, UBV, endometrial cancer, cholestasis, acute porphyria hepatic impairment, severe renal impairment **Possible interaction** with drugs that increase risk of TE	Hot flushes, leg cramps, peripheral oedema, influenza-like symptoms; *less commonly* VTE, thrombophlebitis; *rarely* rash, GI dist. hypertension, arterial TE, headache (incl. migraine), breast discomfort, thrombocytopenia

Table 20.5 Clonidine

Cautions	Contraindications	Side effects
Depression; heart failure; Raynaud's syndrome; antihypertensive therapy; cerebrovascular disease; polyneuropathy; constipation	Severe bradyarrhythmia; **Interacts** with drugs that can cause bradycardia, hypotension or CNS depression	Constipation, dry mouth, N&V; postural hypotension; depression, sleep disorder, dizziness, headache, drowsiness; *less commonly* Raynaud's syndrome, paraesthesia, hallucination, rash, pruritus; *rarely* atrio-ventricular heart block, gynaecomastia, alopecia

* In the UK only found in Femoston® – a *Cyclical HRT*

and *medroxyprogesterone*) and **testosterone analogues** (*norethisterone* and *norgestrel*). The newer progestogens (*desogestrel, norgestimate* and *gestodene*) are all derivatives of norgestrel – the latter 2 are only found in COCs. Although norgestrel isn't used medicinally in the UK, its active isomer *levonorgestrel* is widely available (see Table 20.6). Also used with *ethinylestradiol* in various COCs and with *estradiol* in the HRT product FemSeven®.

Progesterone and its analogues are less androgenic than the **testosterone analogues**, and neither *progesterone* nor *dydrogesterone* cause virilisation.

Dienogest (Table 20.7)

A nortestosterone derivative for **endometriosis**. It has a **progestogenic effect in the uterus, reducing the production of estradiol and thereby suppressing endometriotic lesions**. Although it has been available for many years in the COC Qlaira® this daily 2mg tablet only became available in early 2020.

Dysmenorrhoea and Menorrhagia

Oral progestogens for **menorrhagia** are relatively ineffective compared with *tranexamic acid* or where **dysmenorrhoea** is also a factor – *mefenamic acid*. The *levonorgestrel-releasing intrauterine system* (Mirena® and Levosert®) may be useful for women also requiring contraception. Oral progestogens have also been used for **severe dysmenorrhoea**. But where contraception is also required in younger women, the best choice is a COC.

Tranexamic Acid (Table 20.8)

An **antifibrinolytic** compound which is a potent competitive inhibitor of the activation of plasminogen to plasmin. Licensed for the treatment of **menorrhagia**.

Mefenamic Acid (Table 20.9)

Mefenamic acid is a non-steroidal anti-inflammatory drug (NSAID), indicated for **acute pain (incl. dysmenorrhoea)**, and **menorrhagia**. It *inhibits prostaglandin synthesis and the binding of prostaglandin E2* to its receptor.

Ulipristal (Table 20.13)

This is a **progesterone receptor modulator** characterised by a tissue-specific partial progesterone antagonist effect.

MHRA/CHM Advice

The use of Esmya® (*ulipristal acetate*) for **uterine fibroids** was suspended in March 2020 due to the risk of serious liver injury. It was re-licensed in February 2021 with strict guidelines that it is only to be used for the intermittent treatment of moderate to severe uterine fibroid symptoms before menopause and when surgical procedures are not suitable or have failed and with the patient's informed consent.

Emergency Hormonal Contraceptives (EHC)

Ulipristal is equally effective as *levonorgestrel* (see Table 20.6) as an EHC.

When prescribing or supplying an EHC, women should be advised:

- that their next period may be early or late
- that a barrier method of contraception should be used until their next period
- to seek medical attention promptly if any lower abdominal pain occurs because this could signify an ectopic pregnancy
- to return in 3 to 4 weeks if the subsequent menstrual bleed is abnormal
- regarding future contraception

A *copper intra-uterine contraceptive device (IUCD)* can be inserted up to 120 hours (5 days) after unprotected intercourse and is more effective than hormonal methods (98%); sexually transmitted infections should be tested for and use should be covered by antibacterial prophylaxis (e.g. *azithromycin* 1 g stat). If intercourse has occurred > 5 days previously, the device can still be inserted up to 5 days after the earliest likely calculated ovulation (i.e. within the minimum period before implantation), regardless of the number of episodes of unprotected intercourse earlier in the cycle.

Anti-oestrogens

Clomifene (table 20.10) and *tamoxifen* (table 20.11) are used in the treatment of female infertility due to **oligomenorrhoea** or **secondary amenorrhoea**.

They induce gonadotropin release by **occupying oestrogen receptors in the hypothalamus**, thereby interfering with feedback mechanisms; *chorionic gonadotropin* is sometimes used as an adjunct. Patients should be warned that there is a risk of multiple pregnancy (rarely more than twins).

Table 20.6 *Progesterone, Norethisterone, Levonorgestrel & Medroxyprogesterone Acetate (MPA): non-contraceptive indications*

Cautions	Contraindications	Side effects	Prescribing
Diabetes; **migraine**; (except progesterone) cardiac dysfunction; Hx BC – seek specialist advice (ssa); rheumatoid arthritis; SLE; **positive antiphospholipid antibodies**[5]; (except levonorgestrel) conditions that may worsen with fluid retention; **risk factors for thromboembolism**; *Norethisterone/Levonorgestrel*: multiple risk factors for cardiovascular disease. *Norethisterone/MPA*: liver tumours – ssa. *MPA*: hypertension. *Progesterone*: Hx of depression. *Levonorgestrel*: Hx of VTE / IHD / stroke (incl. TIA). malabsorption states. Key: also a caution with **Oestrogen only HRT or POPs and COCs**.[5] a contraindication for COCs. N.B. these cautions are the same as for POPs except for progesterone add Hx of depression	Acute porphyrias; **breast cancer** (with levonorgestrel only a caution when for EHC); also (except levonorgestrel) **Hx of VTE** and **UVB** For progesterone & norethisterone also history during pregnancy of idiopathic jaundice, pemphigoid gestationis or severe pruritus[b]; For progesterone missed miscarriage, genital cancer. Key: also a contraindication with all oestrogens and progestogens (except conjugated oestrogens, dienogest and estradiol) or **all oestrogens and progestogens (except levonorgestrol)**.[b] all also cautions for COCs (but COCs also incl. chorea). **Significant interactions** that could possibly lead to failure of contraception with antiepileptics; antiretrovirals; rifamycins; aprepitant & fosaprepitant; crizotinib, dabrafenib & vemurafenib; bosentan, griseofulvin, modafinil, selegiline, St John's wort, sugammadex, ulipristal. *Levonorgestrel* - also lumacaftor *MPA* - sugammadex only *Progesterone* - no interactions	Menstrual disturbance, PMS (including bloating, fluid retention, breast tenderness), weight change, N&V, headache, dizziness, insomnia, drowsiness, depression, change in libido; also skin reactions (including urticaria, pruritus, rash, and acne), hirsutism and alopecia. Jaundice and anaphylactoid reactions have also been reported.	*Medroxyprogesterone Acetate* • 2.5–10 mg od for 5–10 days from day 16 to 21 of cycle, repeated for 2 cycles in **dysfunctional uterine bleeding** and for 3 cycles in **secondary amenorrhoea** • **mild to moderate endometriosis**. 10 mg tds for 90 days, start on day 1 of cycle • **progestogenic opposition of oestrogen HRT**, 10 mg od for the last 14 days of each 28-day oestrogen HRT cycle *Norethisterone* • **endometriosis**, 10–15 mg od for 4–6 months or longer, starting on day 5 of cycle (if spotting occurs increase dose to 20–25 mg od reduce once bleeding stops • **dysfunctional uterine bleeding, menorrhagia**, 5 mg tds for 10 days to arrest bleeding; to prevent bleeding 5 mg bd from day 19 to 26 (but see tranexamic acid and mefenamic acid below for more effective treatments) • **dysmenorrhoea**, 5 mg tds from day 5 to 24 for 3–4 cycles • *premenstrual syndrome – not recommended* • **postponement of menstruation**, 5 mg tds starting 3 days before expected onset (menstruation occurs 2–3 days after stopping) *Progesterone* • **opposition of oestrogen HRT**, 200 mg od on days 15–26, or 100 mg od on days 1–25 • **premenstrual syndrome, post-natal depression** by *vagina or rectum*, 200mg od as Cyclogest® pessaries. Can increase to 200–400mg bd. For PMS start on day 12–14 and continue until onset of menstruation (evidence of efficacy is equivocal).[8] • Various preparations of e also available as oral or vaginal formulations for use in infertility. *Levonorgestrel for emergency contraception* – 1.5 mg no later than 72 hours after coitus – 3 mg (unlicensed) if taking enzyme-inducing drugs – repeat if vomiting within 2 hours

Table 20.7 Dienogest

Cautions	Contraindications	Side effects	Prescribing
Diabetes (progestogens can decrease glucose tolerance - monitor patient closely); Hx depression/ectopic pregnancy/ gestational diabetes; risk of osteoporosis/ VTE; **Significant interactions** are with anti-epileptics and a few other uncommon drugs.	Past or present arterial / cardiovascular disease or liver tumours; diabetes with vascular involvement; prolonged immobilisation sex hormone-dependent malignancies (confirmed or suspected); UVB; VTE (active).	*Common*: Alopecia; anxiety; asthenic conditions; breast abnormalities; depression; GI discomfort/disorders; haemorrhage; headaches; hot flush; libido loss; mood altered; nausea; ovarian cyst; pain; skin reactions; sleep disorder; vomiting; vulvovaginal disorders; weight changes.	**Significant interactions:** apalutamide, enzalutamide, fosphenytoin, mitotane, phenobarbital, phenytoin, primidone, rifampicin

Table 20.8 Tranexamic acid

Cautions	Contraindications	Side Effects	Prescribing
Irregular menstrual bleeding (establish cause before initiating therapy); massive haematuria (avoid if risk of ureteric obstruction); patients receiving oral contraceptives (increased risk of thrombosis).	Thromboembolic disease; fibrinolytic conditions following disseminated intravascular coagulation (unless predominant activation of fibrinolytic system with severe bleeding); history of convulsions.	Nausea, vomiting, diarrhoea (reduce dose); *less commonly* dermatitis; *rarely* thromboembolic events, visual disturbances incl. impairment of colour vision (discontinue); *also reported* malaise and hypotension on rapid IV injection, convulsions.	• **Menorrhagia:** (initiated when menstruation has started):, By mouth, 1 g tds for up to 4 days; maximum 4 g daily. − **Local Fibrinolysis:** 0.5–1g by slow IV or infusion (= 0.1 g/min.) 8–12 hrly. − **General Fibrinolysis:** 1 g by slow IV or infusion (= 0.1 g/min.) 6–8 hrly. **No significant interactions.**

Bromocriptine and Cabergoline (Table 20.14)

These *stimulate dopamine receptors in the brain which inhibit prolactin release by the pituitary*. Although licensed, they are <u>not</u> recommended for routine use to **suppress lactation** or **postpartum breast pain due to engorgement**. First-line treatment is simple analgesia and breast support. If dopaminergics are required, then *cabergoline* (with its much longer half life) is preferred at 250 mcg every 12 hr for 2 days with food (to reduce N&V), or as a single dose of 1 mg orally.

Bromocriptine is licensed for **hypogonadism, galactorrhoea** and **infertility** at 1 to 1.25mg nocte, increasing gradually to about 7.5mg per day (max. 30mg per day). For **prevention of lactation** use 2.5mg bd.

Cabergoline is also indicated for the treatment of dysfunctions associated with hyperprolactinaemia, including **amenorrhoea, oligomenorrhoea, anovulation** and **galactorrhoea** at a dose of 0.25 mg to 2 mg once a week.

The licensed brand of *Cabergoline* for the all the above indications is Dostinex® 0.5mg (Pfizer). For Parkinson's it's Cabasar® 1mg or 2mg (also Pfizer). All strengths are also available as generics.

Table 20.9 Mefenamic acid

Cautions	Contraindications	Side effects	Prescribing
Acute porphyria; coagulation defects; connective tissue disorder; Hx of Crohn's or ulcerative colitis; dehydration; elderly; epilepsy; hepatic impairment; in long-term use, reduced reversible female infertility; may mask infection; uncontrolled hypertension; risk factors for CVD; heart failure; cerebrovascular/ ischaemic heart/ peripheral arterial disease.	Severe heart failure; Crohn's or ulcerative colitis active GI ulceration or bleeding; Hx of recurrent or previous NSAID related GI ulceration or haemorrhage (>1 distinct episode); severe liver disease; avoid if possible or use with caution in renal impairment following coronary artery bypass surgery.	Nausea, diarrhoea, and occasionally bleeding/ ulceration; rashes, angioedema, bronchospasm; headache, dizziness, nervousness, depression, drowsiness, insomnia, vertigo, tinnitus, photosensitivity, haematuria; *less commonly* paraesthesia, fatigue; *rarely* hypotension, palpitation, glucose intolerance, thrombocytopenia, haemolytic and aplastic anaemia.	• 500 mg tds. **NSignificant interactions:** anticoagulants; fibrinolytics (e.g. alteplase); heparins; diuretics; oral steroids; quinolones, bevacizumab, bivalirudin, cabozantinib, caplacizumab, cobimetinib, colistimethate, deferasirox, eptifibatide, erlotinib, inotersen, lithium, methotrexate, mifamurtide, nicorandil, nicotinic acid, pemetrexed, ruxolitinib sodium clodronate, tirofiban, trametinib, trastuzumab, trastuzumab, zidovudine.

Table 20.10 Clomifene: Cautions, contraindications and side effects

Cautions	Contraindications	Side effects	Prescribing
PCOS (cysts possibly also increase the risk of exaggerated response), OHSS, fibroids, ectopic pregnancy, multiple births.	Ovarian cysts, hormone-dependent tumours or undiagnosed vaginal bleeding. Avoid in severe liver disease.	Visual disturbances (withdraw), OHSS (withdraw), hot flushes, abdominal pain, nausea & vomiting, depression, insomnia, mastalgia, headache, intermenstrual spotting, menorrhagia, endometriosis, convulsions, weight gain, rash, dizziness, hair loss.	50 mg od for 5 days, starting within 5 days of onset of menstruation (preferably on 2nd day) or at any time if cycles have ceased; if progestin-induced bleeding is planned, or if spontaneous uterine bleeding occurs before therapy, start on day 5. 2nd course of 100 mg daily for 5 days may be given in absence of ovulation; most patients who are going to respond will do so with first course; 3 courses should constitute adequate therapeutic trial; lower dosage or duration recommended if unusual sensitivity to pituitary gonadotropin is suspected, e.g. in PCOS. **No interactions.**

Gonadotrophins

Follicle-stimulating hormone (FSH) and luteinising hormone (LH) together (as in *menotrophin*), follicle-stimulating hormone alone (as in *follitropin*) or *choriogonadotropin alfa* (hCG) are used in the treatment of **infertility in women with proven hypopituitarism** or who have **not responded to clomifene**. *Lutropin alfa* is given in conjunction with FSH. Also used in **superovulation treatment for assisted conception** (such as in vitro fertilisation).

Danazol

A synthetic steroid that ***inhibits pituitary gonadotropins***. Derived from *ethisterone* it has marked affinity for androgen receptors, less so for progesterone receptors with only a minimal affinity for oestrogen receptors. Until its withdrawal from the UK market in May 2020 it was licensed for **endometrosis** and **severe fibrocystic breast pain**. Still available through specialist importers.

Table 20.11 Tamoxifen: Cautions, contraindications and side effects

Cautions	Contraindications	Side effects	Prescribing
Occasional cystic ovarian swellings in premenopausal women; increased risk of TE, especially when used with cytotoxics; porphyria. **Significant interactions:** bupropion, cinacalcet, fluoxetine, paroxetine, rolapitant, terbinafine Coumarins – raised INR.	Personal or family history of idiopathic VTE or genetic predisposition to TE.	Hot flushes, vaginal bleeding and vaginal discharge, pruritus vulvae, GI disturbance, headache, light-headedness, tumour flare, decreased platelet counts; occasionally oedema, rarely hypercalcaemia if bony metastases, alopecia, rash, uterine fibroids; also visual disturbances.	• Anovulatory infertility, 20 mg daily on days 2, 3, 4 and 5 of cycle; if necessary the daily dose may be increased to 40 mg then 80 mg for subsequent courses; if cycles irregular, start initial course on any day, with subsequent course starting 45 days later *or* on day 2 of cycle if menstruation occurs • Breast pain (unlicensed). Used if symptoms can be related to cyclic oestrogen production. Can take just on days when symptoms are predicted.

Table 20.12 Gonadotrophin Preparations

Recombinant Technology		Natural Extracts	
Follitropin alfa / delta	rFSH	**Urofollitropin**	purified extract of HPU containing FSH
Follitropin alfa + lutropin alfa	rFSH + rLH	**Menotrophin**	purified extract of HPU containing FSH and LH in a ratio of 1:1
Lutropin alfa	rLH	**Choriogonadotropin alfa**	Human chorionic gonadotropin (hCG)

r = Recombinant, FSH = follicle-stimulating hormone, LH = luteinising hormone, HPU = human postmenopausal urine

Table 20.13 Ulipristal

Cautions	Contraindications	Side Effects	Prescribing
Repeated use within a menstrual cycle **Significant interactions:** antiepileptics, COCs, progestogens, protease inhibitors e.g. ritonavir, rifamycins, aprepitant, clarithromycin, griseofulvin, efavirenz and nevirapine, itraconazole, ketoconazole and voriconazole, St. John's wort and a few other uncommon drugs.	Breast / cervical / ovarian / uterine cancer; breastfeeding (avoid for 7 days after EHC dose); uncontrolled asthma; undiagnosed vaginal bleeding. For *uterine fibroids*: vaginal bleeding not caused by uterine fibroids.	Abdominal/back pain; diarrhoea; dizziness; fatigue; GI dist. headache; menstrual irregularities; muscle spasms; N&V *Rarely* blurred vision; breast tenderness; dry mouth; hot flushes; pruritus; rash; tremor; uterine spasm	• **EHC** 30 mg stat as soon as possible after intercourse, but ≥ 120 hr. Repeat if vomiting within 3 hr. Risk of EHC failure if contraception started within 5 days of treatment. Additional precautions (barrier methods) required for a further 7 days for parenteral progestogen-only and combined contraceptives (9 days for *Qlaira*®) and 2 days for POPs. • **Uterine Fibroids (under expert supervision):** 5 mg od for up to 3 mths. Start during week 1 of menstruation, may be repeated. Re-treat no sooner than week 1 of the 2nd menstruation after completing the previous course. Max. 4 courses.

Table 20.14 Bromocriptine and Cabergoline

Cautions	Contraindications	Side effects
Previous peptic ulcer*, Raynaud's, cardiovascular disease or Hx serious mental disorders. Excl. pituitary tumour before treatment. **Significant interactions:** clarithromycin/erythromycin and dronedarone. For *bromocriptine* also triazole antifungals (e.g. fluconazole) and ketoconazole, protease inhibitors (e.g. ritonavir), diltiazem, verapamil and some other uncommon drugs.	Pre-eclampsia or postpartum hypertension, severe CVD, cardiac valvulopathy (except in lactation suppression); history of pulmonary, retroperitoneal or pericardial fibrosis and of puerperal psychosis. *For *bromocriptine*: particularly in acromegaly.	Sudden onset of sleep, hypotension, nasal congestion, dyspepsia, angina, depression, hallucinations. Monitor closely for hypertension; pulmonary, retroperitoneal and pericardial fibrosis as well as Impulse Control Disorders e.g. pathological gambling, binge eating and hypersexuality.

Cetrorelix and Ganirelix

These are *gonadotropin-releasing hormone (GnRH or LH-RH) antagonists*, which modulate the hypothalamic-pituitary-gonadal axis by **competitively binding to the GnRH receptors** in the pituitary gland, thus inhibiting the secretion of LH and FSH. Onset of suppression is virtually immediate (without an initial stimulatory effect) and is maintained by continuous treatment.

Side Effects: nausea, headache, injection site reactions and rarely rash, facial oedema and dyspnoea.

Contraindications: moderate to severe renal and hepatic impairment; also in pregnancy and breastfeeding.

Dose: 250mcg sub-cutaneously, starting on day 5 or 6 of ovarian stimulation with gonadotropins. Both continue until the day of induced ovulation.

Gonadorelin Analogues

These produce an initial phase of stimulation; continued administration is followed by *down-regulation of GnRH receptors*, thereby reducing the release of gonadotropins (FSH and LH), which in turn leads to inhibition of androgen and oestrogen production.

They are used in the treatment of **endometriosis, precocious puberty, infertility, male hypersexuality with severe sexual deviation, anaemia due to uterine fibroids (together with iron supplementation), breast cancer, prostate cancer** and **before intra-uterine surgery.** *Leuprorelin* and *triptorelin* for 3 to 4 months before surgery reduce uterine volume, fibroid size and associated bleeding. For women undergoing hysterectomy or myomectomy, a vaginal procedure is made more feasible following the use of a gonadorelin analogue.

Cautions

Non-hormonal, barrier methods of contraception should be used during entire treatment period; also metabolic bone disease because can decrease bone mineral density.

Contraindications

Pregnancy, breastfeeding and UVB. In endometrosis use for >6 months due to risk of osteopenia (do not repeat).

Side Effects

Menopausal-like symptoms (e.g. hot flushes, increased sweating, vaginal dryness, dyspareunia and loss of libido) and a decrease in trabecular bone density; these can be reduced by HRT (e.g. with an oestrogen and a progestogen or with tibolone).

Also headache (rarely migraine) and hypersensitivity reactions including urticaria, pruritus, rash, asthma and anaphylaxis. When treating uterine fibroids, bleeding associated with fibroid degeneration can occur.

Spray formulations can cause irritation of the nasal mucosa and nose bleeds; local reactions at the injection site can occur. Also palpitations, hypertension, ovarian cysts, changes in breast size, musculoskeletal pain or weakness, visual disturbances, paraesthesia, changes to hair, oedema of the face and extremities, weight changes and mood changes including depression.

Preparations

Goserelin, leuprorelin, and *triptorelin* are subcutaneous or intramuscular injections. *Nafarelin* is a nasal spray, while *buserelin* can be injected or used intranasally.

Combined Oral Contraceptives (Table 20.15)

COCs prevent ovulation by *suppressing the release of gonadotropins*. Those that contain a fixed amount of an oestrogen and a progestogen in each active tablet are termed 'monophasic'; those with varying amounts are termed 'phasic'.

Low strength preparations (containing *ethinyloestradiol* 20 mcg) are particularly appropriate for women with risk factors for circulatory disease.

Standard strength preparations (containing *ethinyloestradiol* 30 or 35 mcg or in 30–40 mcg 'phased' preparations) are appropriate for standard use but do carry a risk of VTE. 'Phased' preparations contain are generally reserved for women who either do not have withdrawal bleeding or who have breakthrough bleeding with monophasic products.

For **progestogenic side effects**, e.g. depression, sustained weight gain, loss of libido with mood change, acne, hirsutism, vaginal dryness, breast tenderness:

- Use an oestrogen dominant combination e.g. Gedarel®, Cilest®, Marvelon®, Femodene®, Yasmin®

For **oestrogenic excess**, e.g. nausea, bloating, breast tenderness, cyclical weight gain, vaginal discharge with no infection, loss of libido with no mood change, benign breast disease, fibroids, endometriosis:

- Try a progestogen dominant combination e.g. Rigevidon® or Microgynon® 30 or a low-dose oestrogen COC, e.g. Gedarel® 20/150

Encourage a 3-month trial before switching.

Drospirenone (a derivative of spironolactone) in Yasmin® has anti-androgenic and anti-mineralocorticoid activity, and therefore can increase plasma potassium.

Table 20.15 Combined Oral Contraceptives

Cautions	Contraindications	Side effects
Active trophoblastic disease – ssa; Crohn's disease/ inflammatory bowel disease; gene mutations associated with BC (e.g. BRCA 1); Hx severe depression esp. if induced by hormonal contraceptive; hyperprolactinaemia – ssa; **migraine**; personal or family history of hypertriglyceridaemia (increased risk of pancreatitis)*; **risk factors for arterial disease / VTE**; sickle cell disease; undiagnosed breast mass. *Key:* also a caution for **Oestrogen-only HRT and POPs.** *also a caution for *ethinylestradiol* and *tibolone.*	Acute porphyrias; gallstones; heart disease associated with pulmonary hypertension or risk of embolus; *Hx of BC*[a] (but can be used after 5 years if no evidence of disease and non-hormonal methods unacceptable); Hx during pregnancy of cholestatic jaundice/pemphigoid gestationis/pruritus/chorea[b]; / haemolytic uraemic syndrome; migraine with aura[c]; **Hx of VTE**; sclerosing treatment for varicose veins; Multiple risk factors for TE; SLE[a]; transient cerebral ischaemic attacks without headaches; undiagnosed vaginal bleeding. TIAs; **UVB** *Key:* also a contraindication for all oestrogens and progestogens (except conjugated oestrogens, dienogest and estradiol) or *Oestrogen-only HRT* or **all oestrogens and progestogens (except levonorgesterol)**. [a]also a caution for POPs, [b]also a caution for norethisterone and progesterone, [c]also a caution for desogestrel, [d]also a caution for POPs and HRT.	N&V, abdominal cramps, liver impairment, hepatic tumours; fluid retention, thrombosis, hypertension, changes in lipid metabolism; headache, depression, chorea, nervousness, irritability; changes in libido, breast tenderness, enlargement, and secretion; reduced menstrual loss, 'spotting' in early cycles, absence of withdrawal bleeding, amenorrhoea after discontinuation, changes in vaginal discharge, ectropion; contact lenses may irritate, visual disturbance; leg cramps; skin reactions, chloasma, photosensitivity; *rarely* gallstones and SLE.

Note: The possible small increase in the **risk** of breast cancer and cervical cancer should be weighed against the protective effect against cancers of the ovary and endometrium.

Most COCs contain *ethinyloestradiol* plus a range of progestogens. The estrogen *mestranol* and *norethisterone* are in Norinyl-1®, while *dienogest* (Qlaira®) and *nomegestrol* (Zoely®) are available in combination with *oestradiol* as oral preparations.

Dose: Traditional regimen – 1 tablet od for 21 days starting on day 1–5 of cycle (if reasonably certain woman is not pregnant, first course can be started on any day of cycle); subsequent courses repeated after 7-day tablet-free interval (during which withdrawal bleeding occurs).

Regimen Choice

Information on both 21 day and 'tailored' regimens should be provided. Tailored regimens can only use 'monophasic' ethinylestradiol containing preparations and are <u>unlicensed</u>. Options are;

– 21 days followed by a 4 day HFI (hormone free interval)

– 9 weeks of continuous use followed by a 4 or 7 day HFI (aka tricycling)

– 21 days or more followed by a 4 day HFI when breakthrough bleeding occurs

– continuous use with no HFI

There is no difference in efficacy or safety of the traditional 21 day regimen over tailored regimens. N.B. Withdrawal bleeds do not represent physiological menstruation and cannot be relied on as reassurance of a woman's pregnancy status. Use of the traditional regimen may be associated with disadvantages such as; heavy or painful withdrawal bleeds headaches and mood changes increased risk of incorrect use with subsequent unplanned pregnancy.

Norelgestromin is combined with *ethinyloestradiol* in a transdermal patch (Evra®). Useful in poor compliance but not wanting a long-acting reversible method or if there are concerns with absorption.

Dose: 1 patch to be applied once weekly for 3 weeks, followed by a 7-day patch-free interval.

There is a vaginal contraceptive ring (NuvaRing®) available that contains *etonogestrel* combined with *ethinyloestradiol*.

Dose: Insert 1 ring, remove on day 22; repeat after 7-day ring-free interval. For those > 90kg consider non-topical options or add in additional precautions.

Risk Factors for VTE

Increased risk with COC, particularly during the first year and possibly when restarting after a break of 4 weeks.

But risk is considerably lower than that associated with pregnancy (see Table. 20.13).

Caution if 1 factor is present; **avoid or seek specialist advice** if 2 or more:

- Family Hx VTE in first-degree relative >45 years, if <45 years – seek specialist advice (ssa)*
- Body mass index ≥ 30 kg/m^2 (if ≥ 35 kg/m^2, – ssa*)
- Long-term immobilisation – ssa
- Superficial venous thrombosis
- Age over 40 years (avoid if over 50 years)*
- Smoking

(if >35 years and stopped for 1yr+ otherwise if <15 cigarettes/d. or stopped <1yr. – ssa)*

- 6–26 weeks postpartum, if breastfeeding
- 3–6 weeks postpartum, if non-breast feeding
- Hx of hypertension in pregnancy*
- Major surgery
- Uncomplicated valvular/congenital heart disease, cardiomyopathy or long QT syndrome*
- SLE without antiphospholipid antibodies*
- High altitude (>4500m for 1 week+)

Risk increases with age and in the presence of the above risk factors and also varies depending on the type of progestogen (see Table 20.13).

Risk Factors for Arterial Disease

Caution if 1 is present, but **avoid** if 2 or more:

- All VTE factors marked * plus as follows
- Hypertension – adequately controlled or > 140 mmHg systolic or 90 mmHg diastolic – ssa (avoid if > 160 mmHg or 100 mmHg)
- Hx of hypertension in pregnancy
- Dyslipidaemias
- Headache (non-migrane) during CHC use
- Prior migraine without aura. If it starts on a CHC or if migraine **with** aura >5yr. ago – ssa
- Idiopathic intracranial hypertension
- Rheumatoid Arthritis

The risk associated with air travel may be reduced by appropriate exercise during the journey and possibly by wearing graduated compression stockings.

Table 20.16 VTE risks with combined hormonal contraceptives (CHC)

	Risk of VTE per 10,000 women years
Non–contraceptive users and not pregnant	2
CHC containing ethinyloestradiol plus levonorgestrel, norgestimate or norethisterone	5–7
CHC containing etonogestrel (ring) or norelgestromin (patch)	6–12
CHC containing ethinyloestradiol plus gestodene, desogestrel or drospirenone	9–12
Pregnancy	29
Immediate postpartum period	300–400

Adapted from the Faculty of Sexual & Reproductive Healthcare FSRH Guideline on Combined Hormonal Contraception, November 2020.

UK Medical Eligibility Criteria (UKMEC) is a classification system of risk factors and contraindications for all contraceptive methods. A summary is available at www.fsrh.org/documents/ukmec-2016-summary-sheets/.

Missed Pill

- Critical time – **beginning** or **end** of a cycle (as this lengthens the pill-free interval). So, take as soon as remembered, then take the next pill at the normal time (even if this means taking 2 together).
- If only 1 pill is missed, then take an active pill as soon as remembered and then resume as normal. No additional precautions are necessary.
- If >1 missed pill (especially from the first 7 in a packet), may be unprotected. Take an active pill as soon as possible, then resume normal pill taking. Use additional precautions for 7 days. If these run beyond the end of the packet, the next one should be started at once, omitting the pill-free interval / inactive tablets.

Diarrhoea and Vomiting

- If vomiting < 2 hours of taking a pill, then take another.
- With persistent vomiting or severe diarrhoea lasting > 24 hours, additional precautions should be taken for 7 days.

- If it occurs during the last 7 tablets, omit next pill-free interval / inactive pills.

Interactions

The effectiveness of **all hormonal contraceptives** is considerably reduced by drugs that induce hepatic enzyme activity, e.g. *nevirapine* and *ritonavir*; *carbamazepine*, *eslicarbazepine*, *oxcarbazepine*, *phenytoin*, *phenobarbital*, *primidone* and *topiramate*; *St John's wort*; and especially *rifabutin* and *rifampicin*. (*Lamotrigine* and *griseofulvin* are not thought to be enzyme-inducing. However, they may reduce contraceptive efficacy.) Many other uncommon drugs have significant interactions. For patients with HIV infection a condom together with a long-acting method (such as an injectable contraceptive) may be more suitable.

Strategies for managing interactions include:

- Change contraceptive method (e.g. parenteral progestogen-only contraceptives, intra-uterine devices)
- For **short courses** – use a COC with ethinyloestradiol 30 mcg or more daily in a 'tricycling' regimen (see p.195). Additional precautions also needed i.e. careful and consistent use of condoms, and for 4 weeks after stopping.
- For **long-term courses (>2 months),** increase the dose of a COC to ethinyloestradiol 50 mcg or more od by taking a 30 mcg COC plus a 20 mcg COC, or two 30 mcg COCs (unlicensed use) and use 'tricycling'.

  Additional precautions are not necessary; continue for 4 weeks after stopping enzyme-inducing drug.[1]

  If breakthrough bleeding occurs, ethinyloestradiol can be increased in increments of 10 mcg up to 70 mcg od.

  Alternatively, additional precautions or an alternative method unaffected by the interaction should be used.

  Use of contraceptive patches and vaginal rings (including the concurrent use of 2 patches or 2 vaginal rings) is not recommended.[1,3]

- For long-term courses of *rifampicin* or *rifabutin*, an alternative method (such as an IUCD) is **always** recommended because they are such potent enzyme-inducing drugs. Continue for 4 weeks after stopping the enzyme-inducing drug, as this is the time needed for the enzymes to return to their previous level of activity.

- Since 2011 no additional precautions are required when COCs are taken with antibacterials that **do not** induce liver enzymes, i.e. only need to be careful with rifamycins. (N. B. macrolides, e.g. *erythromycin*, are enzyme inhibitors.)

Surgery

- Oestrogen-containing contraceptives (and HRT) should preferably be discontinued 4 weeks before major <u>elective</u> surgery and <u>all</u> surgery that immobilises a lower limb.
- Recommence (for HRT, once fully mobile) at the first menses > 2 weeks after full mobilisation.
- A progestogen-only contraceptive may be offered.
- In <u>emergency</u> surgery, low molecular weight heparin plus graduated compression stockings is advised.

Reasons to Stop Immediately (Incl. HRT)

- Sudden severe chest pain (even if not radiating to left arm)
- Sudden breathlessness (or cough with blood-stained sputum)
- Severe pain in stomach or in the calf of one leg
- Serious neurological effects including;
  - unusual severe, prolonged headache, especially if 1st time or getting worse
  - sudden partial / complete loss of vision
  - sudden disturbance of hearing or other perceptual disorders or dysphasia
  - bad fainting attack or collapse
  - 1st unexplained epileptic seizure
  - weakness, motor disturbances
  - very marked numbness suddenly affecting one side or a part of the body
- Hepatitis, jaundice, liver enlargement
- BP > 160 mmHg systolic and 95 mmHg diastolic
- Immobility after surgery or leg injury
- Detection of a contraindicating risk-factor

Oral Progestogen-Only Contraceptives (Table 20.17)

Oral progestogen-only pills (POPs) *alter cervical mucus to prevent sperm penetration and may inhibit ovulation* in some women. Oral *desogestrel* consistently inhibits ovulation and this is its primary mechanism of action.

POPs offer a suitable alternative if oestrogens are contraindicated. Available as *desogestrel* 75 mcg, *levonorgestrel* 30 mcg or *norethisterone* 350 mcg tablets.

Dose: One tablet od, on a continuous basis, starting on day 1 of cycle and taken at the same time each day. Additional contraceptive precautions are not necessary when initiating treatment.

Table 20.17 Oral progestogen-only contraceptives i.e. *Desogestrel*, *Levonorgestrel* and *Norethisterone*

Cautions	Contraindications	Side effects
Diabetes (can decrease glucose tolerance); Hx BC[e] – ssa; – SLE[$]; rheumatoid arthritis; multiple risk factors for cardiovascular disease; malabsorption states; **positive antiphospholipid antibodies**[$] *Desogestrel:* also migraine with aura[f]; also (and for *levonorgestrel*) Hx of stroke (incl. TIA); Hx of VTE; ischaemic heart disease; UVB. *Norethisterone:* **also risk factors for TE** conditions that may worsen with fluid retention; hypertension; also (and for *levonorgestrel*) **migraine**; also (and for *desogestrel*) cardiac dysfunction; liver tumours – ssa.	Acute porphyrias; **breast cancer**; *Norethisterone:* also has other contraindications, but these are for non-contraceptive uses.	Menstrual irregularities (oligomenorrhoea, menorrhagia) are more common than with COC but tend to resolve on long-term treatment. nausea, vomiting, headache, dizziness, breast discomfort, depression, skin disorders, disturbance of appetite, changes in libido.

Key: also a caution for **COCs or Oestrogen-only HRT** or just **Oestrogen-only HRT**. [e] a contraindication for COCs and Oestrogen-only HRT. [f] a contraindication for COCs and a caution for *desogestrel*. [$] a contraindication for COCs.

Interactions

Effectiveness reduced by enzyme-inducing drugs (see p. 196) and griseofulvin.

An alternative contraceptive method is recommended during treatment and for at least 4 weeks after stopping the enzyme-inducing drug.

For a short course (<2 months) a POP may be continued in combination with additional precautions for the duration of treatment and for 4 weeks after stopping.

Missed Pill

If the POP is delayed by > 3 hours (12 hours for *desogestrel*), contraceptive protection may be lost.

Continue normal pill-taking but use additional precautions for the next 2 days.

Diarrhoea and Vomiting

If vomiting occurs < 2 hours of taking a POP, another pill should be taken as soon as possible.

If a replacement pill is not taken < 3 hours (12 hours for *desogestrel*) of the normal time, or in cases of persistent vomiting or very severe diarrhoea, additional precautions should be used during illness and for 2 days after recovery.

Risk

There is a small increase in the risk of breast cancer, possibly of a similar magnitude as that associated with COCs – however the evidence is less conclusive. But this should be weighed against the benefits.

Parenteral Progestogen-Only Contraceptives

Medroxyprogesterone Acetate

This is a long-acting progestogen given by intramuscular injection every 12 weeks (*Depo-Provera*®) or by subcutaneous injection every 13 weeks (*SAYANA PRESS*®). At least as effective as the COC preparations.

Likelihood of menstrual disturbance and the potential for a delay in return to full fertility. Waiting until 6 weeks after birth may minimise bleeding problems.

Tends to cause weight gain. During the first 1–2 years, average increase was 5–8 lbs. After 4–6 years an average of 14–16.5 lbs was gained. This is a result of increased fat and is not secondary to an anabolic effect or fluid retention.

If not breastfeeding, can give first dose within 5 days postpartum – but this does increase the risk of irregular vaginal bleeding. Although only licensed in breastfeeding to start after 6 weeks the benefits outweigh any risks.

Specific parenteral *contraindication*: Hx BC. Can use >5 years if no evidence of disease and non-hormonal contraceptive methods unacceptable (Cf. COCs).

No proven effect on VTE, MI or stroke and may

- reduce pain associated with endometriosis
- be protective against ovarian/endometrial cancer
- reduce the severity of sickle crisis pain
- have a weak association with breast cancer and after 5yrs. use cervical cancer which both reduce after stopping.[4]

Specific *cautions* for IM/SC use: cervical cancer, Hx of stroke* / VTE, IHD*, multiple risk factors for CVD*, UVB* (*ssa).

Possible *side effects*: acne, decreased libido, mood swings, headache, hot flushes and vaginitis.[4]

Noristerat®

Norethisterone enanthate is a deep IM injection given on days 1–5 of cycle or immediately after parturition, that provides short-term interim contraception for 8 weeks.

Cautions / contraindications are the same as for oral *norethisterone*. Additional cautions in IM use are cervical cancer, Hx of stroke incl. TIA*, IHD*, multiple risk factors for CVD* or UVB* (*ssa).

Nexplanon®

Etonogestrel-releasing implant is a single, flexible rod inserted subdermally, which provides contraception for up to 3 years. Local reactions such as bruising and itching can occur at the insertion site. Contraceptive effect is rapidly reversed on removal. Correct subdermal insertion by an appropriately accredited healthcare professional is recommended to reduce the risk of neurovascular injury and migration of the implant. Not licensed outside the age range of 18–40 years.

Cautions / contraindications are the same as it's prodrug *desogestrel*, except for the additional caution of cervical cancer.

Interactions

Norethisterone and *MPA* injections are not affected by enzyme-inducing drugs (e.g. see p.196). But they (and *griseofulvin*) may reduce the effectiveness of the *etonogestrel*-releasing implant. For short courses (<2 months) can continue with additional precautions (e.g. condoms) and for 4 weeks after stopping.

Benefits and Risks

- In studies, removal rates due to bleeding problems are 16%–20% over 2–3 years of use (N.B. this may not represent current rates in UK). But 65% to >80% of users are 'satisfied' or 'very satisfied' with their implant[3]

- With progestogen-only injectables amenorrhoea or reduced bleeding is common and may reduce menstrual problems. Any small loss of bone density is usually recovered after discontinuation.[4]

Intra-uterine Progestogen-Only Device (LNG-IUS)

This releases *levonorgestrel* directly into the uterine cavity via a T-shaped plastic frame. Mirena® intra-uterine system (IUS) is licensed for use as a **contraceptive**, **primary menorrhagia** and **the prevention of endometrial hyperplasia during oestrogen replacement therapy**. Levosert® is indicated for **contraception** and **menorrhagia**, while Jaydess® and Kyleena® are only licensed for **contraception**. Licensed effectiveness for these products is between 3 and 5 years. Useful for women who have excessively heavy periods; return of fertility after removal is rapid and appears to be complete.

Contraindications

Specific to IU use: active trophoblastic disease, acute blood malgnancies, emergency contraception, PID, post-abortion / postpartum sepsis, recent STI (if not fully investigated and treated), UVB, uterine / cervical malignancy.

Cautions

Specific to IU use: anatomical abnormalities*, cardiac disease*, cervical intraepithelial neoplasia, epilepsy (risk of seizure at insertion), immunosuppression (risk of infection)*, postpartum*, risk of STI, young age (*ssa).

Avoid intercourse >6 days before removal or use another contraceptive method (FSRH – Faculty of Sexual and Reproductive Healthcare).

Risks

Uterine Perforation (MHRA/CHM advice – June 2015)

- occurs most often during insertion – may not be detected until later
- risks are up to 36 weeks postpartum or breastfeeding
- inform patients that 1 in 1000 perforate and that signs / symptoms include:
    - severe pelvic pain (worse than period cramps)
    - pain or increased bleeding for > a few weeks
    - sudden changes in periods
    - pain during intercourse
    - unable to feel the threads (threads can be seen in partial perforation)

STI and PID

If the woman experiences sustained pain within the first 20 days after insertion, she must attend **immediately**; as this is when a pelvic infection is most likely to occur. It is believed to be related to existing carriage of an STI. Risk factors are;

- < 25 years *or*
- > 25 years *and*

    have a new partner *or*

    have had > 1 partner in the past year *or*

    their regular partner has other partners.

The FSRH advises pre-insertion screening for chlamydia +/- *Neisseria gonorrhoeae*.

Teratogenic Drugs

FSRH (February 2018) and MHRA (March 2019) guidance states that females of childbearing potential should be advised to use highly effective contraception if they or their male partners are taking drugs with known or potential teratogenic effects i.e. male/female sterilisation, IUCD, LNG-IUS or a progestogen-only implant.

Pre-menstrual Syndrome[5]

First line: Exercise, cognitive behavioural therapy, vitamin B6, combined new generation pill containing, e.g. *drospirenone* (cyclically or continuously). Continuous or luteal phase (day 15–28) low dose SSRIs, e.g. *citalopram 20mg/escitalopram* 10 mg.

Second line: *estradiol* patches (100 micrograms) + *progesterone* (100 mg or 200 mg on days 17–28, orally or vaginally) or Mirena® or Levosert® N.B. additional contraceptive methods are required.

Higher dose SSRIs continuously or in the luteal phase, e.g. *citalopram* 40mg/*escitalopram* 20 mg.

Third line: GnRH analogues.

If using for >6 months, to reduce the risk of trabecular bone loss commence add-back HRT i.e. continuous combined oestrogen + progesterone e.g. 50–100 micrograms *estradiol* patches or 2–4 doses of *estradiol* gel combined with *progesterone* 100 mg/day or *tibolone* 2.5 mg.

Fourth line: Surgical treatment ± HRT.

Possible SSRIs side effects are nausea, insomnia, somnolence, fatigue and reduction in libido. SSRIs should be discontinued prior to and during pregnancy as they can cause;

- in the early stages a small risk of congenital heart defects
- neonatal withdrawal symptoms
- persistent pulmonary hypertension in the new-born
- Pregnancy often helps PMS symptoms.

- *Micronised progesterone* is theoretically less likely to reintroduce PMS-like symptoms and should therefore be considered as first line for progestogenic opposition.
- GnRH analogues may be used for 3 months for a definitive diagnosis if the symptom diary alone is inconclusive.
- *Spironolactone* can be used in women to treat physical symptoms.
- Low dose *danazol* (200 mg bd) is effective in the luteal phase for breast symptoms. Must use contraception due to its potential virilising effects on female foetuses.
- Treating PMS with only *progesterone* or progestogens is *not* appropriate.

Polycystic Ovary Syndrome (PCOS)[6]

First-line: lifestyle changes – including diet, exercise and weight loss. These can precede or accompany drug options.

Individual CVD risk factors should be assessed. Hypertension should be treated; however, lipid-lowering should only be prescribed by a specialist.

Metformin

Although unlicensed for PCOS, *metformin* improves;

- insulin sensitivity
- may aid weight reduction
- helps normalise menstrual cycle (by increasing the rate of spontaneous ovulation)
- may improve hirsutism
- initially 500 mg od with breakfast for 1 week, then 500 mg bd, with breakfast and evening meal for 1 week, then 1.5–1.7 g od in 2–3 divided doses.
- caution if eGFR <45 ml/min. and avoid if <30 due to increased risk of lactic acidosis. can also be caused by iodine-containing x-ray media, so need to stop before, and not restart until 48 hours after the test.
- GI side effects are common, but often transient. If troublesome, then the slow release preparation can be of benefit.

NICE guidance acknowledges that;

- the unlicensed use of *co-cyprindiol* (Dianette®) and COCs in PCOS is common
- for acne and hirsutism there is no significant difference between *metformin* and *co-cyprindiol*
- *metformin* is less effective at improving menstrual regularity than *co-cyprindiol*.

Recurrent Miscarriage[8]

Pregnant women with antiphospholipid syndrome and recurrent miscarriages should be considered for treatment with low-dose *aspirin* plus *low molecular weight heparin* to reduce the risk of further miscarriage.

Neither corticosteroids nor intravenous immunoglobulin improve the live birth rate of women with recurrent miscarriage associated with antiphospholipid antibodies as compared with other treatments; their use may provoke significant maternal and foetal morbidity.

Antibiotics

This section is based on the microbial environment in Gloucestershire[7]. Obviously, your institution's guidelines will vary depending on local circumstances.

Pelvic Inflammatory Disease (PID) (Table 20.18)

Ofloxacin and *moxifloxacin* should be avoided in patients at high risk of gonococcal PID because of

Table 20.18 Pelvic inflammatory disease

Severity	1st line oral/iv antibiotics	Penicillin allergy
A Minor infection	CEFTRIAXONE 500 mg intramuscularly stat Followed by: DOXYCYCLINE 100 mg orally bd plus METRONIDAZOLE 400 mg orally bd Duration: 14 days	OFLOXACIN 400 mg orally bd plus METRONIDAZOLE* 400 mg orally bd Duration: 14 days
B/C Severe life-threatening infection, e.g. pyrexia >38°C, clinical signs of tubo-ovarian abscess, signs of pelvic peritonitis. Continue IV therapy until 24 hours after clinical improvement, then switch to oral.	CEFTRIAXONE 2 g intravenously od plus DOXYCYCLINE 100 mg orally bd plus METRONIDAZOLE 500 mg intravenously tds (or 400 mg orally tds if oral antibiotics tolerated and patient absorbing)	CLINDAMYCIN 900 mg intravenously tds plus GENTAMICIN intravenously 7 mg/kg od (or as per local protocol)
Intravenous to oral switch	DOXYCYCLINE 100 mg orally bd plus METRONIDAZOLE 400 mg orally bd To complete 14 days	CLINDAMYCIN 450 mg orally qds plus OFLOXACIN 400 mg orally bd To complete 14 days

*Anaerobes are of relatively greater importance in patients with severe PID. Metronidazole may be discontinued in those patients with mild or moderate PID who are unable to tolerate it.

increasing quinolone resistance in the UK (e.g. when the patient's partner has gonorrhoea, in clinically severe disease or following sexual contact abroad). For more detailed guidance see: https://www.bashh.org/guidelines

Uncomplicated Chlamydial Infection

First line: *Doxycycline* 100 mg bd orally for 7 days

- If poor compliance: *Azithromycin* 1 g orally stat
- If pregnant: *erythromycin* 500 mg orally qds for 7 days OR 500 mg orally bd for 14 days
- Refer to genito-urinary medicine clinic for follow-up and contact tracing.

Uncomplicated Gonococcal Infection

- Penicillin and quinolone antibiotics can no longer be relied upon for empirical treatment.

1st line: *ceftriaxone* 250 mg intramuscularly stat OR if known *ciprofloxacin* sensitive strain and not pregnant or breastfeeding: 500 mg orally stat.

UTI in Pregnancy (Table 20.19)

Avoid *trimethoprim* in the 1st trimester as it has an anti-folate activity (manufacturers advise avoid totally).

Short-term use of *nitrofurantoin* is unlikely to cause foetal problems but avoid at term, as it may increase the risk of neonatal haemolysis.

Surgical Prophylaxis

Hysterectomy, manual removal of placenta, third- and fourth-degree tear, major surgery, extensive oncological surgery.

Intravenous – stat at induction: *co-amoxiclav* 1.2 g

- If penicillin allergy: *clindamycin* 600 mg plus *gentamicin* 3 mg/kg (up to a max. of 300 mg)
- If current / previous MRSA positive: add *teicoplanin* <50 kg: 600 mg 50–100 kg: 800 mg >100 kg: 1200 mg

Vaginal and Vulval Infections

The imidazoles (*clotrimazole, econazole, fenticonazole* and *miconazole*) are effective against candida in short courses of 1 to 14 days according to the preparation used. Treatment can be repeated if the initial course fails to control symptoms or if they recur.

Vaginal applications may be supplemented with antifungal cream for vulvitis and to treat other superficial sites of infection.

Oral treatment of vaginal infection with the triazole antifungals *fluconazole* or *itraconazole* is also

Table 20.19 Urinary tract infection in pregnancy

Severity	1st line oral/iv antibiotics	Penicillin allergy
A/B Minor to severe infection Lower Urinary Tract Infection – (Cystitis) OR Asymptomatic bacteriuria of pregnancy	TRIMETHOPRIM 200 mg orally bd OR NITROFURANTOIN modified-release 100 mg orally bd (NB is contraindicated with eGFR < 45 ml/min) OR CEFALEXIN 500 mg orally bd OR CO-AMOXICLAV 625 mg orally tds Typical duration: 7 days	**Non-severe penicillin allergy:** CEFALEXIN 500 mg orally bd **Severe penicillin allergy:** TRIMETHOPRIM 200 mg orally bd OR NITROFURANTOIN modified-release 100 mg orally bd Typical duration: 7 days
C Severe life-threatening infection; Pyelonephritis	CO-AMOXICLAV 1.2 g intravenously tds for 48 hours minimum, then switch to oral OR If poor response to intravenous co-amoxiclav use: TAZOCIN 4.5 g intravenously tds for 48 hours minimum, then switch to oral OR If poor response to Tazocin OR colonisation with ESBL producing organism OR ESBL producing organism on culture then use: MEROPENEM 1 g intravenously tds Typical duration for pyelonephritis: 14 days total	GENTAMICIN intravenously 7 mg od (as per local protocol) OR if gentamicin is contraindicated, then discuss with Consultant Microbiologist. Maximum recommended duration of gentamicin: 7 days Typical duration for pyelonephritis: 14 days total (including oral switch)

ESBL (extended-spectrum beta lactamase) RISK FACTORS: Recent hospitalisation or broad-spectrum antibiotic therapy (especially cephalosporins or quinolones), recurrent urinary tract infection, urinary catheterisation, previously isolated ESBL producing organism.

effective. Both classes have many interactions, but with single-dose fluconazole, these are not significant. Oral treatment should be **avoided** in pregnancy.

Recurrent infection can occur during antibiotic treatment, diabetes, pregnancy or sometimes with oral contraceptives. Reservoirs of infection need to be treated, e.g. digits, nail beds, umbilicus, GI tract and bladder. Also, any partner may be a source of reinfection – up to 6 months of treatment may be required. Various unlicensed regimens are in the BNF.

Trichomonal infections need oral *metronidazole* or *tinidazole*. *Clindamycin* cream and *metronidazole* gel are used in **bacterial vaginosis**.

Genital ulceration is usually due to **herpes simplex virus-2** and can be treated with oral or topical antivirals such as *aciclovir, famciclovir* or *valaciclovir*.

References

1. British National Formulary https://bnf.nice.org.uk/ last updated 9.8.21 – source of most information.
2. https://www.fsrh.org/documents/ukmec-2016-summary-sheets/ (amended Sept. 2019)
3. UK Medicines Information Q&A 43.7 (Nov. 2016), What is a suitable combined oral contraceptive pill in a patient who is taking hepatic enzyme-inducing drugs?
4. https://www.fsrh.org/documents/cec-ceu-guidance-implants-feb-2014/ (updated Feb. 2021)
5. https://www.fsrh.org/standards-and-guidance/documents/cec-ceu-guidance-injectables-dec-2014/ (updated Oct. 2020)
6. www.rcog.org.uk/globalassets/documents/guidelines/gt48managementpremensturalsyndrome.pdf
7. www.rcog.org.uk/en/guidelines-research-services/guidelines/gtg17/
8. www.nice.org.uk/advice/esuom6/chapter/key-points-from-the-evidence
9. www.rcog.org.uk/globalassets/documents/guidelines/gtg_33.pdf
10. https://viewer.microguide.global/GHNFT/ADULT

Single Best Answer Questions

1.1 When prescribing HRT which of the following is a caution rather than a
   a. Breast cancer
   b. Diabetes mellitus
   c. Recent angina
   d. Endometrial hyperplasia
   e. Abnormal liver function

1.2 Answer the same question for the following:
   a. Breast cancer
   b. Migraine
   c. Recent angina

Table 20.20 Antibiotics

Antibiotic mode of action	Cautions	Contraindications	Side effects
AZITHROMYCIN / ERYTHROMYCIN binds to the ribosomal 50s sub-unit and inhibits peptide translocation.	Predisposition to QT prolongation (electrolyte disturbances and drugs that prolong the QT interval). May aggravate myasthenia gravis. Erythromycin has >150 **significant interactions.** Azithromycin has <10.	In *pregnancy and breastfeeding*, for azithromycin manufacturers advise use only if adequate alternatives not available, while erythromycin is considered safe. In severe renal impairment for erythromycin max. 1.5 g per day.	Hepatotoxicity, pancreatitis, arrhythmias, Stevens-Johnson syndrome, toxic epidermal necrolysis. Generally reversible hearing loss (sometimes with tinnitus).
CEFTRIAXONE / CEFALEXIN / CEFUROXIME inhibits bacterial cell wall synthesis following attachment to penicillin-binding proteins. This interrupts peptidoglycan biosynthesis, leading to bacterial cell lysis.	Sensitivity to beta-lactam antibacterials; false-positive urinary glucose and Coombs' test, renal failure, dehydration – risk of ceftriaxone precipitation in gall bladder. All have **significant interactions** with colistimethate. For Ceftriaxone also anticoagulants and calcium chloride/gluconate.	Cephalosporin hypersensitivity; safe in *pregnancy and breastfeeding*. Cephalexin half normal dose if eGFR 5–20 mL/min. Cefuroxime 750 mg bd if eGFR 10–20 mL/min.	Diarrhoea (rarely antibiotic-associated colitis), nausea and vomiting, abdominal discomfort headache; rashes, anaphylaxis; transient hepatitis and cholestatic jaundice; *rarely* prolongation of prothrombin time, pancreatitis.
CLINDAMYCIN binds to the 50s subunit of the bacterial ribosome and inhibits the early stages of protein synthesis. Mainly bacteriostatic, though high concentrations may be slowly bactericidal.	Discontinue immediately if diarrhoea or colitis develops; monitor liver and renal function if treatment exceeds 10 days.	Diarrhoea, acute porphyria. Safe in *pregnancy and breastfeeding*. Only **interacts** with non-depolarising neuromuscular blocking drugs e.g. Atracurium.	Oesophagitis oesophageal ulcers, taste disturbances, nausea, vomiting, antibiotic-associated colitis; jaundice; leucopenia eosinophilia, thrombocytopenia; polyarthritis.
CIPROFLOXACIN / OFLOXACIN inhibit both type II topoisomerase (DNA-gyrase) and topoisomerase IV, required for bacterial DNA replication, transcription, repair and recombination.	Hx epilepsy, glucose 6 phosphate dehydrogenase deficiency, myasthenia gravis, avoid excessive sunlight, can prolong the QT interval. May impair performance of skilled tasks, effects enhanced by alcohol. Ofloxacin, **interacts** with anticoagulants and NSAIDs. Ciprofloxacin also **interacts** with clozapine and phenytoin, plus a few other uncommon drugs. Ciprofloxacin: 250–500 mg bd if eGFR 30–60 mL/min. Ofloxacin: usual dose stat, then half dose if eGFR 20–50 mL/min.	Hx tendon disorders, damage or even rupture can occur within 48 hr. and up to several months later. Risks are >60 yr or corticosteroid. Ofloxacin **interacts** with anticoagulants and NSAIDs (risk of seizures). Ciprofloxacin also **interacts** with clozapine and phenytoin, plus a few other uncommon drugs. Avoid in *pregnancy* because of arthropathy in <u>animal</u> studies.	Anorexia, sleep disturbances, asthenia, confusion, anxiety, depression, hallucinations, tremor, blood disorders, disturbances in vision / taste; *rarely* hepatic dysfunction, hypotension, vasculitis, dyspnoea, convulsions, psychoses, peripheral neuropathy, renal failure, interstitial nephritis, photosensitivity, disturbances in hearing / smell.

Table 20.20 (cont.)

Antibiotic mode of action	Cautions	Contraindications	Side effects
CO-AMOXICLAV *Amoxicillin* acts similarly to cephalosporins, but can be degraded by beta-lactamases produced by resistant bacteria. *Clavulanate*, structurally related to penicillins, inactivates some beta-lactamase enzymes, thereby preventing inactivation of amoxicillin.	Cholestatic jaundice can occur either during or shortly after treatment and is 6 times > with amoxicillin. More common >65 years and men; usually self-limiting, *very rarely fatal*. Treatment not usually >14 days. **Interactions:** Amoxicillin can cause a rash with allopurinol, toxicity with methotrexate increase INR with warfarin. Clavulanate can cause liver damage with other hepatotoxic drugs.	Penicillin hypersensitivity, i.e. previous anaphylaxis, urticaria, or immediate rash – minor reaction or >72 hr post dose are unlikely to be allergic. Previous penicillin-associated jaundice or hepatic dysfunction. If eGFR 10–30 mL/min. 625 mg bd orally or 1.2 g intravenously, then 600 mg bd. Safe in *pregnancy and breastfeeding.*	Rashes and anaphylaxis and can be fatal. Allergic reactions occur in 1–10%; anaphylactic reactions <0.05%. Those with Hx of atopic allergy (e.g. asthma, eczema, hay fever) are at greater risk of anaphylactic reactions. *Rarely* encephalopathy, usually due to accumulation. Severe skin reactions and vasculitis reported.
DOXYCYCLINE inhibits bacterial protein synthesis by binding to the 30S ribosomal subunit.	Myasthenia gravis, SLE, hepatic impairment. **Significant interactions:** anticoagulants, retinoids, ciclosporin and lithium. Antacids; aluminium, calcium, iron, magnesium & zinc salts decrease absorption. Antiepileptics may decrease levels.	*pregnancy and breastfeeding,* deposition causes staining in bones and teeth and occasionally dental hypoplasia. Avoid with retinoids (benign intracranial hypertension).	*Rare* side effects include hepatotoxicity, pancreatitis, blood disorders, photosensitivity (avoid sunlight and sunlamps); anorexia, dry mouth, flushing, anxiety and tinnitus.
GENTAMICIN affects the integrity of the plasma membrane and the metabolism of RNA, most important effect is inhibition of protein synthesis at the level of the 30s ribosomal subunit.	Assess renal function before starting and during treatment. Correct dehydration before starting. Monitor auditory and vestibular function. **No significant interactions** with common drugs.	Myasthenia gravis. Ototoxic diuretics (e.g. furosemide) should be separated by as long a period as practicable. Avoid unless essential in 2nd and 3rd trimester. Once-daily dosing should be avoided when creatinine clearance < 20 mL/min.	Nephrotoxicity and irreversible ototoxicity, peripheral neuropathy. *Rarely* hypomagnesaemia on prolonged therapy. hypocalcaemia, hypokalaemia and stomatitis, blood disorders, headache, encephalopathy, and convulsions.
METRONIDAZOLE is a prodrug. Un-ionized it is selective for anaerobic bacteria as they intracellularly reduce it to its active form, which covalently binds to DNA, thus inhibiting bacterial nucleic acid synthesis.	Disulfiram-like reaction with alcohol – facial flushing, nausea, headache, vomiting, chest pain, vertigo, sweating, thirst, blurred vision, weakness, confusion and hypotension. In severe liver disease, reduce total daily dose to one-third, and give once daily.	Manufacturer advises avoiding high-dose regimens in pregnancy. **Significant interactions** with busulfan, capecitabine, fluorouracil, lithium and warfarin.	Furred tongue, oral mucositis, anorexia; *very rarely* hepatitis, jaundice, pancreatitis, drowsiness, dizziness, headache, ataxia, psychotic disorders, darkening of urine, thrombocytopenia, pancytopenia, myalgia, arthralgia, visual disturbances, rash, pruritus, and erythema multiforme.
MEROPENEM is a carbapenem with similar actions to penicillins and cephalosporins.	Sensitivity to beta-lactam antibacterials. In hepatic impairment, monitor LFTs. Only **interacts** to lower levels of sodium valproate and valproic acid – therefore avoid.	History of immediate hypersensitivity reaction. In *pregnancy* use only if potential benefits outweighs risks – no information available. Normal dose every 12 hours if eGFR 26–50 mL/min.	Thrombocythaemia, rash, pruritus; *less commonly* paraesthesia, eosinophilia, thrombocytopenia, leucopenia; *rarely* convulsions; haemolytic anaemia, positive Coombs' test and severe skin reactions.

Drug	Cautions / Interactions	Side effects
NITROFURANTOIN is activated by bacterial flavoproteins (nitrofuran reductase) to active reduced intermediates that are thought to modulate and damage ribosomal proteins or other macromolecules, especially DNA, causing inhibition of DNA, RNA, protein, and cell wall synthesis.	Anaemia; diabetes mellitus; electrolyte imbalance; vit. B and folate deficiency; pulmonary disease; on long-term therapy monitor liver function and for pulmonary symptoms, esp. in the elderly susceptibility to peripheral neuropathy; false-positive urinary glucose (if tested for reducing substances); urine may be coloured yellow or brown.	G6PD deficiency, acute porphyria. Avoid if eGFR < 45 mL/min.; may be used with caution if eGFR 30–44 mL/min. antibacterial efficacy depends on renal secretion; risk of peripheral neuropathy; In *pregnancy* avoid at term – may produce neonatal haemolysis. **Significant interactions** with dapsone and prilocaine.	Acute and chronic pulmonary reactions, peripheral neuropathy, angioedema, anaphylaxis, sialadenitis, urticaria, rash and pruritus; *rarely*, cholestatic jaundice, hepatitis, exfoliative dermatitis, erythema multiforme, pancreatitis, arthralgia, blood disorders, benign intracrania hypertension, and transient alopecia.
TAZOCIN® *Piperacillin*, a broad-spectrum, semi-synthetic penicillin inhibits both septum and cell-wall synthesis. *Tazobactam*, is an inhibitor of many beta-lactamases,	History of allergy; false-positive urinary glucose. **May interact** with neuromuscular blockers, warfarin and methotrexate (toxicity).	Penicillin hypersensitivity. Max. 4.5 g every 12 hours if eGFR less than 20 mL/min. In *pregnancy* manufacturers advise use only if potential benefits outweighs risks.	Stomatitis, dyspepsia, constipation, jaundice, hypotension, headache, insomnia, injection-site reactions.
TEICOPLANIN inhibits cell-wall biosynthesis at a site different from that affected by beta-lactams by specifically binding to D-alanyl-D-alanine residues.	Risk of 'red man syndrome' with bolus administration, vancomycin sensitivity, no dose adjustment needed in renal impairment until day 5. **No significant** interactions.	Teicoplanin hypersensitivity. Hx 'red man syndrome' with vancomycin is not a contraindication. In *pregnancy*, manufacturer advises use only if potential benefits outweigh risks.	Rash, pruritus nausea, vomiting, diarrhoea, bronchospasm, dizziness, headache, fever, leucopenia, thrombocytopenia, eosinophilia, tinnitus, mild hearing loss, thrombophlebitis; also renal failure, serious skin reactions.
TRIMETHOPRIM is a dihydrofolate reductase inhibitor which affects the nucleoprotein metabolism of micro-organisms by interference in the folic-folinic acid systems.	Predisposition to folate deficiency; porphyria. Reduce dose if eGFR <30 mL/min. **Significant interactions** with anticoagulants, colistimethate, dapsone, methotrexate and pyrimethamine.	Blood dyscrasias – inform patients on long-term treatment how to recognise signs of blood disorders. In *pregnancy* teratogenic risk in first trimester (folate antagonist); manufacturers advise avoid.	Hyperkalaemia, depression of haematopoiesis; *rarely* severe skin reactions, angioedema, anaphylaxis; aseptic meningitis and uveitis reported.

d. Endometrial hyperplasia

e. Abnormal liver function

2. When prescribing HRT, with which of the following is there not a significant interaction?

a. Thalidomide

b. Raloxifene

c. Pomalidomide

d. Simvastatin

e. Ospemifene

3. When prescribing HRT, there is no proven increased risk of developing:

a. Stroke

b. Breast cancer

c. Cervical cancer

d. Ovarian cancer

e. Venous thromboembolism

4. Which statement is not true? Tibolone

a. has oestrogenic and progestogenic activity and also weak androgenic activity

b. should be used with caution in epilepsy, migraine and diabetes

c. is unsuitable in premenopausal women (unless she is being treated with a gonadotropin-releasing hormone analogue)

d. increases the risk of stroke

e. significantly affects mammographic density

5. For clonidine, which statement is false?

a. It acts centrally by stimulating alpha$_2$-adrenergic receptors and producing a reduction in sympathetic tone

b. Usual dosing is 50 mg twice daily, increased after 2 weeks to 75 mg twice daily if necessary

c. Cautions include depression, heart failure, Raynaud's syndrome and antihypertensive therapy, and it is contraindicated in bradycardia

d. It interactions with tricyclic antidepressants and beta-blockers

e. It diminishes the responsiveness of peripheral vessels to constrictor and dilator stimuli, thereby preventing the vascular changes associated with menopausal flushing

6. Which of the following progestogens is least likely to cause virilisation?

a. Norgestrel

b. Gestodene

c. Norgestimate

d. Desogestrel

e. Dydrogesterone

7. Regarding Ulipristal, which statement is false?

a. It is a receptor modulator characterised by a tissue-specific partial progesterone antagonist effect

b. It is indicated in the pre-operative treatment of moderate to severe symptoms of uterine fibroids

c. It is equally effective as levonorgestrel as an emergency hormonal contraceptive and can be used up to 120 hours after intercourse

d. It may reduce the effectiveness of combined hormonal and progestogen-only contraceptives.

e. It is known to have significant interactions with antiepileptics, rifamycins, ritonavir and St. John's wort

8. Which of the following statements is false? Leuprorelin

a. is a gonadorelin analogue that acts by up-regulation of gonadotropin-releasing hormone receptors

b. when used for 3 to 4 months before vaginal hysterectomy, it reduces the uterine volume, fibroid size and associated bleeding

c. treatment necessitates the use of non-hormonal, barrier methods of contraception during the entire treatment period

d. is licensed for subcutaneous and intramuscular routes, while other gonadorelin analogues are available as nasal sprays

e. when used for endometriosis should not continue for more than 6 months

9. Regarding combined oral contraceptives, which statement is false?

a. They are available in low dose preparations containing only 20 mcg of the synthetic oestrogen ethinyloestradiol

b. Phased preparations are generally reserved for women who *either* do not have withdrawal bleeding *or* who have breakthrough bleeding with monophasic products

c. Risk factors include family history of venous thromboembolism in first-degree relative aged under 45 years, body mass index $\geq$ 30, long-term immobilisation, history of superficial thrombophlebitis, age over 35 years and smoking

d. If the patient vomits within 2 hours of taking then another pill should be taken

e. COCs interact with the potent enzyme inducer rifampicin to such an extent that for long term courses an alternative method (e.g. parenteral progestogen or an IUD) is recommended. This should be continued for 4 weeks after stopping the rifampicin

10. Which of the following statements is false? Tranexamic acid is

a. an antifibrinolytic compound which is a potent competitive inhibitor of the activation of plasmin to plasminogen

b. used in menorrhagia (initiated when menstruation has started) by mouth at 1 g 3 times daily for up to 4 days

c. to be used with caution in patients receiving oral contraceptives and is contraindicated in thromboembolic disease and history of convulsions

d. to be discontinued if patient notices changes in their colour vision

e. licensed to be used intravenously, but not as continuous infusion

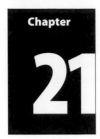

Surgical Site Surveillance

Balpreet Attilia

1 Surgical Site Infection

A surgical site infection (SSI) is a healthcare-associated infection occurring after an invasive or surgical procedure. It is usually localized to the incision site but can extend into deeper structures with presentation delayed up to 30 days. SSI accounts for up to 20% of all healthcare-associated infections [2].

SSI covers a spectrum of conditions ranging from a self-limiting wound discharge to septic shock and multi-organ failure. Approximately 5% of patients undergoing surgery will have an SSI, many of which may be preventable, which represents a substantial cost to the NHS.

1.1 What Is an Infection?

An infection occurs when a micro-organism is found within the host tissue and there is an associated inflammatory response to its presence. Therefore Group B streptococcus isolated on a vaginal swab is not an infection unless there is a concurrent inflammatory response.

Bacteraemia is the presence of viable bacteria in the bloodstream of the host. Usually this is identified from taking blood cultures which grow micro-organisms. Septicaemia is a confusing term, and its use is no longer recommended.

1.2 What Is an Inflammatory Response?

The five cardinal signs of inflammation are *rubor* (redness), *calor* (heat), *tumor* (swelling), *dolor* (pain) and *function laesa* (disturbance of function). An inflammatory response can be localised or systemic within the body.

A systemic inflammatory response includes the cardinal signs above and the addition of two or more of the following:

- Temperature > 38° or < 36°C
- Tachycardia > 90 beats per minute

- Respiratory rate > 20 breaths per minute or $PaCO_2$ < 32 mmHg.
- White cell count more than $12(\times 10^9/L)$, less than $4(\times 10^9/L)$ or greater than 10% mature forms [3].

Systemic inflammatory response syndrome, or SIRS, was defined in 1992 by the American College of Chest Physicians and the Society of Critical Care Medicine consensus conference committee, publishing definitions for sepsis and its sequelae. It can be caused by sepsis but also many other cytokine releasing conditions, for example burns, pancreatitis, trauma and autoimmune conditions.

1.3 Sepsis

Sepsis is the systemic response to infection defined by the presence of two or more SIRS criteria caused by a known or suspected infection. Sepsis can progress to severe sepsis and septic shock, defined as follows:

- Severe sepsis: sepsis in the presence of acute organ dysfunction, for example hypo-perfusion or hypotension
- Septic shock: severe sepsis in the presence of persistent or refractory hypotension or tissue hypo-perfusion despite adequate fluid resuscitation [3]

Septic shock can in turn lead to multi-organ dysfunction such that body homeostasis cannot be maintained without intervention [3]. Examples of this are detailed in Table 21.1.

2 Prevention, Recognition and Management of Infection

2.1 Prevention

Several steps are taken prior to a procedure or surgical intervention to prevent surgical site infection. Many of these steps are universal and have become part of the WHO surgical checklist, for example antibiotic prophylaxis prior to skin incision. Steps can also be

Table 21.1 Examples of organ dysfunction by a system in sepsis

System	Symptoms	Signs
Cardiovascular	Shortness of breath, chest pain, arrhythmias, cardiac arrest	Tachycardia, hypotension, altered central venous pressure, reduced cardiac output
Respiratory	Difficulty in breathing shortness of breath	Tachypnoea $PaCO_2 < 32$ mmHg $saO_2 < 90\%$
Neurological	Confusion	EEG abnormality
Endocrine	Weight loss	Hyperglycaemia, hypalbuminaemia
Haematological	Excessive or unusual bleeding or bruising	Thrombocytopenia, increased D-dimers, abnormal white cell count, abnormal clotting
Gastrointestinal	Abdominal pain, distension, ileus, GI bleeding	Elevated amylase/pancreatitis
Hepatic	Jaundice	Deranged LFTs, hypalbuminaemia
Renal	Oliguria, anuria	Deranged renal function tests

taken intra-operatively and post-operatively to prevent infection.

2.1.1 Pre-operative Prevention

General advice should be given in a written format that they understand to all patients undergoing surgery. All patients should be advised to shower or bathe (or helped to bathe) using soap, either the day before or on the day of surgery. Patients should be advised not to remove hair routinely from the operative site in order to reduce the risk of SSI or to use razors for hair removal as this increases the risk of surgical site infection. If hair has to be removed to perform the operation, electric clippers with a single-use head should be used on the day of surgery [2].

Patients should be given appropriate clothing to wear for the surgical procedure, usually in the form of a non-sterile theatre gown that allows easy access to the operative site but maintains patients' dignity. Patients do not routinely require bowel preparation before surgery but specific procedures may require this if there is a high risk of bowel injury or contamination [2].

All theatre staff should wear specific, non-sterile theatre scrubs in areas where operations are undertaken. Theatre staff should keep their movements in and out of the operating area to a minimum. The operating team should remove all hand jewellery, artificial nails and nail polish before operations, as these can harbour microorganisms such as Serratia marcescens and candida [2].

Nasal decontamination with topical antimicrobial agents to eliminate Staphylococcus aureus is not routinely recommended to reduce the risk of SSI [2].

Consider giving a single dose of antibiotic prophylaxis intravenously on starting anaesthesia and give a repeat dose if the half life of the antibiotic is shorter than the duration of the operation. Consult local trust guidelines for the recommended antibiotics and doses for specific operations.

2.1.2 Antibiotic Prophylaxis

Antibiotic resistance is an emerging concern with increasing multi-resistant strains surfacing. Antibiotic use must therefore be rationed and evidence-based.

Antibiotic prophylaxis is not universally indicated for all surgical procedures. Surgical wounds can be classified as follows:

- **Clean Wound (type 1):** an uninfected operative wound, where the respiratory, gastro-intestinal and genito-urinary tract are not entered
- **Clean-Contaminated Wound (type 2):** the respiratory, gastro-intestinal and genito-urinary tract are entered under controlled conditions, without unusual contamination
- **Contaminated Wound (type 3):** open, fresh or accidental wounds, or surgical procedures where there are major breaks in sterile technique or gross spillage of contaminated body fluids
- **Dirty-Infected Wound (type 4):** old traumatic wounds with retained devitalised tissue or those that involve existing clinical infection or a perforated viscus [4].

Give antibiotic prophylaxis for clean surgery (type 1) if involving a prosthesis or implant, for clean-contaminated surgery (type 2) and for contaminated surgery (type 3). The patient with a dirty infected wound should be receiving treatment antibiotics and therefore prophylaxis may not be required, although consider whether there may be any additional benefit from prophylaxis [2].

2.1.3 Intraoperative Prevention

Many steps taken intra-operatively to reduce SSI may become second nature and risk complacency, for example hand decontamination before surgery. Hand decontamination at the start of the operating list should be performed with antiseptic aqueous or alcohol-based solution (povidone-iodine or chlorhexidine) and a single-use nail brush or nail pick. Subsequent hand decontamination should use alcohol gel or antiseptic aqueous or alcohol-based solution [2].

Wearing sterile gowns and gloves is necessary; however, consider wearing two pairs of sterile gloves if there is a high chance of a break in the glove or serious consequences of possible contamination [2].

The patient's skin should be cleaned with aqueous or alcohol-based solution (povidone-iodine or chlorhexidine), which should be allowed to evaporate dry prior to draping. Incise drapes that are iodophor-impregnated may be used to reduce the risk of SSI. Intra-operative skin disinfection is not recommended [2].

The anaesthetist can also help in reducing SSI by ensuring the patient's homeostasis is maintained during the surgery. Particular emphasis is placed on avoiding hypothermia by checking the patient's temperature throughout surgery, using blankets and warm air devices (Bear-Hugger®). Other parameters that should be maintained include oxygenation greater than 95%, adequate organ perfusion and glycaemic control with insulin in diabetic patients [2].

Appropriate dressing should be used to cover wounds. Intra-cavity lavage is not routinely recommended to reduce the risk of SSI [2].

2.1.4 Post-operative Prevention

Wound dressings should be removed using a sterile non-touch technique and wounds healing by primary intention should be cleaned with sterile water in the first 48 hours. Patients can shower after 48 hours, and tap water should be used to clean wounds after this time.

Patients with wounds healing by secondary intention should be referred to a tissue viability nurse for advice on appropriate dressings and management [2].

Post-operative fever within 48 hours of surgery is almost always cytokine related and usually resolves within 2–3 days. It is therefore important to perform a clinical examination to exclude additional symptoms and signs of infection.

Specific post-operative infections are discussed as follows.

2.2 Recognising Infection

Numerous early warning scores have been devised to help improve the early recognition of sepsis. However, according to both local and national audits, healthcare professionals remain poor at this, for example the Confidential Enquiry into Maternal Deaths 2014, which focused on sepsis [1]. The adoption of 'National Early Warning Score' (NEWS) for surgical patients should standardise the recognition of symptoms and signs of sepsis based on measuring and recording of the vital signs. However, considering sepsis as a diagnosis is the first step to recognising it.

Most infective sources of SSI originate from the patient and the most common cause is the patient's own skin flora.

Healthcare-associated infections include surgical site infections, by definition occurring at the site of the surgery, and post-operative infections distant from the site of surgery, for example urinary tract or lower respiratory infections. Other healthcare-associated infections include bacteraemias (e.g. from IV cannulation sites) and antibiotic-associated diarrhoeas (particularly Clostridium Difficile).

2.2.1 History and Clinical Examination

Do not forget the basics! Take a clinical history from the patient if possible and thoroughly examine the patient if necessary. Do not forget a breast examination, especially in the postnatal woman in whom mastitis is common.

Check the skin beneath surgical dressings and examine the site of any foreign bodies, for example catheters and drains. Take care to protect the patient's dignity, exposing only the area(s) being examined and always have a chaperone present for examinations. A thorough history and examination should give a clue as to the source of infection.

2.3 Management

In 2012 the Surviving Sepsis campaign was launched and, along with the UK Sepsis, Trust developed the 'Sepsis Six'. This is a care bundle or set of six medical interventions which, when performed within the first hour following the recognition of sepsis, has been shown to improve morbidity and mortality. This has been adopted by almost all trusts in the UK into local

Table 21.2 Investigations included in a septic screen

Haematological	FBC (raised WCC common, may be reduced in overwhelming sepsis) Coagulation screen Thick and thin blood film (malarial parasites) Confirm sickle cell / thalassaemia status
Biochemistry	Sodium, potassium, urea, creatinine Glucose (usually *increased* in SIRS) Amylase (raised in pancreatitis, ischaemic bowel, perforated bowel) Liver function tests Cardiac enzymes Creatinine kinase
Microbiology	Cultures of blood, MSU/CSU, sputum, CSF, wound/vaginal swabs
Bedside	ABG, lactate and ECG
Radiology	CXR and other imaging

guidelines and protocols, based on the UK Sepsis Trust recommendations.

2.3.1 Investigations

Investigations are performed to confirm the presence of infection. The threshold of suspicion must therefore be low in order to perform correct and timely investigations. The investigations required will depend on the clinical history and examination: a 'septic screen' may be required in difficult cases (Table 21.2).

Deeper infection may be clinically or radiologically suspected in post-operative patients. Consider sending samples obtained from percutaneous aspiration, surgical drainage or debridement to microbiology and histology.

If the source of infection is unclear, give broad-spectrum antibiotics initially until the source becomes clear or microbiology investigations identify the infective organism.

Give specific antibiotics when an SSI is obvious, for example wound cellulitis. Consult local antibiotic guidelines and resistance patterns. Liaise with microbiology if in doubt or if the patient has allergies.

3. Specific Infections

3.1 Cellulitis

Cellulitis occurs in the superficial layers (dermal or subcutaneous) of the skin and is the most common type of SSI. Severe inflammation of skin causes redness, warmth, pain and swelling around a break in the skin which allows micro-organisms, commonly Streptococcus and Staphylococcus species, to cause infection. Treatment is with antibiotics and regularly checking the affected area in order to ensure it is improving. Often the affected area is marked out with a pen in order to quickly assess whether there is clinical improvement with antibiotics.

3.2 Abscess

Abscess tends to occur in deeper structures than does cellulitis and is an infectious accumulation of purulent material in a closed cavity. Specific clinical findings are a fluctuant, compressible swelling that is very tender. Treatment is with antibiotics, and abscesses usually require surgical drainage.

3.3 Necrotising Fasciitis

Necrotising fasciitis is a surgical emergency. It is a deep infection of the skin and soft tissue that can spread across the fascial planes. There is no diagnostic test, and it is a clinical diagnosis. Characteristic features include a 'dishwater' discharge and a grey colour of the affected tissues. The patient may report pain that is out of proportion to the clinical appearance.

Although rare, it is a rapidly progressing life-threatening infection involving aerobic and anaerobic organisms. The most common cause is Streptococcus, which can cause 'toxic shock' with a β-haemolytic strain.

Deep subcutaneous tissues along the fascial plane are involved first (fasciitis) when the overlying skin initially shows very few changes. The underlying muscle is not usually involved. Clinical examination may reveal crepitus and x-rays of the affected area show air in the soft tissues.

Nectrotising fasciitis has been divided into two groups:
- Polymicrobial (type1): when multiple species are involved, including mixed aerobes and anaerobes
- Isolated (type 2): occurs in 15% of cases, when a single organism is involved [6]

Treatment includes immediate resuscitation followed by urgent surgical debridement. Any pus or affected tissue should be sent to microbiology and histology. Antibiotics should be started empirically and changed depending on clinical response and microbiology results. Re-exploration of the affected area is usually recommended within 24–48 hours to ensure the tissue is healthy [6].

Patient isolation is unnecessary unless the infection is caused by the highly infectious and virulent

Group A Streptococcus. De-isolation of these patients can occur only once biopsies are culture negative.

3.4 Endometritis

Endometritis is an infection of the decidua. It is a common cause of postpartum febrile morbidity. A major risk factor is delivery by emergency Caesarean section when endometritis is almost four times more likely to occur. The symptoms and signs include lower abdominal pain, general malaise, fever, vaginal discharge and uterine tenderness.

The diagnosis is clinical. Approximately 5–20% of patients develop bacteraemia, and treatment may include evacuation of the uterus if there is a suspicion of retained products. Antibiotics should be broad spectrum with anaerobic cover until clinical improvement and no fever for 24–48 hours.

3.5 Antibiotic-Associated Diarrhoea

Antibiotics can cause diarrhoea by disruption of the normal bowel flora (allowing overgrowth of other species), by a direct effect of the antibiotic (by increasing gut motility), or rarely as an allergic response to the antibiotic [7].

The most common species to cause antibiotic-associated diarrhoea is Clostridium Difficile, responsible for 20– 30% of cases [7]. Other reported culprits include Clostridium Perfringens, Staphylococcus Aureus, Candida species, Klebsiella Oxytoca, and Salmonella species.

3.5.1 Clostridium Difficile-Associated Diarrhoea

Clostridium Difficile-associated diarrhoea is a significant cause of morbidity and mortality in hospital patients. Clostridium Difficile is an anaerobic Gram-positive spore-forming bacterium that is spread via the faecal-oral route [8]. Up to 20% of hospitalised patients may be colonised with C. diff; one-third of those colonised will produce toxins. The two main toxins are forms A and B; toxin B is 1000 times more cytotoxic than toxin A [8]. One strain, *toxigenic S-type 5236*, is responsible for 70% of all cases in the UK [8].

The risk factors for developing C. diff infection are:

- Advanced age (>65 years old)
- Antibiotic treatment with clindamycin, cefalosporins, fluoroquinolones and co-amoxiclav
- Underlying morbidity (recent surgery, chronic medical condition)

- Use of a proton-pump inhibitor (PPI) or other acid-suppressive drugs
- Hospitalisation
- Exposure to infected cases
- Long duration of antibiotic use or multiple antibiotics concurrently [7]

When infected, the majority of patients suffer mild, self-limiting symptoms which recover with conservative measures and withdrawal of the causative antibiotic. In symptomatic patients, the diagnosis is two-step: the presence of glutamate dehydrogenase (GDH) in stool is a screening test for the disease, and detection of toxin production is diagnostic.

The treatment involves management of fluid losses, antibiotic treatment to eradicate C. diff (oral metronidazole or oral vancomycin) and actions to minimise the spread to others, including basic hygiene measures and barrier nursing or source isolation if necessary. Antimotility agents and probiotics are not recommended as part of the treatment of antibiotic-associated diarrhoea [7].

In severe cases, GI endoscopy and CT scanning can demonstrate findings of pseudomembranous colitis and toxic megacolon, two of the complications associated with C. diff infection.

References

1. Knight M, Kenyon S, Brocklehurst P, Neilson J, Shakespeare J, Kurinczuk JJ (eds.), on behalf of MBRRACEUK. *Saving Lives, Improving Mothers' Care – Lessons Learned to Inform Future Maternity Care from the UK and Ireland Confidential Enquiries into Maternal Deaths and Morbidity 2009–12.* Oxford: National Perinatal. Epidemiology Unit, University of Oxford, 2014

2. NICE Clinical Guidance 74, October 2008. www.guidance.nice.org.uk/cg74

3. Bone R et al. (1992). Definition for sepsis and organ failure and guidelines for the use of innovative therapies in sepsis. *Chest*;**101**:1644–55

4. Mangram AJ et al. (1999). Guideline for prevention of surgical site infection. *Infect Control Hosp Epidemiol* **1999**;20:247–80

5. The UK Sepsis Trust. www.sepsistrust.org

6. Hasham S. Necrotising fasciitis. *BMJ*(2005);**330**:830–3

7. NICE Clinical Knowledge Summaries. Antibiotic associated diarrhea. www.cks.nice.org.uk/diarrhoea-antibiotic-associated#!topicsummary

8. Starr J. Clostridium difficile associated diarrhoea: Diagnosis and treatment. *BMJ* (2005);**331**:498–501

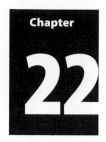

Chapter 22

Data Interpretation in Gynaecology

Andrew Sizer

As in 'Data Interpretation in Obstetrics,' questions can draw on knowledge from the entire Part 1 curriculum. As the new Part 1 exam including the clinical domains is now well established, themes of questions over the past three years have been examined and represented as follows.

Module 6 Post-operative Care

- Questions may involve the interpretation of a scenario or results in a post-operative scenario
- Be familiar with the interpretation of blood gas results; these can feature in both obstetrics and gynaecology
- Be aware of the main electrolytes in the body and the main causes of electrolyte disturbance
- Simple imaging may be given with an accompanying scenario for interpretation, for example an ultrasound scan showing a pelvic collection, or a CT urogram showing ureteric obstruction
- Fluid balance and urine output have been mentioned previously, but be aware of classifications and definitions.

Electrolytes and imbalances are explored in Table 22.1.

Urine output is discussed in Table 22.2.

Module 7 Surgical Procedures

- To date, there have been very few questions about the interpretation of surgical procedures
- In theory, there could be questions about any surgical procedures in gynaecology that would be encountered at the ST2 level. From the current training matrix, this includes:
  - ○ Laparoscopy
  - ○ Hysteroscopy
  - ○ Surgical management of miscarriage

- Surgical images may be presented to interpret the likely pathology
- Histology reports may be presented with a clinical scenario for interpretation

Module 13 Gynaecological Problems

The blueprinting grid states:

Interpret commonly performed investigations for benign gynaecological conditions

Questions in this module tend to fall into one of four main groups:

- Surgical images that may represent normal anatomy or a pathological process (see Module 7 above)
- Ultrasound images that may represent normal anatomy or a pathological process
- Interpretation of normal and abnormal female endocrinology, especially relating to the menstrual cycle
- Interpretation of other blood results, e.g. causes of anaemia

Please see the example questions at the end of this chapter.

Module 14 Subfertility

The blueprinting grid states:

Interpret basic investigations in investigation of infertility.

- Many questions in recent examinations have focussed on the interpretation of male endocrinology and semen analysis (Table 22.3)

Terms used in the interpretation of a semen analysis are given in Table 22.4.

Classification of causes of an abnormal semen analysis is given in Table 22.5.

Interpretation of Acid Base Disturbance

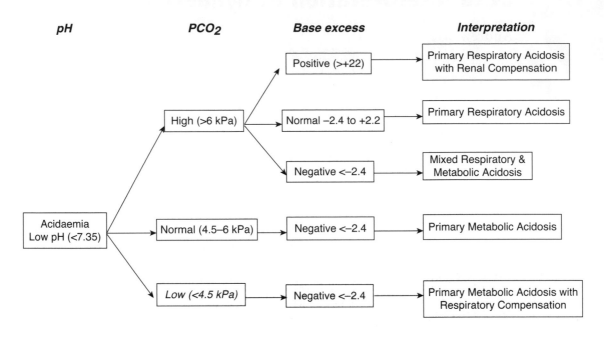

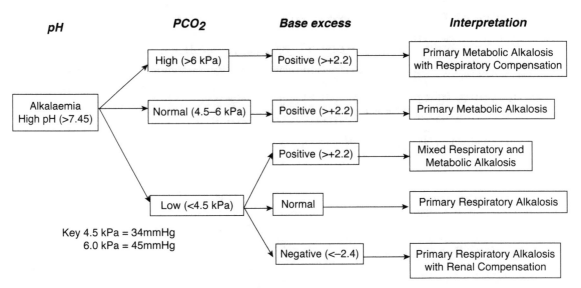

Figure 22.1 Acid-base balance

- There may be images of an oocyte around the time of fertilisation, or in relation to assisted conception
- Imaging may be provided for interpretation, for example

- Ultrasound imaging of ovaries, uterus and fallopian tubes, e.g. hydrosalpinx
- Imaging of tests of tubal patency, e.g. hysterosalpingogram and hystero-contrast-salpingography

Table 22.1 The five most important electrolytes

Electrolyte	Function	Distribution	Disturbance and Causes
Sodium (Na)	Key role in fluid balance Contributes half the osmolarity of the extracellular fluid	Predominantly in extracellular fluid Regulated by antidiuretic hormone, aldosterone and atrial natriuretic peptide	Hyponatraemia: caused by insufficient intake (e.g. inadequate sodium in intravenous fluids), excessive water, diuretic therapy or hypoadrenalism Hypernatraemia: caused by excessive salt intake, excessive water depletion or hyperaldosteronism
Potassium (K)	Maintenance of intracellular fluid volume Regulation of pH Establishes resting membrane potential of cells	Predominantly in intracellular fluid Serum level regulated by aldosterone	Hypokalaemia: caused by dietary insufficiency, inadequate intravenous, therapy, insulin therapy, beta-agonists, vomiting, **diarrhoea** Hyperkalaemia: caused by excessive intravenous administration, blood transfusion. Addison's disease, potassium-sparing diuretics
Calcium (Ca)	Role in excitable cells, neurotransmitter release and blood clotting	Predominantly in bone Mainly extracellular Regulated by parathyroid hormone	Hypocalcaemia: caused by hypoparathyroidism, inadequate vitamin D intake and renal disease Hypercalcaemia: caused by malignancy or hyperparathyroidism
Chlorite (**Cl**)	Balances anions in all fluid compartments	Diffuses easily between extracellular fluid and intracellular fluid **levels** linked to sodium concentration	Hypochloraemia: Found in pyloric stenosis and respiratory alkalosis Hyperchloraemia: caused by excessive intravenous saline administration or **severe** dehydration
Bicarbonate (HCO$_3$)	Major buffer in plasma Helps maintain balance of anions and cations in all fluid compartments	Predominantly or extracellular fluid, although small amounts also found in intracellular fluid Serum level controlled by kidneys	Deficit leads to metabolic acidosis; caused by use of carbonic anhydrase inhibitors, diarrhoea, **fistulae** Excess leads in metabolic alkalosis; caused by excessive bicarbonate administration, chronic vomiting, diuretic use

From *MRCOG Part 1 – Your Essential Revision Guide*, 2016.

Table 22.2 Definition of urine output

Urine output	Numerical definition	Comments
Anuria	<100 ml urine produced in 24 hours	–
Oliguria	<400 ml urine produced per day, but more than 1oo ml/day	Many causes including drugs, dehydration, endocrine disturbance, abnormal renal function
Normal urine output	0.5–1.0 ml/kg/h (In infants 2ml/kg/h)	Dependent upon age and renal function
Polyuria	>3 litres urine production per day	Many potential causes including diuretics, increased fluid intake, diabetes mellitus, diabetes insipidus, Addison's disease

From *MRCOG Part 1 – Your Essential Revision Guide*, 2016.

Table 22.3 Lower reference limits (5th centiles and their 95% confidence intervals) for semen characteristics

Parameter	Lower reference limit
Semen volume (ml)	1.5 (1.4–1.7)
Total sperm number (106 per ejaculate)	39 (33–46)
Sperm concentration (106 per ml)	15 (12–16)
Total motility (PR + NP, %)	40 (38–42)
Progressive motility (PR, %)	32 (31–34)
Vitality (live spermatozoa, %)	58 (55–63)
Sperm morphology (normal forms, %)	4 (3.0–4.0)

Source: WHO (2010) WHO Laboratory Manual for the Examination and Processing of Human Semen, 5th ed., p. 224.
From *MRCOG Part 1 – Your Essential Revision Guide*, 2016.

Table 22.5 Classification of causes of an abnormal semen analysis

Classification	Examples of causes
Pre-testicular	Hypothalamic hypogonadism Hyperprolactinaemia Kallmann's syndrome Anabolic steroid abuse Drugs
Testicular	Cryptorchidism Klinefelter's syndrome Y chromosome microdeletions Testicular tumours Chemotherapy and radiotherapy
Post-testicular	Vasectomy Congenital absence of the vas deferens Diabetes Infection

Table 22.4 Terms used in the interpretation of a semen analysis

Term	Description
Azoospermia	No spermatozoa present
Oligozoospermia	Low sperm count (<15 × 10^6/ml)
Asthenozoospermia	Low sperm motility (progressive motility <32%)
Teratozoospermia	Low sperm normal morphology (<4%)

Table 22.6 Ultrasound finding at different gestational ages

Gestational age	Ultrasound findings
4/40	Thickened endometrium. Usually no ultrasound evidence of pregnancy at this gestation
5/40	Gestation sac visible with hyperechogenic ring
5–6/40	Yolk sac visible
5+ – 6+/40	Fetal pole visible
6–7/40	Fetal heartbeat visible

Module 16 Early Pregnancy Care

The blueprinting grid states:

Interpret ultrasound in early pregnancy and commonly performed investigations including HCG measurement

- Ultrasound images or reports may be provided with a clinical scenario for interpretation (Table 22.6).
- Determination of viability in early pregnancy with transvaginal ultrasound (after NICE 2012; Table 22.7).
- Interpretation of serum HCG levels where there is no ultrasound evidence of pregnancy (after NICE 2012; Table 22.8)

Table 22.7 TVS findings, diagnosis and action in early pregnancy

Ultrasound findings	Diagnosis and action
Intrauterine gestation with visible fetal heartbeat	Viable pregnancy and reassurance
Visible fetal pole but no fetal heartbeat • Crown-rump length <7 mm • Crown-rump length ≥7 mm	• Pregnancy of uncertain viability. Perform repeat scan a minimum of 7 days later • Likely missed miscarriage. Either seek second opinion or repeat scan a minimum of 7 days later
Intrauterine gestation sac but no visible fetal pole • Mean sac diameter <25 mm • Mean sac diameter ≥ 25 mm	• Pregnancy of uncertain viability. Perform repeat scan a minimum of 7 days later • Likely anembryonic pregnancy. Either seek second opinion or repeat scan a minimum of 7 days later

Table 22.8 Interpretation of serum HCG levels

Baseline HCG	HCG level 48 hours later	Interpretation
Grossly elevated	Grossly elevated	Consider the possibility of gestational trophoblastic disease
Normal	Rise in level >63%	Likely early viable intrauterine pregnancy (ectopic pregnancy not excluded)
Normal	Fall in level <50% or rise in level <63%	Pregnancy of unknown location (PUL). Arrange urgent review in early pregnancy service
Normal	Fall in level >50%	Likely complete miscarriage

- Blood results of other hormone levels in pregnancy may be provided, especially thyroid function tests
- Imaging, histology, karyotypes or reports may be provided for interpretation in relation to gestational trophoblastic disease

Module 17 Gynaecological Oncology

- Most of the questions in this module are related to calculation of the Risk of Malignancy Index and/or an understanding of its component parts (Table 22.9)
- RMI I is currently used with the formula RMI = U × M × CA125
- There may be simple imaging to interpret, for example endometrial thickness in postmenopausal bleeding, metastases in gestational neoplastic disease

Module 18 Urogynaecology and Pelvic Floor Problems (Table 22.10)

- Currently there are very few questions in relation to this module
- There may be questions relating to an understanding of simple cystometry

Table 22.9 Risk of malignancy index

Component of RMI I	Description
U (ultrasound score)	5 component parts – score 1 for each feature present • Multilocular cysts • Solid areas • Bilateral lesions • Ascites • Metastases U = 0 (for an ultrasound score of 0) U = 1 (for an ultrasound score of 1) U = 3 (for an ultrasound score of 2–5)
M (menopausal status)	M = 1 (premenopausal) M = 3 (postmenopausal)
CA 125 level	Serum level measured in iu/ml

- There may be questions relating to a bladder diary and the classification of urinary frequency

Short Best Answer Questions

1. Following a difficult therapeutic laparoscopy, a woman is admitted to the gynaecology ward. For analgesia, she is given a morphine patient-controlled analgesia device.

Table 22.10 Definition of urogynaecological terms

Term	Definition (Modified from International Continence Society)
Urinary frequency	Voiding more than 8 times per day with no overall increase in volume
Nocturia	Waking to void more than 1 time per night
Urgency	Sudden compelling desire to void which is difficult to defer
Polyuria	Production of more than 3 litres of urine per day

She is noted to be quite drowsy, and her oxygen saturation is low.

An arterial blood gas is taken with the following result:

pH 7.32

PCO_2 6.5 kPa

Base excess +1

What disturbance of acid-base balance is present?

a. Metabolic acidosis
b. Metabolic alkalosis
c. Normal blood gas
d. Respiratory acidosis
e. Respiratory alkalosis

2. A 38-year-old woman who is 8 weeks pregnant is admitted to the gynaecology unit with protracted vomiting that has not settled with antiemetics. Intravenous access is obtained to administer IV fluids and blood is sent to test for urea and electrolytes. The woman describes palpitations, so an ECG is arranged with the following result:

What is the most likely disturbance of electrolyte balance?

a. Hyperkalaemia
b. Hypernatraemia
c. Hypocalcaemia
d. Hypokalaemia
e. Hyponatraemia

3. On the day following an uncomplicated hysterectomy, an ST2 doctor is asked to check a woman's urine output chart.

The woman has a BMI of 25 kg/m^2

The fluid output chart shows an average urine output of 50 ml/hour since the operation.

How would this urine output be classified?

a. Anuria
b. Normal urine output
c. Oliguria
d. Polyuria
e. Urinary frequency

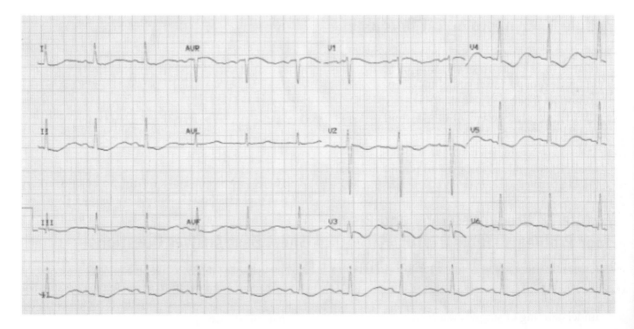

4. Following successful entry for a diagnostic laparoscopy, an ST2 doctor looks down into the pelvis to view the anatomical structures.
   The following view is obtained:

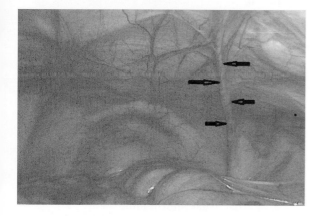

What structure is contained in the anatomical structure identified by the arrows?

    a. Inferior epigastric artery
    b. Obliterated umbilical artery
    c. Urachus
    d. Ureter
    e. Vitelline duct

5. A 25-year-old woman presents to the gynaecology admission unit with acute onset left-sided pelvic pain. She is currently day 16 of a regular 28-day cycle. Pregnancy test is negative. The pain settles with oral NSAIDs.
   An ultrasound scan is performed with the following result:

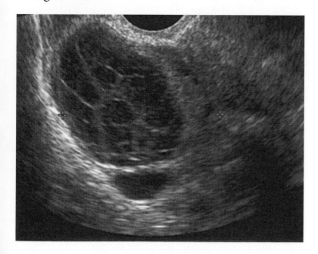

What is the most likely diagnosis?

    a. Ectopic pregnancy
    b. Endometrioma
    c. Haemorrhagic ovarian cyst
    d. Ovarian torsion
    e. Ovarian tumour

6. The image below shows the hormone changes during a 28-day menstrual cycle.

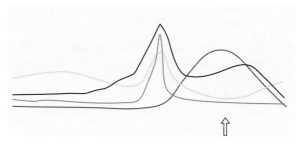

An endometrial biopsy is taken on the day indicated by the arrow.
Histologically, what type of endometrium will be seen?

    a. Atrophic
    b. Follicular
    c. Luteal
    d. Proliferative
    e. Secretory

7. A couple attends the fertility clinic.
   The man's semen analysis gives the following report:

    Volume 2 ml
    Density 20 million/ml
    Progressive motility 25%
    Morphology 5% normal forms

How would this semen analysis be classified?
    a. Asthenozoospermia
    b. Normal semen analysis
    c. Oligoasthenozoospermia
    d. Oligozoospermia
    e. Teratozoospermia

8. A woman attends the early pregnancy unit. It is 7 weeks since her last menstrual period. A pregnancy test is positive. She has experienced moderate PV bleeding.

A transvaginal ultrasound scan is arranged which shows no evidence of an intrauterine pregnancy. Endometrial thickness is 12 mm.
A serum HCG is measured. It is 280 iu/l.
48 hours later the HCG level is 100 iu/l.
What is the most likely diagnosis?

a. Complete miscarriage
b. Early pregnancy of uncertain viability
c. Ectopic pregnancy
d. Incomplete miscarriage
e. Pregnancy of unknown location

9. A 55-year-old woman whose last period was 2 years ago attends the gynaecology clinic with symptoms of bloating.
An ultrasound scan is arranged which shows a bilocular mass with no solid areas or ascites.
Serum CA125 is 20 iu/ml

What is the Risk of Malignancy Index for this woman?

a. 0
b. 10
c. 20
d. 60
e. 120

10. The following diagram shows three different types of fertilisation:
What will be the outcome from fertilisation 'B'?

a. Complete hydatidiform mole
b. Down's syndrome
c. Edward's syndrome
d. Normal pregnancy
e. Partial hydatidiform mole

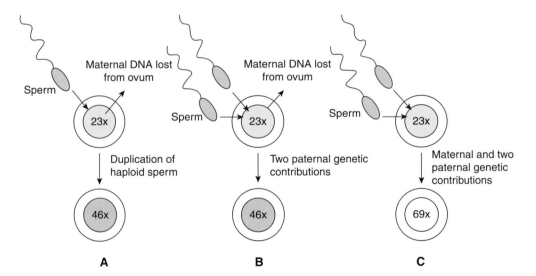

Chapter 23

Clinical Management in Gynaecology

Amy Shacaluga

Contraception

1 Combined Hormonal Contraception (CHC)

Failure rates (perfect use) 0.3%

Failure rate (typical use) 9% per annum.

Less unscheduled bleeding than with progestogen-only methods.

Caution

- Enzyme inducing drugs reduce efficacy of contraception.
- Lamotrigine levels are reduced by CHC and may result in increased seizure frequency.

Risks

Thromboembolism

Stroke (individuals with migraine with aura)

Hypertension

Breast cancer

Prescribing

UK Medical Eligibility Criteria for Contraceptive (UKCMEC) should be consulted when deciding forms of contraception.

BMI, BP and weight should be documented.

History should aim to elicit migraine, thromboembolic risk, cardiovascular risk, hyperlipidaemia and smoking status.

UKMEC categories are given in Table 23.1

Action:

a. COCP

Inhibit the FSH and LH release from the pituitary, alter cervical mucus and endometrial lining potentially contributing to their efficacy.

Table 23.1 UKMEC categories

Category	Definition
UKMEC 1	A condition for which there is no restriction for the use of contraceptive method
UKMEC 2	A condition where the advantages of using the method generally outweigh the theoretical or proven risks
UKMEC 3	A condition where the theoretical or proven risks usually outweigh the advantages of using the method
UKMEC 4	A condition which represents unacceptable health risks is the contraceptive method is used

- Monophasic (same dose); mostly between 20–35 micrograms of ethinylestradiol (EE) or mestranol in combination with progesterone.
- Phasic (variable dose); Mainly 21 active pills (first 7 days inhibit ovulation and the remaining 14 pills maintain anovulation), the following can be either pill-free or placebo and cause withdrawal bleed.

What to do in the event of a missed pill:

What to do in the event of a missed pill [from FSRH.org].

b. Combined Transdermal Patch (CTP)

One patch applied and worn for 1 week to suppress ovulation. Replaced once a week for two further weeks and seven patch-free days. Releases 33.9 micrograms EE and 203 micrograms norelgestromin/ 24 hours.

c. Combined Vaginal Ring

Release EE (15micrograms) and etonogestrel (120 micrograms) per day, for 21 days. Following a ring-free interval of 7 days and a withdrawal bleed a new ring is inserted.

If ONE pill has been missed (48-72 hours since last pill in current packet or 24-48 hours late starting first pill in new packet)	If TWO OR MORE pills have been missed (>72 hours since last pill in current packet or >48 hours late starting first pill in new packet)

Continuing contraceptive cover
- The missed pill should be taken as soon as it is remembered.
- The remaining pills should be continued at the usual time.

Continuing contraceptive cover
- The most recent missed pill should be taken as soon as possible.
- The remaining pills should be continued at the usual time.
- Condoms should be used or sex avoided until seven consecutive active pills have been taken. This advice may be overcautious in the second and third weeks, but the advice is a backup in the event that further pills are missed.

Minimising the risk of pregnancy
Emergency contraception (EC) is not usually required but may need to be considered if pills have been missed earlier in the packet or in the last week of the previous packet.

Minimising the risk of pregnancy		
If pills are missed in the first week (Pills 1-7)	If pills are missed in the second week (Pills 8-14)	If pills are missed in the third week (Pills 15-21)
EC should be considered if unprotected sex occurred in the pill-free interval or in the first week of pill-taking.	No indication for EC if the pills in the preceding 7 days have been taken consistently and correctly (assuming the pills thereafter are taken correctly and additional contraceptive precautions are used).	OMIT THE PILL-FREE INTERVAL by finishing the pills in the current pack (or discarding any placebo tablets) and starting a new pack the next day.

2. Progestogen-Only Methods

a. Progestogen-Only Pill (POP) (Table 23.2)

Altered bleeding pattern most common reason for discontinuation (25% discontinuation <1 year).

A clinical history should identify any UKMEC 3 or 4 criteria. This includes a Hx of breast cancer > 5 years/ongoing (4), Gestational trophoblastic neoplasia, active viral hepatitis, severe cirrhosis (decompensated), liver tumours and use of liver enzyme inducers. New diagnosis of ischaemic heart disease, stroke or migraine with aura should prompt a clinical review of medication.

Action

POPs traditionally work by altering cervical mucus, and for some, ovulation is inhibited.

Efficacy

99% effective with failure rates are 0.3 and 8.0 per 100 woman years, and lower if over age 40.

Missed pills (>3 hours late with traditional POPs) require additional precaution for 48 hours and taking the missed pill ASAP.

Liver enzyme-inducing drugs are not recommended with POPs and can take up to 4 weeks for liver enzymes to return to normal hence additional contraception is needed.

Table 23.2 Progestogen-only pills

Brand name	Type of progestogen	Dose (micrograms)
Cerazette >12 hours before considered a missed pill	Desogestrel (inhibition of ovulation mainly)	75
Femulen	Ethynediol diacetate	500
Micronor	Norethisterone	350
Norgeston	Levonorgestrel	30
Noriday	Norethisterone	350

Long-Acting Reversible Contraception

a. Progestogen-Only Injectable (DMPA IM 150 mg Medroxyprogesterone Acetate in 1 ml) and NET-EN Noristat 104 mg MPA in 65 ml)

Acts mainly by inhibiting ovulation, with the effect of thickening cervical mucus. It is associated with a 6% failure rate in the typical user.

It can be used concurrently with enzyme-inducing drugs.

Risks

There is a small loss of bone mineral density which recovers after discontinuation of use and is thus not recommended after 50 years of age. Return of fertility may take up to 1 year.

Side Effects

Include weight gain especially in BMI<30 and women <18 years, injection site reaction (SC>IM).

Progestogen-Only Implant (Nexplanon)

Subdermal rod licensed for 3 years (38 mg etonogestrel). Primarily preventing ovulation but also altering cervical mucous.

Pregnancy rate < 1 in 1000 over 3 yrs (NICE).

Insertion up to day 5 of menstrual cycle without additional contraception. Alternatively 7 days of extra contraception.

Side Effects

Commonly associated with altered bleeding patterns (especially in first 3 months).

25% have prolonged bleeding.

Efficacy may be altered by enzyme inducers, and additional precautions for 28 days should be used.

b. Levonorgestrel Intrauterine System LNG IUS

T-shaped device with an elastomer core containing levonorgestrel (LNG). The LNG-IUS (Mirena) releases 20 micrograms of LNG per day (10 mcgs >5 yrs). Benefits include use for menorrhagia, endometrial protection during HRT or breast cancer therapy as well as reduce dysmenorrhea from endometriosis adenomyosis.

Pearl index score of 0.52. If pregnancy does occur while IUS is in situ there is a higher rate of ectopic pregnancy.

It is licensed for greater than 5 yrs but not for contraceptive benefit.

Copper IUD (Copper T380A, TT380 Slimline and T-Safe 380)

Non hormonal intrauterine device made of plastic and copper (some also contain noble metals).

They can be used for emergency contraception.

Action

Cu-IUDs interfere with implantation. Owing to the copper, sperm penetration is inhibited, in addition to having an anti-implantation effect.

Pregnancy rates are 0.1%–1% within the first year (copper content >300 mm^2). They generally last for 5 years, but a few with copper-banded arms 380 mm^2 can last for 10 years.

1 Emergency Contraception (EC)

A full history to include the precise risk and timing of unprotected sexual intercourse (UPSI).

Details of contraception failure and use of medications that could affect contraceptive efficacy are important (enzyme inducers). Consideration should be given to medical eligibility and efficacy of methods as well as previous use within the cycle.

A pregnancy test cannot exclude pregnancy if there has been an episode of UPSI less than 3 weeks previously.

Offer testing for STIs including HIV (<25 yrs up to 9.1% chlamydia test positive), and if UPSI has just occurred, retesting is advised.

Future contraceptive options should be discussed as they may influence EC choice and continued contraception following

1. Copper-bearing intrauterine device (Cu-IUD):

   - Efficacy: <120 hours from UPSI event or within 5 days from earliest estimation of ovulation.
   - Copper is toxic to ovum/sperm and has an anti-implantation effect.
   - Failure <1%
   - Consider antibiotics

2. Oral EC:

   Levonorgestrel (LNG)

   - 1.5 mg
   - Primarily ovulation inhibition by prevention of follicular rupture or luteal dysfunction. It can inhibit ovulation by 5–7 days.
   - Efficacy up to 72 hours after UPSI
   - Not effective once ovulation has occurred.
   - Can be used more than once per cycle
   - Advise 7 days additional contraception following
   - Avoid in women taking enzyme inducers as reduces efficacy

   Ulipristal acetate (UPA) (ellaOne)

   - 30 mg single dose
   - Progesterone receptor modulator
   - Inhibits or delays ovulation, suppressing the growth of lead follicles before ovulation. Thought to be ineffective in delaying follicular rupture once LH peak has occurred.
   - Efficacy up to 120 hours after UPSI
   - Advise 14 days of additional contraception following EC
   - Contraindications: severe asthma, hepatic dysfunction and galactose intolerance, lactase deficiency or gluco-galactose malabsorption
   - Avoid in enzyme inducing drugs

Table 23.3 Types of miscarriage

Type	Findings
Threatened	Intrauterine pregnancy, Cervical os = closed
Inevitable	Intrauterine pregnancy Cervical os = open
Incomplete	RPOC with cervical os open +/− products seen
Complete miscarriage	Empty uterus on USS with closed cervical os
Missed miscarriage	CRL >7 mm with no FH or an empty gestation sac with MSD >25 mm

Side-effects: Headache, nausea and altered bleeding. If vomiting occurs within 2 hours, a repeat dose is required with LNG and 3 hours with UPA.

Early Pregnancy Loss

1. Miscarriage (Table 23.3)

Miscarriage is the loss of pregnancy < 24 weeks gestation and occurs in up to 20% of pregnancies.

Causes

- Chromosomal: 50 % of miscarriages in the first trimester have chromosomal abnormalities (12% >12/40).
- Uterine anomalies (second trimester)
- 25% have no known cause

Clinical Examination

Any vaginal bleeding under 24 weeks gestation warrants clinical examination. This should include heart rate, blood pressure, oxygen saturations and temperature, as well as a speculum examination to identify potential local causes of bleeding.

An open cervical os usually indicates an inevitable miscarriage; presence of tissue within it may induce cervical shock (hypotension, bradycardia +/− collapse).

A full septic screen should be undertaken should the woman present unwell, +/− pyrexia +/− PV discharge which may be offensive as this is likely to represent a septic miscarriage.

Rhesus status of the woman should be established, and anti-D given to all non-sensitized RhD negative women presenting with bleeding in pregnancy >12 weeks gestation.

Table 23.4 Management of miscarriage

Type of Management	Treatment	
Expectant	First line. Awaiting for physiological expulsion of products of conception. The woman should have f/up in 2 weeks with an USS to confirm complete miscarriage.	70% will expel POC
Medical	Administer misoprostol to prompt uterine contractions in order to expel POC.	Missed miscarriage = 800 mcg misoprostol Incomplete = 600 mcg misoprostol
Surgical	Evacuation of retained products under general or local anaesthetic using dilatation of the cervix and curettage	

Ultrasound scan (USS) will identify viable pregnancies, provide reassurance for women, location and gestation of pregnancy (as well as chronicity), and aim to diagnose ectopic pregnancy (also heterotopic), and size of retained products of conception to guide management accordingly.

Management (Table 23.4)

Management is dependent on the woman's wishes, gestation and clinical situation.

2   Recurrent Miscarriage

Recurrent miscarriage is defined as the loss of three or more consecutive pregnancies. It affects approximately 1% of women trying to conceive. Risks include maternal age and number of previous miscarriages, as the risk of further miscarriage increases after each consecutive loss.

Investigations

a. Antiphospholipid antibodies: Lupus anticoagulant (viper venom time test) or anticardiolipin antibodies (2 tests 12 weeks apart)
A medium or high titre of IgG +/– IgM
b. Thrombophilia screen: Factor V leiden, Prothrombin gene mutation and Protein S.
c. Karyotyping:
   – Cytogenetic analysis third or further miscarriages
   – Both partners should undergo karyotype of a peripheral blood film where POC reveals an unbalanced structural chromosomal abnormality.
d. Ultrasound scan: may reveal suspected uterine anomalies
e. Hysteroscopy +/– Laparoscopy: uterine synechiae/ septum may be divided

Management

a. APLS diagnosis: offer low dose aspirin and low molecular weight heparin
b. Thrombophilia: heparin during pregnancy may improve birth rate in women with h/o second-trimester miscarriage.
c. Abnormal karyotype warrants a referral to a geneticist +/– Pre implantation genetic diagnosis
d. Uterine malformations: consider removing septae, but no evidence to suggest this improves outcome.
e. Cervical cerclage: h/o one second trimester miscarriage attributable to cervical factors, USS surveillance initially; if cervix <25 mm <24 weeks gestation, a cerclage can be considered.

Management of Ectopic Pregnancy and Pregnancy of Unknown Location (PUL)

Ectopic pregnancy is still a cause of in maternal death in the UK. An ectopic pregnancy is the result of the implantation of a blastocyst on a site other than the endometrium in the uterine cavity.

Location of Ectopics

Fallopian tube 98%

Ampullary 70%

Isthmic 12%

Fimbrial 11%

Ovarian 3.2%

Interstitial 2.4%

Abdominal 1.3%

Risk Factors (Table 23.5)

Table 23.5 Risk factors for ectopic pregnancy

High risk	Other risks
- Previous conservative management of ectopic (15%) - Tubal pathology/ surgery - Sterilization - In-utero diethylstilboestrol exposure (nine-fold increase)	- PID, especially recurrent infection - Intrauterine systems if pregnancy occurs - Cigarette smoking (tubal motility)

Assessment

History taking should include:

LMP in conjunction to the **menstrual cycle (length)**; in order to estimate gestation.

Risk factors (previous ectopic, IUD/IUS, tubal ligation, IVF, PID, progesterone). Up to 50% do not have any risk factors.

Past medical history should be evaluated to include previous abdominal or pelvic surgery, obstetric history and any previous methotrexate treatments.

Clinical examination

a. Presentation

Pain, either generalized or unilateral +/– subdiaphragmatic irritation with shoulder tip pain (peritoneal irritation).

Bleeding per vaginum is the result of decidual shedding with a decidual cast often being passed.

Collapse may indeed be the presenting factor.

b. Clinical observations should be taken to assess haemodynamic stability (pulse, BP, respiratory rate and repeated at intervals to establish any deterioration).

c. Abdominal and pelvic examination

– Acute abdomen; to elicit peritonism +/– distension could indicate haemoperitoneum.

– Pelvic examination; including speculum to reveal the quantity and source of pelvic bleeding, and rule out local sources such as cervical pathology.

– A bimanual would also give an indication of adnexal masses or cervical motion tenderness where there is blood in the pelvis.

Investigations

Urine pregnancy test initially, as well as

BHCG: A level >1500 should reveal an intrauterine gestation on ultrasound scan, failure to identify such would indicate a pregnancy of unknown location. Normal pregnancy will show a doubling of HCG levels. (Use caution, as up to a third of ectopics will show a similar biochemical picture.)

Group and save +/– crossmatch blood plus rhesus status; if Rh-negative and bleeding, will require anti-D immunoglobulin.

Full blood count: A baseline level to compare subsequent levels which may indicate further bleeds/rupture.

Transvaginal Ultrasound

This is the method of choice to locate the ectopic pregnancy, evaluate whether it is a live ectopic (warranting surgery), and whether any further pelvic pathology may be identified.

In the case of an inconclusive scan, BHCG levels may be taken 48 hours apart to verify spontaneous resolution or ongoing pregnancy/ presence of trophoblastic tissue. In the case of haemodynamic instability, management should be expedited to include laparoscopy/ laparotomy.

If a pregnancy is not identified with levels <1500 iu, a repeat scan should be performed when levels are equal or above this.

In the event that no pregnancy is seen >1500 iu level, a laparoscopy should be considered to locate the pregnancy.

Management

a. Expectant management of ectopic:

For asymptomatic women with USS diagnosis less than 100 ml of fluid in pouch of Douglas and decreasing levels of hcg less than 1000 iu/l at presentation. Follow-up should include twice-weekly hcg levels and weekly TVS to ensure decreasing hcg levels and reducing size of adnexal mass within the week.

b. Expectant management of pregnancy of unknown location:

PUL in women who are haemodynamically stable, with minimal symptoms at risk of an ectopic may be managed expectantly with follow-up 48–72 hours to intervene if serum hcg rises or plateaus. This may include a laparoscopy or indeed consideration of medical management.

c. Medical management:

Stable patients, BHCG <3000 iu/l (although has been used >5000 iu/l), women must be willing to be followed up in EPAU or equivalent with serial bhcg levels +/– USS.

A single dose of intramuscular methotrexate calculated by patient body surface (50 mg/m^2). BHCG levels are then taken days 4 and 7.

– 7% may rupture during treatment.

– Inform that a teratogenic risk exists for up to 3 months following treatment, and good contraception should be included in their care plan.

Advise against intercourse and encourage fluid intake during treatment. Side effects include conjunctivitis, GI upset and stomatitis. Any pain warrants readmission for either observation of definitive treatment.

d. Surgical management:

In haemodynamically stable patients, laparoscopy is preferred over laparotomy; if compromised, the quickest approach is advised.

Either salpingotomy or salpingectomy may be performed, but in the presence of contralateral tubal disease, salpingotomy is advised and women informed of risk of future ectopic.

Salpingotomy is performed via a linear incision on anterior mesenteric border of fallopian tube and removal of ectopic. Follow-up to ensure there is no persistent trophoblastic tissue by serum BHCG levels.

Gestational Trophoblastic Disease and Neoplasia

Characterized by abnormal proliferation of trophoblast of the placenta. This includes complete and partial molar pregnancies as well as that of invasive molar disease, choriocarcinoma and rarely placental site trophoblastic tumour.

Incidence is approximately 1 into 710 live births (increased in women from Asian or Far Eastern descent).

Risk Factors

20× more likely if <15 years; 10× increased risk if >40 years

Previous GTD (up to 2.5 %)

Blood group A women with blood group O partners (×10 risk)

Women with blood group AB are more likely to develop GTN

Pathophysiology

Complete mole: 46XX or 46XY, paternal origin, euploid and sex chromatin positive

Arise when an ovum with no genetic material is fertilized by two haploid sperm. Only paternal DNA.

Partial mole: From fertilization of an oocyte by two sperm resulting in triploidy with 2:1 paternal to maternal DNA content. (69XXY = 70%, 69XXX 27%, 69XYY 3%).

Invasive mole: Characterized by the presence of enlarged hydropic villi invading the myometrium. They are different to choriocarcinoma as they contain hydropic villi along with marked trophoblastic proliferation. They may both cause metastatic lesions as can involve the vasculature (vagina and lungs namely).

Clinically

Up to 30% may present with hyperemesis gravidarum

Majority present with irregular bleeding/spotting in the first trimester

Up to 30% have theca lutein cysts on the ovary, which may present as ovarian accidents

Up to 10% biochemical hyperthyroidism

10% will have first- or second-trimester pre-eclampsia

Investigations:
Blood Tests

Serum HCG correlates closely with tumour load and allows for close monitoring to ensure resolution of disease. Usually found > 200 000 IU/L with complete molar pregnancy.

Table 23.6 FIGO 2000 scoring system

FIGO Scoring	0	1	2	4
Age (years)	<40	≥40	-	-
Antecedent pregnancy	Mole	Abortion	Term	
Interval months from end of pregnancy to treatment	<4	4-<7	7-<13	≥13
Pretreatment serum Hcg (iu/l)	$<10^3$	$10^3–10^4$	$10^4 – 10^5$	$≥10^5$
Largest tumour size incl uterus (cm)	<3	3- <5	≥5	-
Site of metastases	Lung	Spleen, kidney	GI	Liver, brain
Number of metastases	-	1–4	5–8	>8
Previous failed chemotherapy	-	-	Single drug	2 or more drugs

Ultrasound scan

'Snowstorm appearance' resulting from hypoechoic cystic structures.

Choriocarcinoma usually fills the uterine cavity with increased vascularity and occasionally will breach the myometrium.

Treatment

Suction evacuation of complete moles is the treatment of choice (no fetal parts). Prostaglandin and oxytocin use should be reserved for uncontrolled bleeding owing to the theoretical risk of trophoblastic tissue being disseminated to lungs. If the size of a partial molar pregnancy precludes the use of suction, a medical termination is advised.

Persistent Gestational Trophoblastic

Gestational trophoblastic neoplasia may develop after a molar pregnancy, a non-molar pregnancy or a live birth. It affects 10% of the GTD population, diagnosed with the persistence or increase of HCG levels. Associated findings are enlarged uterine size and theca lutein cysts.

Any women with GTD should be given information regarding their condition and referral to a trophoblastic screening centre.

If Hcg is normal within 56 days of a pregnancy event, then follow-up for 6/12 from the uterine evacuation date. If this is not normal, then follow-up for 6/12 from normalization of Hcg level. All women should notify their screening centre after any subsequent pregnancies so their Hcg levels can be measured 6–8 weeks following the event to exclude recurrence.

Chemotherapy

Regimens are chosen with regard to the patient's prognostic risk. Assessment via FIGO 2000 scoring system.

Scores <6 are treated with a single agent IM methotrexate alternating daily with folinic acid for 7 days. Cure rates for low risk are nearly 100%. Scores >7 are considered high risk and by contrast treated with IV multiagent chemotherapy, with cure rates of 95%.

Advice

Conception if not advised during treatment and up to a year following.

Barrier contraception until Hcg levels return to normal.

Age of menopause is advanced after receiving chemotherapy.

FIGO 2000 scoring system (Table 23.6)

Sexually Transmitted Infections and Contraception

1 Vaginal Discharge (Table 23.7)

Pathophysiology

The vagina's glycogen-rich environment promotes acid-tolerant organisms. The pH of the vagina is <4.5, owing to the formation of lactic acid from glycogen. Fluctuations in oestrogen make the vaginal flora susceptible to change, often being disrupted by non-organic causes such as soaps, washing detergents and notably vaginal douching.

Causes

- Bacterial vaginosis

  Replacement of normal lactobacilli leads to an overgrowth of mixed anaerobic organisms, leading to an increased vaginal pH (>4.5).

Table 23.7 Classification, investigation and treatment of vaginal discharge

Non-infective causes	Investigation	Treatment
Polyps (uterine/ cervical)	USS/ Histology	Excision
Oestrogen deficiency	? Menopausal/ ? Cyclical	Topical oestrogen or HRT
Foreign body	Clinical assessment	Removal and possible antibiotics
Allergy	Patch testing	Removal of allergen
Fistulae	MRI	Surgical correction
Neoplasm	Urgent referral to oncology	Treatment depending on cancer
Cervical ectropion	Nothing or colposcopy +/–biopsy to rule out CIN or neoplasm	Cryocautery / excision

Table 23.8 Investigation of Candida infection

Investigation	Laboratory preparation	Detection of	Information
High vaginal swab	Microscopy and gram stain	BV:- Gram + and – cocci Clue cells (bacterial cells seen coating epithelial cells)	
From Posterior fornix		Candida: spores and pseudohyphae	
	Saline wet microscopy (dipping HVS into saline)	Trichomonas vaginalis	Need to request specific test in most laboratories
	Culture	Candida: Sabourad agar. TV needs to be requested	

Gardnerella vaginalis is commonly found (but it is also a commensal of 30–40% of asymptomatic women), *Prevotella, Mycoplasma hominis,* and *Mobiluncus* species.

Presentation: 'fishy odour', no itch, no vulval inflammation

O/E: pH > 4.5

Treatment: Oral metronidazole 2 g stat dose first line. Clindamycin is also an option but has been associated with pseudomembranous colitis.

In pregnancy or breastfeeding, metronidazole 400 mg BD for 5–7/7

• Candida

Consider immunocompromised and diabetes if recurrent, recent antibiotic treatment, non-cotton underwear. Caused by overgrowth of yeast *C. albicans (70–90%)* or *C. glabrata.*

Presentation: itching +/– soreness, superficial dyspareunia, dysuria

O/E: 'curdy thick white discharge', satellite lesions, fissuring and oedema

Investigation: Litmus paper pH <4.0–4.5, Microscopy pseudohyphae or HVS.

Treatment: Antifungal – oral and or intravaginal imidazole and triazole antifungals

Treatment: fluconazole 150 mg stat orally and clotrimazole pessary 500 mg PV stat

Investigations (Table 23.8)

Endocervical Swab

- Columnar cells
- Avoid contact with vaginal mucosa
- Nucleic amplification test (NAAT): amplification of DNA that is present in *chlamydia trachomatis*, using PCR. It can also be done on a urine sample (lower sensitivity).

Infective causes (sexually transmitted) (Table 23.9)

Table 23.9 Infective causes of sexually transmitted diseases

STI	Chlamydia
Signs and symptoms	Majority asymptomatic Inc vaginal discharge, post-coital and or inter-menstrual bleeding, dysuria, lower abdominal pain and deep dyspareunia Mucopurulent cervicitis +/– contact bleeding Cervical motion tenderness, Perihepatitis
Investigations	NAAT, or retest in 2 weeks from sexual exposure Vulvovaginal swabs and endocervical swabs
Treatment	Stat dose of 1 g azithromycin or 100 mg BD 7/7 doxycycline (contraindicated in pregnancy) Avoid sexual intercourse until they or partners have completed treatment/ or 7 days if treated with one dose azithromycin
Other	Most common curable STI in the UK Prevalence 15–24-year-olds, 1.5–4.3% Uncomplicated infection does not require removal of IUS/IUD
Complications	Pelvic inflammatory disease, tubal infertility and ectopic pregnancy

STI	Gonorrhoea
Signs and symptoms	Asymptomatic, altered vaginal discharge, dysuria, rarely IMB. Mucopurulent cervical discharge with induced cervical bleeding. Lower pelvic tenderness (<5%)
Investigations	Endocervical swab Microscopy: gram stained specimens show monomorphic Gram-negative diplococcic within polymorphonuclear leukocytes. NAATs: more sensitive than culture, sensitivity >96%. Culture: allows confirmatory identification and antimicrobial susceptibility testing, which is important as antibiotic resistance increases.
Treatment	Ceftriaxone 500 mg IM and azithromycin 1 g oral single dose Complicated: ceftriaxone 500 mg IM and doxycycline 100 mg bd 10–14 days. Other: spectinomycin 2 g IM and azithromycin 1 g PO
Other	Test of cure: confirm compliance, ensure resolution enquire about adverse reactions. Test 2 weeks after completion of antibiotics.
Complications	

STI	Trichomonas
Signs and symptoms	Asymptomatic (10–50%) Commonest is vaginal discharge, vulval itching, dysuria, offensive odour. Occasionally presenting with vulval ulceration. Thick discharge (70%), classically frothy yellow discharge in 10–30% Vulvitis and vaginitis Strawberry cervix (2%) to the naked eye
Investigations	HVS from posterior fornix or urine with NAAT Microscopy: mobile trichomonads (wet slide)
Treatment	Avoid intercourse for a week after treatment Metronidazole 2 g orally single dose Or 400-500 mg BD 5–7 days
Other	Avoid alcohol during treatment and 48 hours following

STI	Syphilis (not including congenital syphilis)
Signs and symptoms	Painless chancre, rash on soles and palms of feet classically. May present with hepatitis, meningitis and neurological symptoms.
Investigations	Dark ground microscopy and PCR Non-specific: Treponemal antibody test (cannot differentiate between T. pallidum, yaws, bejel or pinta – all caused by different subspecies of Treponema). Specific: EIA to detect IgM and IgG AND confirmed with a second different test. Quantitative VDRL once tests are positive. CXR/MRI/CT and lumbar puncture may be needed in patients presenting with neurological, cardiovascular or ophthalmic involvement.
Treatment	Parenteral penicillin treatment of choice Pregnancy: benzathine penicillin G 2.4 mu
Other	Caused by spirochete bacterium Treponema Pallidum. Transmitted by direct contact with an infectious lesion (1/3 will develop disease) or vertical transmission. T. Pallidum invade through mucosal surface or breached skin and produce a chancre. Incubation period is approx. 21 days. Secondary syphilis may develop after 4–10 weeks of appearance of initial chancre (usually mucocutaneous rash and lymphadenopathy). Resolves in < 12 weeks and enters asymptomatic latent stage.

Herpes Simplex Virus

STI	Primary herpes simplex	Non-primary herpes simplex
Pathophysiology	HSV 1 or 2 Following primary infection disease latent in sensory ganglia, with reactivation subsequently	
Signs and Symptoms	Only 1/3 of individuals have recognizable symptoms Painful ulceration, dysuria, systemic infections fever and myalgia Blistering and ulceration, lymphadenitis	Minor symptoms generally Asymptomatic viral shedding
Investigations	NAATs test of choice, by swabbing ulcer base. Serology for type-specific antibodies (IgG HSV1 or 2)	Episodic antivirals or suppressive antiviral therapy (if 6 recurrences/yr)
Treatment	Antivirals: Aciclovir 400 mg TDS 5/7	Aciclovir 800 mg TDS 2/7 (short course) Aciclovir 200 mg five times daily Also valaciclovir or famciclovir
Pregnancy	Greatest risk of transmission in third trimester, <6/52 of delivery 41% risk neonatal herpes if primary lesions present at delivery Daily suppressive acyclovir 400 mg tds from 36 weeks reduces lesions at term Type-specific antibody testing if within 6 weeks of delivery (IgG 1 and 2) when compared with vaginal swab may confirm recurrence or first episode	Recurrent herpes at time of delivery (0.3% risk of neonatal herpes with vaginal delivery) Daily suppressive acyclovir from 36 weeks will reduce recurrence and shedding

Urogynaecology

Lower urinary tract symptoms are common and a targeted history will allow for appropriate investigations to better arrive at a diagnosis. This should include a quality-of-life assessment, which can then be evaluated following treatment.

Urinary Tract Infection (UTI)

UTIs are very common in women, owing to their short urethral length, with up to 50% having at least one episode. They may be due to bacterial or fungal infections of the kidneys, ureters (pyelonephritis) or bladder (cystitis). The most common organism is *E. coli*, followed by *Proteus* species. Fungal infections

233

Table 23.10 Clinical assessment of urinary tract infections

Lower urinary tract infection	Pyelonephritis	Asymptomatic bacteriuria
Dysuria, frequency, urgency, urge incontinence, offensive urine, lower abdominal pain, malaise, strangury, frank haematuria.	Flank pain, fever, rigors, raised inflammatory markers.	Incidental finding in culture despite lack of symptoms, in pregnancy can lead to premature delivery in up to 30%.

are often caused by candida and are rare, usually owing to foreign bodies (catheters, ureteric stents, ureteric stones). A normal vaginal pH protects against uropathogens, and thus with vaginal infections such as bacterial vaginosis, which alter the same, women are at increased risk of contracting UTIs.

Clinical assessment (Table 23.10)

Investigations

Urine dipstick – Usually positive for blood (also due to stones, glomerular bleeding or tumours), leukocytes, nitrites (except gram-positive organisms and low dietary nitrate +/– high ascorbic acid content) and protein.

Urine microscopy, culture and sensitivity – A midstream urine serves to avoid contamination with vaginal discharge and to quantify the number of white cells and culture the main organism.

FBC – Usually a neutrophilia (eosinophilia schistosomiasis).

Management

Encourage fluid intake and alkalizing agents to reduce bladder irritability. (Cranberry juice inhibits binding of E. coli fimbriae to urothelium.)

Oral antibiotics may be started empirically or if the symptoms are severe enough admission for IV antibiotics may be needed.

Urinary Incontinence

Urinary incontinence is the involuntary leakage of urine. This may in turn be subdivided into stress urinary incontinence (SUI), urge urinary incontinence (UUI), mixed urinary incontinence (MUI).

SUI – involuntary leakage on exertion, sneezing or coughing

UUI – involuntary leakage preceded by urgency

MUI – combination of above

Nocturnal enuresis – loss of urine during sleep

Pathophysiology

Due to neuromuscular or connective tissue damage which could be the result of several aetiological factors (age, obesity, parity, pregnancy, menopause and oestrogen deficiency, lower urinary tract infection).

Urinary continence is maintained by keeping a low intravesical pressure usually <10cmH$_2$O, with a higher urethral sphincter resistance. Increased abdominal pressures (cough) are counteracted by increases in the urethral pressure prior to the rise of pressure in the bladder.

Clinical Examination and Evaluation of Urinary incontinence

History

Storage symptoms; frequency, nocturia, urgency, urinary urge incontinence (UUI), stress urinary incontinence (SUI) or constant leakage

Voiding symptoms; hesitancy, straining and flow

Postmicturition symptoms; incontinence or incomplete emptying

Bowel; constipation may exacerbate symptoms and should be treated

Surgery; including previous pelvic/ prolapse surgery, spinal surgery

PMH, DH (diuretics)

Evaluation

1. Bladder diary; 3/7 to document input and output, frequency, timings and incontinence episodes.
2. Quality of life assessment; impact on lifestyle and serves to compare following treatment.

Clinical Assessment

BMI; weight loss helps with incontinence.

Abdominal examination and pelvic examination; rule out any masses, as well as cough stress test.

POP Q scoring to assess pelvic organ prolapse.

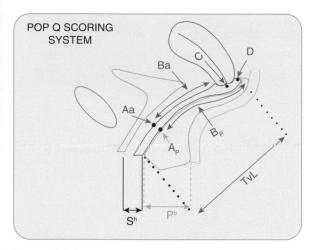

POP Q SCORING SYSTEM

Figure 23.1 Flow rate curve

Vulval skin; oestrogen deficiency, evidence of skin disorder or chronic exposure to urine which may irritate and exacerbate symptoms.

Neurological cause warrants a full neurological exam identifying S2,3,4 knee tendon reflex, sensory innervation S1 of the sole and lateral aspect of toes, S2 posterior aspect of thigh, S3 perineal sensory innervation with abduction and dorsiflexion of toes, S4 perianal area.

Include cognitive examinations if deemed necessary (elderly population).

Investigations
1. MSU; $> 10^5$ organisms/mL is significant as well as nitrites. Blood calculi or CA.
2. Residual volume (ultrasound or catheter); large residuals remaining post void could indicate neurological disease or outlet obstructions
3. Urodynamics;
   a) Uroflowmetry; screening test for voiding difficulty and gives information on flow rate, non-invasive.
   b) Cystometry;

Pressure/volume relationship of the bladder is assessed during filling and voiding. Includes measurement of intravesical (pressure transducer in bladder) and intra-abdominal pressures (pressure transducers in rectum). Intravesical pressure – intra-abdominal pressure = detrusor pressure

$$P_{ves} - P_{abd} = P_{det}$$

Normal Parameters
Filling
Residual urine <50 ml

Capacity >400 ml

Absence of uninhibited detrusor contractions during filling

Negligible rise in detrusor pressure on filling <15cm H_2O for volumes <500 ml

Voiding
No leakage on increased abdominal pressure

No provoked detrusor contractions on precipitating factors

Maximum voiding detrusor pressure <50cmH_2O with a max flow rate >15 ml/s for a volume voided >150 ml.

Video Urodynamics (Gold Standard)
This includes the above with the addition of contrast medium instead of saline to fill the bladder during cystometry, radiologically screening the bladder and urethra throughout the procedure. Looks into bladder morphology, support and function.

Ambulatory Urodynamics
Useful for investigating detrusor overactivity in cases where standard investigations have failed to elicit it. In a similar way to urodynamic studies allowing for event logging and quantifying leakage on an electronic pad.

Management of urinary incontinence (Table 23.11)

Conservative management will help all forms of UI

- Fluid intake <1.5 L per day, avoid caffeinated beverages and alcohol
- Diet changes to avoid constipation and reduce BMI if raised
- Smoking cessation
- Medications evaluated

Pharmacological Treatment of OAB/UUI
1. Antimuscarinic drugs:

   Assess whether on any anticholinergic medications, discuss side effects (constipation, dry eyes/mouth, constipation). Benefits may take a month.

   Mainly M2 and M3 muscarinic receptors in the bladder. Side effects occur owing to their effect on

Table 23.11 Management of urinary incontinence

Type of incontinence	SUI	UUI/OAB	MUI
Conservative management	Pelvic floor exercises (8 × three occasions/ day) +/– physiotherapy input for 3/12 Vaginal cones	Bladder training Biofeedback	Pelvic floor exercises (8 × three occasions/day) +/– physiotherapy input for 3/12

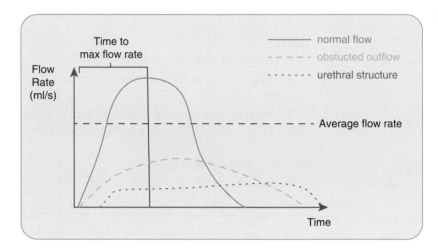

Figure 23.2 Diagram of POP Q and table

other muscarinic receptors in the body (dry mouth, blurred vision, tachycardia, constipation, drowsiness).

Oxybutynin 5 mg TDS if tolerated, or dose reduced (not too old/frail women).

Tolterodine 2 mg higher affinity for bladder receptors (less S/E)

Darifenacin (od)

2. Desmopressin: mainly nocturia (avoid >65 yrs and CF patients, CV disease or hypertension). Can reduce urine by 50%.
3. Duloxetine (SSRI thought to increase urethral sphincter closure)
4. Intravaginal oestrogen

Invasive Procedures for OAB

1. Botulinum toxin A: bladder wall injection to prevent detrusor overactivity
2. Percutaneous sacral nerve stimulation (if unable to perform intermittent catheterization and no response to pharmacological treatment)
3. Augmentation cystoplasty uses a segment of bowel to act as a reservoir by suturing onto the bisected bladder wall (small risk of malignancy)

Surgical Approaches for SUI:

- Synthetic mid-urethral tape (type 1 macroporous tape).
- Open colposuspension
- Autologous rectus fascial sling
- Intramural urethral bulking agents

Pelvic Organ Prolapse

The herniation of pelvic and/or abdominal organs through the vaginal canal occurs as a result of a failure in mechanical support of the vagina.

1. Levator ani muscles contain fast- and slow-twitch fibres which maintain urethral and anal patency during times of raised intra-abdominal pressures.
2. Endopelvic fascia (ligamentous)
   a. Uterosacral and cardinal ligaments aid in vertical suspension at the apex of the vagina
   b. Lateral vaginal attachment (middle third), connecting it to arcus tendinous fascia pelvis
   c. Fusion of vaginal endopelvic fascia to perineal body posteriorly, levator ani laterally and urethra anteriorly

Assessment of POP
Quality of Life Assessment

International continence society uses the POP-Q scoring system. This system uses the hymen as a fixed landmark given the score of 0, with reference to anterior, superior and posterior vaginal compartment. The distance to the vaginal landmarks are given a negative number per cm above the hymen and by contrast a positive number below it.

Types of Prolapse

Anterior vaginal wall prolapse

- A defect in the pubocervical fascia resulting in protrusion of the bladder known as a cystocoele

Posterior vaginal wall prolapse

- Rectocoele from defect in rectovaginal fascia
- Pouch of Douglas hernia
- Enterocoele
- Sigmoidocoele

Vaginal vault prolapse

- Prolapse of the vaginal cuff following hysterectomy (Uterosacral and cardinal ligaments are detached from vaginal apex.)

Management

1. Conservative; lifestyle, pelvic floor muscle training but no evidence for these in POP.
2. Pessaries; avoids surgery, should be changed at least 6/12 and vagina checked to ensure no infections, ulcerations or fibrous band formation have ensued.
    i. Ring pessaries support pelvic organs
    ii. Shelf pessaries for stages III and IV POP
3. Surgery;
    i. Uterine prolapse; vaginal hysterectomy, sacrohysteropexy (fertility preserving), sacrospinous fixation or total vaginal mesh
    ii. Anterior compartment; anterior colporrhaphy (40% recurrence), mesh repairs (limited data on success)
    iii. Posterior vault prolapse; posterior colporrhaphy, vaginal enterocoele repair
    iv. Vaginal vault repair; abdominal sacrocolpopexy (gold standard), SSF, mesh repairs and colposcopies

Carbohydrate Metabolism

Mary Board

1 Glucose Metabolism

Carbohydrates present the most accessible energy source for many tissues. Glucose is the only fuel that can be respired anaerobically, for example by the Type 2 skeletal muscle fibre during intensive exercise or by the erythrocyte which has no mitochondria. It is also the preferred fuel for the central nervous system (CNS). The brain has a sustained high energy requirement to allow continuous ion pumping and maintenance of membrane potentials, and accounts for approximately 20% of resting energy expenditure in the fat-free mass of the adult. In the fed state, the brain consumes only glucose, oxidising it to supply 100% of its energy requirement, accounting for about 120 g glucose per day in the adult. In the starving state, the brain may reduce its glucose requirement by up to 75% by consumption of ketone bodies but the remaining 25% of its energy must always come from glucose. Lipoproteins do not cross the blood-brain barrier, depriving the brain of fat as an oxidative fuel. The dependence of the CNS on glucose justifies the complexities of glucose homeostatic mechanisms designed to maintain availability of this substrate through the bloodstream and explains the potentially coma-inducing consequences of poorly controlled diabetes or excessive alcohol consumption.

1.1 Anaerobic Metabolism (Glycolysis)

The glycolytic pathway (Fig. 24.1) is vital to both anaerobic and aerobic oxidation of glucose and occurs within the cytosol of all cells of the body. The product of the pathway under aerobic conditions is pyruvate which is then converted into the acetyl CoA substrate for the tricarboxylic acid cycle (TCA cycle). Conversion of glucose into lactate by the pathway of glycolysis produces 2 mols ATP/mol glucose and is the primary means of energy generation in anaerobic tissues. The lactate dehydrogenase reaction functions to regenerate NAD^+ for continued glycolytic activity (Fig. 24.1) and the occurrence of anaerobic

respiration in the body is characterised by the appearance of lactate in the blood.

1.1.1 Production of Lactate

Lactate, produced during anaerobic respiration by vigorously exercising muscle, for example, leaves the muscle tissue and travels to the liver via the blood. The liver is able to re-convert lactate into glucose using the pathway of gluconeogenesis. The glucose may then travel back to the muscle to fuel another round of anaerobic energy generation. This relationship between the two tissues is the Cori cycle (Fig. 24.2). Whereas glycolysis yields 2 mols ATP/mol glucose for muscle contraction, gluconeogenesis consumes 6 mols ATP/mol glucose. This energetic imbalance is one of the reasons why anaerobic muscle contraction is of limited duration. When aerobic conditions are restored, any remaining lactate may be fully oxidised to CO_2 and H_2O. The oxygen required for this process is sometimes referred to as the oxygen debt.

Homeostatic mechanisms normally ensure that lactate is removed from the bloodstream to prevent it from accumulating to a level where it might threaten the pH of the blood. Certain disease states are characterised by higher-than-normal levels of anaerobic respiration: cancer, respiratory failure, sepsis, kidney failure. These conditions may cause lactic acidosis where lactate accumulates, the pH of the blood drops below the normal minimum of 7.36 and electrolyte imbalance follows as the kidney attempts to rectify the pH.

Anaerobic metabolism is 15-fold less efficient than oxidative metabolism in terms of mols ATP generated per mol glucose (Table 24.1) but has huge significance for certain tissues of the body (Table 24.2).

1.2 Aerobic Metabolism

Full oxidation of glucose to its combustion products (Fig. 24.3) is much more efficient in terms of ATP yield, producing 30–32 mol ATP/mol glucose compared with

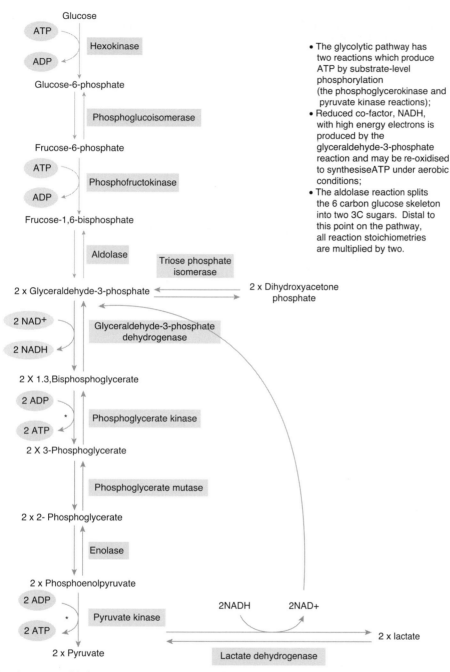

- The glycolytic pathway has two reactions which produce ATP by substrate-level phosphorylation (the phosphoglycerokinase and pyruvate kinase reactions);
- Reduced co-factor, NADH, with high energy electrons is produced by the glyceraldehyde-3-phosphate reaction and may be re-oxidised to synthesiseATP under aerobic conditions;
- The aldolase reaction splits the 6 carbon glucose skeleton into two 3C sugars. Distal to this point on the pathway, all reaction stoichiometries are multiplied by two.

* Reactions responsible for the production of ATP by substrate-level phosphorylation I ADP = adenosine diphosphate I ATP = adenosine triphosphate I NAD$^+$ = oxidised form of nicotinamide adenine dinucleotide I NADH = reduced form of NAD

Figure 24.1 Pathway of glycolysis and the lactate dehydrogenase reaction

2 mol ATP/mol glucose during anaerobiosis (Table 24.1). Other fuels, such as fats, ketone bodies and amino acids, may also be respired aerobically. The aerobic pathway of glucose metabolism follows on from the cytosolic glycolytic pathway and takes place within the mitochondrial compartment when pyruvate

dehydrogenase converts the glycolytic product, pyruvate, into the TCA cycle substrate, acetyl CoA (Fig. 24.4). Reduced co-factors, NADH and FADH₂, produced from TCA cycle activity (Fig. 24.4), have high energy electrons and transfer energy from the oxidation reac-

tions of the cycle to the redox reactions of the electron transport chain (ETC). A supply of oxygen is required to accept electrons following electron transport chain activity, accounting for the consumption of oxygen during aerobic respiration.

1.2.1 Mitochondrial Function

Mitochondria represent the primary site of ATP generation for tissues under aerobic conditions, containing the enzymes of the TCA cycle and carriers of the electron transport chain (ETC), as well as enzymes of the beta-oxidation pathway of fat oxidation. The organelles contain a small amount of DNA, which takes the form of a plasmid and which encodes some proteins for use within the mitochondrion: 13 out of 80 protein subunits for oxidative phosphorylation plus 2 ribosomal and 22 transfer RNA genes for protein expression. Mitochondrial DNA has a mutation rate around 20 times higher than that of nuclear DNA, reflecting the presence of oxygen metabolism within this compartment and the lack of the sophisticated DNA proofreading mechanisms present in the nucleus. This DNA is inherited in a non-Mendelian manner through the maternal line only. The high mutation rate underlies the prevalence of mitochondrial disorders and hence the move toward three-person IVF where healthy mitochondrial DNA is supplied by a donor. Mutations in mitochondrial DNA affect the oxidative metabolism of

Table 24.1 Steps producing ATP during aerobic and anaerobic oxidation of glucose

Reduced co-factors produced (moles per mole glucose)	Route of ATP synthesis	Resulting ATP yield* (moles per mole glucose)
GLYCOLYSIS		
	Substrate-level phosphorylation	2 ATP
2 NADH [b]	Oxidative phosphorylation	5 ATP
PDH REACTION		
2 NADH	Oxidative phosphorylation	5 ATP
TCA CYCLE		
	Substrate-level phosphorylation [c]	2 ATP
6 NADH	Oxidative phosphorylation	15 ATP
2 FADH₂	Oxidative phosphorylation	3 ATP

The red bracket shows the span of anaerobic respiration and the blue bracket shows the span of aerobic respiration.

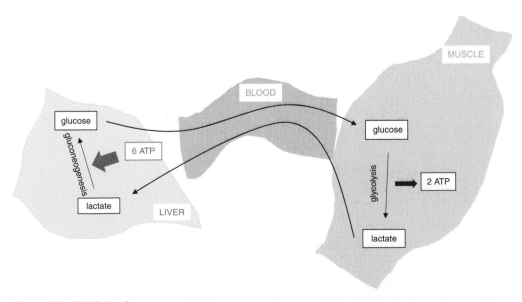

Figure 24.2 The Cori cycle

Table 24.2 Anaerobic tissues

Tissue	Reason for dependence on anaerobic respiration
Type 2 (fast twitch, white) muscle fibre	Used for high power output, short-duration exercise; O_2 diffusion into the fibre is too slow a process to maintain ATP supply; flux through glycolysis can be increased 1000-fold within milliseconds by powerful regulatory mechanisms; fibres have large internal glycogen stores but few mitochondria, little myoglobin and are poorly vascularised.
Erythrocyte	Cells have no mitochondria and therefore no oxidative metabolism; internal volume is preserved to accommodate haemoglobin and to maintain the property of cell-deformability.
Retina	Few mitochondria are present since their cytochromes would impede the passage of light; O_2 metabolism produces reactive oxygen species which might damage light-sensitive pigments.
Kidney medulla	Poorly perfused with blood and a poor oxygen supply.

$$C_6H_{12}O_6 + 6O_2 \rightarrow 6CO_2 + 6H_2O$$

Figure 24.3 Complete oxidation of glucose yields combustion products

the cell and have a greater impact on those tissues with a high, continuous ATP requirement and dependence on fuel oxidation, such as nervous tissue (Table 24.3).

1.2.2 Aerobic Tissues

Some tissues, predominantly those with a sustained high energy requirement, are noteworthy for their highly aerobic metabolism (Table 24.4). These tissues are supremely sensitive to any interruption in oxygen supply and ischaemic conditions rapidly result in tissue damage.

2 Control of Blood Glucose Levels

The importance of the glucose substrate for the CNS, among other tissues, justifies the elaborate nature of homeostatic mechanisms dedicated to maintaining the availability of glucose through the blood. Normal blood glucose varies between approximate limits of 4 mM (fasted state) and 8 mM (post-prandial state) (Fig. 24.5). At 4 mM glucose, there is around 3.6 g of glucose in the adult circulation (based on a total blood volume of 5 L and the molecular weight (MW) of glucose of 180 g). This is a concentration that allows the functionality of all body systems. At 2 mM glucose, there remains 1.8 g of glucose in the circulation but a hypoglycaemic coma is very likely to be the result. This illustrates the significance of the concentration of blood-borne substrates, rather than their absolute quantities. The basis of this significance lies in the transport mechanisms which allow uptake into dependent tissues. The brain, for example, has a proteinaceous glucose transporter, GLUT3, with a Km for glucose of 1.6 mM which allows

uptake of glucose by facilitated diffusion. (The Km represents the concentration of substrate at which the enzyme achieves half-maximal velocity and therefore a low Km indicates high enzyme activity at normal physiological concentrations of substrate.) The value for Km tells us that at 1.6 mM the glucose transporter will be operating at half its maximal velocity (Vmax) and that at any normal physiological concentration of glucose (4-8 mM), the transporter will be saturated and working at Vmax. If the blood glucose concentration drops into the range of 2-3 mM, GLUT3 is no longer operating at Vmax and the brain is unable to satisfy its glucose requirement, resulting in loss of tissue function. GLUT3 has the lowest Km of any glucose transporter, and its presence in nervous tissues gives the brain preferential access to blood glucose over other tissues. The placenta also expresses the GLUT3 transporter, and fetal tissues show a similar reliance on the glucose substrate.

2.1 Hypoglycaemia

Children may tolerate slightly lower fasting limits of blood glucose, as may pregnant women. However, hypoglycaemia can cause disorientation, confusion and coma, as the brain is deprived of ATP, and sweating, as the autonomic nervous system stimulates release of adrenaline. A number of conditions may result in hypoglycaemia, as blood glucose levels drop below the normal range (Table 24.5).

2.2 Glycogen as a Source of Blood Glucose

Blood glucose must be continually replenished to avoid decreases in concentration during fasting or exercise. Glucose is stored as the polymer, glycogen, in the liver (around 100 g glucose as glycogen in the adult) and skeletal muscle (around 200 g in the adult). Glycogen is not a particularly efficient means of storing energy since a considerable degree of hydration is necessary to

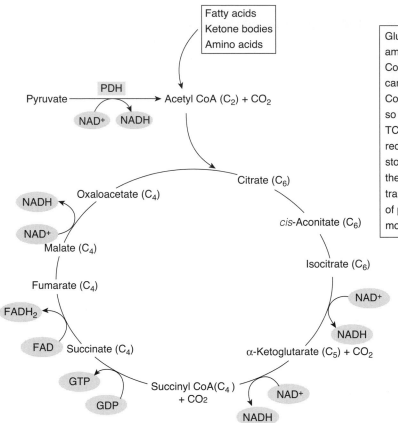

Glucose, fatty acids, ketone bodies and amino acids can all produce the acetyl CoA substrate for the TCA cycle. Two carbons enter the cycle per turn as acetyl CoA and two carbons are evolved as CO_2, so that there is no net synthesis of any TCA cycle intermediate. High energy reduced cofactors, NADH and $FADH_2$, store energy which is redeemed when they are re-oxidised by the electron transport chain. Note that two molecules of pyruvate are produced per glucose molecule, causing two turns of the cycle.

Note that 2 moles of acetyl CoA are produced per mole of glucose and that oxidation of this acetyl CoA requires two turns of the cycle.
CoA=coenzyme A | GDP=guanosine diphosphate | GTP=guanosine triphosphate | FAD=oxidised form of flavin adenine dinucleotide | $FADH_2$=reduced form of FAD | NAD^+=oxidised form of nicotinamide adenine dinucleotide | NADH=reduced form of NAD+ | PDH=pyruvate dehydrogenase | TCA=tricarboxylic acid

Products of the TCA cycle per turn:
Reduced co-factors: $3NADH + 1FADH_2$;
High-energy compound: 1ATP (from GTP);
Decarboxylation products: $2CO_2$.

The pyruvate dehydrogenase reaction is irreversible and two carbons are lost from the TCA cycle as CO_2 for every two carbons that enter the cycle as Acetyl CoA. This means that there is no metabolic route from Acetyl CoA to any intermediate on the pathway of gluconeogenesis; thus acetyl CoA cannot be converted into glucose.

Figure 24.4 The tricarboxylic acid cycle

maintain the branched structure and accessibility of the polymer to degrading enzymes. Glycogen is stored with approximately three times its weight in water, so that total body glycogen stores weigh more than 1.2 kg, at considerable dilution of its energy storage potential. As a result, glucose reserves are very limited compared with the body's glucose requirements (the brain alone consumes around 120 g/day in the adult). Fasting for 24 hours is sufficient to deplete liver glycogen reserves (mobilisation stimulated by glucagon) and intensive exercise of 60 minutes duration to deplete muscle (mobilisation stimulated by adrenaline acting at its muscle β2-adrenoceptor). Thereafter, hepatic gluconeogenesis must supply glucose to tissues via the blood to ensure that the brain's residual glucose requirement is satisfied.

Table 24.3 Mitochondrial disorders

Disorder	Mutated mitochondrial gene	Phenotype
Leber's hereditary optic neuropathy (LHON) *1 in 25,000 births*	Subunits 1, 4 or 6 of NADH dehydrogenase (complex 1 of ETC)	Sudden onset bilateral blindness, largely in males aged 20–30, due to degeneration of optic nerve
Myoclonic epilepsy with ragged red fibres (MERRF) *1 in 400,000 births*	tRNA-lysine (required for protein synthesis)	Epilepsy, abnormal development of Type 1 oxidative muscle fibres
Mitochondrial encephalopathy, lactic acidosis and stroke-like episodes (MELAS) *1 in 185,000 births*	tRNA-leucine (required for protein synthesis)	Encephalopathy and stroke due to nerve degeneration and insufficient energy supply for nerve function; increased anaerobic respiration produces lactate
Neuropathy, ataxia, retinitis pigmentosa (NARP) *Rare*	Subunit 6 of ATPase	Disrupted muscle function, elevated blood lactate, learning difficulties, reports of psychosis

Table 24.4 Highly aerobic tissues

Tissue	Energy consumption rate (kcal/kg/day) [1]	Proportion of REE of FFM (%)	Preferred substrate
Central nervous system	240 (brain)	20	Glucose
Heart	440	20	Ketone bodies, fatty acids
Type 1 skeletal muscle fibre	14.5 (total skeletal muscle)	25	Fatty acids

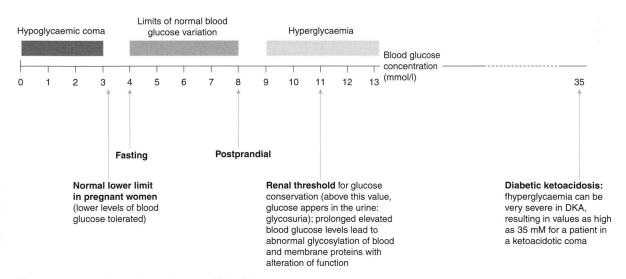

Figure 24.5 Normal and abnormal ranges of blood glucose concentration

3 Metabolism in Starvation

Maintenance of blood glucose levels is a priority to the starving body. Fat stores are large but the acetyl CoA produced from their breakdown may not be converted into glucose. The pyruvate dehydrogenase reaction is irreversible and two carbons are lost from

Table 24.5 Some causes of hypoglycaemia

Cause	Reason
Poorly controlled diabetes (fasting state)	Loss of insulin means poor glycogen deposits and fewer resources for fasting.
Alcohol consumption	Increased NADH/NAD ratio in liver arising from ethanol oxidation suppresses hepatic gluconeogenesis [2]; alcohol stimulates late-phase insulin secretion [3].
Von Gierke's disease (1 in 50,000–100,000 births)	Lack of hepatic glucose-6-phosphatase reduces hepatic glucose output (gluconeogenesis + glycogen mobilisation).
Cori's disease (1 in 100,000 births)	Lack of glycogen debranching enzyme reduces efficiency of glycogen mobilisation.

the TCA cycle when the 2 C molecule, acetyl CoA, is the substrate (Fig. 24.4). The liver converts non-carbohydrate amino acid precursors from the wasting of muscle tissue into glucose, using the pathway of gluconeogenesis (Fig. 24.6). The process of muscle protein breakdown begins after 24 hours of fasting in the adult and accelerates as starvation continues. Release of amino acids is stimulated by the action of the long-term stress hormone, cortisol. Non-essential muscles break down first but, if starvation persists, essential muscles lose mass too, which compromises their function. Death due to starvation occurs after about 60 days in the normal-sized adult, before fat stores of the body have been exhausted, and is commonly due to failure of heart or diaphragm muscle.

4 Carbohydrate Metabolism in the Diabetic

4.1 Role of Insulin

The blood insulin:glucagon ratio is the single most important determinant of blood glucose concentration. Loss or reduction of the insulin signal brings about many changes to carbohydrate metabolism, which tend to be more severe for the Type 1 diabetic (where an autoimmune reaction destroys the insulin-producing pancreatic beta cells) and milder for the insulin-resistant state (where tissues lose their responsiveness to insulin) associated with Type 2 or gestational diabetes mellitus (GDM). (Note GDM is considered to represent a predisposition to develop Type 2 diabetes later in life [4].) The severity of disruption of glucose tolerance in the diabetic (Table 24.6) illustrates the vital role played by insulin in the normal state.

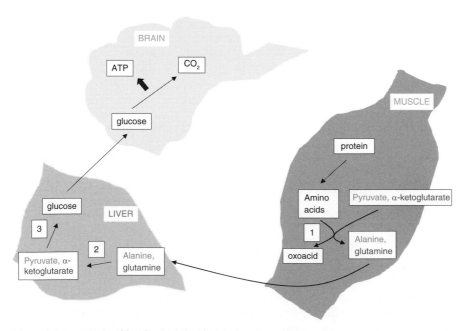

Figure 24.6 Provision of fuel for the brain during starvation

Table 24.6 Changes in carbohydrate metabolism in diabetes

Metabolic disturbance	Result of reduced insulin effect
Hyperglycaemia (fed state)	Failure to recruit GLUT4 glucose transporter in muscle and stimulate muscle glucose uptake; failure to suppress hepatic gluconeogenesis so that liver continues to export glucose into blood despite hyperglycaemia: animal studies have shown significant flux of carbon from muscle protein to blood glucose in order to sustain this process [5]; blood glucose above 11 mM produces a state of osmotic diuresis where glucose is lost in the urine along with water to dilute it.
Poor glycogen reserves	Failure to stimulate glycogen synthesis in muscle and liver in the fed state.
Hypoglycaemia (fasting state)	Poor glycogen reserves leave little to mobilise in the fasting state.

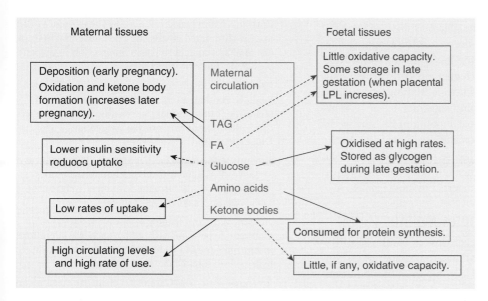

Figure 24.7 Partitioning of fuels between maternal and fetal tissues during pregnancy and gestation

TAG: triacylglycerol; FA: fatty acid; LPL: lipoprotein lipase

4.2 Hyperglycaemia

Hyperglycaemia results from the loss of insulin-stimulated glucose uptake by tissues in the postprandial state. In quantitative terms, the most important factor is the loss of glucose uptake by skeletal muscle due to the failure of insulin to stimulate recruitment of the GLUT4 transporter. Osmotic effects of high blood glucose mean tissues lose water to dilute the blood. Above 11 mM, glucose appears in the urine (glycosuria) and must be diluted, leading to polyuria and dehydration. Prolonged hyperglycaemia in the poorly controlled diabetic leads to abnormal glycosylation of proteins. Advanced glycosylation end products (AGE) appear (e.g. HbA1 c in blood) and glycosylation of membrane proteins contributes to deterioration of tissue function, especially of peripheral nerves and the kidney. High blood glucose levels stimulate rapid fetal growth in GDM, contributing to macrosomia relative to the developmental stage (rate of fetal growth is proportional to maternal blood glucose concentration [6,7]).

5 Carbohydrate Metabolism in Pregnancy

Fetal tissues are dependent on the glucose substrate for energy requirements and probably oxidise little of alternative substrates. The placenta expresses the low Km (high affinity) GLUT3 glucose transporter in a similar manner to nervous tissues. This leads to unequal partitioning of glucose present in the maternal circulation as the fetus has preferential access (Fig. 24.7).

5.1 Insulin Resistance in Pregnancy

Adjustment of the insulin-sensitivity of maternal tissues accompanies normal pregnancy. In early pregnancy, enhanced insulin-sensitivity favours anabolic activities of maternal tissues, such as the synthesis and storage of lipids. However, in later pregnancy, insulin-sensitivity can be reduced by 50–70%, favouring nutrient uptake by the fetus at the expense of that by the mother. Fetal tissues are dependent on the glucose substrate for ATP generation and probably do not oxidise appreciable amounts of fat. Although the loss of insulin sensitivity by maternal tissues leads to higher rates of synthesis and higher circulating levels of ketone bodies, fetal tissues probably cannot oxidise this substrate as an energy source. This leads to clear partitioning of fuels between maternal and fetal tissues during pregnancy and gestation with higher rates of glucose consumption by fetal tissues compared with higher rates of consumption of fats and ketone bodies by maternal tissues (Fig. 24.7).

5.2 Gestational Diabetes Mellitus (GDM)

GDM represents a more severe loss of insulin sensitivity. The loss of sensitivity of maternal tissues to insulin means that hyperglycaemia accompanies the condition and stimulates faster than normal growth of fetal tissues, leading to fetal macrosomia. Hyperketonaemia is also present such that ketone bodies may appear in the urine. This is a harmful situation, since studies have shown that high levels of maternal ketone bodies may have a teratogenic effect, causing elevated rates of birth defects [8,9]. The increasing incidence of GDM (now up to 9.2% of pregnancies in the US [10]), along with its predisposing factor of obesity, illustrates the need for lifestyle and pharmacological agents to treat it. It has been proposed that the criteria for diagnosis of GDM be broadened to include less severe disruptions of glucose tolerance since even milder fluctuations of glucose homeostasis are considered to have adverse effects on pregnancy outcomes [11].

References

1. Elia, M. (1992) Organ and tissue contribution to metabolic rate. In: Kinney J.M., Tucker H.N. (eds.), *Energy metabolism: Tissue determinants and cellular corollaries*. New York: Raven Press, 61–79.

2. Madison, L.L., Lodner, A. and Wulff, J. (1967) Ethanol-induced hypoglycaemia II: Mechanism of suppression of hepatic gluconeogenesis. *Diabetes* **16** 252–8.

3. Huang, Z. and Sjoholm, A. (2008) Ethanol acutely stimulates islet blood flow, amplifies insulin secretion and induces hypoglycaemia via nitric oxide and vagally mediated mechanisms. *Endocrinology* **149** (1) 232–6.

4. Lee, A. J., Hiscock, R. J., Wein, P., Walker, S. P. and Permezel, M. (2007) Gestational diabetes mellitus: clinical predictors and long-term risk of developing type 2 Diabetes – a retrospective cohort study using survival analysis. *Diabetes Care* **30** (4) 878–83.

5. Koopmans, S.J., VanderMeulen, J., Wijdenes, J., Corbijn, H. and Dekker, R. (2011) The existence of an insulin-stimulated glucose and non-essential but not essential amino acid substrate interaction in diabetic pigs. *BMC Biochemistry* **12** 25.

6. Breschi, M.C., Seghieri, G., Bartolomei, G., Gironi, A., Baldi, S. and Ferrannini, E. (1993) Relation of birthweight to maternal plasma glucose and insulin concentrations during normal pregnancy. *Diabetologia* **36** (12) 1315–21.

7. Taslimi, M.M., Navabi, K., Acosta, R., Helmer, A. and El-Sayed, Y.Y. (2008) Concealed maternal blood glucose excursions correlate with birth weight centile *J Diabetes Sci Technol* **2** (3) 456–60.

8. Horton, W.E. and Sadler, T.W. (1983) Effects of maternal diabetes on early embryogenesis: alterations in morphogenesis produced by the ketone body, β-hydroxybutyrate. *Diabetes* **32** 610–6.

9. Jovanovic-Peterson, C.M. (1991) Glucose metabolism in pregnancy In: Cowett, R. (ed.), *Principles of Perinatal-Neonatal Metabolism*. New York: Springer-Verlag.

10. DeSisto,C.L., Kim, S.Y. and Sharma, A.J. Prevalence estimates of gestational diabetes mellitus in the United States, Pregnancy Risk Assessment Monitoring System (PRAMS), 2007–2010 *Prev. Chronic Dis.* 2014 **11** 130415.

11. Cundy, T., Ackermann, E. and Ryan, E.A. (2014) Gestational diabetes: New criteria may triple the prevalence but effect on outcomes is unclear. *British Medical Journal* **348** g1567.

Single Best Answer Questions

1. Type 2 muscle fibre respires anaerobically because:

   a. the pathway for oxidative metabolism is longer than that for anaerobic metabolism

   b. there is no oxygen available for aerobic respiration

c. oxygen diffusion into the muscle fibre is too slow to sustain the muscle's ATP-requirement

d. aerobic respiration produces less ATP than anaerobic respiration

e. delivery of aerobic fuels to the muscle is too slow to sustain the muscle's ATP requirement

2. Lactate, rather than pyruvate, is the product of anaerobic respiration because:

a. the accumulation of pyruvate within the cell would be toxic

b. pyruvate is consumed by other reactions within the cell

c. pyruvate is too unstable to be transported in the bloodstream

d. the production of lactate regenerates NAD^+ for continued glycolytic activity

e. the production of lactate regenerates glucose for continued glycolysis

3. Loss of the insulin signal in diabetes causes:

a. hypoglycaemia

b. hyperglycaemia in the fed state because insulin-stimulated glucose-uptake by muscle does not occur at appropriate rates

c. hyperglycaemia in the fed state, which causes increased rates of glucose-oxidation

d. hyperglycaemia in the fed state, which causes tissues to respire anaerobically

e. hyperglycaemia in the fed state, which causes the liver to stop exporting glucose

4. The brain's dependence on the glucose substrate means that:

a. the brain respires anaerobically

b. the brain has a low Km glucose transporter

c. the brain competes unfavourably with other tissues for blood glucose

d. the brain releases lactate into the blood stream

e. the brain generates ATP at higher rates than other tissues

5. Using the pathway of gluconeogenesis, glucose may be synthesised in the liver from:

a. lactate and certain glucogenic amino acids

b. fatty acids and ketone bodies

c. lactate and fatty acids only

d. all amino acids

e. sucrose, maltose and lactose

6. Alcohol causes hypoglycaemia because:

a. alcohol metabolism inhibits glucose-6-phosphatase

b. it inhibits insulin release

c. it causes higher rates of glucose uptake by tissues, such as skeletal muscle

d. it inhibits hepatic glucose output

e. it stimulates insulin secretion by the pancreas and suppresses gluconeogenesis in the liver

7. Fatty acids are an oxidative substrate for which tissues?

a. Heart, Type 2 skeletal muscle fibre, brain

b. Erythrocytes, CNS, Type 1 skeletal muscle fibre

c. Heart muscle, nervous tissue, Type 2 skeletal muscle fibre

d. Heart, Type 1 skeletal muscle fibre

e. Kidney medulla, heart, CNS

8. The actions of insulin cause:

a. increased uptake of glucose and glycogen synthesis by skeletal muscle; suppressed glycogen mobilisation and gluconeogenesis by liver

b. increased uptake of glucose by all tissues of the body to promote glucose clearance from the blood

c. increased hepatic glucose output as glycogen is mobilised and gluconeogenesis stimulated

d. increased appetite as insulin acts on its hypothalamic receptor

e. increased uptake of glucose and glycogen synthesis by skeletal muscle; increased glucagon secretion by the pancreas

9. Tissues with sustained high energy requirements tend to respire aerobically because:

a. the delivery of oxidative fuels via the bloodstream is more reliable than the delivery of anaerobic fuels

b. full oxidation of fuels to their combustion products releases more chemical energy than partial oxidation of glucose to lactate

c. the production of lactate from anaerobic respiration is toxic to cells

d. the re-conversion of lactate to glucose consumes too much ATP

e. glucose, the only anaerobic fuel, cannot be taken up by aerobic tissues

Chapter 25

Fat Metabolism

Mary Board

1 Roles of Fats

Fats have energy-storing, structural and regulatory roles in the body (Table 25.1). Depots of white adipose tissue (WAT) therefore not only function to store energy but also to provide precursors for synthesis of other species. Specific roles are played by certain fatty acids in this regard. For example, long-chain derivatives of the essential fatty acids of the omega 3 series (which cannot be synthesised *de novo* but must be taken in through the diet and modified) contribute to membrane formation in the CNS and the retina. The importance of the roles played by omega 3 fatty acids in anchoring specific membrane proteins involved in signalling is illustrated by the effects of dietary deficiencies. About ⅔ of the total content of docosahexaenoic acid (22 carbon fatty acid derived from linolenic acid) are assimilated in the final three months of gestation and the remaining ⅓ during the first three months of life. An interruption of supply during these crucial periods produces a measurable adverse effect on the development of cognitive function and of visual acuity. Omega-3 fats are not frequently deficient but are initially synthesised by marine plants and usually enter our diet via fish. Thus, followers of a vegan diet can become deficient during pregnancy and breastfeeding (see Section 7 and Table 25.9).

1.1 Energy Storage

Fats are energy dense compared with carbohydrates and proteins and *in vitro* combustion values shown in Table 25.2 demonstrate that chemical properties of the molecules contribute to this phenomenon, giving a two-fold increase in energy content per unit weight of fat compared with carbohydrate or protein. Fats are highly reduced, releasing a lot of energy during oxidation and may be regarded as rich sources of reduced co-factors, NADH and $FADH_2$ (electron donors which pass electrons along the electron transport chain, leading to ATP-synthesis). Fat is also stored in an anhydrous manner (whereas glycogen is hydrated) and the differential in terms of ATP-production per unit weight of stored fat compared with glycogen in the body is around seven-fold. Energy is stored as fat in the form of the triacylglycerol (TAG) molecule (Fig. 25.1a), in which three fatty acid side chains are esterified to the three carbons of the glycerol molecule. The degree of saturation of the fatty acid side chain has implications for the behaviour of the TAG molecule in mediating the fluidity of the adipocyte TAG depot. Due to the *cis* arrangement of hydrogen atoms, double bonds cause the fatty acid side-chain to adopt an angle of 135°. The resulting kink disrupts the association of fatty acids within the TAG molecule (Fig. 25.1a). TAGs with higher content of unsaturated fatty acids produce

Table 25.1 Major roles of fats

Role	Form of fat	Comments
Energy storage	Triacylglycerol	Inclusion of unsaturated fatty acids mediates fluidity
Membrane formation	Phospholipid	Specialised roles of Ω3 fatty acids in CNS
Hormone synthesis	Essential (unsaturated) fatty acids	Arachidonic acid produces eicosanoids (prostaglandins, prostacyclins, thromboxanes and leukotrienes).
Intracellular signalling	Phospholipid	Breakdown releases second messengers within the cell
Regulation of gene transcription	Fatty acids and fat-soluble vitamins	Growth and development effects

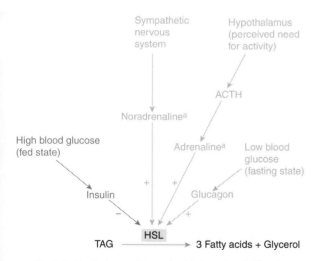

cis-Oleic acid

Stearic acid[b]

Linoleic acid[c]

Glycerol backbone

The presence of a double bond causes the fatty acid side chain to bend and adopt an angle of 135 degrees; such bends disrupt the packing of the side chains and thus the inclusion of unsaturated fatty acids is important in maintaining the fluidity of the TAG depot.

Saturated fatty acid;

Mono-unsaturated fatty acid;

Poly-unsaturated fatty acid

Figure 25.1(a) Chemical structure of a triacylglycerol

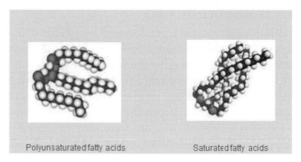

Polyunsaturated fatty acids   Saturated fatty acids

Figure 25.1(b) Space-filling models of triacylglycerol molecules

Sympathetic nervous system

Hypothalamus (perceived need for activity)

ACTH

Noradrenaline[a]

High blood glucose (fed state)

Adrenaline[a]

Low blood glucose (fasting state)

Insulin

Glucagon

+ +

−   +

HSL

TAG ⟶ 3 Fatty acids + Glycerol

[a] Mediated by beta-3-adrenergic receptors | + indicates an increase in HSL activity | −indicates a decrease in HSL activity | ACTH = adrenocorticotrophic hormone | HSL = hormone-sensitive lipase | TAG = triacylglycerol

Figure 25.2 Hormonal control of lipolysis in the adipocyte

a less dense depot with a lower melting temperature than those with saturated fatty acids (Fig. 25.1b) and the inclusion of unsaturated fats is vital in maintaining the fluidity of the TAG depot and its accessibility to degrading enzymes. TAGs are stored as one large droplet in the cytosol of the adipocyte and mobilisation involves lipolysis to release fatty acids for transport. Lipolysis is under hormonal control (Fig. 25.2) and levels of blood fat show large variations according to conditions (Table 25.3).

Energy content is derived from *in vitro* combustion values in a bomb calorimeter (fuels are converted to CO_2 and H_2O and energy evolved as heat is measured).

1.2 Leptin

Fats are stored in white adipose tissue (WAT) and we have recently become aware that this tissue functions as an endocrine organ as well as an energy storage organ. WAT releases a number of adipokines, including leptin, a small peptide which has anorexigenic effects on the CNS as well as increasing fuel uptake and utilisation in peripheral tissues, such as skeletal muscle. That leptin plays a significant role is illustrated by the congenital obesity of the leptin-deficient *ob/ob* mouse. Leptin is released into the plasma to achieve a concentration that is proportional to the fat mass of the body: obese subjects have higher plasma leptin concentrations than lean subjects. There is evidence to suggest that obese subjects may suffer from a degree of leptin resistance and thus the anorexigenic effects of the hormone are diminished. Leptin has multifarious roles, stimulating angiogenesis and haematopoiesis, as well as having effects on appetite and energy expenditure. It also has roles in the reproductive process. It is considered that low levels of leptin, due to the fat mass dropping below a critical volume, are the reason why female athletes and anorexic patients cease to menstruate. Leptin can thus be seen as a signal that fuel stores of the body are sufficient to sustain pregnancy.

2 Transport of Fats

Fats are insoluble and form destructive micellar structures in aqueous solution. Micelles may pass through cell membranes, damaging them and disrupting their function and therefore fats must be buffered in the bloodstream. Buffering takes the form of covalent complexes formed between the fat and specific proteins (Table 25.4). There are a number of different lipoprotein complexes with distinct origins and functions and the lipoprotein profile of the blood has implications for health. We can see from Table 25.4 that both LDL and HDL function to transport cholesterol. LDL collects newly synthesised cholesterol from the liver and takes it to peripheral tissues where it may

be stored. HDL serves the reverse route, scavenging cholesterol from tissues and taking it to the liver where it may be excreted. Thus, high levels of LDL are associated with active storage of cholesterol ('bad fat') and high levels of HDL with active excretion of cholesterol ('good fat'). Moreover, oxidised forms of LDL may contribute to atherogenesis. A low LDL: HDL ratio is therefore considered to have favourable health implications. Various conditions and dietary practices have an impact on the LDL:HDL ratio within the blood and thus on health (Table 25.5).

3 Oxidation of Fats

Tissue-specific lipoprotein lipases release fatty acids from lipoproteins and thus the fat can become an oxidative substrate for the target tissue. Repeated cycles of the four steps of the β-oxidation pathway (Fig. 25.3) convert the fatty acid into acetyl CoA, the substrate for the TCA cycle, and allow full oxidation and ATP-generation from the substrate (Table 25.6). Fats are very significant energy-yielding substrates for a variety of tissues, particularly those with a high,

Table 25.2 Energy content of macronutrients

Macronutrient	Energy content (kJ/g)
Fat	37
Carbohydrate	17
Protein	17

Table 25.3 Levels of blood fat under different conditions

Condition	Hormonal agent	Plasma [fat] (mM)
Fed	Insulin	0.1–0.3
Starved (8 days)	Glucagon	2.2 [1]
Exercise (15 min + 15 min rest)	Adrenaline	1.0 [2]
Stress (racing driver)	Adrenaline	1.7 [3]
Diabetic coma	Loss of insulin signal	3.0 [4]
GDM (fed)	Reduction of insulin sensitivity	0.7 [5]

Table 25.4 Lipoproteins in the blood

Lipoprotein	Main fat constituent	Function
Chylomicron	Dietary TAG	Transports TAG from the intestine to other tissues for oxidation or storage (fed state)
VLDL	Endogenous TAG, cholesterol	Transports TAG produced in the liver to other tissues where it can be oxidised (fasting state)
LDL	Cholesterol and cholesteryl ester	Transports cholesterol from the liver to other tissues
HDL	Cholesteryl ester	Scavenges cholesterol from many tissues and takes it to the liver for excretion
Fatty acid–albumin	Fatty acid	Transports fatty acids from adipose tissue to other tissues where they can be oxidised (fasting state)

HDL – high-density lipoprotein, LDL – low-density lipoprotein, TAG – triacylglycerol, VLDL – very-low-density lipoprotein

Table 25.5 Effects on the lipid profile of the blood of dietary intake

Dietary practice	Active dietary constituent	Effect on LDL:HDL
Diet rich in saturated fats	Fats from meat and dairy	↑↑
Diet rich in trans-unsaturated fats	Partially hydrogenated fatty acids from processed foods	↑↑
Diet rich in polyunsaturated fats	Plant oils	↓
Diet rich in mono-unsaturated fats ('Mediterranean diet')	Olive oil (oleic acid), walnut or almond oils	↓
High fat, low carbohydrate diet ('Atkins diet')	Substantial replacement of carbohydrate by fat	↓
Policosanol (licensed for cholesterol reduction) [7]	Mixture of higher aliphatic alcohols from sugar cane wax extract	↓

See [6] for review of effects of dietary fat on the lipid profile.

sustained energy requirement, such as heart and Type 1 skeletal muscle fibres, and become the predominant fuel for the body after the first 24 hours of starvation. The importance of fat as a fuel can be illustrated by the effects of the inborn error of metabolism, MCAD deficiency (1 in 10,000 births in UK), where a mutation reduces the activity of one of the group of enzymes catalysing the first step of the β-oxidation pathway, medium-chain acyl CoA dehydrogenase (MCAD). This enzyme is responsible for metabolising a proportion of the fatty acids in the diet – those with chain lengths of between 6 and 14 carbons. Symptoms of MCAD deficiency include hypoglycaemia and hepatomegaly which can quickly progress to coma and death [8]. Some studies have shown a high degree of association between MCAD deficiency and sudden infant death syndrome (SIDS), although for MCAD deficiency to be fatal in the infant, usually a viral infection is implicated [9], meaning that the classical pattern of SIDS is not followed. When oxidation of fatty acids is impaired in this way, episodes of fasting impose a greater dependence on the glucose present in the blood, leading to rates of consumption which can cause a drop in blood glucose concentration below the normal minimum with consequent impairment of brain function.

3.1 Fat Metabolism during Starvation

During episodes of fasting and starvation, TAG mobilization is stimulated by the action of the hormone, glucagon, blood fat levels increase (Table 25.3) and so do rates of fat oxidation through the unregulated β-oxidation pathway. After the depletion of glycogen reserves at 24 h of starvation, fat becomes the predominant fuel and high rates of β-oxidation increase the supply of acetyl CoA to the TCA cycle. In order for acetyl CoA to be oxidised, it must condense with oxaloacetate (see Fig. 24.4), and more oxaloacetate is required to accommodate the raised levels of acetyl CoA. Oxaloacetate must be synthesised from a carbohydrate precursor (the loss of $2CO_2$ in the TCA cycle and the irreversibility of the PDH reaction mean that oxaloacetate cannot be synthesised from acetyl CoA). In all circumstances, it is thus the case that fat oxidation requires a supply of carbohydrate. In prolonged starvation, the source of the extra oxaloacetate will be glucogenic amino acids released by wasting muscle (Fig. 25.4).

4 Ketogenesis

In the mitochondria of the starving liver, levels of acetyl CoA are high due to increased rates of β-oxidation, whereas levels of oxaloacetate are low because this intermediate is withdrawn from the TCA cycle to provide precursors for gluconeogenesis (note that the liver is the only tissue in which substantial rates of gluconeogenesis occur). The imbalance between acetyl CoA and oxaloacetate stimulates the liver to produce ketone bodies (Fig. 25.5) and this pathway is not regulated except by the supply of its acetyl CoA substrate. Ketone bodies, acetoacetate (AcAc) and D-3-hydroxybutyrate (HB), are exported by the liver which lacks the enzymes for their utilisation. Concentrations start to increase in the blood after around 24 h of starvation in the adult, when glycogen has been depleted and hepatic gluconeogenesis becomes active (Fig. 25.6). Maximum values are achieved after around 3–4 days starvation and this

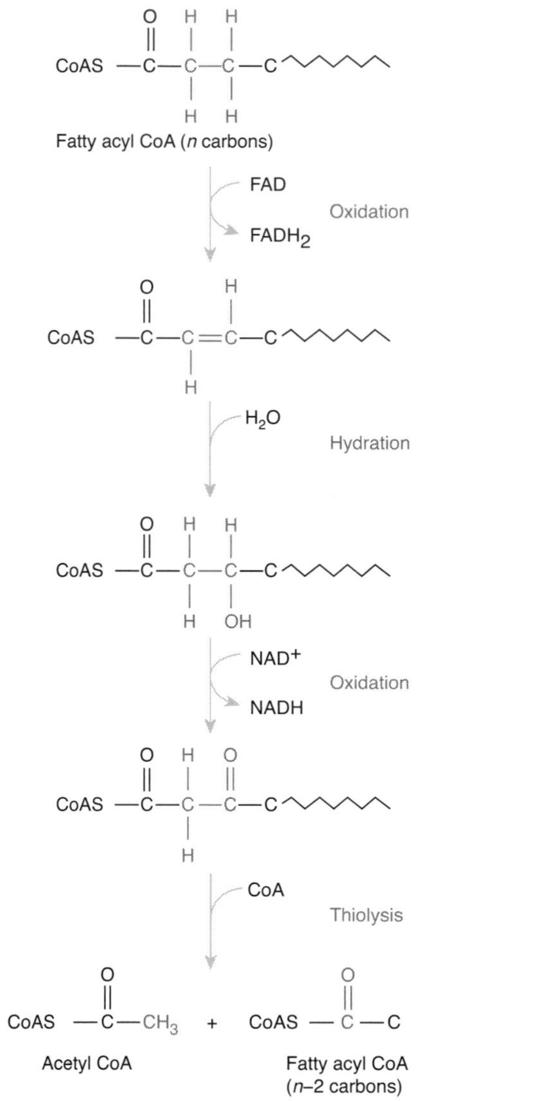

Repeated cycles of these four reactions convert the fatty acid with n carbons into $n/2$ moles of acetyl CoA. CoA = coenzyme A I FAD = oxidised form of flavinadenine dinucleotide I $FADH_2$ = reduced form of FAD I NAD^+ = oxidised form of nicotinamide adenine dinucleotide I NADH = reduced form of NAD

Figure 25.3 The β-oxidation pathway

coincides with the adaptation by the brain to deriving about 75% of its energy from ketone body oxidation. The ketonaemic profile shown in Figure 25.6 is typical of the adult. In the child, with correspondingly smaller glycogen deposits, the onset of ketogenesis and the attainment of maximal ketone body concentrations would occur at an earlier stage after the onset of fasting.

Table 25.6 ATP production from the 16 C fatty acid, palmitate

Reduced co-factors/ GTP produced (moles/ mole palmitate)	ATP produced (moles/ mole palmitate)
7 × β-oxidation	
7 NADH	17.5
7 FADH$_2$	10.5
8 × TCA cycle	
24 NADH	60
8 FADH$_2$	12
8 GTP	8
Fatty acid activation	−2
Total	**106**

4.1 Ketogenic Diet

The ketogenic diet consists of low carbohydrate and high fat intake which mimics the blood levels of these substrates associated with the starved state. The aim is to supply around 90% of calories in the form of fat [reviewed by 10]. It has traditionally been used for the management of epilepsy where it is considered that synthesis of the excitatory neurotransmitter, glutamate, is suppressed and levels of GABA increased while supply of an oxidative substrate to the CNS (ketone bodies) is maintained [reviewed by 11]. More recently, further observations have been made regarding the neuroprotective effects of the ketogenic diet which indicate a role in ameliorating a range of neurodegenerative disorders, such as Parkinson's disease, Alzheimer's disease and stroke (Table 25.7). The action of HB in inhibiting the group of enzymes known as histone deacetylases (HDAC) allows ketone bodies to influence gene expression and may play a role in slowing the ageing process, in general, and neurodegeneration, in particular. HB may also bind specific receptors and fulfil a signalling role to inhibit fat breakdown (feedback inhibition) and lower metabolic rate.

5 Metabolism in obesity: Insulin-resistance

Obesity can be crudely seen as a problem of energy balance, where intake exceeds expenditure. The predisposition to obesity is a more complex situation, comprising genetic and environmental factors. That there is a genetic component, is indicated by the

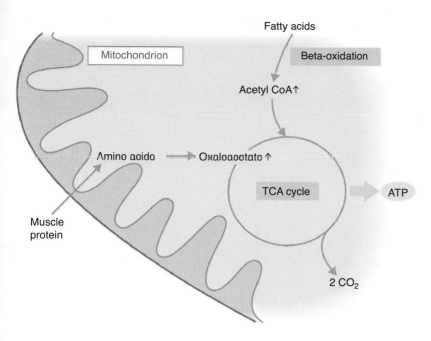

Figure 25.4 Metabolism of fats by peripheral tissues during starvation

↑ = increased I CoA = coenzyme A I TCA = tricarboxylic acid

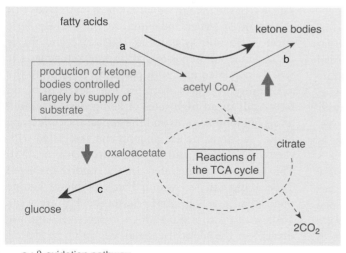

Figure 25.5 Production of ketone bodies by the liver during starvation

a : β-oxidation pathway

b: pathway of ketogenesis

c : pathway of gluconeogenesis

geographical demarcation of obesity with some nations, such as Samoa, having extremely high rates (over 50% in rural areas and over 70% in urban areas). Attempts to link specific polymorphisms with the obese state have been inconclusive, possibly because many mutations of different loci may combine to give the same phenotype.

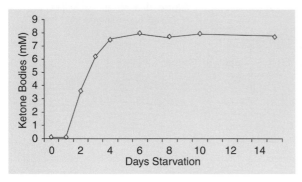

Figure 25.6 Blood concentrations of ketone bodies during starvation in the adult

Table 25.7 Neuroprotective effects of ketogenic diet

Condition	Comments
Epilepsy	>90% decrease in seizure-frequency in children with refractory epilepsy [12]
Alzheimer's disease	Acute administration of medium-chain TAGs improves memory in patients [13]
Parkinson's disease	Patients showed 43% reduction in Unified Parkinson's Disease Rating Scale after 28 days on diet [14]
Stroke	Animal models of ischaemia showed improved outcome and resistance to effects of occlusion [15]

Some polymorphisms, however, occur at sufficiently high rates in the obese population to be considered a consistent contributory factor. One such is a common polymorphism of the Melanocortin 4 receptor (MC4 R). This receptor occurs in the arcuate nucleus of the hypothalamus, where it has a role in mediating the appetite and interacts with other appetite control factors, such as leptin, ghrelin and insulin. Obesity also represents one of the most significant predisposing factors for the development of Type II diabetes. It is considered that the hyperlipidaemic and hyperglycaemic state following from overeating may be a contributory factor. Having high levels of glucose and fat present in the blood at the same time is an abnormal situation and leads to the phenomenon of 'substrate competition' in utilising tissues, such as skeletal muscle. The normal response of muscle to the increased availability of fat is to suppress glucose uptake by this tissue. This is a necessary response to starvation conditions in order to ensure that, when scarce, available glucose is taken up by the brain rather than peripheral tissues. However, this glucose-sparing effect may become exaggerated in the obese individual and prevent the normal clearing of glucose from the bloodstream in the postprandial state, a situation that we equate with loss of glucose tolerance or insulin resistance. The pancreas attempts to compensate for the insulin resistance by increasing its output of the hormone, leading to a prediabetic period of hyperinsulinaemia. When the pancreas can no longer sustain the increased output, insulin levels drop and, in the presence of developing insulin-resistance, diabetes is the result.

It has long been observed that exercise ameliorates the condition of insulin resistance. We have recently become able to explain the mechanism behind this observation. Exercise activates the enzyme, AMP-dependent protein kinase (AMPK), in muscle tissue. The result is that AMPK stimulates the processes of glucose uptake and oxidation and fatty acid oxidation in this tissue. Thus, glucose and fats are cleared from the blood. The well-established anti-diabetic, metformin, operates by a similar mechanism in activating AMPK in liver.

6 Diabetic Ketoacidosis

The loss of the insulin signal in the diabetic leads to a condition of hyperlipidaemia, as the anti-lipolytic effect of insulin is reduced (Fig. 25.2 and Table 25.3). Since neither β-oxidation nor ketogenesis is strictly regulated and both pathways respond to the availability of their substrates, high levels of blood fatty acids mean high rates of ketogenesis. Elevated levels of blood ketones and the appearance of ketone bodies in the urine are phenomena associated with even mild diabetes and can cause problems in GDM. The effect is exaggerated in the poorly-managed Type 1 diabetic, in whom levels of blood ketone bodies can reach 35 mM. AcAc and HB are weak acids with pKas of 3.6 and 4.4, respectively and are present in the bloodstream in a ratio of 10 HB : 1 AcAc. The pH of the blood is normally buffered by the equilibrium between carbonic acid (H_2CO_3) and the bicarbonate ion and proton (HCO_3^- and H^+) (Fig. 25.7). Elevation of blood concentrations of ketone bodies to several times the normal maximum can overwhelm the buffering capacity of the blood and lead to a drop in pH below the normal minimum of 7.36. Acidosis disturbs pH-sensitive processes in the bloodstream, such as the interaction of haemoglobin (Hb) with O_2, causing a progressively more hypoxic

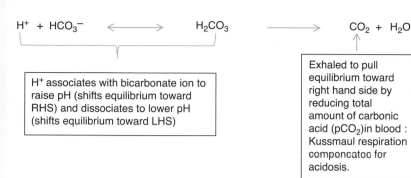

$$H^+ + HCO_3^- \longleftrightarrow H_2CO_3 \longrightarrow CO_2 + H_2O$$

Figure 25.7 Bicarbonate buffering of blood pH

H^+ associates with bicarbonate ion to raise pH (shifts equilibrium toward RHS) and dissociates to lower pH (shifts equilibrium toward LHS)

Exhaled to pull equilibrium toward right hand side by reducing total amount of carbonic acid (pCO_2)in blood : Kussmaul respiration compensates for acidosis.

state of the body. A sequence of events is then triggered, leading to the condition of diabetic ketoacidosis (Fig. 25.8). The kidney responds to acidosis by excreting protons, leading to electrolyte imbalance and respiratory compensation leads to stertorous breathing to exhale CO_2 and displace the bicarbonate buffering equilibrium toward the right-hand side (Fig. 25.7).

7 Neonatal Metabolism

Many pathways become active around the time of birth which allows the neonate to adopt a more fat-centred pattern of substrate consumption compared with the glucose-centred metabolism of the foetus. Such pathways include those of ketogenesis, ketone body utilisation and gluconeogenesis. Both human breast and formula milks have relatively high fat contents (Table 25.8). Note that the content of essential, long-chain fatty acids, vital for membrane-formation in the CNS and retina, varies with diet (Table 25.9). Fats are used as an oxidative substrate for many tissues and to synthesise ketone bodies by the neonatal liver (Fig 25.9). Fats are also the substrate for the specialised thermogenic organ, brown adipose tissue (BAT), present in abundance in the neonate but largely or completely lost by the human adult. BAT consumes fats when stimulated by noradrenaline released by the sympathetic nervous system on the perception of cold. Partially uncoupled mitochondria in BAT mean that the energy of fat metabolism is released as heat, rather than being used to synthesise ATP. The neonate can thus generate heat by the process of non-shivering thermogenesis and maintain core body temperature.

References

1. Albrink, M.J. and Newirth, R.S. (1960) Effect of previous starvation on the response of plasma lipids and free fatty acids to a fat meal. *J. Clin. Invest.* **39**, 441–6.

2. Friedberg, S.J., Harlan, W.R., Trout, D.I. and Estes, E. H. (1960) The effect of exercise on the concentrations and turnover of plasma non-esterified fatty acids. *J. Clin. Invest.* **39**, 215–20.

3. Taggart, P. and Carruthers, M. (1971) Endogenous hyperlipidaemia induced by emotional stress of racing drivers. *Lancet* **I**, 363–6.

4. Watkins, P.J., Hill, D.M., Fitzgerald, M.G. and Malins, J.M. (1970) Ketonaemia in uncontrolled diabetes. *Br. Med. J.* **4**, 522–5.

5. Meyer, B., Calvert, D. and Moses, R. (1996) Free fatty acids and gestational diabetes mellitus. *Aust. N.Z. J. Obstet. Gynaecol.* **36**, 255–7.

6. Yanai, H., Katsuyama, H., Hamasaki, H., Abe, S., Tada, N. and Sako, A. (2015) Effects of dietary fat intake on HDL metabolism. *J. Clin. Med. Res.* **7** (3) 145–9.

7. Castano, G., Mas, R., Fernandez, L., Illnait, J., Gomez, R. and Alvarez, E. (2001) Effects of policosanol 20 versus 40 mg/day in the treatment of patients with type II hypercholesterolemia: A 6 month double blind study. *Int. J. Pharmacol. Res.* **21** (1) 43–57.

8. Matern, D. and Rinaldo, P. (updated March 2015) *Medium chain acyl coenzyme A dehydrogenase deficiency gene.* www.ncbi.nlm.nih.gov/books/NBK1424.

9. Wilson, C.J., Champion, M.P., Collins, J.E., Clayton, P.T. and Leonard, J.V. (1999) Outcome of medium chain acyl CoA dehydrogenase deficiency after diagnosis *Arch. of Dis. in Childhood* **80**, 459–62.

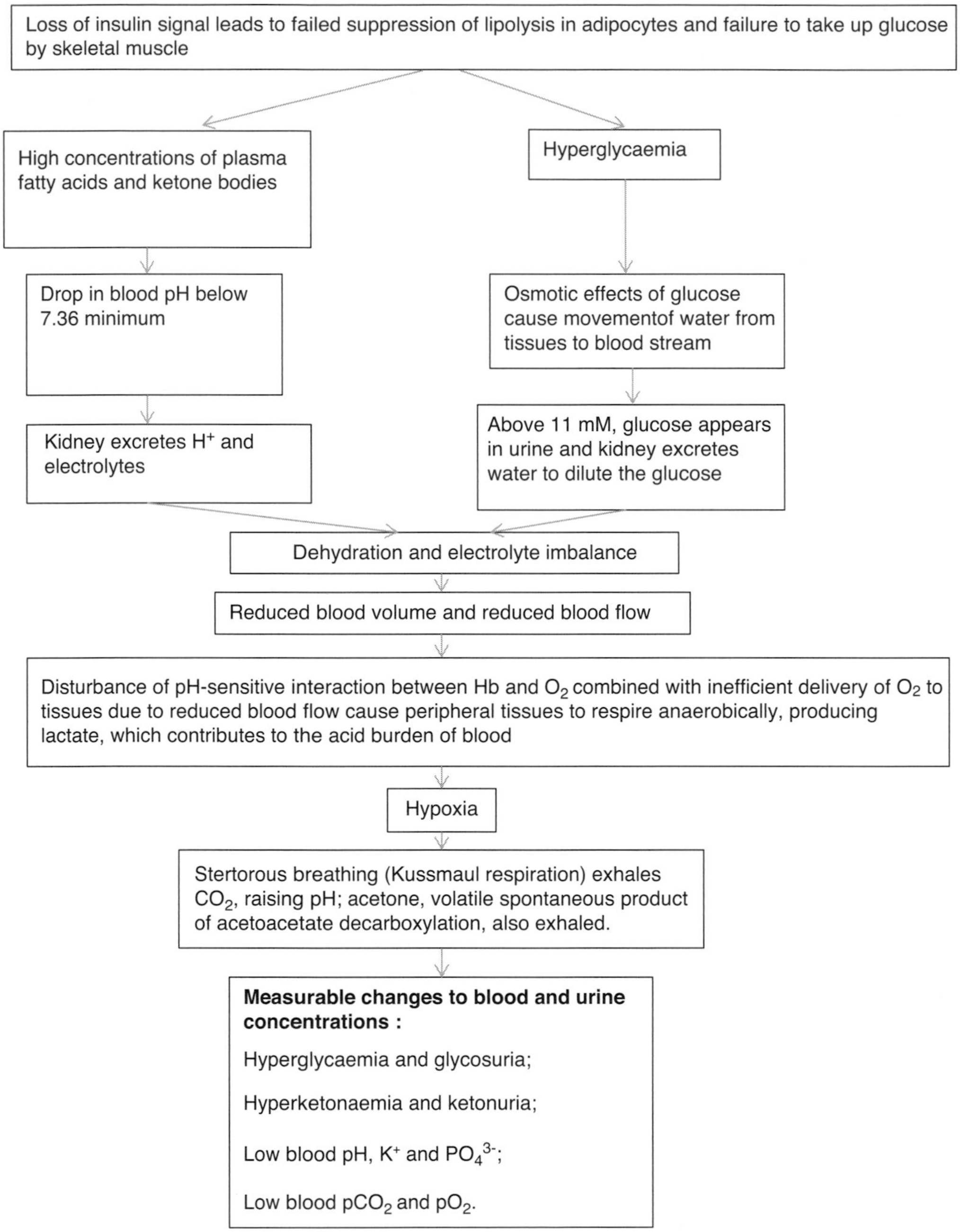

Figure 25.8 M etabolic disturbances in diabetic ketoacidosis

10. Gasior, M., Rogawski, M.A. and Hartman, A.L. (2006) Neuroprotective and disease-modifying effects of the ketogenic diet. *Behav. Pharmacol.* **17** (5–6), 431–9.

11. Bough, K.J. and Rho, J.M. (2007) Anticonvulsant mechanisms of the ketogenic diet. *Epilepsia* **48** (1), 43–58.

12. Freeman, J.M., Vining, E.P.G., Pillas, D.J., Pyzik, P.L., Casey, J.C. and Kelly, M.T. (1998) The efficacy of the ketogenic diet: A prospective evaluation of intervention in 150 children. *Paediatrics* **102**(6),1358–63.

13. Reger. M.A., Henderson, S.T., Hale, C., Cholerton, B., Baker, L.D., Watson, G.S., et al. (2004) Effects of β-

Table 25.8 Macronutrient constituents of human breast, cow and formula milk

Constituent (per litre)	Human breast	Cow	Formula
Protein (g)	9	31	15
Carbohydrate (g)	74	49	72
Fat (g)	42	38	36
% total energy as fat	54	53	49
Energy (MJ)	3	2.8	2.8

Table 25.9 Content of docosahexaenoic acid in human breast milk of vegetarians and omnivores

Essential fatty acid (% of total fatty acids)	Omnivores	Vegetarians
Docosahexaenoic acid	0.3	0.1
Linoleic acid	10.9	22.4
Linolenic acid	0.5	0.7

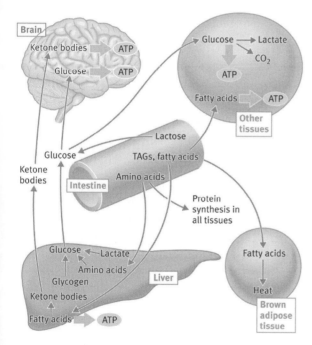

TAG = triacylglycerol

Figure 25.9 Metabolism in the neonate

hydroxybutyrate on cognition in memory-impaired adults. *Neurobiol Aging.* **25**, 311–14.

14. VanItallie, T.B., Nonas, C., Di, R.A., Boyar, K., Hyams, K. and Heymsfield, S.B. (2005) Treatment of Parkinson disease with diet-induced hyperketonemia: a feasibility study. *Neurology.* **64**,728–30.

15. Prins, M.L., Fujima, L.S. and Hovda, D.A. (2005) Age-dependent reduction of cortical contusion volume by ketones after traumatic brain injury. *J Neurosci Res* **82**, 413–420.

Single Best Answer Questions

1. Fats are transported as lipoproteins because:

   a. Fatty acids would otherwise be unable to enter target cells

   b. Fats would otherwise compete with glucose for cell uptake

   c. The insolubility of fats, combined with their amphipathic structures, means that they form micelles when uncomplexed in aqueous solution

   d. Fats would otherwise threaten the pH of the blood

2. Leptin's roles in metabolism include:

   a. Increasing the appetite and causing increased fuel uptake by muscle

   b. Causing the pancreas to secrete glucagon

   c. Preventing glucose uptake by muscle

   d. Decreasing the appetite and increasing fuel utilisation in skeletal muscle

3. Hyperketonaemia causes:

   a. An increase in blood pH

   b. A decrease in pH and increase in pCO_2 of the blood

   c. A decrease in pH, decrease in pCO_2 and a decrease in pO_2 of the blood

   d. Hyperglycaemia and decreased pH of the blood

4. Oxidation of fatty acids:

   a. Occurs in the mitochondria, using the β-oxidation pathway, which is controlled by the supply of its substrate

   b. Occurs in the cytosol and is regulated by phosphorylation of MCAD

   c. Occurs in the mitochondria and is inhibited by glucose oxidation

   d. Occurs in the peroxisomes

5. Factors or conditions which increase the concentration of fats in the blood include:

   a. Actions of glucagon, actions of adrenaline, diabetes and a high-fat diet

   b. Actions of insulin on the adipocyte and resistance to leptin

   c. Hyperketonaemia and hyperglycaemia

   d. Actions of glucagon, actions of insulin and a diet rich in polyunsaturated fatty acids

6. Ketone bodies increase in concentration in the blood when:

   a. Insulin acts on its hepatic receptor

   b. Hepatic glycogen stores have been depleted and gluconeogenic rates increase

   c. Glucagon acts on its hepatic receptor

   d. Glucose is cleared from the bloodstream in the post-prandial state

7. Fats cannot be converted into carbohydrates because:

   a. The reactions of the TCA cycle cannot be reversed

   b. Carbon dioxide is exhaled

   c. Oxaloacetate is an intermediate of the TCA cycle as well as of gluconeogenesis

   d. The pyruvate dehydrogenase reaction is irreversible and CO_2 is lost during reactions of the TCA cycle

8. The significance of fat as an oxidative fuel for the neonate is demonstrated by:

   a. The concordance of SIDS with MCAD deficiency

   b. The use of the fat substrate by BAT

   c. The assimilation of docosahexaenoic acid into membranes of the developing CNS

   d. The presence of the ketogenic pathway in the neonatal liver

9. Fat metabolism produces more energy per unit weight than carbohydrate metabolism in the human because:

   a. Fats are transported as lipoproteins which are taken up by specific tissues

   b. Fat molecules are highly reduced and stored anhydrously

   c. The pathway for carbohydrate metabolism is much longer and more strictly regulated

   d. Fats can be stored in much larger quantities than carbohydrates

10. The molecular disturbances accompanying diabetic ketoacidosis include:

   a. The loss of the anti-lipolytic insulin signal, hyperlipidaemia and the kidney failing to appropriately excrete protons in the presence of insulin resistance

   b. The loss of the anti-lipolytic signal from insulin, hypolipidaemia, hypoketonaemia and excessive glucagon production

   c. The loss of the anti-lipolytic signal from insulin, hyperlipidaemia, hyperketonaemia and increased hepatic gluconeogenesis

   d. The loss of the anti-lipolytic signal from insulin, hyperlipidaemia, hyperketonaemia, elevated pCO_2 and elevated pO_2

Steroid Hormones and Prostaglandins

Anthony E. Michael

Despite both being derived from lipid substrates, steroid hormones and prostaglandins differ fundamentally in their molecular structures, biosynthetic pathways, mechanisms and speed of action. This chapter covers each of these topics in turn, comparing and contrasting the synthesis and actions of steroids versus prostaglandins. In the final section, the functional interactions between these two families of lipid hormones are considered in the physiological control of myometrial contraction at parturition.

1 Steroid Hormone Synthesis and Metabolism

1.1 Classification and Structures of Steroid Hormones

Steroid hormones can broadly be classified as falling into one of two steroid hormone super-families: they are all either corticosteroids, synthesised in specific zones of the adrenal cortex, or gonadal steroids (commonly referred to as 'sex steroids'), synthesised in the ovary, testis and placenta.

Within these two super-families, there are five classes of steroid hormone, defined by (a) the number of carbon atoms and (b) their functional side chains. Those steroid hormones with 21 carbon atoms include the mineralocorticoids (such as aldosterone), glucocorticoids (such as cortisol) and the progestogens (of which the major physiological example is progesterone). The physiological androgens (dehydroepiandrosterone, androstenedione and testosterone) each contain 19 carbons, whereas the physiological oestrogens (estrone, oestradiol and oestriol) each have 18 carbon atoms and a definitive aromatic (phenolic) ring structure with delocalised electrons.

Each of the steroid hormones is synthesised ultimately from cholesterol as a lipid substrate (Fig. 26.1).

Consequently, all steroids share the same cyclohexaphenanthrene ring structure with 3 cyclohexane rings (the A, B and C rings) and a single cyclopentane (D) ring (Fig. 26.1).

Those steroids which possess a carbon-carbon double bond in the B ring (between carbon positions 5 and 6) are termed Δ^5 steroids and have limited physiological actions/low potency. Examples of such weak Δ^5 steroids include pregnenolone and dehydroepiandrosterone (DHEA). In contrast, steroid hormones which possess their carbon-carbon double bond in the A ring (between carbon positions 4 and 5), termed Δ^4 steroids, are strong hormones with profound physiological actions / high potency. Examples of these stronger Δ^4 steroids include progesterone, cortisol, aldosterone and testosterone.

1.2 Intracellular Transport and Metabolism of Cholesterol

In principle, the steroidogenic substrate, cholesterol, could be derived from any of the following four sources:

- *de novo* biosynthesis of cholesterol from acetate (catalysed by hydroxymethylglutaryl-coenzyme A [HMGCoA] reductase)
- plasma membrane cholesterol (reduces the fluidity, and hence impedes the function, of the plasma membrane)
- intracellular lipid droplets (containing esterified cholesteryl oleate)
- plasma lipoproteins

In practice, it is circulating low-density lipoproteins (LDL) and high-density lipoproteins (HDL) that deliver the majority of cholesterol to adrenocortical and gonadal cells as a substrate for the biosynthesis of the steroid hormones.

The rate-determining step in the biosynthesis of all steroid hormones is the initial removal of the 6-

(A)
Cholesterol structure:

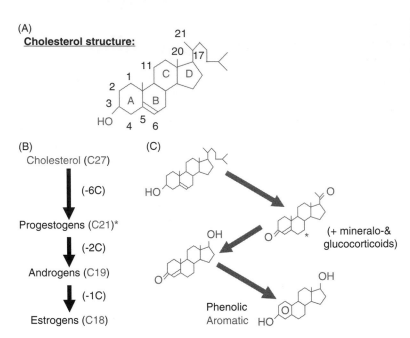

(B)

Cholesterol (C27)

(−6C)

Progestogens (C21)*

(−2C)

Androgens (C19)

(−1C)

Estrogens (C18)

(C)

(+ mineralo-& glucocorticoids)

Phenolic Aromatic

Figure 26.1 Overview of steroid hormone biosynthesis
(A) Structure of cholesterol
(B) Synthesis of steroid hormones from cholesterol
(C) Carbon atom

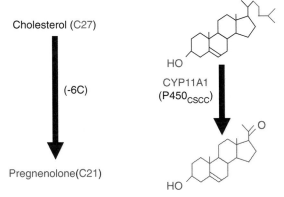

Cholesterol (C27)

(−6C)

CYP11A1
(P450$_{CSCC}$)

Pregnenolone(C21)

Figure 26.2 Metabolism of cholesterol to pregnenolone
CYP11A1 = cytochrome P450 cholesterol side-chain cleavage enzyme

carbon side chain from the D ring of the 27-carbon substrate cholesterol to generate the 21-carbon steroid metabolite, pregnenolone (Fig. 26.2). This reaction is catalysed by cytochrome P450 (CYP)11A1 which acts as a cholesterol side-chain cleavage enzyme on the inner surface of the inner mitochondrial membrane (IMM). This poses a problem since the cholesterol substrate arrives from the outer surface of the outer mitochondrial membrane (OMM), which is separated from the IMM by an aqueous intermembrane space.

Due to its hydrophobic, lipid nature, cholesterol cannot traverse that aqueous space unaided. In the mitochondria of an unstimulated steroidogenic cell, the OMM and the IMM repel each other, maintaining the aqueous intermembrane barriers to mitochondrial cholesterol import, because they carry the same negative membrane potentials, conferred on both the OMM and IMM by the high concentration of chloride ions in the intermembrane space. Although there is an anion channel in the OMM that could export these negatively charged chloride ions (which would then allow the OMM and IMM to come into apposition such that cholesterol could flow in to the mitochondria and act as a substrate for CYP11A1), in the resting steroidogenic cells, this voltage-dependent anion channel (VDAC) is closed (Fig. 26.3A). When gonadal cells are stimulated by gonadotrophins (or adrenocortical cells are stimulated by adrenocorticotrophic hormone), the cells respond by upregulating transcription of the gene that encodes the steroidogenesis acute regulator (StAR) protein (Fig. 26.3B). Furthermore, this short half-life protein is phosphorylated, via protein kinase A, as a consequence of the elevation in intracellular cyclic adenosine-3',5'-monophosphate (cAMP) levels induced by the pituitary (or placental) gonadotrophins. This phosphorylated StAR serves as a ligand for the translocator protein (TSPO) on the outer surface of the OMM and, in so doing, opens the VDAC to liberate the chloride ions from the intermembrane space (Fig. 26.3B). With the consequent change in the electrical potentials of the OMM and IMM, these mitochondrial membranes can form contact sites (equivalent to lowering a drawbridge across the aqueous moat between the two mitochondrial membranes), allowing cholesterol to flux into the mitochondria (by transverse diffusion)

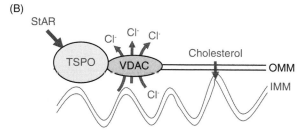

Figure 26.3 Regulation of mitochondrial cholesterol uptake in:
(A) an unstimulated steroidogenic cell
(B) a steroidogenic cell following stimulation by a trophic hormone (LH/hCG, FSH or ACTH)

and be acted upon by CYP11A1 to generate pregnenolone.

The significance of this detailed biochemistry is obvious in pregnancies complicated by lipoid congenital adrenal hyperplasia (LCAH). In this rare condition, mutation of StAR in the fetal adrenal glands prevents the synthesis of all steroid hormones with accumulation of cholesteryl esters within engorged lipid droplets in the adrenocortical cells. This rare condition is usually lethal in utero due to the complete absence of both mineralocorticoids (without which the baby will be unable to maintain sodium and water balance) and glucocorticoids (without which the fetal lungs will have no surfactant and the fetal liver will have no glycogen reserves). The fact that these pregnancies are viable at all indicates that steroidogenesis in the placenta relies not on the same StAR protein as that used in the adrenal and gonadal cells, but on a closely related protein which delivers cholesterol into the placental mitochondria.

1.3 Steroidogenic Enzymes

While steroidogenic pathways can seem overwhelming and complex, they all involve just two families of steroidogenic enzymes: members of the cytochrome P450 (CYP) enzyme family and the hydroxysteroid dehydrogenase (HSD) enzymes. As in the liver, where they detoxify drugs and other xenobiotics, the function of the steroidogenic CYP enzymes is to increase the solubility of the steroid hormones in blood,

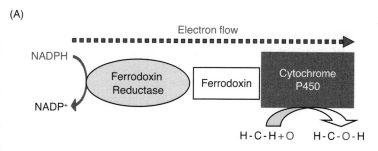

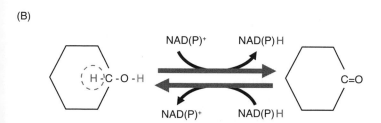

Figure 26.4 Operation of steroidogenic enzymes:
(A) Cytochrome P450 (CYP) enzymes
(B) Hydroxysteroid dehydrogenase (HSD) enzymes

extracellular fluid and urine by catalysing the hydroxylation of substrates to produce more polar (and hence hydrophilic) products.[1] This hydroxylase function of CYP enzymes involves the mediated transport of electrons from NADPH to the haem centre of the CYP enzyme via an electron transport chain which comprises ferredoxin reductase and ferredoxin (Fig. 26.4A). In addition, some of the CYP enzymes are also able to cleave carbon-carbon bonds and, in so doing, to remove side groups from the substrate molecule. Hence, CYP11A1 cleaves the D ring side-chain of cholesterol to convert the 27-carbon cholesterol substrate to the 21-carbon steroid product pregnenolone. Likewise, CYP17A cleaves a further 2 carbons from the D ring of 21-carbon progestogens to generate 19-carbon androgens (e.g. CYP17A converts the 21-carbon progestogen, progesterone, to the 19-carbon androgen, androstenedione).

The steroidogenic HSD enzymes, 3β-HSD and 17β-HSD, both belong to the superfamily of short-chain alcohol dehydrogenase enzymes. As such, these oxidoreductase enzymes catalyse the reversible interconversion of secondary alcohol (hydroxyl) groups with ketone groups on steroid hormones at designated carbon positions (Fig. 26.4B). In addition to oxidising the 3β-hydroxyl group to a ketone at position carbon-3, the 3β-HSD also has an isomerase activity which is responsible for moving the carbon-carbon double bond from the B ring of the weak Δ^5 steroid substrates (pregnenolone and dehydroepiandrosterone) to generate much stronger Δ^4 steroid products (progesterone and androstenedione, respectively). In contrast to the exclusive oxidase direction of action for 3β-HSD, the 17β-HSD enzymes act predominantly as reductase enzymes, reducing a ketone in the D ring of their steroid substrates (on carbon-17) to produce a hydroxyl, thereby increasing steroid potency. It is this reaction which converts the relatively weak androgen androstenedione into testosterone and the weak oestrogen oestrone into oestradiol.

1.4 Tissue-Specific Expression of Steroidogenic Enzymes

The overwhelming general diagram of steroid hormone biosynthesis found in all undergraduate textbooks is misleading: no known steroidogenic tissue expresses all of the enzymes. Instead, the cells of the adrenal cortex express different CYP and HSD enzymes to those found in the ovary which differ again from those expressed in the placenta. As a consequence, different steroidogenic cells produce different steroid hormones, as follows:

- In response to LH, testis Leydig cells produce testosterone because they express CYP11A1, CYP17A, 3β-HSD and 17β-HSD (Fig. 26.5A)

- In response to LH, ovarian theca cells (in a healthy, post-pubertal but pre-menopausal ovary) produce androstenedione (rather than testosterone) because they express CYP11A1, CYP17A and 3β-HSD, but not the 17β-HSD enzyme required to reduce androstenedione to testosterone (Fig. 26.5B)

- In response to FSH, ovarian granulosa cells express the CYP19A1 ('aromatase') enzyme required to covert the 19-carbon substrate androstenedione (generated in the neighbouring theca cells) into the 18-carbon product, oestrone, which can be reduced to oestradiol by the action of 17β-HSD (Fig. 26.5C)

- In response to LH (or hCG in early pregnancy), the cells of the corpus luteum (CL) express the CYP11A1, 3β-HSD, CYP17A, CYP19A1 and 17β-HSD enzymes required to synthesise both progesterone and oestradiol (Fig. 26.5D)

The placenta deserves special mention at this point: it is an 'incomplete endocrine gland' in so far as it does not express all of the enzymes required to synthesise the full repertoire of steroid hormones. Specifically, the placenta does not express the CYP17A enzyme required to metabolise 21-carbon progestogens into 19-carbon androgens and consequently in order to synthesise oestrogens, the placenta has to function in concert with the fetal adrenal gland and maternal liver. Steroid intermediates pass back and forth between the placenta, fetal and maternal circulations. Importantly, 16α-hydroxyandrostenedione, a weak androgen secreted from the fetal zone of the fetal adrenal cortex can be metabolised within the placenta to oestriol: a steroid that is synthesised uniquely by the placenta that serves as a surrogate marker to assess the functional status of the fetal adrenal gland.

1.5 Metabolism and Clearance of Steroid Hormones

On arrival at potential target cells, steroid hormones frequently undergo further metabolism to modulate

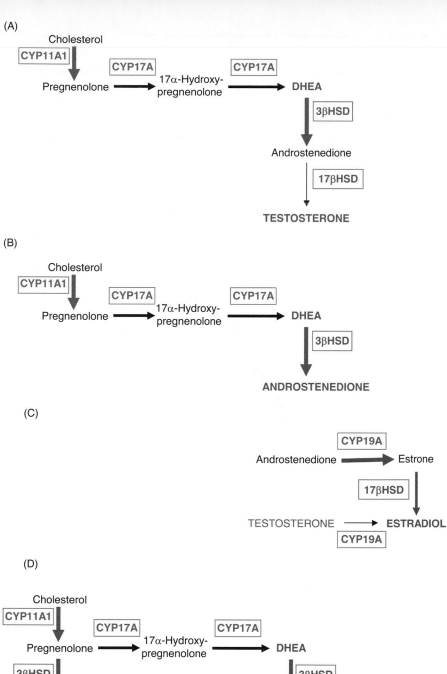

Figure 26.5 Tissue-specific steroidogenic pathways in:
(A) Testis Leydig cells
(B) Follicular theca cells
(C) Follicular granulosa cells
(D) Luteal cells

CYP11A1 = cholesterol side chain cleavage enzyme; CYP17A = steroid 17α-hydroxylase; CYP19A = aromatase; DHEA = dehydroepiandrosterone; HSD = hydroxysteroid dehydrogenase

their potency and physiological actions. As specific examples of this principle, to virilise the external genitalia, testosterone has to be converted within genital skin fibroblasts to the more potent metabolite 5α-dihydrotestosterone (catalysed by the steroid 5α-reductase 2 enzyme) and to cause closure of the epiphyses of the long bones in puberty, testosterone has to be metabolised within the bone by CYP19A to generate oestradiol which acts on the epiphyses via the oestrogen (rather than the androgen) receptor.

In order to be rendered more water-soluble prior to their clearance in the urine or faeces, steroid hormones have to be acted upon by hepatic CYP and/or HSD enzymes, followed by conjugating enzymes that catalyse condensation reactions to add polar or charged chemical groups (e.g. glucuronides and sulphates, respectively) to the polar hydroxyl/alcohol groups created by the CYP and/or HSD enzymes.

2 Steroid Hormone Actions

2.1 Nuclear Receptors

By virtue of their hydrophobicity, steroid hormones pass relatively easily into potential target cells to exert their actions via nuclear receptors which serve as ligand-dependent transcription factors.[2] In the same way as there are five different classes of steroid hormone, there are five corresponding types of steroid hormone receptor (Table 26.1).

Each type of steroid hormone receptor has a common structure comprising the same four functional domains, these being the following:

- ligand-binding domain (binds the steroid hormone ligand in a hydrophobic binding pocket);
- DNA-binding domain (typically comprised of a pair of zinc fingers that can bind the DNA double helix within the nucleus);
- dimerisation domain (located within the ligand-binding domain where it facilitates the dimerization of pairs of ligand-activated steroid receptors);
- transactivating factor (TAF) domains (interact directly or indirectly with proteins in the pre-initiation transcription complex).

In the absence of steroid ligands, steroid hormone receptors can either localise to the cytoplasm or to the nucleus. Following steroid hormone binding, cytoplasmic receptors translocate into the nucleus where they bind DNA to modulate gene transcription.

2.2 Transcriptional Regulation by Steroid Hormone Receptors

Activated steroid hormone receptors always act as dimers, whether as homodimers (e.g. glucocorticoid–glucocorticoid receptor homodimers) or as heterodimers (e.g. glucocorticoid–progesterone receptors). The dimerised receptors bind DNA at either palindromic or tandem repeated pentanucleotide/hexanucleotide sequences, defined as steroid hormone response elements. Such elements are usually located in the upstream (5') promoter region, but due to the 3-dimensional configuration of DNA, they can also occur downstream (3') of the target gene.

Via their TAF domains, the dimerised receptors interact with nuclear-receptor interacting proteins (NRIPs), which either possess or recruit enzymes that modulate the acetylation of histone proteins and so either close or open the DNA double helix to decrease or increase, respectively, the rate of target gene. Hence NRIPs can act either as corepressor or as coactivator proteins. Corepressor proteins possess and/or recruit histone deacetylase (HDAC) enzymes that remove acetyl groups from the histone proteins, which allows the DNA double helix to remain annealed, thus preventing the transcription of the target genes. In

Table 26.1 Classification of steroid hormones

Steroid super-family and class	Number of carbon (C) atoms	Major physiological example
Corticosteroids		
Mineralocorticoids	21	Aldosterone
Glucocorticoids	21	Cortisol
Androgens	19	Dehydroepiandrosterone (DHEA)
Gonadal steroids		
Progestogens	21	Progesterone
Androgens	19	Testosterone
Oestrogens	18	Oestradiol

contrast, coactivator proteins recruit histone acetyl-transferase (HAT) enzymes which acetylate histones causing the DNA double helix to unwind and open to increase the rate of gene transcription.

As a consequence of this complex genomic mode of action, steroid hormones exert relatively slow effects: steroid hormones typically require hours (if not days) to alter cellular functions where those responses rely on changes in target gene expression.

3   Prostaglandins

3.1   Prostaglandin Synthesis and Metabolism

The prostaglandins (PGs) are all derived from the 20-carbon polyunsaturated fatty acid (PUFFA) substrate, arachidonic acid (C20:4), which is a common molecular constituent of phospholipids in the plasma membrane.[3] This PUFFA can be liberated to act as a substrate for PG synthesis by the action of phospholipase A_2 (PLA_2) on the membrane phospholipids. This activity of PLA_2 is inhibited by lipocortin, the gene for which is upregulated by both physiological and pharmacological glucocorticoids (cortisol and dexamethasone, respectively), which accounts for the anti-inflammatory actions of these steroid hormones.

Following its liberation from the plasma membrane, arachidonic acid is oxidised by the cyclooxygenase (COX) enzymes, which metabolise arachidonic acid to PGG_2: an intermediate that is rapidly converted to the endoperoxide metabolite, PGH_2 (Fig. 26.6). There are two COX enzymes: the constitutively active COX-1 isoenzyme and the hormone-responsive/inducible COX-2 isoenzyme. Both of these COX isoenzymes can be inhibited by nonsteroidal anti-inflammatory drugs (NSAIDs) such as aspirin and mefenamic acid. Once generated by the COX enzymes, PGH_2 can be acted upon by the prostaglandin D, E, F and I synthases to generate PGD_2, PGE_2, $PGF_{2\alpha}$ and PGI_2 (prostacyclin), respectively (Fig. 26.6).

The biological function of each PG relies on the presence of an alcohol group at carbon-15 in the PG skeleton such that oxidation of this secondary alcohol to a ketone by 15-hydroxyprostaglandin dehydrogenase (PGDH) causes rapid inactivation of PGs. Due to the high level of expression of PGDH in the lungs, 65% of PG molecules are typically inactivated with each pass through the pulmonary circulation. It is this susceptibility of PGs to oxidative

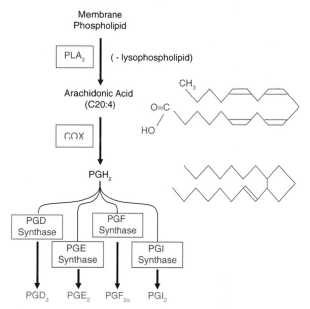

Figure 26.6 Prostaglandin synthesis from membrane phospholipids

COX = cyclooxygenase; PLA_2 = phospholipase A_2.

inactivation which limits these lipid hormones to exerting autocrine and paracrine (rather than endocrine) effects.

3.2   Prostaglandin Actions

Since PGs are synthesised from a PUFFA substrate, they might intuitively be expected to have unrestricted access to the interior of target cells and to exert their actions via intracellular receptors, as for the steroid hormones. However, PGs are actually relatively water-soluble and so exert their actions on target cells via G-protein-coupled receptors (GPCR) in the plasma membrane of target cells.

$PGF_{2\alpha}$ acts via the F-prostanoid (FP/PTGF) receptor to activate the phosphoinositide-specific phospholipase C (PI-PLC) which triggers the inositol trisphosphate (IP_3)–calcium (Ca^{2+}) signalling cascade. In contrast, PGE_2 can activate a series of four different E-prostanoid (EP/PTGE) receptors (EP_1, EP_2, EP_3 and EP_4), most of which are coupled to the adenylyl cyclase-cyclic adenosine monophosphate (cAMP) signal transduction pathway to modulate the activity of the cAMP-dependent protein kinase A (PKA). It is this ability of $PGF_{2\alpha}$ and PGE_2 to activate different signal transduction pathways (centred around Ca^{2+} versus cAMP) which accounts for the fact that, in most tissues, $PGF_{2\alpha}$ and PGE_2 generally exert opposite and antagonistic physiological actions.

However, in the uterus, both PGs activate receptors coupled to mobilisation of intracellular calcium and, as a consequence, analogues of both $PGF_{2\alpha}$ and PGE_2 induce myometrial contractions. Because PGs act on cell surface GPCRs to activate transmembrane signalling cascades culminating in activation of various protein kinases, PGs typically exert cellular actions within seconds to minutes (cf. the much slower genomic actions of steroid hormones).

4 Coordination of Myometrial Contractility

In the introduction to this chapter, a case was made for considering steroid hormones and PGs together on the basis that they are both categories of lipid hormones. In addition to this molecular similarity, these two classes of lipid share a functional convergence in so far as steroid hormones and PGs are both implicated in the molecular and cellular mechanisms of parturition. The molecular co-ordination of myometrial contractions throughout pregnancy and at parturition involves a finely poised balance between, on the one hand, uterotonic molecules that act to induce myometrial contractions and, on the other hand, those physiological tocolytic molecules which inhibit and/or oppose the uterotonic molecules so as to decrease the frequency and/or force of myometrial contractions.

Physiological molecules which stimulate contraction include oxytocin (OT), a neuropeptide hormone secreted both from posterior lobe of the pituitary gland as well as locally from the uterus, and PGs, specifically $PGF_{2\alpha}$. Both of these hormones activate PI-PLC in the plasma membrane of the myometrial myoepithelial cells (via the OT receptor and FP receptor, respectively) to increase the intracellular Ca^{2+} concentration and so activate both myosin light chain kinase and Ca^{2+}/calmodulin-dependent protein kinase, hence increasing the force of myometrial muscle contractions. This stimulation of myometrial contractions is augmented by a synergistic, positive spiral between OT and PG signalling: OT stimulates uterine PG synthesis while $PGF_{2\alpha}$ upregulates the expression of OT receptors (Fig. 26.7).

Steroid hormones can induce and/or accelerate myometrial contractions by impinging on the cellular responses to OT and $PGF_{2\alpha}$ upregulates. Acting via their nuclear receptors, both oestradiol and cortisol up-regulate the expression of the genes encoding OT, the OT and FP receptors, and the COX and PG synthase enzymes required to synthesise PGs.

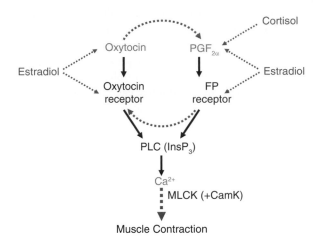

Figure 26.7 The molecular induction of myometrial contractions via the oxytocin–$PGF_{2\alpha}$ positive spiral

CaMK = Ca^{2+}/calmodulin-dependent kinase; IP_3 = inositol trisphosphate; MLCK = myosin light chain kinase; PI-PLC = phosphoinositide-specific phospholipase C

The physiological tocolytic molecules attenuate and/or oppose the cellular responses to OT and $PGF_{2\alpha}$. For example, whereas both OT and $PGF_{2\alpha}$ act via PI-PLC, IP_3 and Ca^{2+} to drive the phosphorylation of the myosin light chain, so increasing myometrial contractions, the natural tocolytic molecules operate primarily via the cyclic-nucleotide second messengers, cAMP and cyclic guanosine monophosphate (cGMP), to activate cAMP-dependent and cGMP-dependent protein kinases culminating in the dephosphorylation of the myosin light chain to limit the force of myometrial contractions.

The major physiological tocolytic is progesterone which decreases the synthesis and attenuates the actions both of OT and of $PGF_{2\alpha}$ through a combination of chronic, genomic and rapid, non-genomic actions.[4] In addition, progesterone is able to elevate the intracellular cAMP concentration and to decrease the operation of gap junctions preventing myometrial myoepithelial cells from acting as a functional syncytium. Other tocolytic molecules include the peptide hormone relaxin and prostacyclin/PGI_2 (both of which elevate intracellular cAMP levels) and nitric oxide (which seems to relax the myometrium independently of its ability to elevate intracellular cGMP concentrations).

At term, the decline in placental progesterone secretion, and hence a fall in the progesterone:estradiol ratio, switches the steroidal control of myometrium contractility from being predominantly relaxant to the pro-contraction signalling pathways required for the onset of labour.

In conclusion, although steroid hormones and PGs are both lipid hormones central to obstetrics and gynaecology, they differ with respect to their molecular substrates and structures, the enzymes required for their biosynthesis, the receptors and signalling mechanisms through which they act, and their mode and speed of action.

References

1. Miller WL, Auchus RJ (2011) The molecular biology, biochemistry and physiology of human steroidogenesis and its disorders. *Endocr Rev* **2**: 81–151

2. Lonard DM, Lanz RB, O'Malley BW (2007) Nuclear receptor coregulators and human disease. *Endocr Rev* **28**: 575–587

3. Capra V, Rovati GE, Mangano P, Buccellati C, Murphy RC, Sala A (2015) Transcellular biosynthesis of eicosanoid lipid mediators. *Biochim Biophys Acta* **1851**: 377–382

4. Mesiano S (2007) Myometrial progesterone responsiveness. *Semin Reprod Med* **25**: 5–13

Further Reading

Arrowsmith S, Wray S (2014) Oxytocin: Its mechanism of action and receptor signalling in the myometrium. *J Neuroendocrinol* **26**: 356–369

Breyer RM, Bagdassarian CK, Myers SA, Breyer MD (2001) Prostanoid receptors: Subtypes and signaling. *Annu Rev Pharmacol Toxicol* **41**: 661–690

Buxton IL (2004) Regulation of uterine function: A biochemical conundrum in the regulation of smooth muscle contraction. *Mol Pharmacol* **65**: 1051–1059

Castillo AF, Orlando U, Helfenberger KE, Poderoso C, Podesta EJ (2015) The role of mitochondrial fusion and StAR phosphorylation in the regulation of StAR activity and steroidogenesis. *Mol Cell Endocrinol* **408**: 73–79

Challis JR, Patel FA, Pomini F (1999) Prostaglandin dehydrogenase and the initiation of labour. *J Perinat Med* **27**: 26–34

Christiaens I, Zaragoza DB, Guilbert L, Robertson SA, Mitchell BF, Olson DM (2008) Inflammatory processes in preterm and term parturition. *J Reprod Immunol* **79**: 50–57

Miller WL (2013) Steroid hormone synthesis in the mitochondria. *Mol Cell Endocrinol* **379**: 62–73

Pasqualini JR (2005) Enzymes involved in the formation and transformation of steroid hormones in the fetal and placental compartments. *J Steroid Biochem Mol Biol* **97**: 401–415

Rone MB, Fan J, Papdopoulos V (2009) Cholesterol transport in steroid biosynthesis: role of protein-protein interactions and implications in disease states. *Biochim Biophys Acta* **1791**: 646–658

Sfakianaki AK, Norwitz ER (2006) Mechanisms of progesterone action in inhibiting prematurity. *J Matern Fetal Neonatal Med* **19**: 763–772

Stocco DM (2002) Clinical disorders associated with abnormal cholesterol transport: mutations in the steroidogenic acute regulatory protein. *Mol Cell Endocrinol* **191**: 19–25

Sugimoto Y, Inazumi T, Tsuchiya S (2015) Roles of prostaglandin receptors in female reproduction. *J Biochem* **157**: 73–80

Xu L, Glass CK, Rosenfeld MG (1999) Coactivator and corepressor complexes in nuclear receptor function. *Curr Opin Genet Dev* **9**: 140–147

Single Best Answer Questions

1. Which of the following statements is true both of steroid hormones and prostaglandins?

    a. Steroid hormones and prostaglandins act via seven-transmembrane domain, G-protein receptors (GPCR) on the cell surface.

    b. Steroid hormones and prostaglandins exert acute effects mediated via second messenger molecules or ions.

    c. Steroid hormones and prostaglandins act via intracellular receptors to modify the rate of gene expression.

    d. Steroid hormones and prostaglandins are synthesised from a lipid substrate.

    e. Steroid hormones and prostaglandins are proteins translated from mRNA transcripts.

2. What is the major steroid hormone secreted from the zona reticularis of the adrenal cortex?

    a. Aldosterone

    b. Cortisol

    c. Dehydroepiandrosterone

    d. Dihydrotestosterone

    e. Progesterone

3. How many carbon atoms are there in the physiological oestrogens: oestrone, oestradiol and oestriol?

    a. 27

    b. 21

    c. 20

    d. 19

    e. 18

4. Other than the number of carbon atoms, what is the structural hallmark of the A-ring of

physiological oestrogens (and most of their pharmaceutical analogues)?

a. Cyclohexane ring
b. Cyclopentane ring
c. Ketone at position C-3
d. Phenolic ring
e. Sulphate esterified at position C-3

5. What is the predominant source of cholesterol for steroid biosynthesis in the gonads and placenta?

a. De novo cholesterol synthesis from acetate
b. Intracellular lipid droplets
c. Plasma membrane cholesterol
d. Plasma lipoproteins (LDL and HDL)
e. Subcellular membrane cholesterol

6. Which enzyme catalyses the rate-determining reaction in the synthesis of steroid hormones from cholesterol?

a. CYP11A1
b. CYP11B1
c. CYP11B2
d. CYP17A
e. CYP19A

7. Which enzyme catalyses the aromatisation of androgen substrates to oestrogens in ovarian granulosa cells and in the placenta?

a. CYP11A1
b. CYP11B1
c. CYP11B2
d. CYP17A
e. CYP19A

8. Which enzyme mediates the release of arachidonic acid from membrane phospholipids as a substrate for prostaglandin synthesis?

a. PLA_1
b. PLA_2
c. PLB
d. PLC
e. PLD

9. At which of the 20 carbon positions must prostaglandins have an alcohol (OH) group if they are to bind receptors and exert a physiological action?

a. C-3
b. C-5
c. C-11
d. C-15
e. C-17

10. Via which structural domain do steroid hormone receptors form either homo- or heterodimers?

a. DNA-binding domain
b. Ligand-binding domain
c. Nuclear localisation domain
d. Transactivating factor-I domain
e. Transactivating factor-II domain

11. Which enzyme has to be recruited by ligand-bound, active steroid hormone receptors to increase the rate of target gene transcription?

a. DNA helicase
b. DNA ligase
c. Histone acetyltransferase
d. Histone deacetylase
e. RNA polymerase

12. Through which second messenger molecule or ion do oxytocin and prostaglandins induce myometrial contractions?

a. Calcium
b. Chloride
c. Cyclic adenosine 3',5'-monophosphate
d. Cyclic guanosine 3',5'-monophosphate
e. Diacylglycerol

13. Through which second messenger molecule or ion can nitric oxide (NO) act to suppress myometrial contractions?

a. Calcium
b. Chloride
c. Cyclic adenosine 3',5'-monophosphate
d. Cyclic guanosine 3',5'-monophosphate
e. Diacylglycerol

14. Through which second messenger molecule or ion can progesterone and relaxin act to suppress myometrial contractions?

a. Calcium
b. Chloride
c. Cyclic adenosine 3',5'-monophosphate
d. Cyclic guanosine 3',5'-monophosphate
e. Diacylglycerol

Calcium Homeostasis and Bone Health

Sadie Jones

1 Calcium Homeostasis

Calcium is essential for many body processes and, consequently, its concentration needs to be tightly regulated at 2.5 mmol/l. Forty-five percent of plasma calcium is bound to albumin, the remainder is either free and active or a component of other compounds. Calcium is important for:

- Muscle contraction
- Nerve conduction
- Enzyme activity
- Bone formation
- Hormone release
- Clotting factor activity

There are three important hormones involved in calcium homeostasis:

- Parathyroid hormone
- Vitamin D
- Calcitonin

1.1 Parathyroid Hormone

Parathyroid hormone (PTH) is made by chief cells in the parathyroid glands and is released into the circulation in response to low plasma calcium levels (Fig. 27.1).

PTH acts on bone and kidneys to increase plasma calcium levels. In bone, PTH directly causes release of stored mineral calcium through *bone resorption* via *increased osteoclast* activity. In kidneys, not only does it directly increase Ca^{2+} absorption from the *distal convoluted tubule*; it also stimulates an enzyme called 1 alpha hydroxylase, which causes the conversion of 25, hydroxyl vitamin D_3 (from the liver) to 1, 25, hydroxyl vitamin D_3 – the *active form of vitamin D*. Active vitamin D increases plasma calcium levels via several mechanisms, discussed as follows.

1.2 Vitamin D

- A sterol hormone (synthesised from cholesterol)

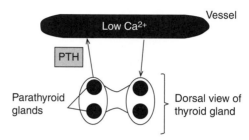

Figure 27.1 Parathyroid hormone secretion

- 90% is synthesised in skin by photo-isomerisation of cholecalciferol (cholesterol) to 25, hydroxyl vitamin D_3 (inactive, stored in the liver)
- 10% is absorbed by diet
- Active vitamin D_3 has a negative feedback effect on PTH ensuring calcium levels are not raised too high

Vitamin D acts to increase plasma calcium levels through *increased osteoclast* activity in bone causing calcium resorption. It also acts on the *proximal convoluted tubule*, causing increased calcium absorption. Finally, it acts on the *GI tract* (jejunum and ileum) to increase calcium absorption. Figure 27.2 summarizes the functions of PTH and vitamin D_3 in calcium homeostasis.

1.3 Calcitonin

- Produced by the parafollicular cells of the thyroid gland
- The function of calcitonin is to decrease plasma calcium levels
- Primarily acts on the bone, reducing osteoclast activity
- Also acts on renal tubules to reduce calcium absorption

1.4 Problems with Calcium Homeostasis (Table 27.1)

1.4.1 Vitamin D Deficiency

Vitamin D deficiency can result from:

- Inadequate dietary intake
- Gut malabsorption
- Liver disease
- Inadequate sun exposure.

If your body has low levels of vitamin D, you are unable to absorb calcium effectively from the gut and therefore PTH is stimulated in order to maintain adequate plasma levels. It is the effects of PTH stimulation that manifest clinically:

Children = rickets (bowed legs, chest deformity and hypocalcaemia)

Adults = osteomalacia (bone pain/fractures, hypocalcaemia)

1.4.2 Osteoporosis

Unlike in osteomalacia, bone mineralisation is not affected in osteoporosis. Osteoporosis is the result of an imbalance in normal bone remodelling. Bone resorption (osteoclast activity) occurs more readily than bone formation (osteoblast activity). This is a condition that post-menopausal women are prone to because a lack of oestrogen results in increased bone resorption while at the same time reducing the amount of new bone that gets deposited. Potential therapeutic/preventative measures include hormone replacement therapy; calcium

Table 27.1 Problems with calcium homeostasis

Hypocalcaemia (e.g. PTH deficiency)
Chvostek's sign (facial twitch when facial nerve is tapped)
Paraesthesia
Tetany carpo-pedal spasm
Prolonged QT interval

Hypercalcaemia (e.g. excess PTH) ('Bones, stones, moans and groans')
Painful **bones** due to resorption
Renal **stones** (excess urinary calcium)
Headaches, abdominal pain, anorexia and constipation cause **groans**
Moans caused by weakness and fatigue

NB: Hypercalcaemia is also associated with sluggish reflexes, polyuria, confusion, coma, shortened QT interval and cardiac arrhythmias.

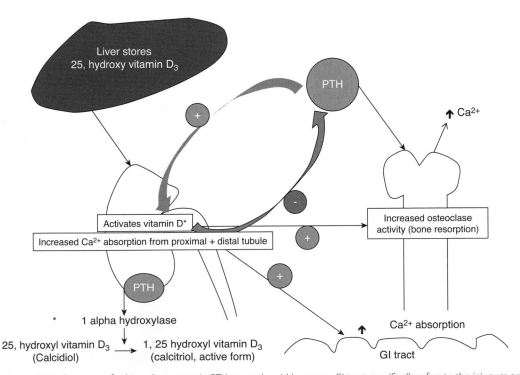

Liver stores 25, hydroxy vitamin D_3

PTH

$\uparrow Ca^{2+}$

Activates vitamin D*

Increased Ca^{2+} absorption from proximal + distal tubule

Increased osteoclase activity (bone resorption)

PTH

* 1 alpha hydroxylase

25, hydroxyl vitamin D_3 (Calcidiol) → 1, 25 hydroxyl vitamin D_3 (calcitriol, active form)

Ca^{2+} absorption

GI tract

Figure 27.2 Summary of calcium homeostasis. PTH = parathyroid hormone. GI tract specifically refers to the jejunum and ileum.

supplementation with vitamin D; bisphosphonates and weight-bearing exercises.

1.5 Suggested Reading

- Alberts B, Johnson A, Lewis J, Raff M, Roberts K, Walter P. *Molecular Biology of the Cell.* 2002. Garland Science.
- Berg JM, Tymoczko JL, Stryer L. *Biochemistry.* 7th edition. 2011. WH Freeman and Company.
- https://m.youtube.com/watch?v=EEM0iRJNhU8. Endocrinology, calcium and phosphate regulation. Armando Hasudungan.

Questions

1. Which of the following organs does not significantly contribute to calcium homeostasis?
   a. Intestine
   b. Kidney
   c. Liver
   d. Skin
   e. Spleen

2. Which of the following confers negative feedback on the secretion of PTH?
   a. Calcitonin
   b. 25, hydroxy vitamin D_3
   c. 1, 25 hydroxy vitamin D_3
   d. PTH
   e. 1 alpha hydroxylase

3. PTH has which of the following effects?
   a. Photo-isomerisation of cholecalciferol to 25, hydroxyl vitamin D_3
   b. Increases absorption of calcium from the proximal convoluted tubule
   c. Decreases absorption of calcium from the distal convoluted tubule
   d. Decreases osteoclast activity
   e. Increases osteoclast activity

4. Which of the following is a typical sign of hypercalcaemia?
   a. Prolonged QT interval
   b. Shortened QT interval
   c. Chvostek's sign
   d. Tetany carpo-pedal spasm
   e. Brisk reflexes

5. Calcitonin is secreted from:
   a. Thyroid gland
   b. Parathyroid gland
   c. Anterior pituitary
   d. Posterior pituitary
   e. Hypothalamus

Chapter

28

Cell Structure and Function

Neil Chapman

1 Introduction

Generally speaking, the cell is the basic functional unit of any tissue. While individual tissues and organs have specific roles, it is the cells that ultimately undertake those activities. Within the cell itself, there are numerous structures and proteins that are required to ensure the cell can successfully perform its tasks [1]. These are listed in Tables 28.1 **and** 28.2.

Table 28.1 List of key cell structures and their associated functions

Structure	Cellular function
Cell membrane	To maintain the cell's integrity; to keep the insides in and the outside out! Semi-permeable barrier. Contains many receptors, ion channels and adhesion molecules for signal transduction (see Table 28.2).
Cytosol/cytoplasm	Area where cell organelles are stored; separated from the nucleus by the nuclear envelope.
Nucleus	Largest organelle in the cell. Location of the genome; site of DNA replication, transcription.
Nucleolus	Sub-structure within the nucleus. Site of ribosomal RNA (rRNA) synthesis.
Lysosomes	Effectively the cell's dustbin. This is a bag of biological nasties (enzymes/ acidic pH) that can degrade old organelles and proteins. Processing of foreign proteins during immune response – presentation of antigen in Major Histocompatibility (MHC) molecules – occurs here in immune cells.
Peroxisomes	Site of hydrogen peroxide generation
Rough endoplasmic reticulum (RER)	A large network of highly convoluted membrane structures that can be continuous with the nuclear envelope. The cytosolic-facing surface is studded with ribosomes which facilitates protein synthesis (mRNA translation) – hence its 'rough' appearance under the electron microscope. Generates glycoproteins/secretory proteins. Cells which make significant amounts of proteins have a rich RER network – for example plasma cells of the immune system
Smooth endoplasmic reticulum (SER)	The SER is similarly convoluted as the RER. The SER, however, lacks any ribosomes – hence its 'smooth' appearance. Site of lipid synthesis, fat metabolism and steroid hormone synthesis. Site of drug detoxification (including alcohol and barbiturates). Certain cells of the liver have an extensive SER.
Golgi body	Responsible for the sorting and trafficking of newly synthesised proteins to their correct cellular location. Has a role in adding complex sugars (glycosylation) onto newly-synthesised proteins.
Mitochondria	Site of oxidative phosphorylation and ATP synthesis – the cell's power station. The enzymes required for the tricarboxylic acid (TCA or Krebs) cycle are located here. Site of TCA cycle and fatty acid oxidation. These organelles contain their own genome, which is ONLY inherited from the mother. Mitochondria also have a function in the final stages of the apoptotic pathway.
Cytoskeleton	A collective term for micro-filaments, composed of actin; micro-tubules composed of tubulin and intermediate filaments. Give structure to the cell. Responsible for the formation of the mitotic spindle prior to cell division (cytokinesis). Facilitates movement of vesicles through the cell (effectively a cellular tram system).
Ribosomes	To translate mRNA (poly-nucleotides) into amino acids (peptides and proteins).
Receptors	To transduce extra-cellular signals into cellular actions.

Table 28.2 Illustrative list of cell membrane proteins

Protein	Illustrative examples

Hormone receptors	• Adrenergic receptors
	  ◦ α1, α2, β1 and β2 subclasses
	• Cholinergic receptors
	  ◦ Muscarinic-1 (M1), Muscarinic-2 (M2), Nicotinic
	• Tyrosine kinase-based receptor
	  ◦ Epidermal growth factor receptor
	  ◦ B- and T-cell receptors

Cell adhesion molecules	All integral membrane proteins so they span the full thickness of the plasma membrane of the cell. Groups include:
	• **Cadherins**
	  ◦ Bind to other cadherins in Ca^{2+}-dependent process
	  ◦ Linked to cytoskeleton
	• **Inter-cellular adhesion molecules (ICAMs)**
	  ◦ Includes vascular cell adhesion molecule (VCAM)-1 glycoproteins
	• **Integrins**
	  ◦ Large family glycoproteins
	  ◦ Facilitate cell signalling between the cytoskeleton (intra-cellular) and the extra-cellular (external) environment
	  ◦ Have an important role in inflammation and immune responses
	• **Selectins**
	  ◦ Three main members – E-, L- and P-selectin
	  ◦ Predominantly found in leucocytes and endothelial cells
	  ◦ Mediate 'cell rolling' – the process of leucocyte binding and subsequent extravasation through the vascular endothelium during an acute inflammatory reaction

Ion channels	• Ca^{2+} channels (L- and T-types), K^+ channels, K^+-activated Ca^{2+} channels (BKCa), Na^+ channels, Cl^- channels
Gap junctions	• Connexin-43 ◦ Facilitates cells sharing common metabolite/signalling pool to give a uniform tissue outcome – uterine contraction

Self: non-self-recognition molecules	• Major histocompatibility molecules
	  ◦ MHC-I: HLA-A, HLA-B and HLA-C
	    ▪ HLA-G only found on fetal cytotrophoblasts
	  ◦ MHC-II: HLA-DR, HLA-DQ, HLA-DP
	    ▪ MHC-II molecules NOT expressed in trophoblast population

Hormones, Signal Transduction Mechanisms and Drug Targets

Cells are continually exposed to a complex and rapidly changing milieu of signalling factors. Within this broad grouping are hormones. Hormones can also be broadly sub-divided into three types of molecules:

1. Protein/peptide hormones (ACTH, growth hormone, hCG, FSH LH)

2. Water-insoluble lipid-based hormones: steroids (progesterone, oestrogen and testosterone) all of which are ultimately derived from cholesterol and eicosanoids (products of arachidonic acid metabolism – the prostaglandins and leukotrienes)

3. Monoamines (adrenaline, dopamine, melatonin and nor-adrenalin).

Further details of this subject can be found in [2].

How is the message conveyed by these signalling molecules converted into a controlled cellular response? Essentially, cells use protein molecules that specifically interact with a given hormone or signal to generate a definitive cellular output. These proteins are called *receptors* and the specificity arises through the inherent shape of the hormone being able to interact with a similarly-shaped pocket on the receptor – an often-cited analogy being that of a hand fitting into a glove. Binding of a signal to a receptor protein is the first step in the pathway that allows the cell to *transduce* the external signal into a specific cellular action. There are many types of receptor proteins, each with differing functions and agonist specificities (Fig. 28.1). A selection of salient examples is also listed in Table 28.3.

There are many receptor types and many mechanisms by which the initial transduction event occurs. The endpoint of the initial transduction event is the generation of small molecule messengers within the cell. Such intra-cellular compounds are termed second messengers. The initial extra-cellular hormone signal is the first message; this is transduced by the receptor into a second messenger which will propagate the signal further. Examples of commonly used second messengers would include Ca^{2+}

ions, cyclic adenosine mono-phosphate (cAMP), cyclic guanosine mono-phosphate (cGMP), Inositol-1,4,5-triphosphate (IP3), Di-acyl glycerol (DAG) and nitric oxide (NO) [1]. Consequently, the overall final cellular response to a given agonist will be the sum of these second messenger pathways and this illustrates why many drugs also have numerous side-effects.

While an in-depth discussion on the molecular physiology of these molecules is beyond the scope of this text and the Part-1 MRCOG exam, there are some fundamentals principles of cell signalling that one should appreciate. This chapter will, therefore, focus on one family of receptors, the G-protein-coupled receptor (GPCR), to illustrate these points.

G-Protein Coupled Receptors

GPCRs are ubiquitous throughout the cellular genome, and more than 800 DNA sequences encoding

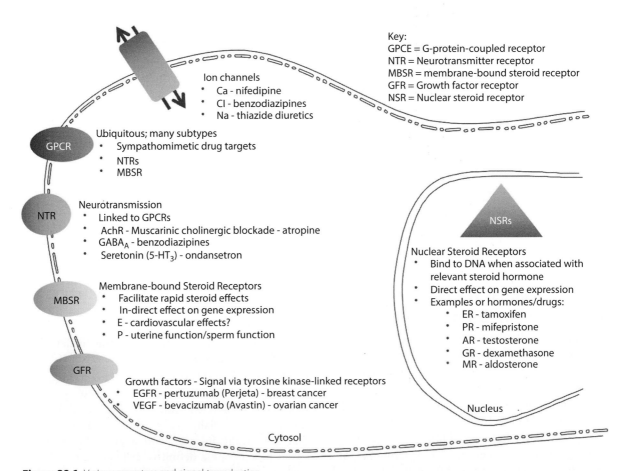

Figure 28.1 Various receptors and signal transduction

Table 28.3 List of different cellular receptors

Receptor type	Transduction mechanism
β2-adrenergic receptors	• G-protein coupled receptor • Utilises the Gαs subunit to induce cAMP formation and increase intra-cellular phosphorylation events which inhibit smooth muscle contraction • Basis of use of β2 agonist therapy (ritodrine; salbutamol)

α2-adrenergic receptors	• G-protein coupled receptor
	• Utilises the Gαi subunit to inhibit cAMP formation and reduce intra-cellular phosphorylation events leading to:
	  ◦ Increased vascular smooth muscle contraction (increase tone)
	  ◦ Increased uterine smooth muscle contraction – basis for use of ergot alkaloids such as ergometrine

Prostaglandin-E receptors: Type-1 (EP1) and Type-3 (EP3)	• G-protein coupled receptor • Utilises the Gαi subunit to inhibit cAMP formation and reduce intra-cellular phosphorylation events leading to: ◦ Increased uterine smooth muscle contraction – basis for use of synthetic prostaglandin analogues such as misoprostol (via EP1-receptor)
Prostaglandin-F2a receptor: FPR	• G-protein coupled receptor • Utilises the Gαp subunit to generate IP3 leading to elevated intra-cellular calcium levels ◦ Increased uterine smooth muscle contraction – basis for use of synthetic prostaglandin analogues such as carboprost

α-, μ-, δ-, k-opioid receptors	• G-protein coupled receptor
	• Utilises the Gαi subunit to inhibit cAMP formation and reduce intra-cellular phosphorylation events leading to:
	  ◦ Reduced Ca^{2+} entry via L and T-type Ca^{2+} channels into nociceptive neurones
	  ◦ Induction of K^+ efflux (hyperpolarisation) of nociceptive neurones
	  ◦ Inhibition of nociceptor pain fibres, e.g. opioid analgesics

GABA$_A$ receptor	• Receptor linked to chloride ion channel • Activation opens Cl⁻ channel causing: ◦ Cl⁻ influx into nerve cell and hyperpolarisation (becomes more difficult to fire impulses) • Site of action of benzodiazepine drugs, e.g. diazepam

different types of GPCR have been described [1]. Significantly, in a clinical context, more than 50% of all drugs used mimic or inhibit various GPCRs, and examples of some important drugs whose actions are mediated by GPCRs are listed in Table 28.3.

The GPCR utilises five cell components to form a receptor complex associated with the inner (cytosolic) side of the cell membrane (Fig. 28.2). Briefly, the complex contains a given receptor protein, in the illustrated example this is the β2-adrenergic receptor. This receptor is closely linked to three guanosine triphosphate (GTP) binding proteins termed Gα, Gβ and Gγ. The fifth component is usually an enzyme required to generate the second messenger; in this example, it is called adenylyl cyclase, although others, such as phospholipase-C (PLC), do exist. Note that for some signals inhibition of such an enzyme is equally important, as detailed in the following discussion.

The receptor protein provides the initial level of specificity of the given signal. Employing the hand-in-glove analogy highlighted previously, the receptor is the glove and the hormone (adrenaline or other β2-specific drugs) is the hand. Very few other 'hands' will fit the β2 glove well enough to cause a biological response.

Of this trimer of GTP-binding proteins, Gα is the key factor because it binds to and then hydrolyses (breaks down) GTP into GDP. Importantly, when Gα binds to GTP, this event allows it to activate the enzyme adenylyl cyclase. Adenylyl cyclase then catalyses the conversion of ATP into the required second messenger, in this case cAMP.

The Gα subunits also give further specificity to the signal (Fig. 28.3):

GPCR – five parts:

- **Receptor protein**
  - ➤ This gives specificity to the signal
  - ➤ It allows the cell to discriminate between different signalling molecules, for example adrenaline will only bind specifically to adrenergic receptors, steroid hormones will only bind specifically to steroid receptors

- **Three G -proteins -α, β, γ**
  - ➤ Gα protein gives specificity

- **Enzyme to make a second messenger**
  - ➤ Adenylyl cyclase synthesises cyclic adenosine monophosphate (cAMP) from ATP

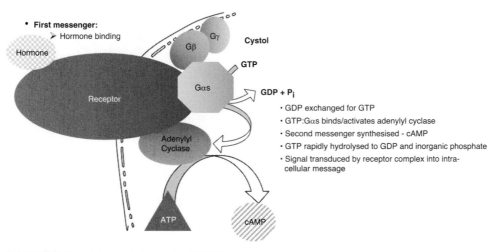

- **First messenger:**
  - ➤ Hormone binding

- GDP exchanged for GTP
- GTP:Gαs binds/activates adenylyl cyclase
- Second messenger synthesised - cAMP
- GTP rapidly hydrolysed to GDP and inorganic phosphate
- Signal transduced by receptor complex into intra-cellular message

Figure 28.2 G-protein coupled receptors (GPCRs)

Gαs – binds to and activates adenylyl cyclase and generation of cAMP promoting a hormone signal.

Gαi – binds to and inhibits activation of adenylyl cyclase. No cAMP is formed; signal is repressed.

Gαρ – binds to and activates phospholipase-C (PLC). This initiates intra-cellular signalling via the phosphoinositide pathway.

The initial signal is terminated when cAMP is hydrolysed to adenosine monophosphate (AMP) by an enzyme called phosphodiesterase. Phosphodiesterase enzymes can be inhibited by methylxanthine-based drugs. This group includes theophylline. As such, theophylline will prevent cAMP degradation and thereby prolong its signalling ability. This illustrates how different families of drugs can induce congruent biological outcomes by utilising different cell signalling pathways.

Signal Cascades

An intra-cellular 'signal cascade' leads to cellular effects. Such cascades serve to *amplify* the original signal input; for example, one molecule of hormone may generate 10 molecules of the second messenger, which, in turn, generates 100 molecules of activated kinase. Consequently, the sum of effects can be:

- Rapid – seconds/mins (nerve impulse; haemostasis)
- Delayed – hours/days (cell division)

Importantly, in terms of medicine, knowledge about such signal cascades facilitates drug (medical) intervention at several levels – for example, those that concern pre-term labour. While the aetiology of pre-term labour remains ill-defined and a discussion of this is beyond the scope of this particular chapter, the (limited) medical interventions are targeted at different intra-cellular signalling pathways. Four examples are provided in

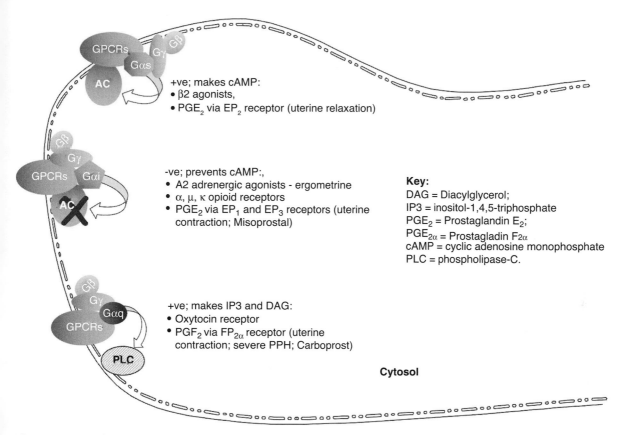

+ve; makes cAMP:
- β2 agonists,
- PGE$_2$ via EP$_2$ receptor (uterine relaxation)

-ve; prevents cAMP:,
- A2 adrenergic agonists - ergometrine
- α, μ, κ opioid receptors
- PGE$_2$ via EP$_1$ and EP$_3$ receptors (uterine contraction; Misoprostal)

Key:
DAG = Diacylglycerol;
IP3 = inositol-1,4,5-triphosphate
PGE$_2$ = Prostaglandin E$_2$;
PGE$_{2α}$ = Prostagladin F$_{2α}$
cAMP = cyclic adenosine monophosphate
PLC = phospholipase-C.

+ve; makes IP3 and DAG:
- Oxytocin receptor
- PGF$_2$ via FP$_{2α}$ receptor (uterine contraction; severe PPH; Carboprost)

Cytosol

Figure 28.3 Gα subunit determines second messenger

the following discussion: signalling cascades and myometrial quiescence, signalling cascades and myometrial contractility, signalling cascades – oxytocin and intra-cellular calcium, and signalling cascades – NF-κB and the genome.

Signalling Cascades and Myometrial Quiescence (Figs 28.3 and 28.4)

While the number of drugs available to treat this condition is limited, β2-sympathomimetics have been used in the past. Briefly, ritodrine binds to β2-adrenergic receptors on myometrial smooth muscle cells. These receptors are linked to a number of effector molecules:

- A GPCR using Gαs. This generates cAMP, which activates protein kinase-A (PKA).
  - PKA is a kinase molecule.
    - A kinase is an enzyme which adds a phosphate group (PO$_4$) to other molecules to modify their function. It is similar to binary (on/off) switch.

  - PKA, in turn, ultimately phosphorylates the acto-myosin ATPase within the muscle cell. This phosphorylation event stops the contraction machine working, thereby stopping the uterine contractions.

- A Ca-activated potassium channel (BKCa).
  - The BKCa channel is linked to β2-adrenergic receptors in human myometrium [3].
  - Activation of these adrenergic receptors by ritodrine induces K$^+$ efflux causing myocyte hyperpolarisation by a poorly-defined mechanism involving changes in intracellular Ca^{2+} ions [Fan et al. https://doi.org/10.1016/j.bbamem.2016.07.016] [4].
  - Hyperpolarisation makes the womb cell refractory to further contractile-stimuli.

At present, the RCOG suggest such drugs, including ritodrine are not used for tocolysis because they still have numerous unwanted systemic side-effects, most notable on the cardiovascular system [5].

277

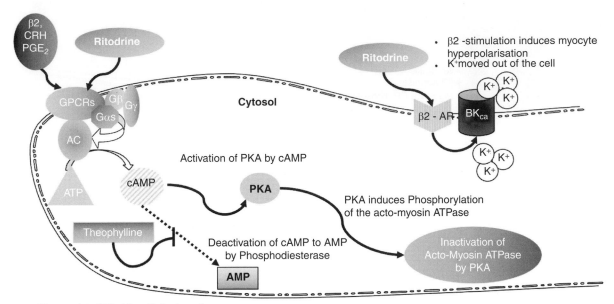

- β2 -stimulation induces myocyte hyperpolarisation
- K+moved out of the cell

- β2 -agonists (Ritodrine; Salbutamol):
  - ➤ increases cAMP; promotes smooth muscle relaxation (quiescence?)
  - ➤ promote myocyte hyperpolarisation - open K+ channels
  - ➤ tocolytic activity??

- Methylxanthin drugs - theophylline:
  - ➤ Inhibit phosphodiesterase enzymes
  - ➤ Prevents cAMP degradation
  - ➤ cAMP signal perpetuated

Key:
GPCR = G-protein-coupled receptor
AC = Adenylyl cyclase
ATP = Adenosine triphosphate
cAMP = cyclic adenosine monophosphate
AMP = adenosine monophosphate
PKA = Protein Kinase A

Figure 28.4 Signalling cascades and myometrial quiescence

Signalling Cascades and Myometrial Contraction (Figs 28.3 and 28.5)

Clinically, it is useful to be able to induce therapeutic myometrial contractions (essentially giving the womb a physiological 'squeeze'). There are a number of drugs able to do this, notably α2-adrenoceptor drugs and ergot alkaloids such as ergometrine, which mediate some actions via α2-adrenergic receptors. Importantly, synthetic prostaglandin analogues, such as misoprostol, acting via prostaglandin E1 and E3 receptors (EP1 and EP3), will also induce myometrial contraction. Alpha2, EP1 and EP3 receptors are GPCRs utilising the Gαi subunit:

- A GPCR using Gαi. In contrast to the Gαs:GTP complex listed previously, the Gαi:GTP complex inhibits adenylyl cyclase prevent cAMP synthesis.

  ○ PKA is therefore not activated.

○ Since PKA is not activated, the acto-myosin ATPase within the myometrial muscle cell remains active and can mediate uterine contractions.

Signalling Cascades – Oxytocin and Intra-cellular Calcium (Figs 28.3 and 28.6)

- Myometrial contractions can be induced by oxytocin (OT) and prostaglandin $F_{2\alpha}$ ($PGF_{2\alpha}$) by elevating levels if intra-cellular Ca^{2+} ions. The receptors for these molecules are GPCRs that utilise the Gαp protein instead of Gαs used by β2-adrenergic receptors. As such, a different activating enzyme, phospholipase-C (PLC), is required.

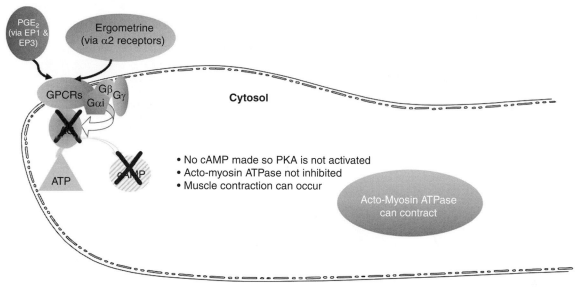

- No cAMP made so PKA is not activated
- Acto-myosin ATPase not inhibited
- Muscle contraction can occur

Acto-Myosin ATPase can contract

- Gαi: GTP inhibits cAMP synthesis:
  - α2-agonists and ergot alkaloids (ergometrine)
  - PGE$_2$ and synthetic prostaglandin analogues (misoprostol) via EP1 and EP3 receptors
  - promotes smooth muscle (uterine) contraction

Key:
α2 - α2-adrenergic receptor
EP1/EP3 = Prostaglandin-E$_2$ receptors sub-type-1 and -3
GPCR = G-protein-coupled receptor
AC = Adenylyl cyclase
ATP = Adenosine triphosphate
cAMP = cyclic adenosine monophosphate

Figure 28.5 Signalling cascades and myometrial contraction

- Once activated by Gαp, PLC stimulates the formation of second messengers by the hydrolysis of a large molecule, called phosphoinsitol-4,5-bisphosphate (PIP$_2$).
- The two second messengers are:
  - a lipid message (diacylglycerol; DAG)
  - a water-soluble sugar molecule called inositol-1,4,5-triphosphate (IP3)
- IP3, binds to its receptor on the muscle endoplasmic reticulum (the sarcoplasmic reticulum; SR). The SR stores intra-cellular Ca^{2+} ions.
- When IP3 binds to the SR, Ca^{2+} is released into the cell. The elevated intra-cellular Ca^{2+} has two main effects:
  - It is bound by calmodulin which causes the concomitant amplification of the signal ultimately activating the acto-myosin ATPase causing myometrial contractions
  - The Ca^{2+} ions, together with DAG, then bind to and activate a second protein kinase called protein kinase-C (PKC), which can enter the nucleus and phosphorylate a number of transcription factors thereby altering which genes the myometrium expresses.

- Knowledge of this pathway permitted an oxytocin receptor (OTR) antagonist to be developed: that drug is called *Atosiban*.
  - Atosiban is a tocolytic (labour-splitting) drug.
  - It has a better safety profile than β2-mimetics.
  - But, as with all tocolytic drugs, it does not stop myometrial contractions indefinitely – it buys you, as a clinician, some time to prepare the fetus for a premature birth [6–8].
- Figure 28.6 also illustrates potential reasons why such tocolytics are not particularly effective. Atosiban is specific for the OTR. It will not have any effect on other pro-contractile pathways such as those mediated by PGF$_{2\alpha}$.

279

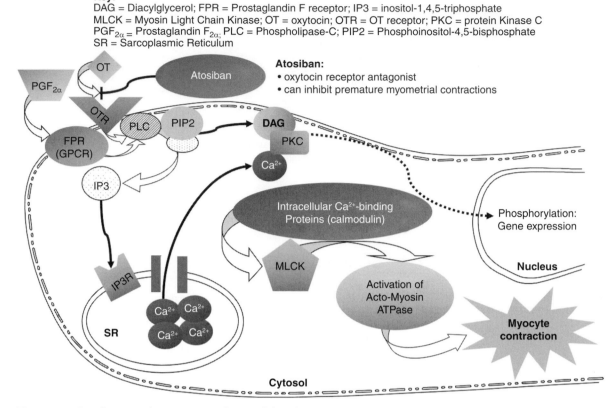

Key:
DAG = Diacylglycerol; FPR = Prostaglandin F receptor; IP3 = inositol-1,4,5-triphosphate
MLCK = Myosin Light Chain Kinase; OT = oxytocin; OTR = OT receptor; PKC = protein Kinase C
$PGF_{2\alpha}$ = Prostaglandin $F_{2\alpha}$; PLC = Phospholipase-C; PIP2 = Phosphoinositol-4,5-bisphosphate
SR = Sarcoplasmic Reticulum

Atosiban:
• oxytocin receptor antagonist
• can inhibit premature myometrial contractions

Figure 28.6 Signalling cascades – oxytocin and intra-cellular calcium

Signalling Cascades – NF-κB and the Genome

There is growing evidence indicating that in the human myometrium, the cessation of uterine quiescence and the onset of normal labour are associated with a number of pro-inflammatory cytokines, including IL-1β, IL-8 and TNF [9], all of which are inducers of, and regulated by, a family of transcription factors collectively referred to as nuclear factor-kappaB (NF-κB; [9,10] Fig. 28.7).

An in-depth discussion of NF-κB biology is beyond the scope of this chapter, but one can be found in [10]. It does, however, provide a good example of a signalling pathway that has rapid effects upon gene expression. Activation of NF-κB causes expression of its own inhibitor, IκB, causing a negative feedback cycle which can occur in seconds to minutes. A simplified version of events is given here:

• Briefly, NF-κB complexes are retained within the cytosol by their inhibitory protein IκB.
• Inflammatory agents, including IL-1β, IL-8, TNF and bacterial products such as lipopolysaccharide (LPS), bind to their cognate receptors and induce various second messenger signals.
• These signals converge at a multi-protein complex called the IκB kinase (IKK) composed of four subunits – IKKα, IKKβ and two copies of IKKγ.
• Once activated the IKK complex phosphorylates IκB at two conserved serine amino acids.
• This phosphorylation serves to tag IκB for a second label called ubiquitin (Ub).
• Two Ub molecules are then added. Ub serves as a means by which a cell can highlight proteins needing to be degraded.
• Once IκB is ubiquitinated, it is degraded leaving NF-κB free to enter the nucleus, where it can modulate expression of many genes involved in inflammation such as cyclo-oxygenase-2 (COX-2) [9].

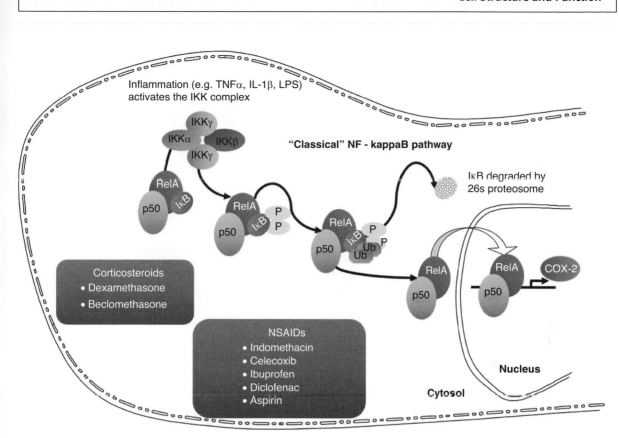

Figure 28.7 Signalling cascades – NF-kappaB and the genome

- COX-2 is one of the key enzymes involved in arachidonic acid metabolism and is important in the synthesis of prostaglandins.
- Non-steroidal anti-inflammatory drugs (NSAIDs) inhibit COX-1 and COX-2 and may also inhibit parts of the NF-κB cascade. Anti-inflammatory steroids (corticosteroids) are also thought to inhibit aspects of the NF-κB activation pathway.

The Cell Division Cycle
Cycle Phases

Hyperplasia (Greek – over formation) can occur within any organ system of the body; for example endometrial hyperplasia – uncontrolled growth of the endometrial lining resulting in a thickened endometrium. Clearly, such an overgrowth of cells is abnormal, so what does constitute normal cell growth? There are five aspects or phases to the normal eukaryotic cell division cycle (Table 28.4; Fig. 28.8), each governed by different families of cyclin-dependant kinases (CDKs) and their associated activator subunits, called cyclins [1]:

Cycle Phase Checkpoints

To ensure the fidelity of genome replication, the cell division cycle has evolved a number of checkpoints. These checkpoints are governed by key cellular proteins including p53, Retinoblastoma (Rb), c-Myc, ataxia telangiectasia mutated (ATM), as well as various cyclin and cyclin-dependant kinase proteins. Table 28.5 describes the salient event at each checkpoint and how they can be subverted by infectious agents (viruses) and manipulated by certain drugs (chemotherapy) (Fig. 28.9).

Summary

A cell signalling system has many points of redundancy. This means if one system fails, there is a backup system to ensure a given response can still be delivered. As we begin to understand the true complexities of many

Table 28.4 Phases of the eukaryotic cell division cycle

Phase	Function
G1	First gap phase. The cell determines if there are sufficient nutrients or resources for it to commit to a cycle of cell division. Mitogens and growth factors stimulate the expression of proteins called cyclins and cyclin-dependent kinases (CDKs). CDKs phosphorylate and activate many proteins required to synthesise DNA during the S phase of the cycle.
S	S-phase CDKs activate those proteins needed to bind DNA and form pre-replication complexes. Replication of DNA occurs in this phase. It is tightly regulated so replication and doubling the chromosome complement can only happen once per cycle. The cell is now temporarily tetraploid.
G2	Second gap phase. The cell grows some more.
M	Mitotic phase – at this stage, the cells actually divide and restore the chromosome complement to a diploid state. This phase is sub-divided into prophase, metaphase, anaphase and telophase. Metaphase is that stage often illustrated in biology texts as this is where the chromosomes have lined along the central axis of the cell ready for division. Contrast mitosis with meiosis. Meiosis is the reductive cell division seen in germ cells during oogenesis and spermatogenesis. Germ cells undergo a second round of cell division to reduce the chromosome complement to single copies – the haploid state. The diploid state is restored at successful fertilisation.
G0	This phase is often described as one where the cell is quiescent. This is only true in terms of cell division: the cell is no longer dividing and may, indeed, be resting. Equally, it may have undergone terminal differentiation to undertake a given function (myoblast becoming a muscle cell)

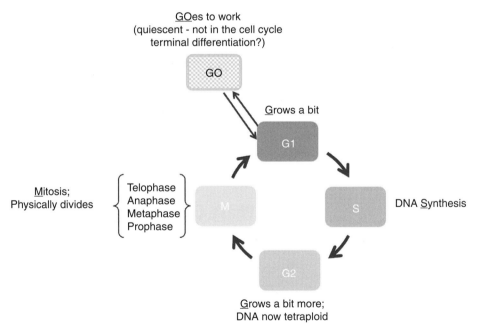

Figure 28.8 Cell division cycle

human diseases, we realise there are few, if any, magic bullets in the medical armoury.

- Cells are a functional unit of a tissue – contain many organelles
  - Organelles have specific functions within a cell
  - Cell-specific organelles – Weible-Paldae body – endothelial cells

- Cells have many protein receptors within plasma membrane
  - Transduce specific endocrine signals
  - Many varieties
- G-protein-coupled receptors are most ubiquitous
  - Gα-subunit specifies which second messenger is made

Table 28.5 Cell cycle checkpoints and associated events

Cell cycle phase	Event
G1:S	This checkpoint regulates the progress of cells through the restriction point of the cycle and into S-phase. DNA damage is sensed by proteins including ATM. Other proteins including p53, stimulate expression of proteins which stop the cell cycle before it is fully committed to replication. This allows the cell to either repair the DNA (using proteins such as BRACA-1 and -2) or to commit to apoptosis. Viruses such as HPV can inhibit the G1:S phase checkpoint and thus facilitate the passage of damaged DNA into the daughter cells. Ultimately this forms the basis of neoplastic transformation.
G2/M	This checkpoint prevents cells with damaged DNA from entering the mitotic (M) phase of replication and passing on damaged DNA to both daughter cells. The p53 protein is closely involved in this checkpoint. Metabolite chemotherapy works at this level. Drugs such as azacytidine or fluorouracil can be incorporated into the DNA. This interferes with the normal double helix structure causing tumour cells to stop dividing.
Spindle	This checkpoint ensures the microtubule spindle is correctly attached to the kinetochores of both nascent sister chromatids in preparation for cytokinesis (actual cell division). Etoposide is a drug which inhibits the formation of the cell spindle. As such, sister chromatids cannot be separated and the Spindle checkpoint is activated which shuts down the cell cycle.

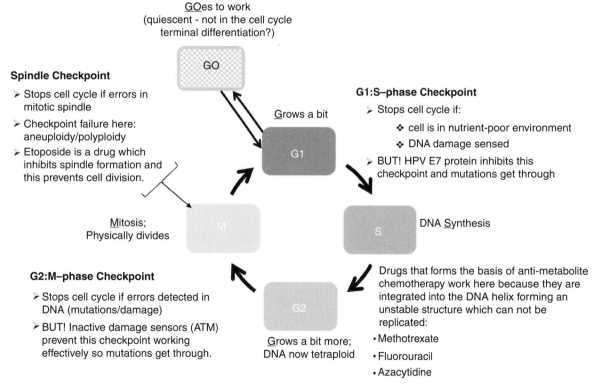

Figure 28.9 Cell division cycle – checkpoints

- Signalling cascades occur in the cell
  - Immediate responses
  - Delayed responses (gene transcription; mRNA translation)
  - Increased intracellular second messengers – cAMP, IP3, Ca^{2+}

- Cell cycle
  - Four phases: G1, S, G2, M
  - G0 – cell not dividing (quiescent) but may be working
  - Checkpoints prevent genome mutations being carried forward

References

1. Alberts, B., Johnson, A., Morgan, D., Raff, M., Roberts, K. Walter, P., Wilson, J. and Hunt, T. (2015). *Molecular Biology of the Cell*. 6th ed. Garland Science, Abingdon.

2. Johnson, M.H. (2007). *Essential Reproduction*. 6th ed. Blackwell, London.

3. Chanrachakul, B., Broughton-Pipkin, F. and Khan R. N. (2004). *Am. J. Physiol. – Cell Physiol.* 287, C1747–C1752 DOI: 10.1152/ajpcell.00236.2004.

4. Fan, Z., Lin, W., Lv, N., Ye, Y. and Tan, W. (2016) R- and S-terbutaline activate large conductance and Ca^{2+} dependent K^+ (BKCa) channel through interacting with β2 and M receptor respectively. *Biochimica et Biophysica Acta (BBA) – Biomembranes*. **1858**, 2745–2752. Doi https://doi.org/10.1016/j.bbamem.2016.07.016

5. RCOG Green-Top 1B. *Tocolytic Drugs for Women in Pre-term Labour* (Feb. 2011).

6. Kenyon, A.P. and Peebles, D. (2011). Myth: Tocolysis for prevention of preterm birth has a major role in modern obstetrics. *Semin. Fetal Neonatal Med.* **16**, 242–246. DOI: 10.1016/j.siny.2011.04.008.

7. Haas, D.M., Deborah M Caldwell, D.M., Page Kirkpatrick, P., McIntosh, J.J. and Welton, N.J. (2012). Tocolytic therapy for preterm delivery: systematic review and network meta-analysis (2012) *BMJ* 345, e6226; DOI: http://dx.doi.org/10.1136/bmj.e6226.

8. Alfirevic, Z. (2012) Tocolytics: Do they actually work? *BMJ* 345: e6531; DOI: http://dx.doi.org/10.1136/bmj.e6531.

9. Cookson V.J. and Chapman, N.R. (2010). NF-κB function in the human myometrium during pregnancy and parturition. *Histol. Histopathol.* 25, 945–956.

10. Cookson, V.J., Waite, S.L., Heath, P.R., Hurd, P.J., Gandhi, S.V. and Chapman, N.R. (2015). Binding loci of RelA-containing nuclear factor-kappaB (NF-κB) dimers in promoter regions of PHM1-31 myometrial smooth muscle cells. *Mol. Hum. Reprod.* 21, 865–883. DOI: 10.1093/molehr/gav051

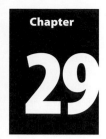

Chapter

29

Cellular Responses in Disease

Raji Ganesan and Josefa E. O. Vella

1 Cellular Adaptations, Cellular Injury and Cell Death

The normal cell maintains a steady state, termed *homeostasis*, in which the internal milieu of the cell is kept within physiological parameters. The response of a cell to any change in its environment constitutes the pathophysiological basis of clinical symptoms. When cells are faced with physiological or pathological stress they respond in several ways, collectively known as *cellular adaptation*. When the capacity of the cell to adapt is exceeded, then the cell undergoes a series of changes referred to as *cell injury*. The degree of injury dictates whether the cell will recover (i.e. reversible cell injury) or progress to *cell death* (i.e. irreversible cell injury). The effect on the tissue will depend on the duration of the injury, the nature of the injurious agent, the proportion and types of cells affected and the ability of the tissue to regenerate.

1.1 Cellular Adaptation (Table 29.1)

Cells may undergo the following reversible adjustments (or adaptation) in response to changes in their environment:

- *Hypertrophy*: increase in cell size leading to an increase in tissue/organ size.
- *Hyperplasia*: increase in cell numbers by cell division leading to an increase in tissue/organ size.
- *Atrophy*: decrease in the size or number of the constituent cells leading to a decrease in the size of an organ.
- *Metaplasia*: replacement of one differentiated cell type with another differentiated cell type.

1.2 Cell injury

There are many causes of cell injury, including simple physical injury, as well as more complex forms of injury such as immunological reactions; these are listed in Table 29.2. These causes can be interrelated; for example, physical injury can result in hypoxic damage secondary to loss of blood. Whatever the cause of injury, the damage occurs intracellularly. The most vulnerable intracellular processes are glycolysis, the citric acid cycle and oxidative phosphorylation. The main biochemical changes are:

- ATP depletion resulting in cell swelling and lowering of the pH
- Release of oxygen-derived free radicals

Table 29.1 Examples of physiological and pathological cellular adaptation

Cellular adaptation	Examples
Hypertrophy	*Physiological:* skeletal muscle hypertrophy in athletes *Pathological:* cardiac muscle hypertrophy in hypertension
Hyperplasia	*Physiological:* uterine muscle in pregnancy *Pathological:* bone hyperplasia in Paget's disease of bone
Atrophy	*Physiological:* involution of the thymus with age *Pathological:* muscle atrophy in paralysis secondary to loss of innervation
Metaplasia	*Physiological:* squamous metaplasia in the uterine cervix in response to change in pH of the vagina *Pathological:* squamous metaplasia in the bronchus secondary to cigarette smoke

Table 29.2 Causes of cell injury and examples

Causes of cell injury	Examples
Hypoxia	Pulmonary embolus, cardiac failure, carbon monoxide poisoning
Chemical	Paracetamol overdose, cyanide poisoning, alcohol
Physical injury	Mechanical trauma, thermal trauma, ionising or UV radiation
Infectious agents	Viruses, bacteria, fungi
Immunologic reactions	Graft versus host disease, autoimmune diseases
Nutritional imbalances	Dietary insufficiency of proteins, vitamins or minerals (e.g. scurvy – vitamin C deficiency), dietary excess (e.g. fat)
Genetic derangements	Cystic fibrosis

Table 29.3 Cell death: Apoptosis versus necrosis

Feature	Apoptosis	Necrosis
Process	Pathological or physiological	Pathological
Number of cells	Single cells	Groups of cells
Cell membrane integrity	Maintained	Lost
Morphology	Cell shrinkage and fragmentation	Cell swelling and lysis
Inflammation	No inflammatory response	Inflammatory response
Fate of dead cells	Ingested (phagocytosed) by neighbouring cells	Phagocytosed by neutrophils and macrophages
Biochemical mechanism	Energy-dependent; endonuclease activity	Energy-independent; loss of ion homeostasis

- Increase in cytoplasmic calcium resulting in activation of intracellular enzymes that damage intracellular organelles
- Disrupted cell membrane permeability
- Irreversible mitochondrial damage that triggers apoptotic cell death

1.3 Cell Death

Cell death is a state of irreversible cell injury and may occur by autolysis, apoptosis or necrosis.

- *Autolysis:* This refers to death of cells post-mortem or after removal from the body at surgery. Autolysis can be seen in organs and tissues removed at surgery if they are not preserved/fixed adequately.
- *Apoptosis:* This is a regulated genetic event designed for cell death; it is also termed 'programmed cell death'. It is seen during embryogenesis and physiological events such as ovarian follicular atresia during the menopause. A cell undergoing apoptosis shows condensation of chromatin followed by fragmentation of the nucleus. Pro-inflammatory mediators are not released during the process of apoptosis and thus there is no associated inflammation (Table 29.3).
- *Necrosis:* It is the death of cells in living tissue and is characterised by swelling of cells, death of cell organelles and release of mediators of the inflammatory response. Necrosis is, therefore, accompanied by inflammation. The cytoplasm appears more eosinophilic and the nucleus can show karyolysis (dissolution), pyknosis (shrinkage) and karyorrhexis (fragmentation) (Table 29.3). There are several types of necrosis resulting in varying morphological changes in the tissue (Table 29.4).

Table 29.4 Types of necrosis: Morphological features and examples

Type of necrosis	Morphological features	Example
Coagulative necrosis	Outlines of tissue preserved on microscopy	Myocardial infarction
Liquefactive necrosis	Tissue morphology lost on microscopy; liquefaction visible macroscopically	Cerebral infarction
Caseous necrosis	Tissue morphology preserved on microscopy; cheesy material visible macroscopically	Tuberculosis
Gangrenous necrosis	Tissue morphology lost on microscopy; gaseous/frothy appearance macroscopically	Clostridial infection
Fat necrosis	Outline of tissue preserved on microscopy	Acute pancreatitis

2 Inflammation

Inflammation is the response of vascularised tissue to injury. It is composed of a complex series of events that start with tissue injury and progress to vascular, chemical and systemic responses, all aimed at restoration of the tissue to normalcy. There are five classical signs of inflammation:

1. Redness (*rubor*) – due to dilatation of vessels
2. Heat (*calor*) – due to increased blood flow
3. Pain (*dolor*) – due to stretching of tissues and/or effect of chemicals released in inflammation
4. Swelling (*tumour*) – due to oedema
5. Loss of function (*functio laesa*)

The non-specific systemic effects of inflammation include raised erythrocyte sedimentation rate (ESR), raised C-reactive protein (CRP), leucocytosis and fever.

Inflammation is divided into acute and chronic patterns.

2.1 Acute Inflammation

Acute inflammation is the immediate response to tissue injury and has an early onset (seconds to minutes). Causes include mechanical injury (e.g. a cut), chemical injury (e.g. acid burns), micro-organisms (e.g. bacteria) and deposits of immune complexes. It is of short duration, lasting from hours to weeks. There are three main components of acute inflammation, namely:

1. Dilatation of small blood vessels
2. Increased vascular permeability
3. Emigration of white blood cells (leukocytes) from blood vessels into the damaged tissues

Following injury, the vessels supplying the injured area dilate, leading to an increase in blood flow. In

Table 29.5 Chemical mediators of acute inflammation

Chemical mediator	Sources
Histamine	Mast cells, platelets, basophils
Serotonin (5HT)	Platelets
Prostaglandins Leukotrienes Platelet-activating factor	Mast cells, leukocytes
Cytokines Nitric oxide	Macrophages, endothelial cells
Kinins (e.g. bradykinin) Complement products (e.g. C3)	Plasma

addition, the vessels become more permeable, resulting in loss of protein-rich fluid from the vessels (*exudation*) and accumulation of fluid in tissues (*oedema*). This leads to an increase in blood viscosity and slow movement of the red blood cells. As a consequence, the leukocytes adhere to the endothelial cells (*margination*) and then migrate through the vessel wall by a process termed *diapedesis (or transmigration)*. Movement toward the area of injury is mediated by chemical messengers such as bacterial products, denatured proteins and cytokines (*chemotaxis*). Destruction of foreign material/removal of damaged tissue occurs by a process known as *phagocytosis* whereby the foreign material/damaged tissue is engulfed by the leukocytes. The main white blood cells involved are, first, *neutrophil polymorphs* and, later, *monocytes* (called histiocytes or macrophages when they are in tissue).

Acute inflammation is mediated by chemical substances referred to as *chemical mediators* (Table 29.5).

Broadly speaking, the chemical mediators of inflammation originate either from plasma or from cells (e.g. mast cells, platelets). The production of these chemical mediators is triggered by microbial products or by factors released by necrotic tissues. The mediators are generally short-lived and removed by phagocytes. This system of checks and balances generally results in the avoidance of potential excess damage by these chemicals.

Acute inflammation may resolve completely, heal by fibrosis or progress to *chronic inflammation* (Fig. 29.1).

2.2 Chronic Inflammation

Chronic inflammation has a late onset (days) and is of long duration, lasting from weeks to years. Typically, the persistent inflammatory changes are combined with attempts at healing. Chronic inflammation is characterised by mononuclear cell infiltration (macrophages, plasma cells and lymphocytes), tissue destruction and granulation tissue formation, resulting in fibrosis. B lymphocytes transform into plasma cells which produce antibodies. T lymphocytes release inflammatory mediators. Chronic inflammation can

Table 29.6 Comparison of histological and immunological features of tuberculosis and sarcoidosis

	Tuberculosis	Sarcoidosis
Bacilli	Present	Absent
Granulomas	Caseating	Non-caseating
Mantoux test	Positive	Negative
Kveim test	Negative	Positive

be a continuation of acute inflammation or start de novo. Causes of primary chronic inflammation include persistent infection, foreign body reactions, autoimmune diseases and chronic granulomatous diseases.

Granulomatous inflammation is a specific type of chronic inflammation characterized by the presence of granulomas in the diseased tissue. Granulomas are collections of macrophages referred to as epithelioid cells. When the granulomas show loss of cellular detail with cheese-like material centrally, they are called caseating granulomas, classically seen in *tuberculosis* (TB). Acid-fast bacilli may be demonstrated in TB by the Ziehl-Neelsen histological stain. A positive Mantoux test, in which intradermal injection of tuberculin evokes an immune response, is indicative of TB exposure. *Sarcoidosis* is the prototypical example of a disease in which non-caseating granulomas are seen. Sarcoid granulomas can occur anywhere in the body, with lymph node, lung and skin being commoner sites. A positive Kveim test, in which granulomas are induced by injection of sterile sarcoid tissue homogenate, is indicative of sarcoidosis. In nearly a third of patients with sarcoidosis, the serum level of angiotensin-converting enzyme is raised. A comparison of tuberculosis and sarcoidosis is given in Table 29.6. A comparison of acute and chronic inflammation is given in Table 29.7.

3 Healing

The process of healing is the body's response to injury in an attempt to restore normal structure and function. Healing may occur by *regeneration* or by *repair*:

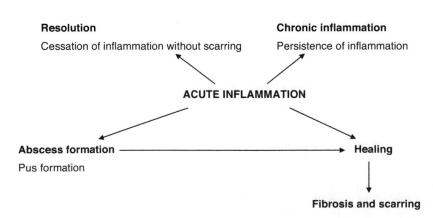

Figure 29.1 Potential outcomes of acute inflammation

Resolution
Cessation of inflammation without scarring

Chronic inflammation
Persistence of inflammation

ACUTE INFLAMMATION

Abscess formation
Pus formation

Healing

Fibrosis and scarring

Table 29.7 Comparison of acute and chronic inflammation

	Acute inflammation	Chronic inflammation
Response	Immediate reaction of tissue to injury	Persisting reaction of tissue to injury
Onset	Rapid (seconds to minutes)	Slow (days)
Immunity	Innate	Cell-mediated
Predominant cell type	Neutrophil	Lymphocytes, plasma cells, macrophages
Duration	Hours weeks	Weeks/months/years
Vascular response	Prominent	Less important

Regeneration involves proliferation of parenchymal cells to replace those which have been destroyed, resulting in complete restoration of the original tissue. Regeneration occurs only when surviving cells of a tissue are capable of cell division.

Repair involves proliferation of mesenchymal cells, resulting in replacement of the injured tissue by fibrous tissue. During the process of repair, specialised tissue called granulation tissue is formed which involves the proliferation of fibroblasts and the formation of new blood vessels at the site of injury (neovascularisation). The fibroblasts contract, leading to wound contraction and the laying down of collagen fibres, resulting in scar formation. Healing by repair is inevitable in tissues which do not have the ability to regenerate.

Tissues may be divided into three groups on the basis of their capacity to regenerate:

- *Labile cells:* proliferate continuously throughout life, replacing those cells which have been destroyed (e.g. skin, intestinal epithelium).
- *Stable or quiescent cells:* normally have a low level of replication but can undergo rapid division in response to stimuli and are therefore capable of reconstituting the tissue of origin (e.g. parenchymal cells of the liver and kidneys).
- *Permanent or non-dividing cells:* lack ability to proliferate (e.g. nerves, cardiac myocytes, skeletal muscle).

Healing of Cutaneous Wounds

Skin wounds are described as healing by primary intention or secondary intention. Wounds with

Table 29.8 Factors which adversely affect wound healing

Local factors	Systemic factors
Blood supply	Drugs (e.g. steroids)
Infection	Extremes of temperature
Foreign bodies	Systemic infection
Mechanical stress	Malnutrition (e.g. vitamin C deficiency)
Necrotic tissue	Diabetes

opposed edges (e.g. clean surgical incisions) heal by primary intention. Larger wounds with separated edges (e.g. a cutaneous ulcer) heal by secondary intention. These differ from each other mainly by the phenomenon of *wound contraction* (Table 29.8).

4 Disturbances in Body Fluids and Blood Flow

4.1 Oedema

Oedema refers to an abnormal accumulation of fluid in tissues. Oedema fluid may be transudate (low protein content) or exudate (high protein content).

Causes of oedema:

- Increased hydrostatic pressure (e.g. congestive cardiac failure, cirrhosis)
- Decreased plasma osmotic pressure (e.g. nephrotic syndrome)

Table 29.9 Factors predisposing to thrombosis, with examples

Predisposing factor	Causes
Changes in the vessel wall	Diabetes mellitus, cigarette smoking, endotoxins, hypertension
Changes in blood constituents	*Congenital:* Factor V Leiden mutation *Acquired:* prolonged immobilisation, tissue injury, cancer, smoking, obesity
Changes in blood flow	Atherosclerotic plaques, arrhythmias, mitral valve stenosis, myocardial infarction, aneurysms, varicose veins

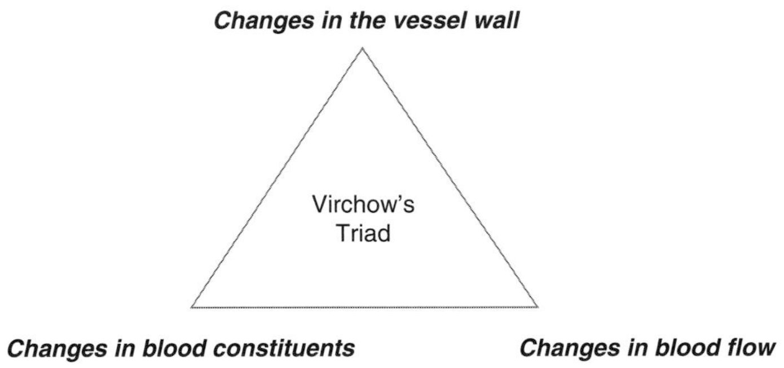

Changes in the vessel wall

Virchow's Triad

Figure 29.2 Virchow's triad

Changes in blood constituents   **Changes in blood flow**

- Obstruction (e.g. malignancy, post-surgery such as following removal of axillary lymph nodes for breast carcinoma)
- Increased vascular permeability (e.g. in inflammation)

4.2 Thrombosis

Thrombosis is the pathological process by which a blood clot forms within the uninterrupted vascular system by a complex process involving the endothelium lining the vessels, platelets and the coagulation or clotting cascade. Three factors predispose to thrombus formation, namely *changes in the vessel wall* (e.g. endothelial injury), *changes in the constituents of the blood* (e.g. increased platelet number, increased prothrombin time) and *changes in blood flow* (e.g. stasis or turbulence). These three factors are known as Virchow's triad (Fig. 29.2; Table 29.9).

Thrombi may undergo dissolution by fibrinolytic activity, then organisation (transformation of the thrombus into vascular connective tissue); re-canalisation of vessels occurs with re-establishment of blood flow. Thrombi can also extend and block the vessel further. In addition, they can detach from the site of original formation and embolise to distant sites.

4.3 Embolus

An embolus is a detached intravascular fragment of material, whether solid, liquid or gas, which is carried by the bloodstream to a point distant from its site of origin or entry. Most emboli arise from thrombi (Table 29.10)

4.4 Infarction

Infarction is the process of tissue necrosis due to ischaemia resulting from occlusion of the arterial supply or venous drainage. The localised area of infarction is called an infarct. Most infarcts occur as a result of thrombi or emboli. Other causes include extrinsic compression of a vessel (e.g. by a tumour) and twisting of vessels (e.g. testicular and ovarian torsion). Infarcts are described as either red (or haemorrhagic) or white (or pale or anaemic). Red infarcts occur in soft loose tissues (e.g. lung) and in tissues with dual circulations (e.g. intestines). White infarcts occur in solid organs with end-arterial circulations (e.g. spleen, heart, kidneys).

The process of infarction is as follows:

Localised hyperaemia due to a local lack of oxygen in the blood

Swelling of the affected part due to oedema and haemorrhage

Cell swelling and degeneration followed by cell death by necrosis (within 12–48 hours)

Autolysis of necrotic tissue and haemolysis of red blood cells

Acute inflammation and hyperaemia in surrounding tissues in response to products of autolysis

Blood pigments (e.g. haemosiderin) deposited in the infarct as a result of haemolysis

Ingrowth of granulation tissue from infarct margin so that infarct is replaced by a fibrous scar

Table 29.10 Types of emboli and their origin

Type of embolus	Origin
Pulmonary embolus	Usually from deep venous thrombosis of the limbs
Amniotic fluid embolus	Amniotic fluid in maternal vessels following a tear in placental membranes
Air embolism	Rapid decompression in deep-sea divers
Fat embolism	From fatty marrow of long bones following fractures

Table 29.11 Types of shock and examples of precipitating factors

Type of shock	Examples of precipitating factors
Cardiogenic shock	Myocardial infarction, cardiac tamponade
Hypovolaemic shock	Severe haemorrhage, burns
Toxic shock	Microbial infection

4.5 Shock

Shock is a condition of circulatory failure characterised by reduced effective circulating volume and consequential tissue hypoxia. In *hypovolaemic* shock, there is an actual loss of blood volume, whereas in *cardiogenic* and *septic* shock, there is decreased cardiac output without actual loss of blood volume. The resulting hypoperfusion and hypoxia of tissues can lead to irreversible neuronal injury, acute renal tubular necrosis, cerebral damage and eventual death (Table 29.11).

Suggested Reading

(1)   Vinay Kumar, Abul K. Abbas and Jon C. Aster. *Robbins and Cotran Pathologic Basis of Disease.* 9th ed. Elsevier Saunders, 2014.

(2)   J.C.E. Underwood and Simon S. Cross. *General and Systemic Pathology.* 5th ed. Churchill Livingstone, 2009.

Single Best Answer Questions

1. Which one of the following refers to an increase in the size of an organ without an increase in the number of constituent cells?

   a. Hypertrophy

   b. Atrophy

   c. Metaplasia

   d. Hyperplasia

   e. Dysplasia

2. Which one of the following is not applicable to necrosis?

   a. Involves groups of cells

   b. Energy-dependent

    c. Accompanied by an inflammatory response

    d. Cells increase in size

    e. Dead cells are phagocytosed by neutrophils and macrophages

3. Which one of the following is the main cell type involved in the acute inflammatory response?

    a. Macrophage

    b. Lymphocyte

    c. Neutrophil

    d. Eosinophil

    e. Plasma cell

4. Which one of the following refers to a collection of epithelioid macrophages?

    a. Granulation tissue

    b. Granuloma

    c. Giant cell

    d. Granular cell

    e. Glomerulus

5. Which one of the following tissue types undergoes healing by regeneration following injury?

    a. Glandular epithelium lining the gastrointestinal tract

    b. Urothelial cells lining the bladder

    c. Haemopoietic cells

    d. Smooth muscle

    e. Skeletal muscle

6. Which one of the following characteristics differentiates a transudate from an exudate?

    a. High specific gravity

    b. Low protein content

    c. Clear in appearance

    d. Low cholesterol content

    e. Caused by increased hydrostatic pressure

7. Which one of the following does not predispose to thrombus formation?

    a. Smoking

    b. Breast cancer

    c. Atrial fibrillation

    d. Asthma

    e. A BMI of 40 kg/m^2

8. Which one of the following features is not associated with septic shock?

    a. Cortisol production

    b. Increased thrombotic tendency

    c. Decreased nutrient delivery to tissues

    d. Hypoglycaemia

    e. Growth hormone production

Pathology of Non-neoplastic and Neoplastic Gynaecological Diseases

Raji Ganesan and Josefa E. O. Vella

1 Non-neoplastic Gynaecological Pathology

Non-neoplastic disease of the female genital tract can be the underlying cause of morbidity. Common gynaecological symptoms include vaginal discharge, bleeding (irregular periods, heavy periods, post-coital bleeding and postmenopausal bleeding), pelvic pain and prolapse. The pathological conditions underlying some of these symptoms include infections, endometriosis, polyps and ovarian cysts.

1.1 Sexually Transmitted Infections and Tubal Damage

A number of organisms can be sexually transmitted (Table 30.1). Some of these organisms are usually spread by sexual contact (e.g. *Chlamydia trachomatis*), while others are typically spread by other routes but can also spread by sexual contact (e.g. *Entamoeba histolytica*). Sexually transmitted infections (STIs) cause inflammation followed by scarring, increase the risk of other STIs and can cross the maternal-fetal barrier to affect the unborn fetus.

Condyloma acuminatum is a sexually transmitted, benign condition caused by the human papillomavirus (HPV) and can affect the vulva, vagina or cervix.

Tuberculous salpingitis is common in areas of the world where the disease is prevalent and is an important cause of infertility in these populations.

Neisseria gonorrhoeae and *chlamydia trachomatis* are the main causes of pelvic inflammatory disease (PID). The infection usually begins in the Bartholin's gland or in other glands in the perineum, then spreads upwards to involve the other genital tract structures. Involvement of the fallopian tubes may cause persistent inflammation (pyosalpinx) or chronic damage (hydrosalpinx). The alterations in the tube can result in infertility or ectopic pregnancy.

1.2 Endometriosis and Adenomyosis

Endometriosis is a common disorder that affects up to 4% of all women and up to 50% of women with symptoms such as infertility or pelvic pain. It is defined as the presence of endometrial glands and/or stroma outside the uterine corpus. The commonest sites (in descending order of occurrence) are ovaries, rectovaginal septum, pelvic peritoneum, laparotomy scars and rarely the umbilicus or appendix or lungs. The presence of endometrial glands and/or stroma in the uterine wall is termed *adenomyosis*. Various theories have been postulated to explain the presence of endometrial tissue outside the uterus[1]:

1. *Retrograde menstruation theory*: this postulates that during menstruation endometrial tissue passes through the fallopian tube and implants in the peritoneal cavity.
2. *Metaplastic theory*: this implies that the lining of the peritoneal cavity can change to endometrial tissue.
3. *Vascular dissemination theory*: this suggests that endometrial tissue is disseminated by blood and lymphatic vessels. This could explain endometriosis in distant sites such as the lungs and nasal cavity.

Endometriosis and adenomyosis can be the underlying cause of pelvic pain, menstrual irregularities and infertility. Malignancies, notably clear cell carcinoma and endometrioid carcinoma, can arise in endometriosis.

1.3 Polyps

Polyps can be seen commonly in the cervix and endometrium and are localised protrusions of glands and stroma into the endocervical canal (and sometimes extending through the cervical os) or uterine cavity, respectively. They may cause abnormal uterine bleeding. They can be removed by simple surgery but tend to recur. Most polyps are non-neoplastic; however,

Table 30.1 Micro-organisms and the diseases they can cause

Organism	Disease caused	Other effects
Trichomonas vaginalis	• Vaginitis	–
Treponema pallidum	• Syphilis	Congenital syphilis in the fetus
Neisseria gonorrhoea	• Gonorrhoeal cervicitis • Bartholinitis • Mixed acute and chronic endometritis • Salpingitis • Pelvic inflammatory disease	Sequelae such as infertility and ectopic pregnancy following salpingitis
Chlamydia trachomatis	• Urethral syndrome • Bartholinitis • Cervicitis • Chronic endometritis • Salpingitis • Pelvic inflammatory disease	Sequelae such as infertility following salpingitis
Low-risk human papillomavirus	• Genital warts or Condylomata	
Mycobacterium tuberculosis	• Chronic endometritis • Salpingitis	–
Herpes simplex virus	• Genital herpes	–
Human immunodeficiency virus (HIV)	• AIDS	Other infections and unusual malignancies

some low-grade malignancies, such as adenosarcomas, may occasionally present as recurrent polyps.

1.5 Fibroids

Fibroids are benign, hormone-sensitive tumours arising from uterine smooth muscle. The pathological microscopic term for a fibroid is leiomyoma, and they may be single or multiple. Macroscopically they are seen as discrete, spherical, firm masses with a uniform whorled white cut surface. On microscopy, they are seen to consist of smooth muscle fascicles without significant mitotic activity or necrosis. Fibroids can undergo a variety of changes including infarction, hydropic degeneration, calcification and ossification. A number of hormone modulating drugs and embolization procedures are used as treatment and this can result in changes in the microscopic appearance. Fibroids may rarely undergo sarcomatous transformation. A variant of leiomyoma, known as intravenous leiomyoma, is capable of spread beyond the uterus through vascular channels.

1.6 Ovarian Cysts

Ovarian cysts may be functional, endometriotic or neoplastic.

Functional cysts are those which form as part of the normal ovarian changes during the menstrual cycle; they include follicular and corpus luteum cysts.

Follicular Cysts

Follicular cysts are common and are found at any age from infancy to the menopause. They form as a result of the accumulation of fluid within follicles, which leads to its distension. Most follicular cysts are asymptomatic, but some may cause acute abdominal pain as a result of rupture and bleeding into the peritoneal cavity.

Corpus Luteum Cysts

Corpus luteum cysts occur frequently during the reproductive years and develop at the end of the menstrual cycle or in pregnancy. Following ovulation, small physiological haemorrhages occur within the corpus luteum which usually organise rapidly. However, if the bleeding is excessive, the corpus luteum becomes distended with blood, resulting in the formation of a cyst. Similar to follicular cysts, most corpus luteum cysts are asymptomatic, but some may cause acute abdominal pain as a result of rupture and bleeding into the peritoneal cavity.

Endometrioma ('Chocolate Cyst')

An endometrioma is a form of endometriosis which is most commonly seen in the ovary and has a characteristic central cystic space which may be filled with altered blood (fancifully likened to liquid chocolate, hence the alternative name of 'chocolate cyst'). The cystic space is lined by endometrial epithelium, beneath which is endometrial stroma and fresh or old (haemosiderin-containing) haemorrhagic foci. Symptomatic patients typically present during the reproductive years with menstrual-associated pain, infertility or a pelvic mass.

Serous Cystadenomas and Cystadenofibromas

Serous cystadenomas and cystadenofibromas may occur at any age but most commonly in the reproductive age group. They are bilateral in approximately 20% of cases and range from 1 cm to 10 cm in diameter. These cysts are usually asymptomatic and discovered incidentally during ultrasound investigation of another gynaecological disorder. On microscopic examination, the cyst is lined by a single layer of epithelial cells which may be ciliated.

Mucinous Cystadenomas

Mucinous cystadenomas typically occur in the third to sixth decades. They are unilateral in 95% of cases and are often large (mean diameter 10 cm). On microscopic examination, the cyst is lined by a single layer of columnar epithelial cells which contain mucin within the cytoplasm.

Mature Cystic Teratomas (Dermoid Cysts)

Mature cystic teratomas, commonly known as ovarian dermoids or dermoid cysts, are the commonest ovarian germ cell tumour. They are most commonly seen in adult women of reproductive age but can occur at any age. They are asymptomatic in around half of patients and may present with abdominal pain as a result of torsion or rupture, or abdominal swelling. It is believed that they are of parthenogenetic origin (a form of asexual reproduction from an unfertilised egg) that occurs in a single oocyte after the first meiotic division. They are composed of mature tissues derived from any of the three germ cell layers. Tissues derived from the ectoderm or neuroectoderm include skin and its appendages, glial tissue and cerebellar tissue. Tissues derived from mesoderm include smooth muscle, bone, teeth, cartilage and fat. Tissues derived from the endoderm include respiratory epithelium, gastrointestinal epithelium and thyroid tissue. Macroscopically, these neoplasms are commonly cystic and filled with keratin, fat and hair. This is reflected on microscopic examination when the commonest structures seen are skin and appendages. Sometimes there may be only one component and such tumours are termed monodermal teratomas (when the component is thyroid tissue it is termed struma ovarii). Although mature teratomas are

benign tumours, malignant transformation may occur in approximately 1–2% of cases, usually in postmenopausal women. Almost any component may become malignant, but squamous cell carcinoma accounts for 80% of malignancies.[1]

2 Neoplasia – Benign and Malignant Gynaecological Pathology

2.1 An Introduction to Neoplasia (Table 30.2)

Neoplasia has been best defined by the eminent British oncologist Sir Rupert Willis as follows: 'a neoplasm is an *abnormal* mass of tissue, the growth of which *exceeds* and is *uncoordinated* with that of the normal tissues and *persists* in the same excessive manner *after the cessation* of the stimuli which evoked the change.' Neoplasms can be benign or malignant. Benign neoplasms can grow but are incapable of spread beyond the structure of origin. Malignancy is defined by the ability of a neoplasm to spread beyond its site of origin; this phenomenon is known as *metastasis*. The notable exceptions are basal cell carcinomas and gliomas which have limited or no capacity to metastasise. Conversely, intravenous leiomyomas are phenotypically benign tumours that can spread through vessels.

Tumour nomenclature (Table 30.3)

The suffix '-oma', derived from Greek and Modern Latin, denotes a noun meaning tumour or abnormal growth. Malignant tumours derived from epithelium are suffixed as '-carcinoma' and those derived from connective tissues as '-sarcoma'.

Degree of Differentiation (Tumour Grade)

Malignant tumours are graded according to the degree to which the neoplastic cells reflect their normal counterparts. Tumours may be:

- Well differentiated
- Moderately differentiated
- Poorly differentiated
- Undifferentiated or anaplastic

Well-differentiated neoplasms are at one end of the spectrum and most closely resemble the tissue from which they arise. In contrast, undifferentiated or anaplastic neoplasms at the other end of the spectrum show no resemblance to the tissue from which they have arisen. Poorly differentiated tumour cells show

Table 30.2 Characteristics of benign and malignant neoplasms

	Benign tumours	Malignant tumours
Growth pattern	Expansive	Infiltrative
Growth rate	Slow	Rapid
Duration	May cease growing	Rarely cease growing
Capsule	Well-developed capsule often present	Usually non-encapsulated and infiltrate into surrounding tissue
Differentiation	Closely resemble tissue of origin (i.e. well differentiated)	Variable between tumours; may have little resemblance to the tissue of origin (i.e. poorly differentiated)
Mitoses	Infrequent	Frequent
Necrosis and ulceration	Unusual	Common
Capacity for metastasis	No	Yes
Effect on host	Usually local (e.g. compression of surrounding tissues, cosmetic effects)	Often kills host due to spread to vital organs such as liver and brain.

Table 30.3 Tumour nomenclature

Tumour type	Definition	Examples
Papilloma	Benign tumour arising from squamous, basal or transitional type epithelium	Urothelial papilloma
Adenoma	Benign tumour of glandular epithelium	Villous adenoma of the colon
Carcinoma	Malignant epithelial tumour	Squamous cell carcinoma from squamous epithelium Adenocarcinoma from glandular epithelium
Sarcoma	Malignant mesenchymal tumour	Rhabdomyosarcoma from skeletal muscle Liposarcoma from fat
Melanoma	Malignant melanocytic tumour	Malignant melanoma
Lymphoma	Malignant tumour of lymphoid tissue	Hodgkin's lymphoma
Leukaemia	Malignant tumour of blood cells	Chronic lymphocytic leukaemia

exaggeration of microscopic features that define malignancy: cellular pleomorphism (variation in size and shape), hyperchromasia (dark staining nuclei), loss of polarity (loss of orientation to a basement membrane with disorganisation of architecture) and increased mitotic activity, including abnormal mitotic forms. In general, well-differentiated tumours grow slowly compared to tumours that are less differentiated.

Metastasis

Malignant neoplasms can spread to sites distant from the primary neoplasm to establish secondary neoplasms known as metastases. Metastases may arise via a number of routes[2,3]:

- *Lymphatic spread* – tumour cells may permeate lymph vessels and be carried in the lymph flow to lymph nodes. Metastases are first seen in the local draining lymph nodes and subsequently in more central lymph nodes. The 'sentinel' lymph node is the hypothetical first lymph node or group of nodes draining a cancer. It is postulated that the sentinel lymph node/s is/are the site of first spread by cancer cells from a tumour. Lymphatic spread is more common with carcinomas than with sarcomas.

- *Haematogenous spread* – tumour cells may permeate blood vessels and be carried in the circulation to distant sites. Common sites for the occurrence of haematogenous metastases are lung, liver, bone and brain. Sarcomas usually spread via the haematogenous route.

- *Transcoelomic spread* – tumours that involve the serosal surface of organs may disseminate

Table 30.4 General principles of tumour staging

Stage	Degree of tumour growth/spread
I	Tumour confined to the organ of origin
II	Local extension of the tumour beyond the site of origin to involve adjacent organs or structures
III	More extensive local involvement or infiltration of neighbouring organs
IV	Tumour with distant metastases

throughout the serous cavity and become implanted on other surfaces. For example, ovarian carcinomas frequently spread throughout the peritoneal cavity by this route.

- *Implantation metastases* – this may occur iatrogenically when malignant cells are left behind in the biopsy tract following biopsy of the tumour.

Staging of Malignant Tumours

The stage of a tumour is the measure of tumour growth and spread and is used to help determine treatment and prognosis. There are different staging systems for each type of tumour; however, for each system, there are general principles which are applied (Table 30.4).

Carcinoma in-situ: An intraepithelial proliferation of neoplastic cells that appear malignant on the basis of their cytological features but are confined within the epithelium by the basement membrane, i.e. there is no invasion and therefore currently no possibility of metastasis.

2.2 Cancer Biology: Pathogenesis of Neoplasms

Neoplastic change, especially malignant transformation, of cells occurs with disruption of cell cycle regulation. The cell cycle is regulated by growth factors which are soluble factors – autocrine when they affect the cell itself and paracrine when they affect neighbouring cells. Cancer cells can control this regulation by secreting growth factors or by increased expression of growth factor receptors. For example, HER2 (a type of epidermal growth factor) is over-expressed in some breast cancers and can be treated by blocking its receptor by trastuzumab (Herceptin).

The cell cycle is a series of highly regulated steps that lead to cell division and duplication of DNA to produce two daughter cells. There are four phases. G1 phase is when the cell undergoes changes to prepare for cell division. At a certain point – R or restriction point – the cell is committed to divide and moves to the S phase. S phase is defined by DNA synthesis that replicates genetic material. In the next phase – G2 – there is a check of the duplicated material to make repairs, if any, in readiness for division. The last phase – M (mitotic segregation) – cell division occurs.

Cyclin and cyclin-dependent kinases control progression in the G1 phase by phosphorylation of regulatory proteins. The regulators of the cell cycle are commonly mutated in cancers. Genes that stop cell cycle progression (tumour suppressor genes) are often downregulated or missing, and genes that promote the cell cycle (proto-oncogenes) are often upregulated or made constitutionally active. The end result is the ability of tumour cells to progress without restraint.

The accumulation of damaged DNA in a cell triggers intrinsic pro-apoptotic pathways. This is a self-protective pathway that is evaded by cancer cells; they do so by upregulation of anti-apoptotic proteins such as BCL-2 or downregulation of pro-apoptotic proteins such as p53.

Normal cells can divide only a limited number of times before they become senescent. The process of cell ageing is governed by telomere shortening such that, once the shortened telomeres reach a threshold, cell arrest is induced, thus allowing ageing cells to stop growing. Tumours contain an enzyme called telomerase that allows lengthening of telomeres. Such a cell evades senescence and continues to divide despite accumulated DNA damage.

In summary, a cancer cell acquires self-sufficiency in growth signals, insensitivity to anti-growth signals, evasion of apoptosis, limitless replicative potential, sustained angiogenesis and an ability to invade and metastasise.

2.3 Cancer Genetics

Cancer arises when a normal cell accumulates genetic mutations until a fully malignant cell is formed. This mutation may be acquired (e.g. caused by chemicals, viruses, irradiation, etc. – Tables 30.5 and 30.6) or inherited. There are two main categories of genetic change leading to cancer: the inactivation of tumour suppressor genes and the activation of proto-oncogenes.

Inactivation of Tumour Suppressor Genes

Tumour suppressor genes act to inhibit inappropriate cell growth and proliferation. p53 is an important

Table 30.5 Physical and chemical agents and the neoplasms they cause

Carcinogen	Neoplasm
Aflatoxin B1	Hepatocellular carcinoma
Asbestos	Mesothelioma
Aniline dyes	Bladder cancer
Anabolic steroids	Hepatocellular carcinoma
Wood dust	Adenocarcinoma of nose and nasal sinuses
Diethyl stilboestrol	Vaginal clear cell carcinoma in offspring
Alkylating agents	Leukaemias, lymphomas

Table 30.6 Oncogenic viruses and the neoplasms they cause

Virus	Neoplasm
HPV 16, 18	Cervical carcinoma
Epstein Barr virus	Nasopharyngeal carcinoma Burkitt's lymphoma
Hepatitis B virus	Hepatocellular carcinoma
HTLV-1	T-cell leukaemia/lymphoma

tumour suppressor gene, sometimes termed 'guardian of the genome'. Normally, DNA damage activates p53, which causes arrest of the cell cycle so that growth and proliferation of the damaged cell are inhibited. p53 may be rendered inactive by mutations or by binding to altered host gene products or viral gene products (e.g. the human papillomavirus (HPV) E6 protein). In the absence of p53 activity, cells with abnormal DNA replicate undisrupted. As they replicate they accumulate mutations which may eventually lead to cancer. Mutations of p53 are the most common type of mutation found in human cancer cells.[4] There are other genes that repair damaged DNA; BRCA and mismatch repair genes are examples of such caretaker genes. BRCA1 and 2 are the most commonly mutated genes in familial breast and ovarian cancer. Mismatch repair gene mutations are implicated in colorectal and endometrial cancer pathogenesis.

Activation of Proto-oncogenes

Proto-oncogenes (e.g. Ras) are host genes that stimulate cell growth and proliferation. As a result of mutations or the action of certain viruses, proto-oncogenes can be converted into carcinogenic oncogenes which promote excessive growth and proliferation.

Inherited Cancers

There are well-defined cancers in which inheritance of a single mutant gene increases the risk of developing a tumour. These are referred to as *inherited cancer syndromes*, and they include familial retinoblastomas, familial adenomatous polyps of the colon, multiple endocrine neoplasia syndrome and von Hippel

Lindau syndrome. Cancers that run in families are referred to as *familial cancers*; these include breast, ovarian and colon cancers. The role of the inherited risk cannot always be clearly defined in an individual case. A small group of autosomal recessive disorders is collectively characterised by chromosomal or DNA instability, and these individuals are predisposed to malignancies. These include xeroderma pigmentosum, ataxia-telangiectasia and Bloom's syndrome.

2.4 Tumour Markers (Table 30.7)

Tumour markers are biochemical indicators of the presence of a tumour and usually refer to a substance that can be detected in blood, plasma or other body fluids. These substances cannot be the primary modalities for the diagnosis of cancer; however, they can be used for:

- Screening for cancers
- Locating the primary in cases of disseminated disease
- Indication of response to therapy
- An early indicator of relapse

2.5 Paraneoplastic Syndromes

Paraneoplastic syndromes are symptom complexes in cancer patients. They may represent the earliest manifestation of an occult neoplasm or mimic metastatic disease. Some of the syndromes are characteristic of certain tumours (Table 30.8). Hypercalcaemia is probably the most common paraneoplastic syndrome.

2.6 Neoplasms of the Female Genital Tract

2.6.1 Cervix

Cervical Carcinoma

The two main malignant diseases arising within the cervix are *squamous cell carcinoma* and *adenocarcinoma*.

Table 30.7 Characteristic tumour markers used in clinical practice

Tumour marker	Neoplasm
Human chorionic gonadotropin (hCG)	Trophoblastic tumours, e.g. choriocarcinoma Non-seminomatous germ cell tumours
Alpha-feto protein (AFP)	Hepatocellular carcinoma Yolk sac tumour
Prostate-specific antigen (PSA)	Prostatic carcinoma
CA 125	Ovarian carcinoma Primary peritoneal carcinoma
Calcitonin	Medullary carcinoma of the thyroid
Immunoglobulins	Multiple myeloma
CEA	Colonic, pancreatic, lung, stomach carcinoma

Table 30.8 Paraneoplastic syndromes and their associated cancers

Syndrome	Associated neoplasm
Cushing's syndrome	Small cell lung carcinoma Pancreatic carcinoma
SIADH	Small cell lung carcinoma Intracranial neoplasms
Carcinoid syndrome	Bronchial adenoma Pancreatic carcinoma Gastric carcinoma
Polycythaemia	Renal cell carcinoma

The incidence of cervical carcinoma in developed countries is low in comparison to developing countries where cervical carcinoma is more common. This may be attributed to cervical screening programmes which enable early identification and treatment of precursor lesions before an established cancer has developed. The precursor lesion of cervical squamous cell carcinoma is *cervical intraepithelial neoplasia (CIN)* and that of adenocarcinoma is *cervical glandular intraepithelial neoplasia (CGIN)*.

The major risk factor for cervical carcinoma is HPV infection.[5] There are more than 100 subtypes of HPV. Some of these show a predilection for infecting the lower female genital tract, notably HPV 6, 11, 16 and 18. HPV 6 and 11 are implicated in benign condylomata and are rarely implicated in malignancy. HPV 16 and, to a lesser extent, HPV 18 are associated with an increased risk of high-grade CIN and cervical carcinomas. In addition to HPV infection, other factors which increase the risk of cervical carcinoma are smoking, concomitant sexually transmitted infections, greater number of sexual partners, lower age at first intercourse, high parity and oral contraceptives.

The area of the cervix where cancers arise is called the transformation zone. CIN and CGIN can be recognised in cervical smears and this forms the basis of the cervical screening programme. The aim of the programme is to reduce cervical carcinoma by detection and treatment of the pre-neoplastic disease. Treatment of pre-invasive conditions reduces the incidence of cervical carcinoma. Since 2012, *HPV testing* has been used

to triage borderline and low-grade abnormalities detected on cervical smears.[6] Triage allows HPV-negative women to revert to routine recall, as their risk of having significant disease is very low, and allows selection of the higher-risk women (i.e. HPV positive) to be referred for colposcopy. HPV testing is also used as a test of cure after treatment of high-grade abnormalities to check reversion to negative after treatment of CIN. In 2008 an *HPV vaccination programme* was introduced in the UK and is offered to girls from 12 to 18 years of age.[6]

2.6.2 Uterus

Endometrial Carcinoma

This is emerging as a disease of more affluent populations. Endometrial carcinomas are broadly categorised as Type 1 and Type 2 (Tables 30.9 and 30.10). Type 1 endometrial carcinoma is the commoner of the two and is associated with oestrogen excess. It is preceded by a condition known as endometrial hyperplasia. Endometrial hyperplasia can be typical and atypical. Atypical hyperplasia has a definite association with endometrioid carcinoma.

Carcinosarcoma (Malignant Mixed Müllerian Tumour)

These are biphasic malignant neoplasms composed of high-grade epithelial and high-grade mesenchymal components, i.e. carcinomatous and sarcomatous elements. They typically occur in postmenopausal women who usually present with abnormal vaginal bleeding. The carcinomatous component is usually serous or endometrioid in type. The sarcomatous component may comprise homologous elements (e.g. undifferentiated endometrial sarcoma, leiomyosarcoma) or heterologous elements (e.g. rhabdomyosarcoma, chondrosarcoma). Homologous sarcomatous elements are more common than heterologous elements. Regarding the histogenesis of these tumours, the malignant stromal

Table 30.9 Characteristics of type 1 and type 2 endometrial carcinoma

	Type 1	Type 2
Incidence	More common	Less common
Age predilection	Younger (pre- and peri-menopausal)	Older (post-menopausal)
Unopposed oestrogen stimulation	Yes	No
Other associations	Diabetes, hypertension, obesity, long-standing tamoxifen use	N/A
Precursor lesion	Endometrial hyperplasia	Serous endometrial intraepithelial carcinoma (SEIC)
Molecular abnormalities	PTEN and k-RAS mutations	p53 mutations
Prognosis	Relatively good	Relatively poor (more likely to present at an advanced stage)
Examples	Endometrioid carcinoma and its variants, mucinous carcinoma	Serous carcinoma, clear cell carcinoma, squamous cell carcinoma

Table 30.10 Types of endometrial hyperplasia and their microscopic features

Type	Microscopic features	Notes
Endometrial hyperplasia without atypia	• Proliferation of glands of varying size and shape • Increased gland-to-stroma ratio • No cytological atypia	• Old terminology: Simple hyperplasia without atypia; complex hyperplasia without atypia.
Atypical endometrial hyperplasia	• Similar features to those described above with superadded cytological atypia	• Old terminology: Simple atypical hyperplasia, complex atypical hyperplasia • Associated with a greater risk of carcinoma than endometrial hyperplasia without atypia

component is thought to be derived from the malignant epithelial component.[7] These tumours are associated with a poor prognosis.

Endometrial Stromal Sarcomas

Endometrial stromal sarcomas are divided into low-grade endometrial stromal sarcomas (low-grade ESSs) and high-grade ESSs. LGESSs are composed of cells which resemble those of proliferative phase endometrial stroma and show permeative growth into the myometrium. They often contain chromosomal rearrangements that result in JAZF1-SUZ12 fusion.[8] These tumours most commonly occur in peri-menopausal women and present with non-specific symptoms such as vaginal bleeding, pelvic pain and dysmenorrhoea. High-grade ESSs are rare malignant tumours of the endometrial stroma which are composed of cells with high-grade, round cell morphology. They often show destructive invasion into the myometrium. These tumours often harbour YWHAE-NUTM2A/B genetic fusions.[8] High-grade ESSs most commonly occur in pre- and post-menopausal women, and most often present with abnormal vaginal bleeding. High-grade ESS are clinically more aggressive than low-grade ESSs.

Undifferentiated Uterine Sarcoma

These tumours are rare and typically occur in post-menopausal patients. They lack any resemblance to proliferative phase endometrial stroma, have high-grade cytological features and show no specific type of differentiation. These are highly aggressive malignant tumours and have a very poor prognosis (< 2 years).[1]

Leiomyosarcoma

This is a malignant smooth muscle tumour and represents the malignant counterpart of leiomyoma. They account for 1–2% of all uterine malignancies and most commonly occur in women over the age of 50. The incidence is increased in patients who are taking tamoxifen therapy for breast cancer. Common symptoms include abnormal vaginal bleeding, pelvic pain and a pelvic mass. Leiomyosarcomas have a poor prognosis even when confined to the uterus at the time of initial diagnosis.[1]

2.6.3 Ovary

A plethora of tumour types is seen in the ovary. These include epithelial tumours, sex cord-stromal tumours, germ cell tumours, miscellaneous tumours and metastatic tumours.

Primary Epithelial Ovarian Carcinomas

These are the commonest ovarian malignancy and can be of many different epithelial types. Ovarian carcinomas are divided into two groups, designated type I and type II:

Type I tumours are slow growing, generally confined to the ovary at diagnosis, and develop from well-established precursor lesions that are termed *borderline tumours*. They are genetically stable and are characterized by mutations in a number of different genes, including KRAS, BRAF, PTEN and alpha-catenin.[1] Type I tumours include mucinous, endometrioid carcinomas and low-grade serous carcinomas.

Type II tumours are rapidly growing highly aggressive neoplasms for which well-defined precursor lesions have not been described. Type II tumours have a high level of genetic instability and are characterized by mutation of the tumour suppressor gene, p53.[1] They often present late, and spread to the omentum is common. Type II tumours include high-grade serous carcinoma, which is the most common ovarian epithelial carcinoma. High-grade serous carcinoma is a distinct entity from low-grade serous carcinoma and does not arise from the transformation of low-grade serous carcinoma. There is an increasing acceptance that most ovarian high-grade serous carcinomas arise from a precursor lesion called serous tubal intraepithelial carcinoma (STIC), usually found in the fimbriae of the fallopian tube, and from there spreads secondarily to the ovary.[9,10]

Risk factors for ovarian cancers include nulliparity and family history. Women from families with the BRCA gene are monitored with imaging and serum CA125 studies because of the increased risk of ovarian cancer. These families also have an increased risk of cancers of the fallopian tube and the peritoneum.

Sex Cord-Stromal Tumours

The commonest malignant sex cord-stromal tumour is the adult type of granulosa cell tumour. They are usually unilateral tumours and can be haemorrhagic. These tumours are characterised by their propensity for late recurrence.

Germ Cell Tumours

Germ cell tumours constitute 15% to 20% of all ovarian tumours. Benign mature cystic teratomas, also known as ovarian dermoid cysts, are common ovarian neoplasms and occur at all ages. Other tumours in this category are seen mainly in children and young adults.

Metastatic Tumours

The ovary is a common site for metastatic tumours, some of which can closely mimic primary ovarian cancers and pose problems for the pathologist. The commonest tumours presenting as metastatic carcinomas are from the uterus, colon, stomach, biliary tract and pancreas. The classic example of metastatic gastrointestinal neoplasia to the ovaries is termed Krukenberg tumour and defines bilateral ovarian enlargement with diffuse infiltrating malignant cells containing intracellular mucin.

2.6.4 Fallopian Tube

High-Grade Serous Carcinoma

High-grade serous carcinoma is the most common subtype of fallopian tube carcinoma and, as mentioned previously, arises from a precursor lesion known as STIC. These carcinomas show mutation of the p53 gene, resulting in an aberrant immunophenotype with p53 immunohistochemistry (i.e. diffuse, strong positive staining or a complete absence of staining). As mentioned previously, most high-grade serous carcinomas in the ovary are now thought to arise within the fallopian tube.[9,10]

2.6.5 Vulva

Squamous cell carcinoma (SCC) is the commonest epithelial malignancy of the vulva. The appearances are similar to squamous carcinomas elsewhere in the body. The prognosis is determined by the size, depth of invasion, degree of differentiation and the presence and extent of nodal metastases. The inguinal lymph nodes are commonly affected. Carcinomas invading to a depth of less than 1 mm are sometimes referred to as superficially invasive and have virtually no risk of metastasis.

The pre-invasive condition of vulval SCC is termed *vulvar intraepithelial neoplasia (VIN)*. Two distinct types of VIN are recognised: classical VIN (also sometimes referred to as uVIN or usual type VIN) and differentiated VIN (dVIN).

Paget's disease of the vulva is a rare disease occurring almost exclusively in post-menopausal women and histologically characterised by the presence of mucin containing malignant cells within the epithelium of the vulva. In most cases, there is no association with invasion, although rarely it may be a spread from an underlying adnexal malignancy.

2.6.6 Vagina

The pre-invasive condition of vaginal squamous cell carcinoma is termed *vaginal intraepithelial neoplasia (VaIN)*. VaIN is much less common than CIN or VIN. It is associated with high-risk HPV infection and may co-exist with VIN (of classical type) and CIN, reflecting the multicentric nature of the viral associated disease.

Sarcoma botyroides is the term given to embryonal rhabdomyosarcoma of the vagina that occurs in children before the age of five. The term refers to the macroscopic appearance of a polypoid mass that fills the vagina of the affected child and bears a resemblance to a bunch of grapes (*botyroides* means 'grape-like' in Greek).

References

1. Mutter G, Prat J, eds. *Pathology of the Female Genital Tract*. 3rd ed. Churchill Livingstone, 2014.

2. Kumar V, Abbas AK, Aster JC. *Robbins and Cotran Pathologic Basis of Disease*. 9th ed. Elsevier Saunders, 2014.

3. Underwood JCE, Cross SS. *General and Systemic Pathology*. 5th ed. Churchill Livingstone, 2009.

4. Lane DP. p53 and human tumours. *Br Med Bull*. 1994;**50**:582–599.

5. Stoler MH. Human papillomaviruses and cervical neoplasia: a model for carcinogenesis. *Int J Gynaecol Pathol*. 2000;**19**:16–28.

6. Pignatelli M, Gallagher P, eds. Molecular testing for human papilloma virus. In *Recent Advances in Histopathology 23*, ed. Denton K, pp. 159–167. JP Medical Ltd, 2014.

7. Sreenan JJ, Hart WR. Carcinosarcomas of the female genital tract. A pathologic study of 29 metastatic tumours: further evidence for the dominant role of the epithelial component and the conversion theory of histogenesis. *Am J Surg Pathol*. 1995;**19**:666–674.

8. Lee C-H, Nucci MR. Endometrial stroma sarcoma – the new genetic paradigm. *Histopathology*. 2015;**67**:1–19.

9. Kurman RJ, Shih I-M. The origin and pathogenesis of epithelial ovarian cancer: a proposed unifying theory. *Am J Surg Pathol*. 2010;**34**:433–443.

10. Salvador S, Gilks B, Kobel M, Huntsman D, Rosen B, Miller D. The fallopian tube: primary site of most pelvic high-grade serous carcinomas. *Int J Gynecol Cancer*. 2009;**19**:58–64.

Single Best Answer Questions

1. Which one of the following statements is not correct?

   a. A leiomyoma is a benign tumour of skeletal muscle

   b. A liposarcoma is a malignant tumour of adipose tissue

   c. A tubular adenoma is a benign tumour of the large bowel

   d. A transitional cell carcinoma is a malignant epithelial tumour

   e. A seminoma is a malignant testicular tumour

2. Which one of the following is not a characteristic of a malignant neoplasm?

   a. Capacity to metastasise

   b. Show invasion through the basement membrane

   c. Well-defined capsule

   d. Rapid growth rate

   e. Infiltrative

3. Which one of the following conditions has a higher than average risk of developing cancer?

   a. Human papillomavirus infection of the cervix

   b. Hepatitis B

   c. Schistosomiasis of the bladder

   d. Inflammatory bowel disease

   e. Addison's disease

4. Which one of following combinations of ovarian tumours and their histogenesis is incorrect?

   a. Adult granulosa cell tumour – sex cord-stromal tumour

   b. Embryonal carcinoma – surface epithelial tumour

   c. Mature teratoma – germ cell tumour

   d. Brenner tumour – surface epithelial tumour

   e. Krukenberg tumour – metastatic tumour

Implantation and Placental Structure and Function

Karin Leslie

1 Overview

Human pregnancy is characterized by haemomono-chorial placentation (where only a single layer of trophoblast tissue separates the mother's and fetal blood), with earlier and deeper invasion into the maternal decidua and myometrium than in any other mammalian species.

- The placenta is fetal in origin
- An organ unique to pregnancy
- Vital during pregnancy for waste exchange, oxygen delivery and fetal nutrition
- 500–1000 kg at term
- Acts as an endocrine organ releasing hormones into the maternal circulation

2 Decidualization and Implantation

Highly orchestrated events that occur in a narrow window of endometrial receptivity.

Failure of normal decidualization linked to miscarriage, recurrent pregnancy loss, failed IVF cycles.

2.1 Decidualisation

- Occurs in the late secretory phase of the menstrual cycle
- 6 days before implantation
- In contrast, in most other mammalian species, decidualization is triggered by implantation

2.2 Cellular Changes of Decidualization

2.2.1 Epithelial Cells

- Lose polarity and develop pinopodes
- Become more secretory
- Secrete a number of factors to signal the blastocyst: LIF, IL-11 (known as the Gp130 cytokines), EGF, HB-EGF
- Develop a number of proteins for blastocyst attachment: integrins $\alpha V\beta 3$, $\alpha 4\beta 1$
- Express mucins: a barrier to trophoectoderm

2.2.2 Stromal Cells

- Grow in size
- Become secretory
- Start making cytokines, growth factors and extracellular matrix
- Secrete a number of factors that will control trophoblast invasion after implantation: IGFBP-1, prolactin
- Key in determining depth of invasion of trophoblast

2.2.3 Immune Cells

- Influx of natural killer cells, T cells and macrophages

2.2.4 Uterine Blood Vessels, Including Spiral Arteries

- Become more permeable
- New angiogenesis
- Essential to support the developing fetus and to prepare for the invading placenta

3 Implantation (Fig. 31.1)

3.1 Pre-attachment

Blastocyst hormonal signals:

- Endocrine: βHCG signalling to mother. Acts on corpus luteum to maintain pregnancy by progesterone production
- Paracrine: crosstalk between mother and blastocyst: secreted signals and adhesion signals (integrins, HSPGs, MUC1). A number of maternal signals are produced which both contribute to

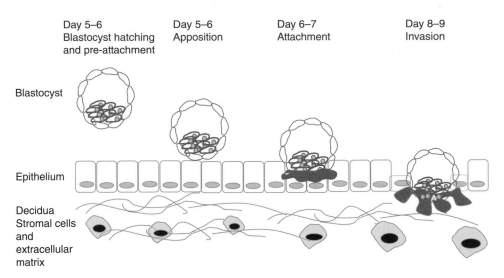

Day 5–6
Blastocyst hatching
and pre-attachment

Day 5–6
Apposition

Day 6–7
Attachment

Day 8–9
Invasion

Blastocyst

Epithelium

Decidua
Stromal cells
and
extracellular
matrix

Figure 31.1 Implantation

decidualisation and signal to the blastocyst: LIF, IL-11, prokineticins

3.2 Apposition

The initial unstable adherence of the outer layer of the blastocyst (trophoblast) to the decidualised epithelial cells.

- Embryonic pole (inner cell mass – ICM) orientates toward endometrium
- Maternal factors play a role in adhesion: LIF, IL11, integrins

3.3 Attachment

Stabilisation of the attachment of the blastocyst to the uterine wall by the outer layer of the blastocyst.

- Integrins and other factors 'cellular glue' → firm attachment
- The beginning of the penetration of the syncytiotrophoblast through the endometrial epithelial cells

3.4 Invasion

Described later in this chapter.

4 Oxygen Tension in Early Pregnancy

- Up until 12th week, the uterine spiral arteries are plugged with trophoblasts

- Placental development therefore occurs under relative hypoxia (2–3% O_2)
- Doppler ultrasound, hysteroscopy and perfusion of pregnant hysterectomy specimens all support highly restricted maternal blood flow to the placenta prior to 10–12 weeks of gestation
- May protect embryo during organogenesis from teratogenic free radicals

5 Early Embryonic Nutrition

- Free-living blastocyst reliant on cytoplasm inherited from the oocyte (maternal)
- Histotrophic; blastocyst is bathed in uterine secretions (from implantation day 8–9)
- Haemotrophic; vascular contact between mother and fetus (from week 10–12)

6 Development of the Placenta

Four Key Steps

- Differentiation of the trophoblast
- Trophoblastic invasion of decidua and inner third of myometrium
- Remodelling of the maternal vasculature in the utero-placental circulation
- Development of mature villous structure and fetal vasculature within villi

6.1 Trophoblast Cell Lineage (Fig. 31.2)

6.2 Invasion

- Interstitial extravillous trophoblast (EVT) invade through the decidua and inner myometrium
- Endovascular EVT migrate up the lumen of spiral arteries
- Trophoblast migrate through the extracellular matrix produced by stromal cells by producing digestive proteases
- Up-regulate a number of matrix metalloproteases (MMPs)
- MMP-2 and MMP-9 are important for movement through the decidua
- MMPs are inhibited by tissue-inhibitors of metalloproteases (TIMPs)
- TIMPs produced by stromal cells to control invasion

6.3 Spiral Artery Remodelling

- EVT invade the vessel interstitially and from the lumen

- Replace the maternal endothelium and break down the vascular smooth muscle layer
- EVT 'switch' from an epithelial to endothelial phenotype
- Leads to a loss of smooth muscle and endothelial lining
- Results in dilation of the vessel and loss of vasoreactivity
- Converts vessel into low pressure, high capacity, flaccid conduit
- Failure of conversion is associated with complications such as preeclampsia and growth restriction

6.4 Villous Structure

- Highly branched to increase surface area for exchange
- Growth is regulated by a number of factors, including IGF I and II

6.4.1 Syncytiotrophoblast (STB)

- Multinucleated and terminally differentiated

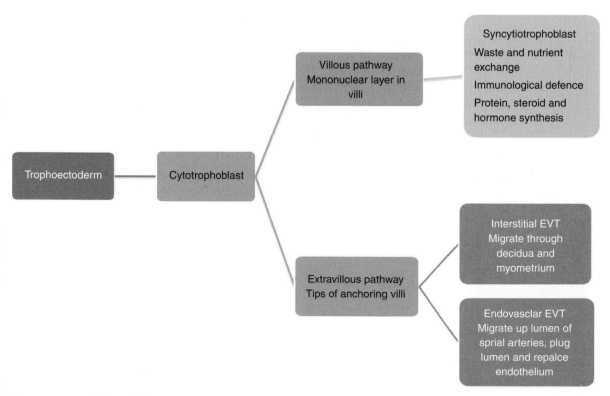

Figure 31.2 Trophoblast cell lineage

- STB forms a single layer – derived from the underlying cytotrophoblast stem cells
- Formed by cell fusion; requires Glial Cells Missing 1 (GCM1), syncytin-1 and -2 and caspase-8
- Endocrine and paracrine organ, syncytium secrete hormones, including hCG into maternal circulation

6.4.2 Cytotrophoblast

- Uninucleated
- Progenitor cells that differentiate and fuse with the syncytium

6.4.3 Types of Villi

- Stem villus – supporting framework
- Intermediate villus – distributing framework
- Terminal villus – functional unit

Large increase in surface area over gestation (10–16 m2) facilitates exchange.Microvilli provide further amplification by a factor of ~ 7.

6.4.4 Fetal Vasculature Development

- Early gestation – branching angiogenesis driven by vascular endothelial growth factor (VEGF)
- Followed by non-branching angiogenesis driven by placental growth factor (PlGF)
- Fetal circulation separated from maternal blood by STB
- Poor vascular development is associated with fetal growth restriction, pre-eclampsia and early pregnancy loss

7 The Mature Placenta

- The villi are arranged into 40–60 lobules
- Each lobule is centred over the opening of a spiral artery
- Each lobule acts as an independent materno-fetal exchange unit
- 500–1000 kg at term

8 Functions of the Placenta

- Materno-fetal transport and vice versa
- Hormone synthesis
- Barrier to vertical transmission of pathogens

8.1 Placental Transport (Fig. 31.3 and Table 31.1)

8.1.1 Gaseous Exchange

- Syncytiotrophoblast is highly active metabolically and occurs down a concentration gradient
- The placenta consumes at least one-third of the O2 supplied to the feto-placental unit
- The development of specialised regions allows the demands of placenta and fetus to be arranged in parallel rather than in series, thereby improving fetal oxygenation
- Rate proportional to surface area and inversely proportional to the thickness of the villous membrane

8.1.1.1 How Is Efficient Oxygen Transfer Achieved?

- Large surface area (16 m^2 at term) with microvilli
- Very thin villous membrane
- Higher oxygen affinity of fetal haemoglobin (HbF) than adult Hb
- Placental double Bohr effect
  - Bohr effect: oxygen dissociation curve shifts to right with fall in pH

8.1.2 Facilitated Diffusion

- Occurs down concentration gradient
- Proteins embedded in the plasma membrane increase the rate of transport
- ATP-independent

8.1.3 Active Transport

Amino acid transport is ATP-dependent.

For most AA, the fetal/maternal plasma ratio is greater than 1, so the amino acids are actively transported against the gradient.

Three main carrier systems:

Table 31.1 Placental transport

Passive diffusion	Respiratory gases, free fatty acids, urea
Facilitated diffusion	Glucose
Active transport	Amino acids
Receptor-mediated endocytosis	IgG

Maternal side

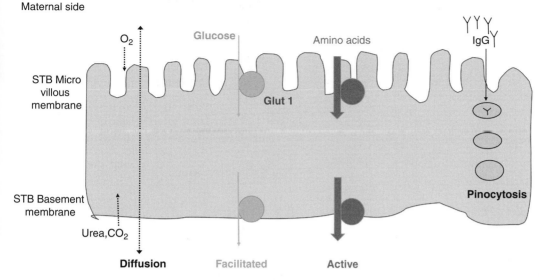

Figure 31.3 Placental transport

- Systems A and ASC
  - Na+-dependent
  - open to neutral AA such as alanine, glycine
- System XAG
  - Na+-dependent
  - selective for acidic AA such as aspartate and glutamate
- System L
  - Na+-independent
  - open to neutral AA such as leucine and phenylalanine
- Na+/H+ exchange pumps restore sodium balance

8.1.4 Receptor-Mediated Endocytosis

- Immunoglobulin transport selective for IgG
- Occurs from 35 weeks onwards against a concentration gradient
- Receptors on microvilli bind IgG and concentrate in the coated pits
- Which are nipped off and move into cytoplasm
- Also known as pinocytosis

9 Placental Hormone Synthesis

9.1 Progesterone

- Placental from 6–9 weeks onwards

- 200 mg/day by late pregnancy
- Maternal cholesterol complexed to LDL receptor on STB
- Metabolised in STB to pregnenolone, then progesterone
- No known regulatory pathway, though oestrogen may promote
- Effects
  - decidualization (the progesterone comes from the corpus luteum at this stage)
  - smooth muscle relaxation – uterine quiescence
  - mineralocorticoid effect – cardiovascular changes
  - breast development

9.2 Oestrogens (Fig. 31.4)

- Placenta cannot synthesise oestrogens alone and operates in concert with the fetal adrenal glands
- E3 > E2 > E1 (oestriol > oestradiol > oestrone)
- Rely on androgens from fetus and maternal adrenals
- DHEAS and 16 OH DHEAS metabolised by STB
- Effects
  - development of uterine hypertrophy
  - metabolic changes (insulin resistance)
  - cardiovascular changes
  - breast development

307

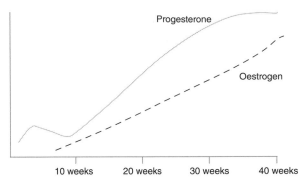

Figure 31.4 Progesterone and oestrogen concentration

Levels reflect placental mass and are not a reliable test of placental function.

9.3 Human Chorionic Gonadotrophin (hCG)

- Glycoprotein with two non-covalently linked subunits
- Alpha subunit as in FSH, LH and TSH
- Beta subunit very similar to LH
- Synthesised in the syncytium
- Control unknown but synthesis of beta subunit is rate-limiting
- Acts on LH receptors in corpus luteum and fetal testis – maintains progesterone levels

9.4 Human Placental Lactogen (hPL)

- 96% sequence homology with growth hormone but less growth-promoting effects
- Synthesised in the syncytium
- Raises maternal FFAs
- Antagonises peripheral effects of insulin and thus raises blood glucose levels
- Induces differentiation of mammary glandular tissues

9.5 Placental Growth Hormone (PGH)

- Differs from pituitary growth hormone by only 13 amino acids
- Synthesised in syncytium and suppresses maternal pituitary growth hormone secretion by 10–20 weeks
- Strong growth-promoting effects
- Key regulator of maternal IGF I levels

10 Umbilical Cord

- Formed at 5 weeks' gestation
- Normally contains 3 vessels
  - 2 arteries (away from fetus)
  - 1 vein (toward fetus)
- Vessels surrounded by Wharton's jelly
- Arteries arise from internal iliac arteries
- Veins drain into ductus venosus, then IVC to RA
- At term, mean length 50 cm, diameter 2 cm

10.1 Funisitis

- Neutrophils present in cord
- Usually migrated from fetal circulation toward infected amniotic fluid
- Associated with chorioamnionitis

10.2 Variations/Pathology

- Eccentric cord insertion
- Velamentous cord insertion (cord inserts into membranes rather than placental surface)
- Vasa praevia – fetal vessels run in the membranes in the lower segment. Associated with a previously low lying placenta, succenturiate lobe; incidence higher in IVF pregnancies

11 Placental Pathology

- Abruption
  - Premature separation of the placenta
  - Occurs in approximately 1% of pregnancies
  - Haemorrhage into the decidua basalis
  - More common in pregnancies with impaired placentation (preeclampsia, growth restriction, chronic hypertension)
- Infarction
  - Ischaemic villous necrosis
  - Interruption of maternal blood supply to a localized area
  - Small infarcts common at term
  - Loss of larger areas causes placental insufficiency
  - Associated with diabetic microangiopathy, hypertension, autoimmune disease, malaria, post mature pregnancies

11.1 Molar Pregnancy

- Oedematous villi – 'bunch of grapes' appearance
- 'Snowstorm' on early ultrasound
- Trophoblastic hyperplasia
- Possible embryonic fragments
- Proliferation correlates with outcome

11.2 Morbidly Adherent Placentation

Abnormally adherent chorionic villi. Associated with previous Caesarean section or uterine surgery.

- Placenta accreta
  - ○ Chorionic villi penetrate into the myometrial layer
- Placenta increta
  - ○ Villi penetrate deep into the myometrial layer to the serosa
- Placental percreta
  - ○ Villi penetrate through the myometrium into subperitoneum/other organs (bladder, etc)

Single Best Answer Questions

1. Which remodelling changes occur in the spiral arteries during pregnancy?
   a. Spiral arteries lose their smooth muscle layer, increase their lumen and are converted into high resistance vessels
   b. Spiral arteries lose their smooth muscle layer, increase their lumen and are converted into low resistance vessels
   c. Spiral arteries lose their smooth muscle layer, reduce their lumen and are converted into low resistance vessels
   d. Spiral arteries relax their muscle tone, increase their lumen and are converted into low resistance vessels
   e. Spiral arteries increase their muscle tone, reduce their lumen and are converted into high resistance vessels

2. Which structure is the primary chorionic villi derived from?
   a. Extraembryonic mesoderm
   b. Cytotrophoblast
   c. Syncytiotrophoblast
   d. Decidua
   e. Decidua basalis

3. Which structure is the secondary chorionic villi derived from?
   a. Extraembryonic mesoderm
   b. Cytotrophoblast
   c. Syncytiotrophoblast
   d. Decidua
   e. Decidua basalis

4. By which mechanism is the placental uptake of glucose carried out?
   a. Sodium exchange pump
   b. Sodium and potassium exchange pump
   c. Facilitated diffusion
   d. Carried molecule co-transport
   e. Simple diffusion

5. By which mechanism does immunoglobulin (IgG) cross the placenta from mother to fetus?
   a. Active transport
   b. Facilitated diffusion
   c. Osmosis
   d. Pinocytosis
   e. Simple diffusion

6. Which placental structure is the intervillous space derived from?
   a. Extraembryonic mesoderm
   b. Cytotrophoblast
   c. Syncytiotrophoblast
   d. Decidua
   e. Lacunae

7. How many layers does the amnion consist of?
   a. One
   b. Two
   c. Three
   d. Four
   e. Five

8. Which type of HLA antigen is predominantly expressed on trophoblast?
   a. HLA B1
   b. HLA G
   c. HLA F
   d. HLA B12
   e. HLA E

Basic and Reproductive Immunology

Karin Leslie

1 Overview (Table 32.1)

2 Innate Immune System

2.1 Mechanisms of Innate Immunity

2.1.1 Barriers

- Mechanical barriers: skin, mucous membranes, cilia
- Surface secretions: gastric acid, sebaceous secretions/sweat
- Bactericidal substances secreted
  - lysozyme-tissue fluids (tears, sweat, urine; not CSF) and in cytoplasmic granules of polymorphic neutrophils. Split polysaccharides of bacterial cell walls
  - Spermine/spermidine cleave NH2 groups

2.1.2 Normal Bacterial Flora ('Microbiota')

Commensal organisms

- 10^{12} in skin (staphs/streps)
- 10^{14} in gut (bacteroides + others)
- Cause opportunistic infection

Lactobacilli in vagina

- reduce pH (pH = 4) by fermenting glycogen

Table 32.1 Overview of basic immunology

Innate	Acquired
Non-specific	Specific and diverse
No memory	Has memory
Immediate maximal response	Time lag to max response (days)
Cell-mediated components: Phagocytes and natural killer cells	T cells, B cells
Humoral components: Complement	Antibody

2.2 Complement

- Humoral component of the innate immune system (can be recruited by the acquired)
- Serum proteins
  - Approximately 20 in number
  - Glycoproteins, abundant, make up 5% of serum proteins
  - Abundant in the liver, intestinal epithelium, spleen, macrophages
- Enzyme cascade (analogous to the coagulation cascade)
  - Circulate as inactive proenzymes with cleavage, resulting in the active form and amplification at each step

2.2.1 Functions of the Complement Cascade

- Makes bacteria more susceptible to phagocytosis
- Directly lyses some bacteria and foreign cells
- Produces chemotactic substances (attracts phagocytes)
- Increases vascular permeability
- Causes smooth muscle contraction, promoting mast cell degranulation

2.2.2 Three Pathways

- Classical
  - Requires antigen-antibody binding
  - Highly efficient
  - Links to acquired immune system
- Alternative pathway
  - Antibody not required
  - Activated by amine and hydroxyl groups on cell surface of pathogens
  - Inefficient, as high concentrations of components needed

- Lectin (mannose-binding lectin) pathway
- Antibody not required
- Activated by glycoprotein groups on cell surface of pathogens (many Gram-positive and -negative bacteria)
- More efficient than the alternative

All three pathways generate C3 convertase

- Cleaves the most abundant circulating complement protein C3
- Sequential interaction with C5-9
- Formation of a membrane attack complex
- Lyses target cells

2.3 Cells of the Innate Immune System

Phagocytes – derived from bone marrow

- Engulf particulate or soluble material (pinocytosis)
- Bind microorganisms by membrane receptors
- Contain digestive enzymes
- Attracted by chemokines and activated by cytokines secreted by antigen-specific T cells
- Link between innate and acquired systems

2.3.1 Monocyte/Macrophage Lineage

Monocytes

- Short-lived cells (few hours) circulating in the blood
- Express 3 different receptors for the Fc region of IgG and also complement receptors
- Migrate into tissues and differentiate into mature macrophages

Tissue macrophages

- Long-lived
- Bind microorganisms that are coated with antibodies (Fc receptors) or complement (complement receptors)
- Then phagocytose, kill, break down and process pathogens
- Present internalized broken down pathogens as peptides to T cells, triggering the adaptive response

2.3.2 Granulocytes

- Neutrophils
  - Found in blood, most abundant circulating leucocyte (50–70% of total)
  - Short-lived (days)
  - Activated through Fc (for IgG) or complement receptors
  - Recognize and kill pathogens (mainly bacteria) by phagocytosis or by releasing cytotoxic granules
- Dendritic cells
  - Professional antigen presenting cells (APC)
  - Capture, process and present antigen to T cells
- Mast cells
  - Found in skin, mucosal surfaces and around blood vessels
  - Express receptors specific for Fc region of IgE
  - Release prostaglandins, histamine, heparin, variety of cytokines and chemokines and other mediators
  - May induce or control inflammation in surrounding tissues
- Basophils
  - Found circulating in blood
  - Similar to mast cells; express receptors for IgE
  - May not be phagocytic
- Eosinophils
  - Found near respiratory and gut epithelia
  - Highly specialized response to parasitic invaders such as schistosomes
  - Attach to surface of parasite and then degranulate
  - Release proteins that damage the parasite cell membrane and cytokines to amplify the immune response

2.3.3 Natural Killer Cells

- Large granulocyte lymphocytes
- Distinct cell population expressing killer-cell immunoglobulin-like receptors (KIRs) and classification determinant (CD) receptors
- Cytotoxic against virally infected cells and tumour cells
- Healthy cells expressing normal 'self' class 1 MHC molecules protected from NK cytotoxicity
- Activated by cytokines secreted by activated T cells
- Peripheral NK cells CD16 bright
- Decidual NK cells CD56 bright CD16 dim

3 Acquired (Adaptive) Immunity

Four fundamental features:

- Memory (do not get the same infection twice)
- Specificity (differentiate between different organisms)
- Diversity (mount a response to many different pathogens)
- Self-tolerance (able to distinguish between self and foreign antigens; breaks down in autoimmune disorders)

3.1 Major Histocompatibility Complex (MHC)

- Genes coding for MHC map to chromosome 6 (6p21.3)
- Encode the HLA antigens (glycoproteins) found on the surface of cells
- Responsible for recognition of 'self'

3.1.1 Class I

'Classic' HLA-A, B and C

- Constitutively expressed
- All nucleated cells
- Highly polymorphic (300–900 alleles)

'Non-classical' HLA E, F and G

- Restricted expression
- Limited polymorphism
- HLA-G expression limited to invasive cytotrophoblast

Role in acquired immunity:

- Present protein fragments to CD8+ cytotoxic T cells
- Short peptides (8–9 amino acids long)
- Derived from inside the cell (cytoplasm)
- Endogenous Ag, e.g. viruses

3.1.2 Class II MHC

HLA-DR, DQ and DP

Highly polymorphic (>800 alleles)

Expressed on specialised antigen-presenting cell (APC) (see next section)

Role in acquired immunity:

- Present Ag fragment to CD4+ helper T cells
- Longer peptides (15–24 amino acids long)
- Derived from outside the cell
- Exogenous Ag, e.g. bacteria

3.2 Antigen-Presenting Cells (APC)

- Express class II MHC on cell surface
  - Macrophages
  - Dendritic cells of lymphoid tissue
  - Langerhans cells in skin
  - B lymphocytes
- Produce interleukin-1
- Take up and process the antigen into peptides which form a complex with class II MHC
- Then present to T helper cells and trigger immune response

3.3 B Cells

- Develop in bone marrow and found in all lymphoid tissue
- Express class II MHC on cell surface
- Produce interleukin-1
- Take up and process the antigen
- Presented to Ag-specific T cells which secrete cytokines and induce clonal B cell proliferation and differentiation into antibody-producing plasma cells

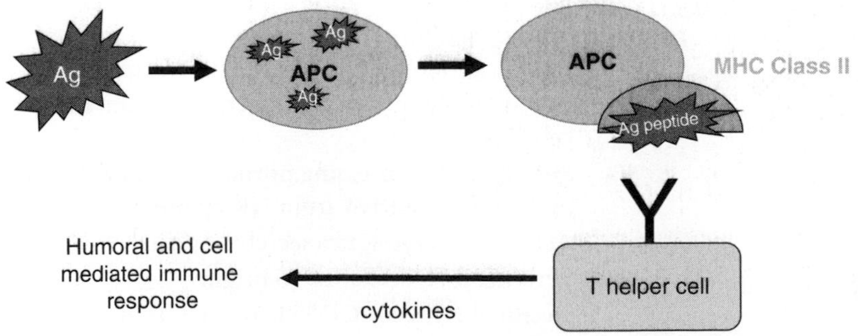

Figure 32.1 Antigen-presenting cells

Table 32.2 The five classes of antibodies in mammals.

Type	IgG	IgA	IgM	IgD	IgE
Heavy chain	Gamma	Alpha	Mu	Delta	Epsilon
Mol weight	150,000	160,000–400,000	900,000	180,000	190,000
Serum (mg/ml)	13.5	3	1.5	0.03	0.0003
Placental transfer	Yes	No	No	No	No
Notes	Binds to phagocyte Fc receptors	In mucosal secretions	Pentamer, largely confined to intravascular pool	Functions as transmembrane Ag receptor on mature B cells	Induces mast cell degranulation, involved in allergic reactions
Proportion of serum immunoglobulin pool (%)	70–80	10–20	5–10	<0.5	Very low in serum

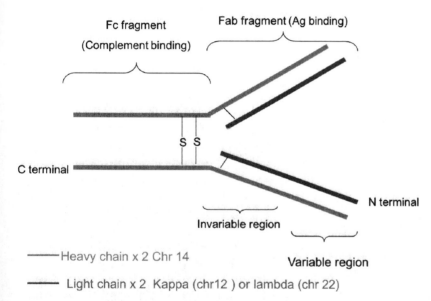

Figure 32.2 Antibody structure

3.4 Antibodies

- Also known as immunoglobulins
- Effective against extracellular bacteria and circulating viruses
- Five classes in mammals (see Table 32.2)
- All made up of two identical light chains and two identical heavy chains (Fig. 32.2)

3.5 Vaccination

- Pathogens modified so they are innocuous
- Primary antibody response triggered by epitope of modified pathogen
- Vaccine replaces initial infection and generation of memory B cells occurs

3.6 T Cells (Fig. 32.3)

- Principal mediators of acquired immunity
- May directly lyse target cells or activate other immune cells via cytokine release
- Immature T cells generated in the bone marrow and mature in the thymus to either helper or cytotoxic T cells
- Then migrate to secondary lymphoid tissue or circulating/peripheral tissues

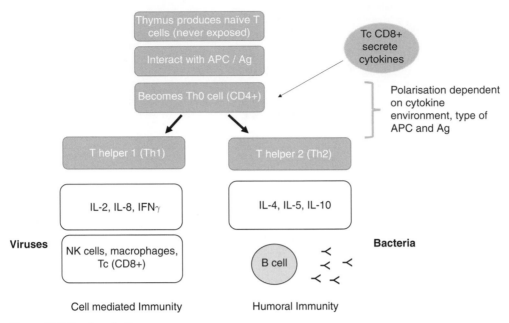

Figure 32.3 T cell production

3.6.1 T Helper Cells (CD4 Positive)

- CD4 transmembrane protein serves as cell adhesion molecule on binding T cell receptor (TCR) to MHC II complex with APC
- Either T helper 1 (Th1) or T helper 2 (Th2); type dependent on the environment around the cell

In pregnancy, a shift to Th2 cells occurs (placenta produces IL-4 and IL-10, promoting shift), resulting in:

- Suppression of cell-mediated immunity
- Increased susceptibility to viral (influenza, varicella) and intracellular pathogens

3.6.2 T Cytotoxic Cells (CD8 Positive)

- Cytolytic function
- Kill tumour and virally infected cells
- MHC Class I restricted
- Secrete patterns of cytokines that can promote either Th1 or Th2 polarization

4 Transplant Immunology

4.1 Types of Grafts

- Autologous (self), e.g. skin grafts
- Syngeneic (identical twin)
- Allogeneic (another human except identical twin), e.g. cadaveric or live donor renal transplant
- Xenogeneic (one species to another), e.g. pig heart transplant in human

4.2 Graft versus Host Disease

Donor T cells in the graft (e.g. bone marrow) initiate an immune response against the host.

Systemic effects:

- Skin – maculopapular rash, skin bullae and necrosis
- Hepatic – transaminitis, hyperbilirinaemia
- Gastrointestinal – mucositis, diarrhoea and vomiting

Prerequisites:

- Immuno-incompetent host
- Infusion of competent donor T cells
- HLA disparity between host and donor

4.3 Rejection

Methods to prevent rejection (Table 32.3)

- HLA matching between donor and recipient
- Immunosuppressive drugs

Table 32.3 Types of rejection

Type of rejection	Time scale	Cells involved	Mechanism
Hyperacute	Minutes to hours	Preformed antibodies react to antigens on donor cells (ABO incompatibility or sensitization to donor MHC)	Antibody binding initiates immunological cascade, complement and coagulation activation, vascular leakage. Rapid destruction of graft
Acute	Days to weeks	Donor leukocytes migrate out of graft and initiate a primary immune response	Activated recipient T cells migrate to the organ and cause graft damage by delayed (type IV) hypersensitivity reactions
Chronic	Months to years	Poorly understood	Vessel occlusion by macrophage infiltration and smooth muscle proliferation leads to graft ischaemia

Table 32.4 Immunosuppressive drugs

Drug	Mechanism
Methotrexate	Folate antagonist
Prednisolone	Inhibits cytotoxic effector cells, anti-inflammatory
Azathioprine	Inhibition of nucleic acid synthesis in mitotic cells
Cyclosporin	Blocks T cell activation
Tacrolimus	Blocks T cell activation
Mycophenolate Mofetil (MMF)	Inhibits IMPDH and hence nucleic acid synthesis, selective for lymphocytes

4.4 Immunosuppressive drugs (Table 32.4)

5 Hypersensitivity reactions

Excessive or inappropriate immune response (Table 32.5).

6 Pregnancy

6.1 Immunological Problems to Solve in Pregnancy

- Fetal tissue is half foreign, a 'semi-allograft' – has to be protected from rejection
- Mother's immune defence must be sufficient during pregnancy to ensure survival
- Fetus immunologically immature at birth – must have maternal antibodies to ensure survival

6.2 Maternal-Fetal Interfaces

Mother and fetus are in direct contact at two sites.

6.2.1 Extravillous Trophoblast with Maternal Immune Cells in the Decidua

Extravillous trophoblast (EVT) invades into the decidua and maternal spiral arteries.

Maternal decidua rich in immune cells (>40% decidual cells are leukocytes in early pregnancy)

- 70% decidual NK cells
- 20% macrophages
- 10% T cells
- Small number dendritic cells, virtually no B cells

Decidual NK cells

- Distinct cell population from peripheral NK cells
- *Not* cytotoxic
- Important role in facilitating/regulating trophoblast invasion by release of cytokines and angiogenic factors

6.2.2 Syncytiotrophoblast and Placental Debris within Maternal Blood

- Syncytiotrophoblast (STB) and maternal blood are in direct contact at the placental surface
- Shedding of placental debris (STB microparticles, DNA, mRNA) into the maternal circulation
- Fetal red blood cells and leukocytes also leak into maternal blood through small haemorrhages

6.3 How Does the Fetus Evade the Maternal Immune Response?

6.3.1 Expression of MHC

Fetal cells express MHC Class I, as do adult cells (HLA-A, HLA-B, HLA-C and HLA-E).

Table 32.5 Hypersensitivity reactions

Type	Name	Example	Ig	Cells	Time
I	Immediate/ anaphylactic	Asthma Penicillin anaphylaxis	IgE	Mast cell, basophil	Mins
II	Antibody mediated	Transfusion reactions	IgM, IgG, complement	Phagocytes, K cells	Min-Hrs
III	Immune complex	SLE, rheumatoid arthritis	IgG±IgM	Neutrophils, complement	Hrs
IV	Delayed / cell mediated	TB	None	Monocytes, lymphocytes	Days

SLE = systemic lupus erythematosus, TB = tuberculosis.

Fetus separated from maternal circulation by the placenta.

Only trophoblast cells (STB and EVT) need to avoid immune detection.

STB completely negative for class I MHC expression (therefore cannot stimulate maternal immune response).

EVT does express class I MHC but a unique pattern compared with other human cells.

Express classical HLA-C and non-classical HLA-E and G.

Does *not* express HLA-A or HLA-B (highly polymorphic and responsible for graft rejection).

HLA-G particularly important.

Extremely limited polymorphism; hence paternal alleles almost identical to maternal.

HLA-G reduces the maternal T cell response to trophoblast

- induces CD8+ T cell apoptosis
- inhibits CD4+ T cell proliferation

HLA-G, HLA-E and HLA-C principally interact with dNK rather than T cells. Binding to dNK receptors inhibits cytotoxic function and leads to the release of beneficial cytokines and angiogenic factors that promote invasion.

6.3.2 Mechanisms That Prevent Maternal IgG Damage

IgG can pass across the placenta (vital for fetal and neonatal immunity).

Fetal leukocytes express HLA-A, HLA-B and HLA-C and leak into the maternal circulation.

Maternal antibodies (IgG) form against these paternal alleles, so why is the fetus not damaged?

- Potentially harmful anti-paternal HLA are filtered by the placenta and do not reach the fetal circulation (cross the STB, then bind to paternal HLA Ag expressed by macrophages and endothelium in the villous tissue; immune complexes then cleared by macrophages).
- Most HLA antigens are widely distributed on both tissues and within the amniotic fluid. Maternal IgG is mopped-up or diluted-out, so no tissue damage occurs.

These mechanisms break down in haemolytic disease of the newborn.

Rhesus antigen is unique; present only on erythrocytes; therefore not widely distributed and not present in amniotic fluid.

6.4 Haemolytic Disease of the Newborn

- 15% of Caucasians are rhesus (Rh) D negative
- Disease usually of second and subsequent pregnancies
- Caused by sensitisation of Rh-negative mother by an Rh-positive baby
- Memory IgG response
- Crosses placenta and leads to haemolysis of fetal red blood cells in utero
- Rhesus antigens: C, D, E, c and e
- Greatest risk of anaemia: anti-D, c and K (Kell)
- Others that can cause significant fetal anaemia: anti-E, Fya (Duffy), Jk and Ce
- Anti-Lewis Ab are not haemolytic (antigens are found in body fluids and are absorbed onto red cell membranes)

6.5 Maternal Immune System

- Complex immunology – tolerate fetal semi-allograft
- Generally state of immunosuppression
- Increased white cell count (30%):
  - increase in neutrophils
  - no change in lymphocytes
- Increased susceptibility to infection:
  - especially viral and intracellular infection
  - polio, influenza, malaria, chickenpox

6.5.1 The Th2 Shift in Pregnancy

- Th0 precursor T cells differentiate into Th1 or Th2 cells in response to cytokine stimulation
- Placental production of cytokines and progesterone promotes a Th2 balance in normal pregnancy
- Th1 type reaction in placenta mainly generates inflammatory responses, activates T cells and NK cells and is correlated with miscarriages, e.g. IFNγ, IL-2
- Th2 type reaction generates non-inflammatory reactions that are consistent with the survival of the fetus, e.g. IL-4, IL-6, IL-10, IL-13

6.6 Fetal Immune System

- Yolk sac first site of immune cells
- T cells develop in thymus from 8/40
- B cells develop in liver and spleen from 12/40
- Immunoglobulins in amniotic fluid from 12/40

IgG crosses the placenta

- Placental receptor bind Fc portion
- Cross via endocytosis from 6/40
- At term fetal IgG > maternal
- Fetal complications arising from maternal IgG include neonatal thyrotoxicosis, myasthenia gravis, neonatal lupus, autoimmune thrombocytopenia, Rhesus disease

6.7 Breast Milk

Rich in secretory IgA, provides protection to the newborn for the first few months of life.

Also contains

- Lysozyme, lactoperoxidase and lactoferrin
- Complement
- Neutrophils

6.8 Hepatitis Immunology and Antenatal Screening

Antenatal patients are tested for hepatitis B surface antigen (HBsAg).

HBsAg positive:

- Acute infection – Anti-HBc IgM positive (often raised ALT)
- Chronic infection (more common) – Anti-HBc IgM negative, Anti-HBc IgG positive
- (NB HBsAg negative, Anti-HBc negative, Anti-HBs positive = immunisation)

6.9 Reproductive Immunology in Pregnancy Disorders

HLA-G expression appears to be important for normal implantation.

Failed IVF cycles are more common with embryos that fail to produce soluble HLA-G.

Recurrent miscarriage and pre-eclampsia are both associated with an increased maternal inflammatory response:

- Failure of the normal shift to Th2 balance
- Increased IFNγ and TNFα levels

Aberrant trophoblast and dNK interactions may be important in failed invasion and preeclampsia:

- dNK receptors may be KIR type A or B, and trophoblast receptors may be type HLA-C1 or HLA-C2.
- If the match is KIR-A and HLA-C2, pre-eclampsia risk is increased.

6.9.1 Immunotherapy for the Treatment of Pregnancy Disorders

Recurrent miscarriage (associated with antiphospholipid syndrome):

- Low dose aspirin, alone or in combination with heparin, may improve reproductive outcomes

Pre-eclampsia:

- In women at increased risk, low dose aspirin reduces the risk by 10–15%
- Statins (anti-inflammatory) currently subject of research trials

Other forms of immunotherapy, including paternal leucocyte immunization, intravenous immunoglobulins and anti-TNFα antibodies, remain highly controversial and may be associated with adverse effects.

Chapter 33

Molecular Biology

Sadie Jones

1 Molecular Biology

Molecular biology concerns the molecular basis of biological activity within a cell. It specifically includes the regulation of interactions between DNA, RNA and protein, as well as how these molecules are bio-synthesised. Understanding this subject is important to all doctors to enable them to:

- Better understand disease processes, e.g. cancer
- Improve their understanding of mechanisms of drug action and other therapeutics
- Understand how certain diagnostic tests work and their limitations

1.1 DNA – Deoxyribose Nucleic Acid

- Most complex molecule known to man
- Two strands of DNA make up a double helix DNA molecule
- Basis of human diversity
- Instructions for molecular and cellular processes
- Instruction to make all molecules that make up the human body
- If all DNA from a human being was laid end to end, it would stretch to the sun and back four times!

DNA is a polymer of nucleotides (Fig. 33.1). A nucleotide is comprised of:

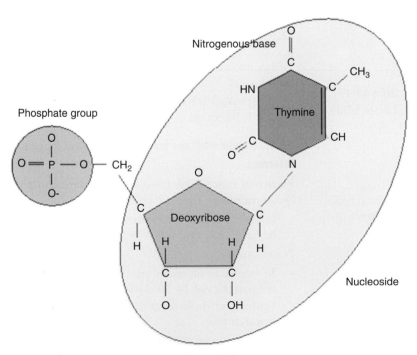

Figure 33.1 A DNA nucleotide (thymine). Comprised of a 5′ carbon sugar (deoxyribose), a phosphate group (bound to the 5′ carbon of the sugar) and a nitrogenous base (bound to the 1′ carbon of the sugar).

- 5' carbon sugar called deoxyribose from which a
- *Nitrogenous base* is bound to the 1' carbon (this subunit is described as a nucleoside), and a
- *Phosphate group* joined to the 5' carbon.

Multiple nucleotides are joined together by phosphodiester bonds to make polymers. The sugar-phosphate chain bound by phosphodiester bonds makes up the DNA backbone.

Two DNA strands are required to make the final DNA molecule that is found in a chromosome. These two strands are bound together by hydrogen bonds that form between complementary nitrogenous bases found on each strand (Fig. 33.2). The nitrogenous bases that make up DNA are:

- Guanine
- Cytosine
- Adenine
- Thymine

Guanine always pairs with *cytosine* with 3 hydrogen bonds

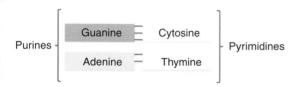

Figure 33.2 Base pairing in DNA. Lines between bases represent hydrogen bonds.

and

Adenine always pairs with *thymine* with 2 hydrogen bonds

1.2 Ribose Nucleic Acid (RNA)

RNA is also a polymer of nucleotides but the nucleotides differ in two ways from those that make up DNA (Fig. 33.3):

- The 5' carbon sugar is biochemically different and called *ribose*.
- The nitrogenous bases are *Guanine, Cytosine, Adenine* and *Uracil* (uracil instead of thymine) (Fig. 33.4).

RNA also differs from DNA in that it is always a single-stranded molecule.

1.3 DNA Replication

DNA replication occurs while a cell is in *interphase*. Interphase is the metabolic phase in which a cell spends the majority of its time. During interphase, a cell carries out its normal 'day-to-day' activities, makes proteins and also replicates its DNA in preparation for mitosis when it divides.

DNA replication involves four key enzymes:

- *Helicase* – DNA unzipper
- *DNA polymerase* – polynucleotide maker

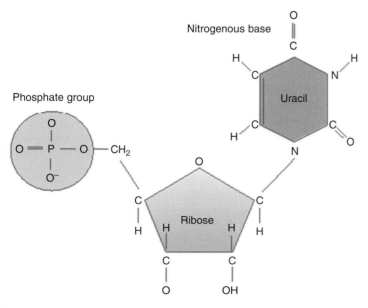

Figure 33.3 An RNA nucleotide. Comprising a 5' carbon sugar (ribose), a phosphate group (bound to the 5' carbon of the sugar) and a nitrogenous base (bound to the 1' carbon of the sugar).

- *Primase* – guider and anchor
- *Ligase* – fixer-upper

DNA replication is initiated at specific points in the DNA known as *origins*. At the origins, initiator proteins bind, forming a replication complex including the crucial enzyme *helicase* which unzips the double helix into its two individual strands. DNA strands are given direction based on the order in which the sugar carbon atoms 5' (bound to phosphate) and 3' (bound to a hydroxyl group) run from left to right. The strand running in the 5' to 3' direction is known as the *leading strand*, and the strand running in the 3' to 5' direction is known as the *lagging strand*. Once

separated, *primase* adds an RNA primer to the DNA strand, guiding DNA polymerase to a point from which to start elongating the new strand of DNA. The leading strand (5' to 3') is replicated quickly and continuously, as this is the direction in which DNA polymerase works, gradually adding complementary nucleotides to the growing DNA polymer. The lagging strand is replicated slowly and discontinuously, requiring multiple RNA primers to be added by primase. This enables short fragments, called *Okazaki fragments,* to be replicated at a time. The Okazaki fragments are then bound together by *DNA ligase* to form a single polymer. The new DNA polymers are then proofread by DNA polymerase and automatically wind up into a new double helix in combination with the original strand from which it was replicated. The result of this process is two DNA molecules consisting of one old and one new chain of nucleotides. This is why DNA replication is referred to as a semi-conservative process (Fig. 33.5).

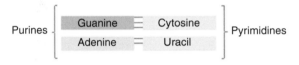

Figure 33.4 Base pairing in RNA. Lines between bases represent hydrogen bonds.

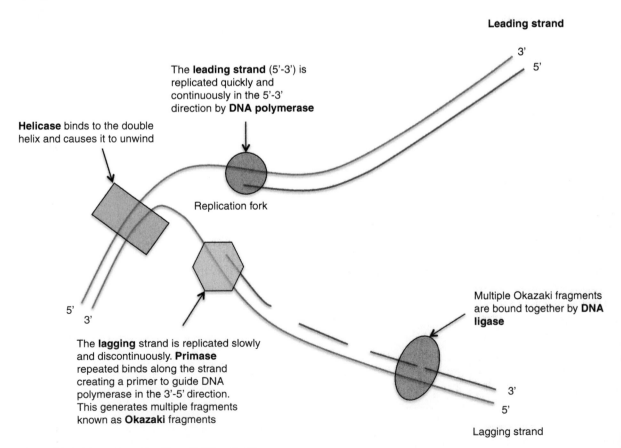

Figure 33.5 Schematic presentation of DNA replication

1.4 Protein Synthesis

Protein synthesis also occurs when a cell is in interphase. Each gene encodes a specific protein. Protein synthesis describes the process by which this code is translated into the protein end product. Protein synthesis can be broadly split into two parts: transcription and translation (Fig. 33.6).

The following play a key role in protein synthesis:

- Transcription factors
- Co-activators
- Helicase
- RNA polymerase
- Ribosomes
- Transfer RNA

1.4.1 Transcription

Transcription takes place in the *nucleus* (Fig. 33.7). *Transcription factors* and *co-activators* indicate that a certain protein is required in the cell and marks the appropriate gene for synthesis. Initially, *helicase* binds to the section of DNA containing the gene of interest and unwinds that section of DNA only. *RNA polymerase* then reads the bases on the DNA in the 3' to 5' direction and generates a complementary messenger RNA (*mRNA*) strand. Remember that the

Figure 33.6 Overview of protein synthesis

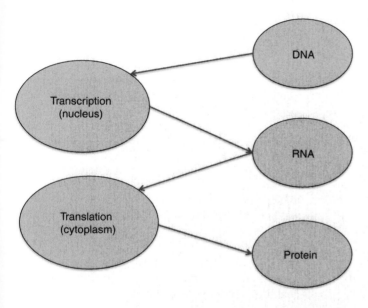

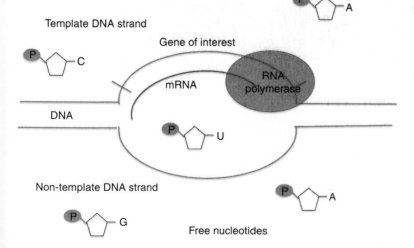

Figure 33.7 Schematic presentation of transcription

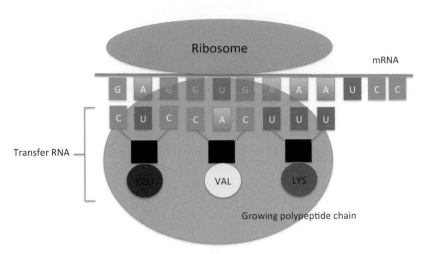

Figure 33.8 Schematic presentation of translation

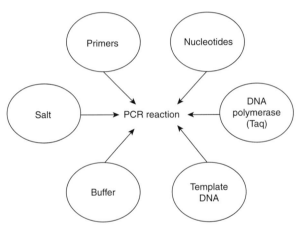

Figure 33.9 Requirements for a successful PCR reaction

nucleotides required to make the mRNA are in constant circulation in the nucleus. The single strand of mRNA is then transported to the cytoplasm through pores in the nuclear membrane known as nucleopores.

1.4.2 Translation

Translation occurs in the *cytoplasm* where *ribosomes* are located (Fig. 33.8). Ribosomes are made of two subunits – one large and one small. The strand of mRNA is fed through the ribosome in order for the code of bases to be translated into a polypeptide made up of amino acids. Every *three* bases (referred to as a *triplet codon*) encode a specific amino acid. Each triplet codon is read by the ribosome and then the appropriate transfer RNA (*tRNA*) molecule, attached to the specific amino acid is recruited into the growing polypeptide chain. Remember, the tRNA molecules

are constantly circulating in the cytoplasm. Once the entire sequence is translated, the complete polypeptide (polymer of amino acids) forms the final protein molecule by undergoing a series of *four folds*.

1.5 Molecular Techniques

This section provides a brief synopsis of some of the more commonly used molecular techniques, including PCR, FISH, DNA sequencing, northern blotting, western blotting and southern blotting.

1.5.1 Polymerase Chain Reaction (PCR)

PCR permits the detection and analysis of any short sequence of DNA, even when it is present in very low quantities. Examples of its use include:

- HIV testing
- HPV testing
- Group B streptococcus testing
- Amniocentesis/chorionic villus sampling

The following components (Fig. 33.9) are required at the correct concentration for a PCR reaction to work optimally:

A PCR reaction involves a machine known as a thermocycler that runs many cycles of repeated heated and cooling of the reaction in order to replicate the DNA in exponential amounts. PCR comprises three stages:

1. *Denaturation* – unwinding of existing DNA template
2. *Annealing* – primer binding
3. *Extension* – production of new DNA polymers (via DNA polymerase)

1.5.2 Fluorescent *in situ* Hybridisation (FISH)

FISH uses a variety of chromosome and gene-specific probes that are fluorescently labelled to identify certain chromosomes, genes, deletions and rearrangements. This technique is used in prenatal diagnosis using samples obtained from amniocentesis and chorionic villus sampling.

1.5.3 DNA Sequencing

DNA sequencing is a relatively new and fast-developing technique that enables the detection of the precise order of nucleotides within an unknown DNA molecule. This technique ultimately permits the precise sequencing of a full human genome. DNA polymerase is used to incorporate fluorescently labelled nucleotides into a growing sequence across the genome. Fluorophore excitation identifies the nucleotide. It is used in new generation prenatal diagnostic testing using free, circulating fetal DNA.

1.5.4 Other Techniques

- *Western blot* – uses fluorescent antibodies to test for *proteins*
- *Northern blot* – uses fluorescent probes to test for *RNA sequences* (gene expression)
- *Southern blot* – uses fluorescent probes to test for *DNA sequences*
- *ELISA* (enzyme-linked immunosorbent assay) – mainly used in immunology to detect *antibodies*

Further Reading

Alberts B, Johnson A, Lewis J, Raff M, Roberts K, Walter P. *Molecular Biology of the Cell.* 2002. Garland Science.

Allison LA. *Fundamental Molecular Biology.* 2007. Blackwell Publishing.

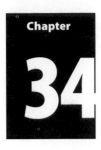

Single-Gene and Chromosome Abnormalities

Sahar Mansour

1 Introduction to Genomic Variation

Chromosomes are thread-like structures located in the nucleus of almost every cell. They are made up of deoxyribonucleic acid (DNA). Less than 2% of human DNA codes for specific genes which transcribes into RNA, and many are then translated into amino acids and proteins (Fig. 34.1)

In humans there are usually 23 pairs of chromosomes: 22 pairs of autosomes and a pair of sex chromosomes.

Males have an X and a Y chromosome.

Females have two X chromosomes.

The human genome is made up of approximately 20,000 to 25,000 genes packaged into 46 chromosomes. All humans have variation or variants in their genome which may be normal or pathogenic.

Large-scale variants include whole chromosome duplications (e.g. trisomy 21) or deletions (e.g. Monosomy X, Turner syndrome).

Medium-scale variants include microdeletions or microduplications (e.g. 22q11 microdeletion)

Small-scale variants include single point variants within the gene with a change in just one or two base pairs (e.g. Noonan syndrome) – These are single-gene disorders. (Fig. 34.2).

2 Chromosomal Abnormalities

Chromosomal imbalances result in abnormalities which may present as recurrent miscarriages, structural abnormalities or intellectual disability.

Balanced chromosomal rearrangements (or translocations) may not cause any problem to the carrier of the translocation but may result in infertility, recurrent miscarriages or fetal abnormalities as a result of chromosomal imbalance in the fetus.

Definitions

Acrocentric chromosome – a chromosome with a very small p arm so the centromere is close to one end. This includes chromosomes 13, 14, 15, 21, 22

Aneuploidy – The occurrence of one or more extra or missing chromosomes leading to an unbalanced chromosome complement e.g. trisomy 21, monosomy X

Autosome – all chromosomes except the sex chromosomes (X and Y)

Centromere – the 'waist' of the chromosome

Chromosomal imbalances – include deletions, duplication, triplication

Euploid – Having a balanced set of chromosomes

Monosomy – one copy of a chromosome instead of two

p arm of the chromosome – the short arm (with 'p' standing for 'petit')

q arm of the chromosome – the long arm (q follows p!)

Telomere – the ends of the chromosome

Triploidy – three copies of every chromosome (i.e. 69 chromosomes)

Trisomy – three copies of one chromosome

Image adapted from: National Human Genome Research Institute.

Figure 34.1 Chromosomes in the cell nucleus

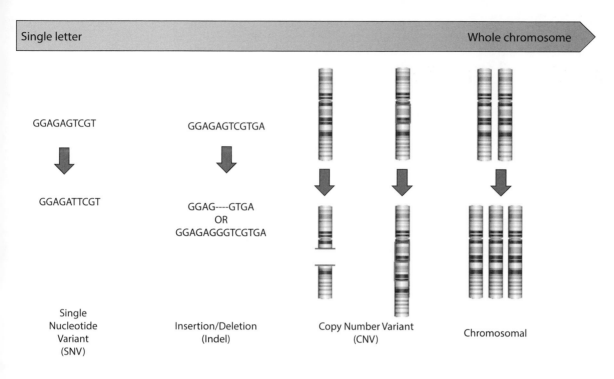

Single letter   Whole chromosome

GGAGAGTCGT

GGAGAGTCGTGA

⬇

⬇

GGAGATTCGT

GGAG----GTGA
OR
GGAGAGGGTCGTGA

Single
Nucleotide
Variant
(SNV)

Insertion/Deletion
(Indel)

Copy Number Variant
(CNV)

Chromosomal

Courtesy of Prof Matt Hurles, Sanger Institute,UK

Figure 34.2 Types of genomic variation

2.1 Chromosome Analysis

Karyotyping

Until recently, traditional karyotyping by G-banding was the main method for looking at the chromosomes. The lymphocytes from a blood sample, chorionic villous sample or amniocentesis are cultured. The cells are arrested in metaphase (see Chapter 28). The nucleus is burst to release the chromosomes and the chromosomes are stained with a Giemsa stain to demonstrate the bands on the chromosomes (Fig. 34.3).

This method is the preferred method to look for aneuploidies, triploidites, structural rearrangements (e.g. ring or marker chromosomes) and translocations. It will also detect large imbalances, deletions or duplications (usually more than 4 MB = 4,000,000 base pairs).

It is not the method of choice to detect small deletions/duplications.

qfPCR

Quantitative fluorescent polymerase chain reaction is a real-time PCR and designed to examine the dosage of the chromosomes to detect the common

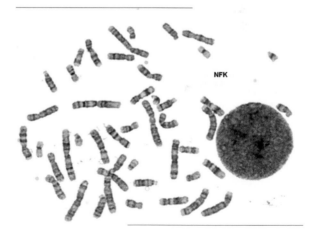

Figure 34.3 G-banding karyotype

trisomies, i.e. 13, 18, 21 and also for monosomy X (Turner syndrome). The advantage is that it is rapid and reliable for the common aneuploidies. It does not look at the structure of the chromosomes, so a traditional karyotype is still required to look at the underlying mechanism (e.g. a Robertsonian

325

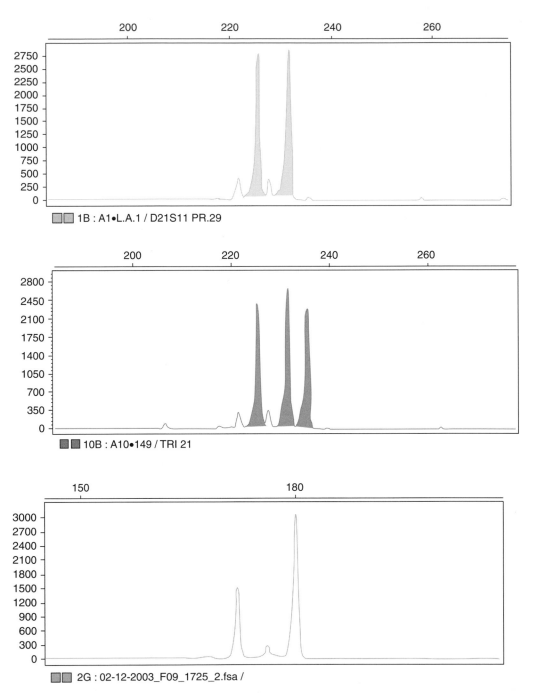

Figure 34.4 qfPCR results

translocation resulting in trisomy will not be detected using this method; Fig. 34.4).

Array Comparative Genomic Hybridization (Array CGH)

The array CGH is a relatively new technique for looking at chromosomes. It compares patient/fetal DNA with reference DNA. It has a much higher resolution than traditional karyotyping, but it only looks at chromosomal dosage so it is not helpful for the detection of balanced rearrangements and will not detect triploidy.

It will detect very small copy number variants (deletions and duplications) (<30KB).

Figure 34.5 Trisomy 21

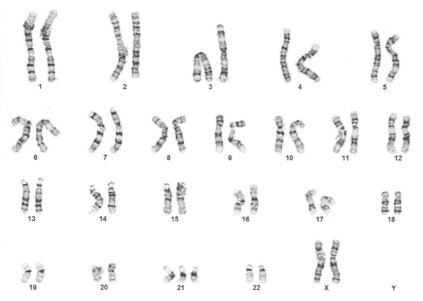

These may be:

- Pathogenic
- Benign
- Unknown significance

It is advisable to read the report carefully.

The array CGH is now recommended for prenatal diagnosis if the nuchal translucency is >3.5 mm or if there are structural abnormalities.

This has resulted in an increased detection of smaller chromosomal imbalances of about 6%.[1]

2.2 The Common Aneuploidies

Trisomy 21

Trisomy 13

Trisomy 18

Turner syndrome

Most aneuploidies will result in a miscarriage and rarely produce a viable pregnancy. The common aneuploidies occur with a high frequency of 0.1–0.2% of all pregnancies. Although the common aneuploidies (listed previously) frequently result in miscarriage, they may produce a viable fetus. For this reason, these conditions are described in more detail here.

Trisomy 21 (Down Syndrome)

This is the most common aneuploidy as the risk of miscarriage is lower. It occurs with an incidence of approximately 1 in 500 pregnancies. It is usually caused by nondisjunction – failure of the chromosomes to separate in meiosis, resulting in an ovum with two copies of chromosome 21, which becomes trisomy 21 when fertilized by the sperm (Fig. 34.5). A small proportion of trisomy 21 (<5%) may result from a Robertsonian translocation which may have been inherited from one of the parents. The full karyotype should therefore always be checked in an affected fetus or baby (Fig. 34.5). Occasionally there is an extra copy of chromosome 21 in only some of the cells (mosaic trisomy 21). These children are usually less severely affected.

Antenatally, Down syndrome can often be detected by an increased nuchal translucency, absent nasal bone, short femurs or congenital heart disease.

Children with trisomy 21 have intellectual disability with characteristic facial features with a mongoloid slant to the eyes (up slanting palpebral fissures), malar hypoplasia and a protruding tongue. The skull shape is brachycephalic (i.e. flat at the back). There is clinodactyly (curved) of the little fingers with brachydactyly (short fingers) and single palmar creases (this can be also seen in the normal population). There is often a sandal gap between the first and second toes (Fig. 34.6). There is marked infantile hypotonia.

Other complications include:

Congenital heart disease (particularly Atrioventricular septal defect)

Jejunal atresia

Trachea-oesphageal atresia

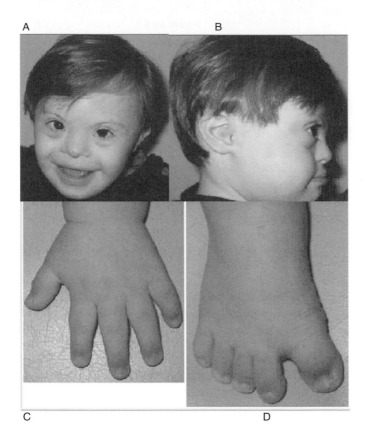

Figure 34.6 Down syndrome (trisomy 21)

A: Typical facial features with up-slanting palpebral fissures, protruding tongue,
B: facial profile with brachycephalyand malar hypoplasia.
C: Hands showing brachydactyly. Feet with sandal gap between hallux and
second toe.

Hirschsprung's disease

Later, there is an increased risk of leukaemia and presenile dementia.

Trisomy 18 (Edward Syndrome)

This condition is due to an extra copy of chromosome 18, trisomy 18. It may present antenatally with an increased nuchal translucency. The fetus may be growth retarded, with congenital heart disease of any form, rocker bottom feet and overlapping fingers. There is a very high rate of spontaneous miscarriage and a high mortality in liveborn infants; 90% of live-born babies die within the first year of life (Fig. 34.7).

Trisomy 13 (Patau Syndrome)

Trisomy 13 also carries a high mortality with a high incidence of spontaneous miscarriage during pregnancy. The vast majority of live-born babies do not survive the first year of life. They may present in utero with an increased nuchal translucency, intrauterine growth retardation, postaxial polydactyly, bilateral cleft lip +/– alveolus, congenital heart disease or holo-prosencephaly of variable severity (Fig. 34.8).

Monosomy X (Turner Syndrome)

Turner syndrome may be due to monosomy X in all or some (mosaic) of the cells. There are also variations with the presence of an abnormal X chromosome (e.g. ring X chromosome) or mosaicism, with some cells with monosomy X and others with 47,XXX, or even mosaicism with 46,XY. The vast majority of babies with Turner syndrome are female (the rare exception is if there is 45,X/46,XY mosaicism, which may result in a male or female or a baby with ambiguous genitalia).

This condition often presents with a very increased nuchal translucency, cystic hygroma or hydrops fetalis at 11 to 13 weeks. There is a very high mortality, with more than 98% resulting in *in utero* demise. Surprisingly, the

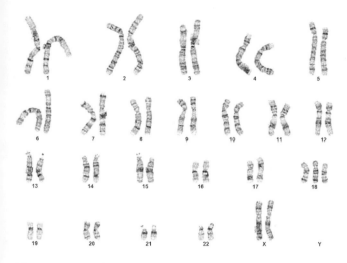

Karyotype – trisomy 18

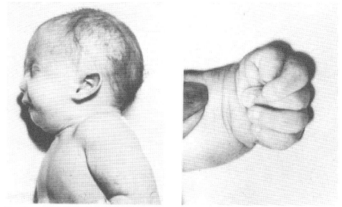

Profile – subtle dysmorphic features with prominent occiput, low set ears. Overlapping fingers are characteri

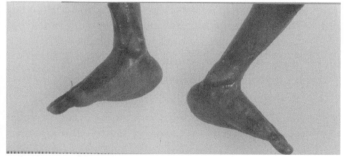

Rocker bottom feet in a fetus

Figure 34.7 Trisomy 18

babies surviving with Turner syndrome do relatively well. The incidence is about 1 in 2500 live births, but much higher at conception.

The following are associated with Turner syndrome:

Normal intelligence

Short stature

Figure 34.8 Trisomy 13

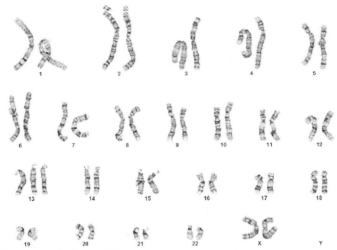

Karyotype of trisomy 13

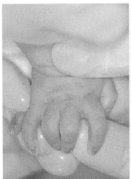
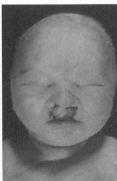
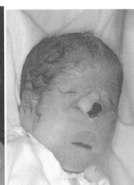

Postaxial polydactyly

Bilateral cleft lip and alveolus

Holoprosencephaly with proboscis

Webbed neck

Wide carrying angle

Lymphoedema at birth or later in childhood

Congenital heart disease particularly bicuspid aortic valve, coarctation of the aorta or rarely hypoplastic left heart

Kidney abnormality especially horseshoe kidney, duplex or pelvic kidney

Infertility

Autoimmune problems, e.g. diabetes, hypothyroidism (see Fig. 34.9)

2.3 Chromosomal Translocation

Approximately 1 in 500 people (i.e. 1 in 250 couples) carries a balanced rearrangement of the chromosomes.

If balanced, there is no loss of genetic material, so this usually causes no problems to that individual but causes reproductive risks, which include:

- offspring with chromosomal imbalance
- recurrent miscarriage
- infertility (particularly in males)

Balanced reciprocal translocation is a rearrangement between any two (or more) chromosomes wherein one portion of a chromosome is transferred to another and vice versa (Fig. 34.10).

Robertsonian chromosomal translocation – the joining of any two acrocentric chromosomes (i.e. chromosomes 13, 14, 15, 21, 22). The acrocentric chromosomes have a very small p arm with very little genetic material, so the centromere is close to one end. The two chromosomes are 'stuck together' at the

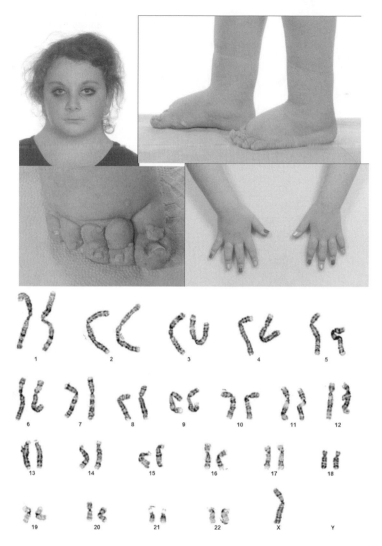

Female with monosomy X, demonstrating webbed neck and four-limb lymphoedema
Photographs taken from :
Atton G, Gordon K, Brice G, Keeley V, Riches K, Ostergaard P, Mortimer P, Mansour
S. The lymphatic phenotype in Turner syndrome: an evaluation of nineteen patients
and literature review.
Eur J Hum Genet. 2015 Dec;23(12):1634-9.

Figure 34.9 Turner syndrome

centromere, so there are only 45 chromosomes instead of 46. This type of translocation increases the risk of trisomy in the fetus (Fig. 34.11).

3 Single Gene Disorders

Point mutations within a significant gene may result in fetal abnormalities. These cannot be detected by normal karyotyping or even array CGH. The testing is targeted to the gene of interest. The most common technique for identification of these variants is Sanger sequencing of the gene of interest. However, massive parallel sequencing of the whole genome is becoming cheaper and more reliable.

A mistake in one base pair within a gene will result in faulty transcription to RNA and then translation into

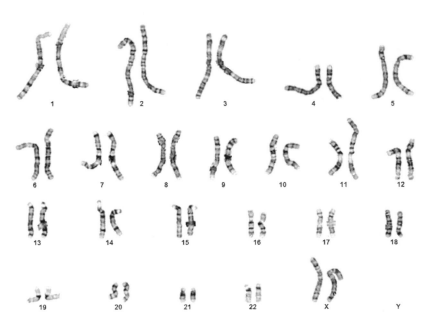

Figure 34.10 Balanced reciprocal translocation between chromosomes 4 and 11

amino acids/proteins leading to a defective protein. The problem may be due to a lack of protein (haploinsufficiency) or interference of a faulty protein (dominant negative) or even gain of function of a protein.

3.1 Mendelian Inheritance

Autosomal Dominant

A point mutation in only one copy of a gene is sufficient to cause an autosomal dominant condition.

If a parent is affected, the offspring has a 50% chance (1 in 2) of being affected (Fig. 34.12).

The mutation can occur as a new event in the egg or sperm (i.e. neither parent is affected)

A dominant condition affects males and females equally.

Examples of autosomal dominant conditions:

Noonan syndrome

Marfan syndrome

Achondroplasia

Neurofibromatosis type 1

Tuberous sclerosis.

Autosomal Recessive

An autosomal recessive condition occurs when there is a mutation in both copies of the gene (biallelic).

In the vast majority of cases, the parents are both carriers but not affected.

If both parents are carriers, the offspring risk is 25% or 1 in 4 (Fig. 34.13).

Examples of autosomal recessive conditions include:

Cystic fibrosis

Sickle cell anaemia

Thalassaemia

Spinal muscular atrophy

If the mutation is known, prenatal diagnosis can be offered by CVS at >11 weeks or amniocentesis >15 weeks. Preimplantation genetic diagnosis may also be an option.

X-Linked Recessive

Females have two X chromosomes; males have an X and a Y. The Y chromosome has very few genes. If a female carries a mutation in one copy of a gene on the X chromosome, she is usually not affected as she has a healthy copy of the gene. Males with one faulty copy will have an X linked recessive condition.

If a woman is a carrier, 50% of her sons will be affected (Fig. 34.14).

If a man is affected by an X-linked disorder (e.g. haemophilia), all his daughters will be carriers (they will inherit his only X chromosome) and all his sons

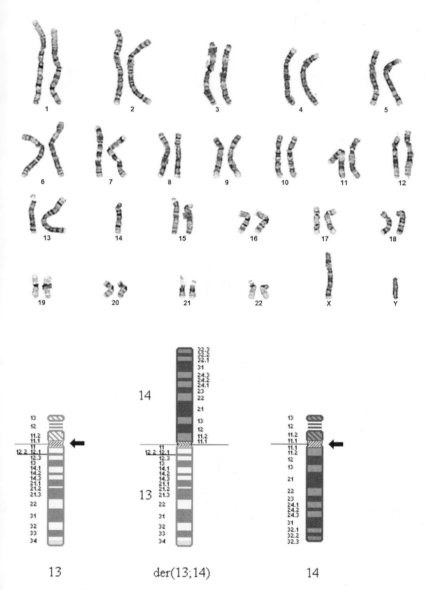

Figure 34.11 Robertsonian chromosomal translocation of chromosomes 13 and 14

will be unaffected (they will inherit his Y chromosome).

The mother is not always a carrier of an X linked condition, as the mutation may occur as a new event in the egg.

Examples of X linked recessive conditions:

Duchenne muscular dystrophy

Haemophilia

G6PD deficiency

Colour blindness

3.2 Non-mendelian

Triplet Repeat Expansion

There are a few genetic conditions due to an expansion of a triplet repeat sequence of the nucleotides within the gene. Triplet repeat sequences are normal in some genes; however, if they increase in size, they interfere with the function of that gene and can become unstable. The expansion may increase from one generation to the next. This causes an increase in

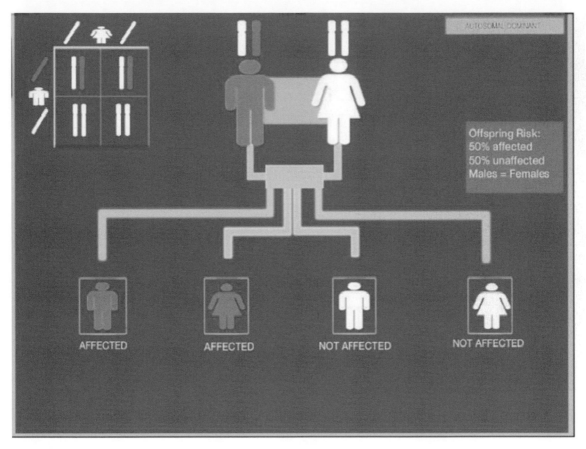

Figure 34.12 Autosomal dominant inheritance

the severity of the condition in each generation – a phenomenon called 'anticipation'.

They may be inherited in an autosomal dominant, recessive or X-linked manner.

Examples of triplet repeat expansions are:

Myotonic dystrophy (autosomal dominant)

Fragile X (X-linked recessive)

Huntington disease (autosomal dominant)

Friedreich's ataxia (autosomal recessive)

Imprinting

In some conditions, the parent of origin of a gene is very important. Some genes are expressed only on the paternal or maternal chromosome. The genes are 'imprinted' with the parent of origin. Any imbalance may result in a genetic disorder that is not necessarily inherited.

This can occur by a number of mechanisms:

1. Microdeletion of an imprinted gene

2. Uniparental disomy of an imprinted chromosome (i.e. both copies of the same chromosome are inherited from one parent)

3. A mutation in the gene controlling imprinting.

Examples of imprinting disorders:

Beckwith Wiedemann syndrome

Russell silver syndrome

Angelman syndrome

Prader Willi syndrome

Multifactorial

There are a number of congenital abnormalities that are not due to a single gene disorder, but there is a slightly higher recurrence risk in families who have had one affected child. These conditions are thought to be due to a combination of a genetic susceptibility (probably more than one gene) and environmental factors.

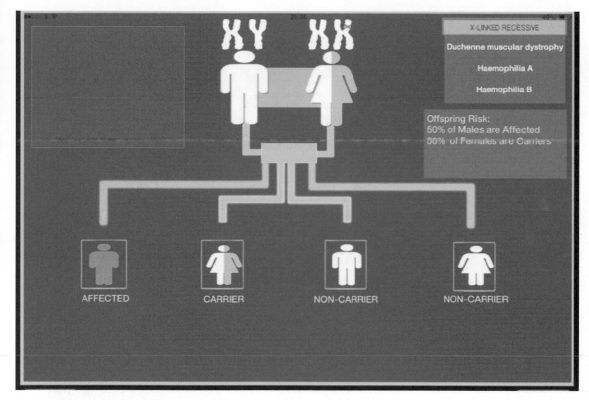

Figure 34.13 Autosomal recessive inheritance

Examples include:

Spina bifida

Cleft lip and/or palate

Congenital heart disease

Autism

4 Prenatal Diagnosis

Targeted prenatal diagnosis can be offered in the following situations:

Familial chromosomal translocation (balanced reciprocal or Robertsonian in one parent)

Known genetic problem in the family – mutation identified

Previously affected child with known genetic defect

Testing by:

Chorionic villous sampling (>11 weeks)

Amniocentesis (>15 weeks)

Non-invasive prenatal diagnosis

Fetal ultrasound

Preimplantation Genetic Diagnosis

PGD is now available for single-gene disorders, parents with a balanced chromosomal translocation, and fetal sexing for X-linked disorders.

It involves the process of in vitro fertilisation. The embryos are tested by removal of one cell at a few days post-conception. Only unaffected embryos are implanted.

The limitations are that it is expensive, a licence is required for each new genetic condition and currently there is only a 20% success rate.

It is now possible and permissible for adult-onset genetic disorders (e.g. breast cancer susceptibility or Huntington's disease)

Acknowledgement

I should like to thank Karen Marks, Senior Scientist in the Cytogenetics laboratory at St George's

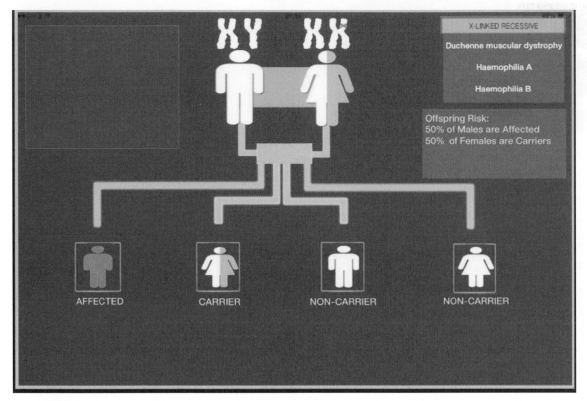

Figure 34.14 X-linked inheritance

University Hospitals, for providing the chromosome images.

References

1. Wapner, et al., Chromosomal microarray versus karyotyping for prenatal diagnosis. *N Engl J Med*. 2012; **367**:2175–2184

2. The Unique Rare Chromosomal Disorders Support Group provides a number of helpful, informative and accurate leaflets: www.rarechromo.co.uk/html/home.asp

3. Robertsonian translocations leaflet: www.rarechromo.org/information/Other/Robertsonian%20Translocations%20FTNW.pdf

4. Array CGH leaflet:www.rarechromo.org/information/Other/Array%20CGH%20FTNW.pdf

5. FutureLearn runs a MOOC (Massive Online Open Course) on 'The Genomics Era: The Future of Genetics in Medicine': www.futurelearn.com/courses/the-genomics-era/3/register

Genetic Screening and Diagnosis

Tessa Homfray

Disorders of Sexual Development

1. Complete sex reversal
2. Ambiguous genitalia

   Note: Depending on the mutation, many syndromes may present with complete or partial sex reversal

   Male internal sex organs derived from Wolffian ducts

   Female internal sex organs derived from Mullerian ducts (Fig. 35.1)

Complete Sex Reversal

46XX Male

1. Translocation of SRY on to X chromosome (Fig. 35.2)
2. SOX9 overexpression

46XY Female

1. Deletion of SRY on Y chromosome
2. Androgen insensitivity syndrome (AIS) (X-linked sex limited)

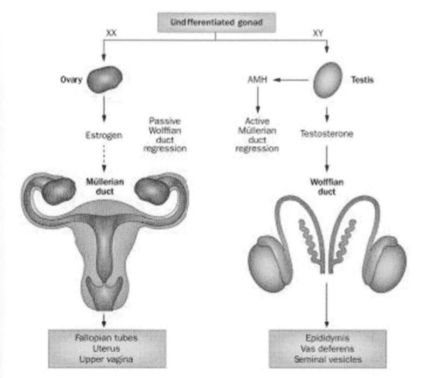

Figure 35.1 Wolffian and Mullerian structures in female and male genital tract

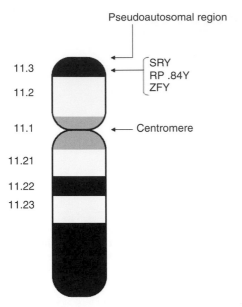

Pseudoautosomal region

11.3

SRY
RP .84Y
ZFY

11.2

11.1 — Centromere

11.21

11.22

11.23

Figure 35.2 Translocation of SRY gene onto an X chromosome will lead to a 46XX normal but infertile male. Genes in pseudo-autosomal region undergo crossing over between X and Y chromosomes.

Mutation in Androgen receptor

Wolffian internal structures

Failure to develop 2° sex characteristics

Short vagina – will require vaginal lengthening with vaginal dilators for sexual intercourse

3. Steroidogenic factor 1 (SF1) (new dominant)

Regulator of endocrine development

Mullerian internal gonads

May have adrenal failure as well

4. WT1 (new dominant)

Denys-Drash syndrome

Diffuse mesangial sclerosis, nephrotic syndrome, Wilms's tumour

Frazier syndrome

Diffuse mesangial sclerosis, nephrotic syndrome, gonadoblastoma

Ambiguous Genitalia

46xx	46xy
Congenital adrenal hyperplasia	AIS
	5α reductase deficiency
	WT1
	Smith Lemli Opitz

Campomelic dysplasia
Chromosome deletions
46X0/46XY

Congenital Adrenal Hyperplasia (CAH) (AR)

≈ 90% 2° 21 hydroxylase deficiency

External genitalia masculinized, normal female internal genitalia

May develop salt-losing crisis; must exclude before discharge from hospital

Autosomal recessive can screen for common mutations

≈ 5% 11β hydroxylase deficiency

Ambiguous/complete XX sex reversal, precocious puberty, short stature, hypertension

Other forms of CAH

Lipoid congenital adrenal hyperplasia – steroidogenic acute regulatory protein (STAR) (46XY sex reversal)

Associated Features for 46XY Ambiguous Genitalia Syndromes

1. 5α reductase deficiency (AR)

$$\text{Testosterone} \xrightarrow{\text{5α reductase}} \text{dihydrotestosterone (DHT)}$$

DHT required for development of the male external genitalia

Virilization at puberty

2. Smith Lemli Opitz (AR) syndrome

Multiple congenital abnormality (MCA) syndrome associated with mental retardation, microcephaly, short stature

7 dehydrocholesterol deficiency

3. Campomelic dysplasia

Short limbs, bent tibia cleft palate frequently lethal

SOX9 deficiency or chromosome inversion 17q separating SOX 9 from its promoter

Other DSDs

1. MURCS Mullerian duct aplasia, unilateral renal agenesis, cervicothoracic somite anomalies

2. Mayer-Rokitansky syndrome

Utero vaginal atresia in otherwise normal females (ovaries, fallopian tubes normal)

3. Cloacal abnormalities

Single common channel for rectum, urethra +/– vagina

Severity of the abnormality variable

Infertility and Miscarriage

Infertility Female

1. Sex chromosome disorders

   45X

   47XXX (premature menopause)

2. Other chromosome disorders

   Translocations infertility more common with male carriers

3. Fragile X premutation (premature menopause)
4. Other single-gene disorders

   Congenital adrenal hyperplasia (maybe atypical presenting as polycystic ovarian syndrome)

   LH/FSH mutations

   Many others poorly understood

Infertility Male

1. Sex chromosome disorders

   47XYY

   ?45X/46XY

2. Other chromosome disorders

   13:14 translocation often causes severe infertility in some males; others normal

3. Y chromosome deletion (Fig. 35.3)

Miscarriage

1. Chromosome translocation

   Unbalanced from:

   - X:Autosome
   - Balanced reciprocal (Figs 35.4 and 35.5)
   - Robertsonian

   If a woman has three miscarriages, then products of conception (POC) should be sent for aCGH to ascertain if there is a chromosomal cause for this.

   - >50% first-trimester miscarriages have a chromosomal abnormality
   - <5% of recurrent miscarriages are secondary to an inherited unbalanced translocation

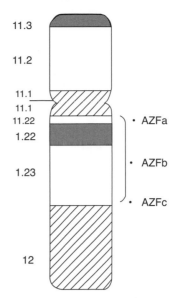

Figure 35.3 Y chromosome deletion of AZfa-c causes infertility

2. Chromosome breakage syndromes (affected male or female)
3. Recurrent hydatidiform mole (maternal only – initially development of the mammalian zygote under control of maternally inherited proteins)
4. Myotonic dystrophy
5. Other

Congenital Abnormalities

High-Risk Pregnancies

1. Family history

   Known genetic disorders

   Mental retardation

   Recurrent miscarriages

   Consanguinity (3% risk in first-cousin marriage in absence of any known abnormalities)

2. Personal obstetric history
3. Abnormal screening tests

   Hb electrophoresis (β globin abnormalities only identified; thalassemia mutations need to be identified prior to PND)

   Rhesus status

   Infection immunity/exposure (variable according to country policy)

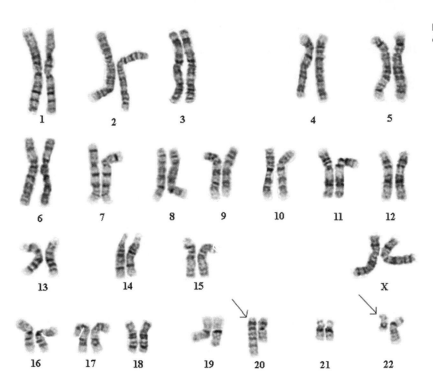

Figure 35.4 Balanced 20:22 chromosome translocation

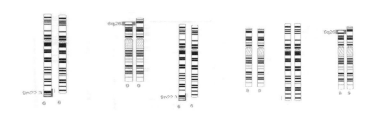

Figure 35.5 Possible viable abnormal unbalanced karyotype resulting from a balanced translocation

A. Balanced Reciprocal Translocation between Chromosome 6q and 9p

B. Unbalanced Chromosome translocation, trisomy tip of 9p, monosomy tip of 6q

C. Unbalanced chromosome translocation,,trisomy of tip6q and monosomy tip of 9p

Major trisomy screening (13, 18, 21)

Combined test: maternal age, nuchal translucency, βHCG, PAPP-A (M0 Ms)

Non-invasive prenatal testing (discussed later)

4. Maternal drug ingestion

Prescribed

Anti-epileptics, particularly valproate

Retinoic acid analogues

Recreational drugs

Cocaine

Alcohol

Smoking

5. Maternal disease

Diabetes mellitus

Maternal autoimmune disease

Systemic lupus erythematosus (SLE)

- Placental function affected with severe recurrent IUGR
- Anti-Rho and Anti-La antibodies destroy fetal cardiac conduction system and cause heart block

Maternal genetic disease

- Effect on maternal health

- ○ Marfan's syndrome
- ■ Risk of aortic rupture during pregnancy/ labour
  - ○ Familial dilated cardiomyopathy
- ■ De-compensation of cardiac function, particularly in third trimester
  - • Effect on pregnancy
  - ◦ Polycystic kidney disease with maternal hypertension
- ■ Pre-eclampsia
  - • Effect on fetus
  - ○ Myotonic dystrophy
- ■ Disease showing anticipation and fetus can be congenitally affected, talipes, polyhydramnios
  - • Risk of fetus having similar disease in future (AD disease)
  - • May effect pregnancy ex polycystic kidney disease, Ehlers Danlos and may pass to fetus

Non-invasive Prenatal Testing (NIPT)

- • Short fragments of free apoptotic DNA present in the maternal plasma derived from the placenta (Fig. 35.6)
- • Can be identified from 5 weeks gestation
- • Fetal fraction of free DNA is 5–10% and increases with gestation; low fetal fraction will lower the accuracy of the test, and if there is a fetal trisomy, the proportion of abnormal DNA will be lower
- • Small placentas may produce less DNA

Screening for major triomies

- • Most methods use next-generation sequencing (NGS) and look for dosage difference of chromosomes 13, 18, 21
- • Analysis of sex chromosome number is unreliable
- • Screening test – needs confirmation by CVS/ amniocentesis

Diagnostic test for single gene disorders

1. Fetal sexing for sex-linked disorders
2. Confirmation of ultrasound abnormalities with new dominant disorders achondroplasia, thanatophoric dysplasia, Apert syndrome (expanding at present)
3. Paternal dominant disease
4. Recessive disease where parents have different mutations and can identify maternal mutation

Identification of maternally inherited mutations remains problematic in view of predominance of maternal free DNA over free placental DNA and dosage and recognising fetal fraction of mutation difficult

5. Rhesus blood group

   For management of pregnancy/postnatal for anti-D

   15% of people are Rh negative; Anti-D only required if baby is Rh positive; typing of fetal blood by NIPT will reduce the number of babies requiring Anti-D. (Anti-D is obtained from ORh

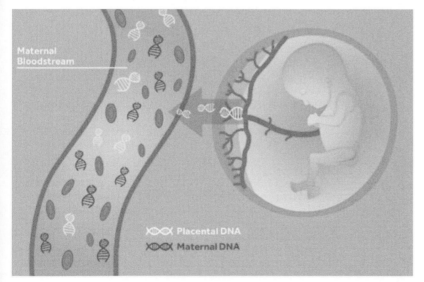

Figure 35.6 Origin of DNA in NIPT is placental DNA

negative male donors who have been isoimmunized with Rh positive cells)

Raised Nuchal Translucency with Normal T13, 18, 21

↑NT ↓Risk of fetal abnormality/pregnancy loss

NT>6 mm 15% chance of a normal baby

Turner syndrome NT >5 mm lethality >99%

Other chromosomal disorders (discussed later)

Congenital heart disease

Diaphragmatic hernia

Fetal akinesia

Rasopathies and other lymphatic disorders

Severe skeletal dysplasias

Very rare genetic syndromes – cannot exclude in pregnancy

Chromosome Disorders Other than Trisomy 13, 18, 21

1. Unbalanced chromosome translocation (Fig. 35.5)
   - Risk of fetal abnormality dependent on the size of the translocated segments
     - Small translocated segments more likely to result in a viable fetus and therefore result in the birth of an abnormal infant
     - Large translocated segments more likely to result in miscarriage as the size of the resulting chromosomal imbalance will be large and therefore the fetus will be non-viable

2. Chromosome deletions and duplications
   - A microdeletion syndrome is a recognised gene deletion syndrome that cannot be identified by a standard karyotype; this would be identified by FISH and aCGH (see Table 35.1)

3. Chromosome mosaicism (Fig. 35.7)
   The presence of more than one population of cells with different numbers of chromosomes.
   - Confined placental mosaicism
     - May cause placental insufficiency and unexplained IUGR
     - May lead to trisomic rescue if present at conception
       - Trisomic rescue is where there is loss of one copy of a chromosome in an embryo that started with three copies of that chromosome so that it now has only two copies
   - May lead to imprinting disorders

An imprinting disorder occurs when there is a parent of origin affect of a loss or gain of genetic material.

   - Trisomic rescue of chromosome 15 maternal disomy –Prader Willi, paternal disomy Angelman syndrome
   - Only certain chromosomes have been associated with imprinting disorders; these are 6, 7, 11, 14, 15

True mosaicism
   - Baby affected and has two different chromosome populations

Table 35.1 Common microdeletion syndromes

Syndrome name	Microdeletion	Prenatal features	Additional features postnatally
Di George	22q11.2 2-3Mb	Conotruncal defects, absent thymus	Cleft palate, immunodeficiency, MR
Williams	7q11.23 1.5–1.8Mb deletion	Supravalvular aortic stenosis, pulmonary stenosis	MR Dysmorphic
Prader Willi	15q11.2, 5.3Mb + deletion (pat)	None	Hypotonia, poor feeding, MR
Angelman	15q11.2, 5.3 Mb + deletion (mat)	None	MR, ataxic gait, happy disposition
Miller Dieker	17p13.3 350Kb+	Ventriculomegaly, MRI lissencephaly	Severe MR, wrinkled skin over the glabella
TAR	1q21.1, 200Kb	Absent radius	Thrombocytopenia
Wolf Hirschhorn	4p16.3 2.5Mb+ deletion	CHD, IUGR, cleft lip/palate	Severe MR

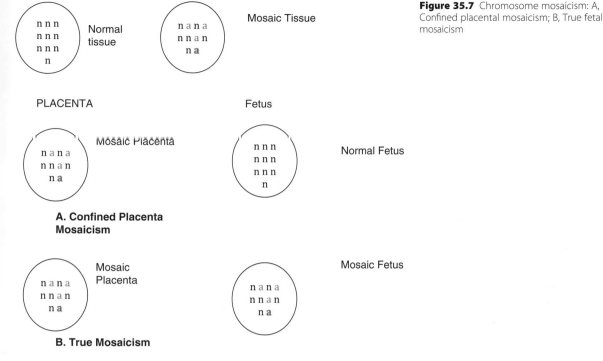

Figure 35.7 Chromosome mosaicism: A, Confined placental mosaicism; B, True fetal mosaicism

- Variable affects depending on the amount of cells with abnormal cell line
- Cannot predict effects on % of cells identified as variable between tissues
- Amniocytes more reliable to identify mosaicism than fetal blood
- Need to correlate result with ultrasound findings
- Well-recognised chromosome mosaic syndrome
  - Isochromosome 12p – Pallister Killian syndrome
  - Mosaic trisomy 8

4. Triploidy

Whole extra set of chromosomes (69 total; Fig. 35.8)

1% of all conceptions

10% of spontaneous abortions

- Paternal origin of extra chromosomes two-thirds (diandry)
  - Result from dispermy
  - Commonly result in spontaneous abortion
  - Large placenta
  - May develop partial mole
- Maternal origin of extra chromosomes one third (digyny)
  - Errors in meiosis II

- Early embryonic demise or late demise with small well-formed fetus
- Small placenta
- Baby often small by 12 weeks and redated
- High risk of preeclampsia if pregnancy continues

Chromosome Analysis In Pregnancy

1. QFPCR (Fig. 35.9)
   - Rapid analysis by DNA dosage of chromosome 13, 18, 21 may look at X and Y but maybe more difficult to interpret; additional chromosomes occasionally may be added to this test (16, 22)

2. Standard karyotype (Fig. 35.10)
   - Cells are cultured and then examined down the light microscope in a metaphase spread
   - 7–14-day analysis
   - Can identify deletions of 5Mb and duplications of 8Mb; quality of preparation may vary

3. Array comparative genomic hybridization (aCGH) (Fig. 35.11)
   - DNA analysis
   - Dosage of DNA measured against a normal person

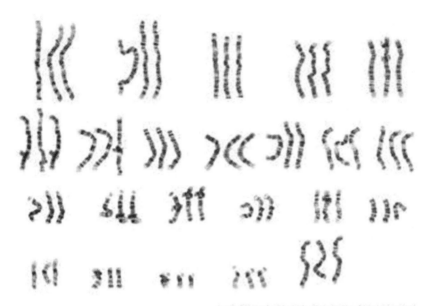

Figure 35.8 Triploid karyotype

(c) 2005, Janet M. Cowan, Ph.D.

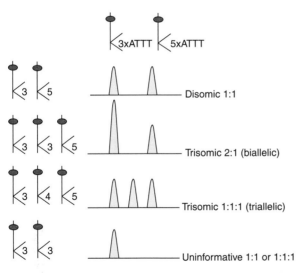

Figure 35.9 QFPCR for rapid analysis of chromosome 13, 18 and 21

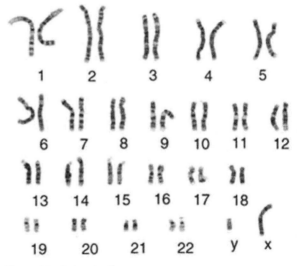

Figure 35.10 Standard karyotype

- Identifies abnormalities down to about 100Kb or less
- Different arrays platforms will identify different size abnormalities
- Nomenclature
  - Standard P short arm Q long arm bands numbered from centromere followed by

sub-bands that require chromosome elongation to identify (Fig. 35.12)

- Chromosome number followed by base-pair abnormality from the beginning of imbalance (base pair 1 is at the top of the P arm and highest number at bottom of Q arm); X1 if deletion; X3 if duplication (except sex chromosome as males only

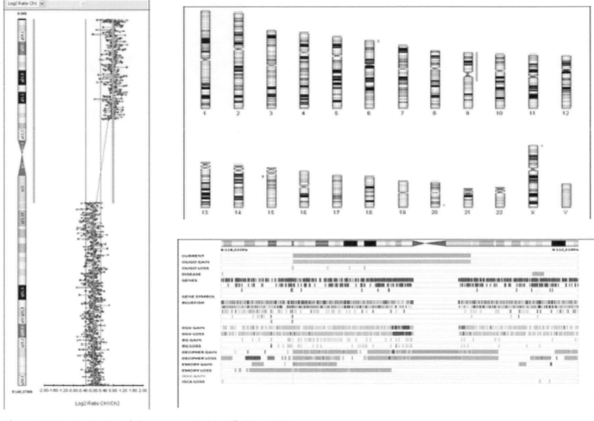

Figure 35.11 Duplication of chromosome 9p identified by aCGH

have 1X), i.e. different from standard karyotype but report might quote both

○ Only tells you about an imbalance

■ Will not indicate if the imbalance is attached to a different chromosome as would be the case with an unbalanced reciprocal chromosome translocation

■ Will not tell you if a trisomy is 2° to a Robertsonian translocation; only that there is an extra copy

■ Will not identify triploidy, as all chromosome areas are abnormal and thus there is no obvious imbalance

• Standard method of analysis in most units in the UK

Common microdeletion syndromes (Table 35.1)

4. Fluorescent in-situ hybridization (FISH) (Fig. 35.13)

• Can count chromosome number but rarely used for this

• Identify microdeletion syndrome but answers a specific question (not a screening test)

• Can use specific probes to chromosomes involved in the translocation and identify an unbalanced translocation

Identification of Single Gene Disorders in Pregnancy

1. Known family history

• Identify by early ultrasound

• Invasive testing if known mutation within the family

○ In absence of ultrasound/MRI abnormalities, this will be the only method of analysis

345

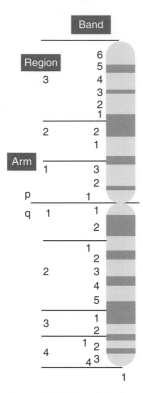

Figure 35.12 Standard chromosome nomenclature

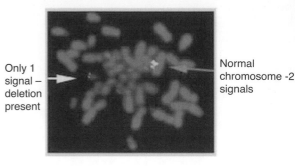

Figure 35.13 Fluorescent in-situ hybridization

2. Absence of family history
   - Identify on screening blood tests ex Hb electrophoresis
   - Ultrasound abnormalities

Importance of identifying fetal abnormalities during pregnancy:

I. Management of pregnancy
   - Short long bones may need to induce early as risk of placental insufficiency
   - Short long bones 2° to achondroplasia – normal pregnancy care

II. Management of labour
   - Osteogenesis imperfecta, avoiding traumatic delivery

III. Neonatal care
   - Duct-dependent congenital heart disease – prostin Rx required in neonatal period prior to surgery

IV. Termination of pregnancy
   - Serious abnormality associated with neonatal lethality

- Short long bones associated with thanatophoric dysplasia
- Serious abnormality associated with long-term disability
  - Cerebellar hypoplasia secondary to Cri-du-Chat syndrome
  - Many brain abnormalities will not be diagnosed with a specific syndrome, but empiric data may suggest a high risk of intellectual disability
  - Agenesis of the corpus callosum (ACC) if isolated; 30% risk of intellectual disability; if associated with other brain abnormalities, >95% risk of intellectual disabilities
- Multiple abnormalities involving different organs will have risk of an associated intellectual disability, even in the presence of a normal brain ultrasound

Investigation of Genetic Disorders in Pregnancy

Non-invasive prenatal diagnosis (NIPD) (as discussed previously)

Chorionic villus sampling (CVS) 10 weeks+

Amniocentesis 16 weeks+

Fetal blood sampling (FBS) 18 weeks+

Limitations at present for the diagnosis of single-gene disorders are the ability to undertake rapid screening of genes in the absence of a known mutation at the beginning of the pregnancy.

Underlying aetiology of many ultrasound features has a large differential diagnosis, and therefore one needs a large number of genes to be screened at the same time to diagnose the specific cause of the abnormalities accurately and rapidly.

Rapid analysis of single genes now becoming possible using next-generation sequencing (NGS)

Exome sequencing – Sequencing of protein-coding regions of a gene

Gene panels – exome sequencing of genes that have been known to have been associated with the phenotype of the fetus/baby

Whole exome sequencing – exome sequencing of all known genes

May be limited to a clinical exome which is all the genes that have been associated with a disease gene (MORBID genes)

Whole genome sequencing – sequencing of all the genome

Variant interpretation of large amount of data very challenging and requires bioinformatics pathways, followed by analysis of remaining possible variants.

Common Ultrasound Abnormalities

Fetal hydrops (Table 35.2)

Short long bones (Table 35.3)

Isolated limb abnormality (Table 35.4)

Brain abnormalities (Table 35.5)

Gynaecological Tumours

Germline mutation

- Present at conception and therefore present in every cell in the body

Somatic mutation

- Occur after conception and therefore only a proportion of cells carry the mutation
- May initiate or drive cancer
- Multiple mutations required for a tumour to become a metastatic cancer
- Patients with a 46XY DSD will need to have remaining gonads removed as at risk of developing Gonadoblastoma
- Patients with a previous hydatidiform mole need to be screened for Choriocarcinoma with AFP and βHCG

Endometrial Cancer

Germline mutations in mismatch repair genes (hereditary non-polyposis colon cancer, HNPCC)

1. 50% risk of uterine cancer in gene mutation carriers
2. Associated with other cancers; most frequently bowel cancer but also ovarian cancer + pancreatic, uro-epithelial
3. Genes MSH2, MLH1 MSH6 (PMS2), MSH6 may be uterine cancer only families

Ovarian Cancer

BRCA1 ovarian cancer risk 30–50%; lifetime risk breast cancer up to 80% (female only)

BRCA2 ovarian risk 10–20% breast cancer 40% + pancreatic and melanoma male breast cancer risk

Table 35.2 Causes of fetal hydrops

		Associated features	Investigations
Chromosomal		Norm only feature in first trimester, later MCA	Invasive testing for qfPCR & aCGH
Isolated CHD		——	Invasive testing aCGH (Isolated CHD rarely associated with FH
Fetal akinesia		Polyhydramnios, micrognathia	aCGH but rare store DNA lethal malformation
Fetal anaemia		Evidence of bleeding may be present, MCA	Fetal Hb, platelets Maternal & fetal blood group
Fetal infection		Symmetrical IUGR, hyperechogenic bowel	CMV, toxoplasmosis, Zika, rubella, varicella, syphilis
Fetal heart failure		Enlarged heart, fetal ↑/↓	Fetal echo
Lung cysts		Nil	Nil
Lymphatic disorders	Rasopathy	Hydronephrosis, mild polyhydramnios, CHD, absent DV	PTPN11 pre-screen, full rasopathy test
	Other	Pedal oedema No other features for majority	VEGF3 No other investigations at present possible

Table 35.3 Causes of short long bones

Diagnosis	Earliest gestation	HC	Chest size	Polydactyly	Other
Osteogenesis imperfecta II	12–14	Clear view of brain	↓	No	Asymm. shortening
Short rib polydactyly	12–14	N	↓	Yes	Exomphalos, CHD
Thanatophoric dysplasia	13	↑	↓	No	Bent femur
Ellis van Creveld	14	N	↓	Yes	CHD
Jeune	16		↓	Yes	
Diastrophic dysplasia	12–14	N	N	No	Hitchhiker thumb, talipes
Hypophosphatasia					
Type 2 collagen					
OI type I, III, IV	20	N	N	N	Asymm shortening
SHOX related	20	N	N	No	None
Robinow	20	↑		No	Wide-open ant fontanelle
Cleidocranial	20	↑	N	No	Wide open ant fontanelle, absent clavicles
Placental insufficiency	20	N	N	No	Hypospadias
Achondroplasia	24+	↑	N	N	↑ femoral shaft/neck angle

Table 35.4 Causes of isolated limb abnormalities

Limb abnormality	Cause	Further investigation
Radial aplasia	Trisomy 18 VATER TAR Fanconi	Karyotype Exclusion other causes and associated fetal anomalies aCGH Chromosome breakage on cultured cells
Ectrodactyly	Isolated Cornelia de Lange	No other features IUCR symmetrical, facial features on US, low PAPP-A
Terminal transverse defect	?Vascular/amniotic band	Follow-up scan but nothing expected
Unilateral short II long bone	? vascular Fracture	Follow-up scan to look for evidence of further fractures. Possible DNA analysis of ColA1/A2
Talipes	Isolated Fetal constraint Arthrogryposis	Offer amnio, rarely abnormal, repeat scan and look for further contractures. If progression, maternal DNA for myotonic dystrophy and blood for acetyl choline receptor antibodies
Polydactyly	Isolated common in black population Skeletal dysplasias Other syndromes	Full ultrasound and further investigations dependent on findings

BRCA1 & BRCA2 may cause 1° peritoneal cancer and fallopian tube cancer

Eligibility for testing for BRCA1 & 2 in patients with ovarian cancer/ovarian cancer risk

1. All serous ovarian cancers irrespective of age, Stage 3 &4 tumours more likely to be mutation positive
2. Known mutation within the family
3. Strong family history of histologically confirmed serous ovarian cancer but no alive family member for testing can test unaffected woman

May have obligate male carriers who can be tested

Prophylactic oophorectomy recommended after childbearing.

Screening is ineffective and should not be recommended

Table 35.5 Causes of major brain malformations

US abnormality	Possible causes	Other investigations
Holoprosencephaly	Trisomy13 Chromosome deletions 13q, 7q Mutations in SHH	Karyotype by aCGH Look for other US abnorm (Smith Lemli Opitz – 7 dehydrocholesterol) Store DNA All severe MR /death
Absent septum pellucidum	Septo optic dysplasia Vascular disruption	Fetal MRI to look for Schizencphaly
Agenesis of corpus callosum	Isolated; many syndromic associations	Karyotype with aCGH, third trimester fetal MRI to look for gyral and neuronal migration abnormality, 30% mental retardation if isolated
Cerebellar vermis hypoplasia/agenesis	Nearly all ciliopathy disorders, Meckel Gruber, Joubert etc.	Look for polydactyly, polycystic kidneys encephalocele Fetal MRI not very helpful; store DNA
Cerebellar hemisphere hypoplasia	Unilat norm vascular origin and if isolated good outcome Bilateral poor outcome	Fetal MRI to check isolated Karyotype with aCGH 5p – commonest Other syndromes no PND possible store DNA
Ventriculomegaly	Many viral screen, bleed, genetic syndromes (Normal outcome in mild 10–12 mm in 97% of cases) Increasing severity, poorer prognosis	Fetal MRI in third trimester to look for neuronal migration and gyral malformation Viral screen, platelet Abs genetic syndromes, Karyotype
Microcephaly	Chromosome and many syndromes	Overall fetal growth, fetal MRI and karyotype, earlier identified more severe MR
Macrocephaly	Normal, CFC, overgrowth (achondroplasia) Hemimegaloencephaly	Full scans; other signs of overgrowth; only MRI if other brain abnormalities suspected

BRCA1 & BRCA2 involved in DNA repair, treatment options in mutation carriers

Other germline mutations recognised in ovarian cancer risk: BRCA1 & 2 include mismatch repair genes risk 4%

RAD51C and RAD51D

References

1. Achermann, JC, Jameson, JL. Disorders of sex development. In *Harrison's Principles of Internal Medicine*, 18th ed., Longo, DL, Fauci, AS, Kasper, DL, Hauser, SL, Jameson, JL, Loscalzo, J (eds.), pp. 3046–55. McGraw-Hill, 2011.

2. Ahmed SF, Achermann JC, Arlt W, Balen AH, Conway G, Edwards ZL, Elford S, Hughes IA, Izatt L, Krone N, Miles HL, O'Toole S, Perry L, Sanders C, Simmonds M, Wallace AM, Watt A, Willis D. UK guidance on the initial evaluation of an infant or an adolescent with a suspected disorder of sex development. *Clin Endocrinol (Oxf)*. 2011 Jul;**75**(1):12–26.

3. Bilgin EM, Kovanci E. Genetics of premature ovarian failure. *Curr Opin Obstet Gynecol*. 2015 Jun;**27**(3):167–74.

4. Krausz C, Escamilla AR, Chianese C. Genetics of male infertility: from research to clinic. *Reproduction*. 2015 Nov;**150**(5):R159–74.

5. Gardner RJMK, Sutherland GR, Shaffer LG. *Chromosome Abnormalities and Genetic Counseling*. Oxford University Press, 2011.

6. Homfray T. Diagnosis of hydrops and multiple malformation syndromes. In *Twining's Textbook of Fetal Abnormalities*, Coady AM, Bower Churchill Livingstone S (eds.), pp. 161–81. Elsevier, 2015.

7. Jones KL, Jones MC, Campo M Del. *Smith's Recognizable Patterns of Human Malformation*. 2013

8. Firth HV, Hurst JA. *Oxford Desk Reference: Clinical Genetics* (Oxford Desk Reference Series), *Pregnancy and Fertility*, pp. 566–644. Oxford University Press, 2005.

9. Kobayashi H, Ohno S, Sasaki Y, Matsuura M. Hereditary breast and ovarian cancer susceptibility genes (review). *Oncol Rep*. 2013 Sep;**30**(3):1019–29.

10. Firth HV, Hurst JA. *Oxford Desk Reference: Clinical Genetics* (Oxford Desk Reference Series), *BRCA1 & 2*, pp. 426–29, *HNPCC*, pp. 454–58. Oxford University Press, 2005.

Useful Websites

Gene Reviews www.genetests.org
OMIM www.omim.org
Orphanet www.orpha.net/
UNIQUE www.rarechromo.co.uk

Biophysics

Neil Pugh and Nazar Amso

Introduction

The modern obstetrician and gynaecologist is increasingly using a wide range of equipment and instruments in their clinical practice, for both diagnostic and therapeutic purposes. With the introduction of the new curriculum, a basic understanding and use of ultrasound imaging are mandatory for all, in addition to a knowledge of conventional diagnostic and therapeutic techniques. However, not all practitioners fully appreciate the background principles on which these techniques are based. It is not so much the complex knowledge of physics and formulae that is required, but rather a knowledge of how the principles of physics are applied in clinical practice. This is fundamental to a better understanding of the techniques as well as their safe, optimal and efficient use. This chapter will consider the scientific foundations and uses of a procedure frequently encountered in obstetric and gynaecological practice.

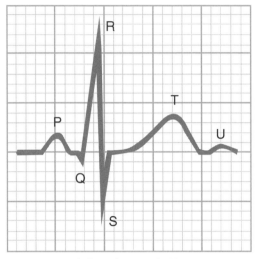

Figure 36.1 Labelling of a normal ECG trace

Principles and Use of Electrocardiography

Electrocardiography is a commonly used non-invasive procedure for the recording of electrical changes in the heart. The trace, called electrocardiogram (ECG or EKG), documents the electrical impulses that are generated during each cardiac cycle. The waves in a normal record are labelled P, Q, R, S and T (Fig. 36.1). The test evaluates cardiac function and identifies any problems that might exist in the frequency and rhythm of the heart rate or in the size and position of the heart's chambers; the test also assesses whether there is any myocardial damage.

Relationship between the Cardiac Cycle and the Electrocardiogram

Electrical stimulation of the myocardium (depolarisation) is followed by restoration of the electrical potential of the myocardial cell (repolarisation). The electric stimulation starts at the sinoatrial node, which acts as the natural cardiac pacemaker. The electrical signal then propagates through the internodal tracts of the atria to the atrioventricular node and subsequently activates the ventricles via the His-Purkinje system. This system consists of a bundle of fibres that divides into right and left branches. The left branch further divides into left anterior and posterior hemifascicles (Fig. 36.2).

In an ECG, the P wave represents atrial depolarization, while atrial repolarisation occurs during ventricular depolarization and hence is not visualised. The QRS wave represents ventricular depolarisation, while the T ventricular repolarisation. The ECG can be either displayed digitally or recorded onto conventional paper.

ECG Planes and Electrode Placement

The heart can be thought of as a generator of electrical signals enclosed in a volume conductor. The body and heart have three dimensions and the electrical signals recorded from the skin will vary depending on the position of the electrodes. Standardization of electrode position is essential.

ECG lead electrodes are placed either in a bipolar or in a unipolar arrangement. In the bipolar lead arrangement, the electrical activity at a single positive electrode is compared with that at a single negative electrode. In the unipolar lead arrangement, the electrical potential at a single positive electrode, the so-called exploring electrode, is compared with the average electrical activity at several other electrodes, which serve as negative pole.

The limb leads (I, II, III) are bipolar leads, while the augmented voltage leads (aVR, aVL, aVF) are unipolar leads. These six leads explore the electrical activity of the heart in the frontal plane (the orientation of the heart seen when looking directly at the anterior chest; see Figure 36.3).

The chest leads (V1, V2, V3, V4, V5, V6) explore the electrical activity of the heart in the horizontal plane (Fig. 36.3). The reference point for the chest leads is obtained by connecting the left-arm, right-arm and left-leg electrodes together. The position of

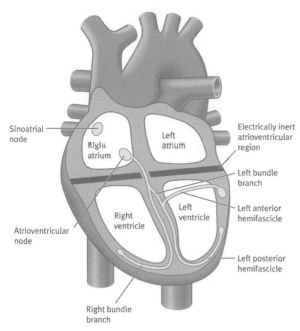

Adapted by permission from: BMJ Publishing Group Ltd. Meek S, Morris F. ABC of clinical electrocardiography. Introduction. I – Leads, rate, rhythm, and cardiac axis. *Br Med J* 324:415–8.

Figure 36.2 Characteristics of lasers commonly used in endoscopic surgery

Figure 36.3

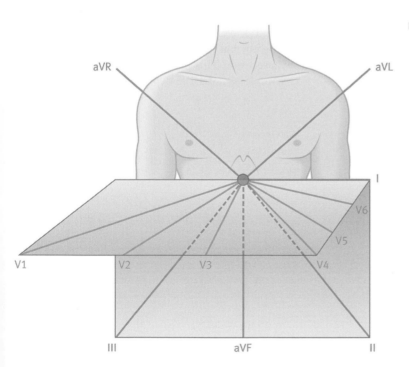

Red = frontal plane of the heart; green = horizontal plane of the heart.

Adapted by permission from: BMJ Publishing Group Ltd. Meek S, Morris F. ABC of clinical electrocardiography. Introduction. I – Leads, rate, rhythm, and cardiac axis. *Br Med J* 324:415–8.

the 6 chest electrodes for standard 12-lead electrocardiography is depicted in Figure 36.4.

In a standard 12-lead ECG:

- Leads II, III and aVF 'view' the inferior surface of the heart

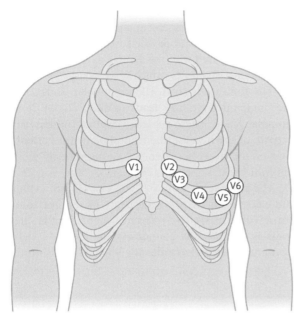

Adapted by permission from: BMJ Publishing Group Ltd. Meek S, Morris F. ABC of clinical electrocardiography. Introduction. I – Leads, rate, rhythm, and cardiac axis. *Br Med J* 324:415–8.

Figure 36.4

- Leads V1 to V4 view the anterior surface to the heart
- Leads I, aVL, V5 and V6 view the lateral surface of the heart
- Leads V1 and aVR view the right atrium and the cavity of the left ventricle

The shape of the QRS complex in any lead depends on the orientation of that lead to the vector of depolarization (Fig. 36.5).

To obtain good electrical contact, the skin is cleaned and gel is applied before placing the electrodes. After removal of the electrodes at the end of the procedure, the skin should be thoroughly cleaned again to avoid skin irritation from the salty gel. No special precautions are required and no complications from this procedure have been observed.

Features of a Normal Electrocardiogram

Normal sinus rhythm on an ECG has the following cardinal features:

- The heart rate is 60–99 beats/minute.
- The cardiac rhythm is regular except for minor variations with respiration.
- The P wave is upright in leads I and II.
- The normal duration of the PR interval is 0.12–20 seconds. This is the time required for the completion of atrial depolarisation, conduction

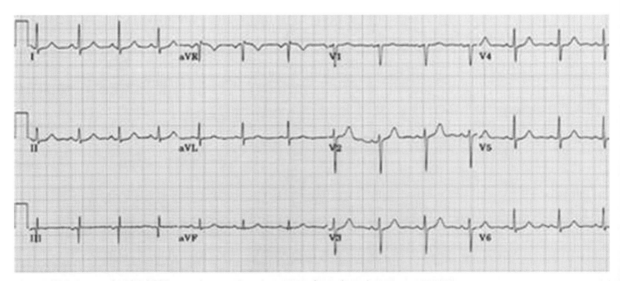

Figure 36.5 A normal 12-lead ECG trace showing the relevant waveforms from the various orientations

through the atrioventricular node and His-Purkinje system and arrival at the ventricular myocardial cells.

- Each P wave is usually followed by a QRS complex.
- The normal duration of the QRS interval is 0.060.10 seconds. This represents the time required for ventricular cells to depolarize.
- Normal values for the QT interval are between 0.30 and 0.43 seconds (0.30 0.45 seconds for women). This is the time required for depolarization and repolarization of the ventricles.

Young healthy individuals, especially athletes, may also display various other rhythms, especially during sleep. For example, respiration may cause sinus arrhythmia, characterized by beat-to-beat variation in the RR interval, with the heart rate increasing during inspiration. This is a vagally mediated effect in response to the increased volume of blood that returns to the heart during inspiration. Other normal findings noted in healthy individuals include tall R waves, prominent U waves (reflecting repolarization of the papillary muscles or His-Purkinje fibres), ST-segment elevation, exaggerated sinus arrhythmia, sinus bradycardia and first-degree heart block.

Principles and Use of Ultrasound

Diagnostic ultrasound uses the transmission of mechanical vibrations through tissue to obtain some information about that tissue. Ultrasound allows us to:

- determine the nature of a tissue (e.g. cystic or solid)
- assess the movement of tissues (such as fetal heart, bowel)
- measure blood flow (e.g. in the ovarian/ follicular circulation, fetal circulation)
- measure structures (such as follicular diameter, femur length)

Ultrasound has an advantage over other imaging modalities because it is non-invasive and does not use ionizing radiation. For these reasons, ultrasound can be used as a screening test and repeated examinations can be made with relative safety. Therefore, ultrasound is ideally suited for use in obstetrics and gynaecology.

The Sound Wave and Its Generation

Sound is a pulsating pressure wave (i.e. a mechanical disturbance of a medium) that passes through the medium at a fixed speed. Any sound wave can be defined by two main parameters, namely its amplitude, which is related to its acoustic power and its frequency. Sound waves with frequencies above 20 kHz are termed ultrasound, with medical ultrasound operating in the low MHz range. Figure 36.6 shows the range of ultrasound frequencies used in the medical environment.

To produce ultrasound, there is the need to generate a pressure wave. This is achieved by incorporating a piezoelectric crystal within a transducer that is placed in contact with the tissue under investigation. The piezoelectric crystal converts electrical energy into mechanical energy and vice versa. When excited by a high-voltage current, the crystal oscillates at a given frequency, which is determined by the thickness of the crystal.

Two types of ultrasound can be produced, namely continuous-wave ultrasound and pulse-wave ultrasound. For imaging purposes, pulse-wave ultrasound is used. It consists of bursts or 'packets' of ultrasound that are sent out at a given frequency. The rate at which these bursts of ultrasound are sent out is known as the pulse repetition frequency. Figure 36.7 shows the temporal profile of pulsed-wave ultrasound. The advantage of this type of ultrasound is that it is possible to obtain spatial information and therefore imaging is possible.

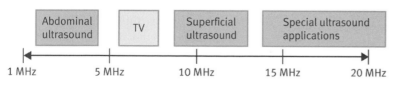

Figure 36.6

TU = transvaginal ultrasound

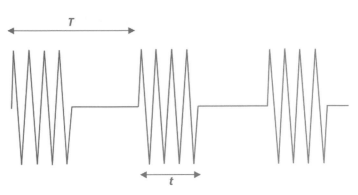

Figure 36.7

T = pulse repetition period | t = pulse length

Interactions of Ultrasound with Tissue

To build up an ultrasound image, the ultrasound pressure wave needs to interact with the tissue under investigation. The pressure wave then needs to return to the piezoelectric crystal to be converted from mechanical into electrical energy. There are three principal interactions with tissue:

- reflection
- scatter
- absorption.

Reflection occurs at interfaces between tissues with different characteristics. The tissue property that determines the degree of reflection is called the acoustic impedance (Z), which is related to the density (p) of the tissue and the velocity (c) of ultrasound in that particular tissue:

$$Z = \rho \times c$$

The greater the difference in acoustic impedance between two tissues, the greater the degree of reflection.

Scatter occurs when ultrasound interacts with a structure whose dimensions are similar to, or smaller than, the wavelength of the ultrasound wave. This is known as Rayleigh scattering, and the resulting wave is scattered in all directions (360^0 scattering). This type of interaction typically occurs when ultrasound interacts with very small structures such as blood cells or parenchyma. The intensity of the scattered wave depends primarily on the dimensions of the target tissue and the wavelength of the ultrasound wave. Generally, the intensity of the scatter increases very rapidly with the frequency of the ultrasound pressure

wave, which puts an upper limit on the frequency of ultrasound that can be used in clinical practice.

Absorption is the conversion of mechanical (ultrasound) energy into heat or internal molecular energy. This can obviously have detrimental results in that the heating effect can produce unwanted bio-effects. In addition, energy is lost from the ultrasound beam, reducing the penetration of the beam. Absorption increases with frequency, which effectively puts an upper limit of 20 MHz on the frequency of ultrasound that can be used.

It is the echoes generated from the reflection at tissue boundaries and scattering within tissues and organs that give rise to the complex echo trains from which the diagnostic information is derived.

Real-Time B-Mode (Brightness Mode) Ultrasound Scanning

Ultrasound scanning is a highly operator-dependent technique. To produce a B-mode ultrasound image, the ultrasound beam needs to be swept across the field of view (Fig. 36.8A). Typically, up to 200 effective ultrasound beams will be used to produce an image (Fig. 36.8B).

Figure 36.9 illustrates the main components of a typical B-mode ultrasound scanner. We will now discuss the role of these components in image formation.

The transducer houses the piezoelectric crystal and generates the ultrasound beam. Modern transducers tend to be broadband transducers with selectable frequencies. Transducers come in different shapes and sizes, depending on the frequencies used and the specific applications.

Figure 36.8

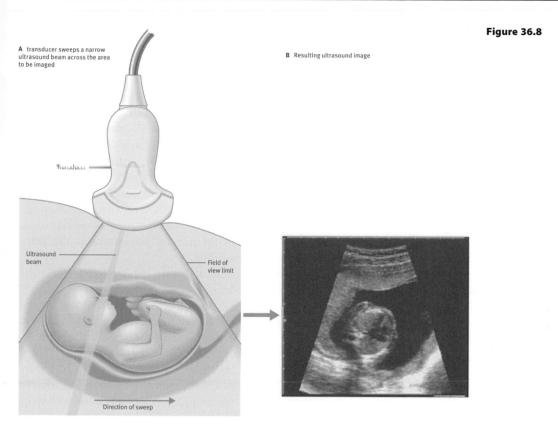

A transducer sweeps a narrow ultrasound beam across the area to be imaged

B Resulting ultrasound image

Transducer

Ultrasound beam

Field of view limit

Direction of sweep

TGC = time-gain compensation

Figure 36.9

The power control allows adjustment of the amount of electric voltage that is applied to generate the ultrasound pulses.

The echoes received from the tissues are converted into electrical signals by the transducer. However, the received signal is much weaker than the transmitted signal, and therefore a receiver amplifier boosts the returning signals to useful levels. As an analogy, the gain control acts like the volume control on a radio.

Owing to the attenuation of ultrasound pulses with depth, echoes from similar reflectors reduce in amplitude as the tissue depth increases. To ensure that echoes from similar reflectors at different depths are displayed at the same amplitude, it is necessary to compensate for attenuation. This is achieved using a technique called time-gain compensation, which essentially employs a series of amplifiers that can be adjusted to increase the image amplification at specific depths.

The scan converter controls the way in which the image is presented. It basically consists of computer memory elements that store greyscale information and produces a digital image that is comprised of tiny picture elements (pixels). Each pixel has a unique address where the value of the echo amplitude is stored. This allows the appropriate shade of grey for each pixel to be displayed on the screen. In the scan converter, various parameters such as reprocessing and post-processing curves can be altered, which can improve image quality.

Flat screens are now generally used to display the images.

Limitations of Real-Time B-Mode Scanning

B-mode ultrasound scanning has several practical limitations, including:

- inadequate spatial resolution
- inadequate penetration
- poor image quality (greyscale)
- low frame rate
- compromised field of view
- low line density

Spatial resolution is the minimum distance between two reflectors or scattering surfaces that is necessary to be able to distinguish two separate echo signals. There are two main components to spatial resolution. Firstly, axial resolution, which is the minimum distance between two points that are located along the beam axis. The axial resolution is determined by the pulse length, which is shorter at higher frequencies. In fact, the axial resolution is equal to half the pulse length and this is why higher frequencies are used to give better axial resolution. The second component of spatial resolution is lateral resolution, which is the minimum distance between two points that are

located at the same range or depth within the tissue (objects side by side in the image). The lateral resolution is determined by the beam width and is highly dependent on beam focusing. The spatial resolution also depends on the slice thickness, which is determined by the thickness of the transducer and is therefore inherent in the transducer's design.

Penetration is reduced by the attenuation of ultrasound. The main factors influencing penetration are absorption and scatter. As alluded to earlier, both absorption and scatter increase with increasing frequencies. Hence, lower frequencies have to be used to achieve greater penetration. As a result, better penetration comes at the price of poorer resolution.

Image quality depends on several factors: the contrast resolution, which is influenced by the pre-processing and post-processing carried out in the scan converter; the dynamic range (the range of echo strengths that can be handled by the amplifiers), which dictates how the echo train is converted to a greyscale; and the temporal resolution, which depends on the number of frames displayed per second (frame rate). All of these factors need to be optimized to obtain the best possible image quality.

Frame rate, line density (the number of scan lines in the image) and field of view (the size of the image displayed) are all interrelated. Ideally, one would like to have a fast frame rate, a high line density and a large field of view to obtain the best possible image. Unfortunately, the interrelation of these factors means that something has to be compromised and, depending on the scan being performed, one has to decide which of the factors are the most important to optimize.

Doppler Ultrasound

The wavelength recorded by an observer depends on the movement of the source and the observer relative to one another. This phenomenon can be used in medical ultrasound to give two pieces of useful information:

- the speed at which the target is moving
- the direction of the motion

The difference in frequency between returning echo and the transmitted ultrasound wave is known as the Doppler frequency shift; in medical ultrasound, it is particularly used to assess blood flow.

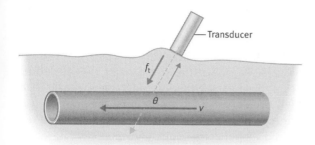

An ultrasound wave is transmitted towards a blood vessel; the ultrasound echo reflected by the red blood cells moving through the vessel incurs a Doppler frequency shift that is proportional to the velocity of the blood flow. | f_t = frequency of the transmitted ultrasound wave | v = velocity of the red blood cells | θ = angle between the transmitted ultrasound wave and the direction of the blood flow

Figure 36.10

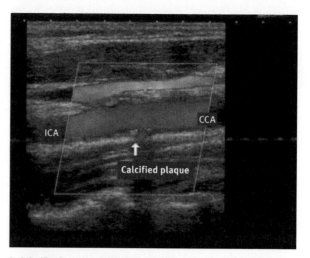

Red signifies flow towards the direction of the colour box; blue signifies flow away from the box; the hue of each colour represents the mean velocity. | CCA = common carotid artery | ICA = internal carotid artery

Figure 36.11

Doppler Equation

If the red blood cells are moving through a blood vessel at velocity v and the angle of insonation between the red blood cells and the ultrasound beam is θ degrees (Fig. 36.10), then the Doppler frequency shift (f_d) is given by the following equation:

$$f_d = \frac{2f_t v \cos\theta}{c}$$

where c is the velocity of ultrasound in soft tissue and (f_t) is the frequency of the ultrasound wave transmitted by the ultrasound transducer.

Doppler Instrumentation

The simplest way to detect blood flow is by use of continuous-wave ultrasound. Instruments of this kind will give us no imaging capability, and the devices thus tend to be fairly basic, designed to assess the pulse or the fetal heartbeat.

To get more information about the nature of blood flow, the Doppler information needs to be coupled with an imaging device. To this end, the main instrument now available is a colour flow scanner, which combines a B-mode real-time greyscale imaging system with pulsed-wave Doppler and colour flow imaging. Colour flow images display direction and velocity information pictorially (Fig. 36.11). Information on the direction of blood flow is colour-coded; generally, flow toward the transducer is red and flow away from the transducer is blue. Information on the velocity of red blood cells is also colour-coded, with dark hues representing low velocities and bright hues representing high velocities.

Safety of Diagnostic Ultrasound

Diagnostic ultrasound has been used for many years with no proven adverse effects, so why should we worry? Modern ultrasound often uses greater acoustic powers than older generation machines, and ultrasound manufactures are using new techniques such as pulse coding, tissue harmonic imaging and contrast-enhanced imaging. These newer techniques undoubtedly increase diagnostic capabilities, but they may also influence the safe use of ultrasound.

Along with developments in ultrasound machines, imaging techniques have changed over the years. Pulsed wave Doppler is used a great deal more than in the early years, and in general terms, their intensities are greater than B-mode imaging (1). Also, the advent of transvaginal scanning has placed sensitive tissues and the fetus closer to the transducers, with a general increase in ultrasound intensities (2). Finally, ultrasound contrast agents are also used in many areas of diagnostic imaging. These produce strong echoes and concentrates mechanical activity in the local area which can lead to localized biological effects (3) as well as the generalized bio-effects.

It is clear, therefore, that there is the potential for ultrasound to produce bio-effects in human tissue, and since most epidemiologic evidence comes from studies using B-mode scanning 20–25 years ago when output powers were lower, we should re-acquaint ourselves with the concept of ultrasound safety in the modern era. As practitioners of ultrasound, we have a duty of care to the patient, and therefore we need to understand the potential bio-effects and up-to-date guidelines relating to ultrasound safety.

The interactions of ultrasound with tissue can give rise to potentially harmful bio-effects, the most important of these being heating and mechanical effects.

Heating

As stated earlier, absorption of ultrasound energy can lead to the heating of tissue. Heating is more likely to occur at sites in the body where the absorption is higher than in the surrounding tissue. For example, bone absorbs energy more strongly than soft tissue does and therefore the surrounding soft tissue can experience secondary heating as a result of conduction from the bone. This is particularly important as fetal bone matures, when large increases in absorption have been documented. Consequently, heating effects during routine fetal assessment need to be considered. Diagnostic ultrasound can produce rises in temperature that are hazardous to sensitive organs and the developing embryo.

To this end, the thermal index has been developed in an attempt to account for the possibility of bio-effects resulting from heating. This index is an estimate of the rise in tissue temperature that might be possible under 'reasonable worst-case conditions' and is defined as the ratio of the acoustic power emitted to the power required to heat a particular target tissue by 1 C. As heating is tissue-specific, there are in fact three thermal indices: the thermal index in soft tissues (TIS), the thermal index in bone (TIB) and the thermal index in the cranium (TIC).

The responsibility for safety issues is with the operator. The operator should therefore continually monitor the thermal index and keep it as low as is consistent with achieving a diagnostic result. Regarding the safe use of ultrasound in obstetric investigations, the British Medical Ultrasound Society (BMUS) recommends monitoring of the TIS during scans carried out in the first 8 weeks following conception and monitoring of the TIB during subsequent scans.

Cavitation

Since the early days of ultrasound, it has been known that ultrasound can lyse or otherwise damage cells in suspension. This effect is not a result of the thermal properties of ultrasound; instead, it is attributable to the presence of gas-filled cavities in tissue exposed to ultrasound waves. These cavities can either oscillate or collapse under the pressure of the ultrasound beam, producing either considerable shear forces or high pressures and temperatures that can damage cell membranes or produce highly reactive free radicals. This phenomenon is known as cavitation. Gas in the lung, in the intestine and in contrast agents increases the likelihood of cavitation and mechanical damage.

Once again, an index has been developed in an attempt to account for the possibility of bio-effects resulting from mechanical effects. This is known as the mechanical index and is related to the maximum negative pressure and frequency in an ultrasound field.

At present, there is considerable debate as to whether exposures at diagnostic ultrasound levels are able to induce cavitation effects in the absence of exogenous bubbles (such as those that are used as ultrasound contrast agents). The consensus of opinion is that they are unlikely to occur at significant levels, but the possibility of low-level activity cannot be altogether ruled out (4).

Guidelines and Recommendations for the Safe Use of Diagnostic Ultrasound

There are a number of guidelines and recommendations for the safe use of diagnostic ultrasound and these change or are updated at regular intervals. A good review of the current guidelines and recommendations can always be found on the website of the BMUS (www.bmus.org). The BMUS also provides recommended thermal and mechanical index values. The EFSUMB (www.efsumb.org), the American Institute of Ultrasound in Medicine (www.aium.org) and the World Federation of Ultrasound in Medicine and Biology (www.wfumb.org) also publish their latest documents on their websites.

Principles and Use of X-Rays, Computed Tomography and Magnetic Resonance Imaging X-Rays

X-radiation is a form of electromagnetic radiation. X-rays have a wavelength in the range of 10–0.01 nm, corresponding to frequencies in the range of $0.03–30 \times 10^{18}$ Hz and energies in the range of 120 eV to

120 keV. They are longer than gamma rays but shorter than ultraviolet rays. X-rays with energies below 12 keV are classified as soft X-rays and those above as hard X-rays, owing to their penetration abilities.

Radiography is considered to be a non-invasive medical test method that is primarily used for diagnostic purposes. It is the oldest and most frequently used form of medical imaging. As a result, the term *X-ray* is used to refer to a radiographic image produced using this method as well as to the method itself. X-rays are a form of ionising radiation and as such can be dangerous. X-rays were listed as a carcinogen by the US government in 2005.

The sievert (Sv) is the SI unit of measure of radiation and denotes the amount of energy delivered to a human body by gamma radiation or X-radiation (ionising radiation). Commonly, the radiation exposure from an X-ray is in the microsievert range. The average person living in the United States receives approximately 3 mSv annually from background sources alone.

Beam Formation and Detection

X-rays are produced by accelerating electrons, which are then made to collide with a metal target; the precise nature of the metal target depends on the type of application. In the X-ray tube, the electrons suddenly decelerate upon collision with the metal target and can knock out an electron from the inner shell of the metal atom. Electrons from higher energy levels then fill up the vacancy, and X-ray photons are emitted as a result. The process is extremely inefficient, and a considerable amount of energy and heat has to be wasted to produce a reasonable flux of X-rays.

X-rays were originally detected by use of a photographic plate and later by use of an X-ray film in a cassette. These devices are generally referred to as image receptors. Plates and films have been largely replaced in hospitals by computed and digital radiography, although film technology is still used in some countries and for industrial applications. Computed and digital technologies have several advantages: they do not require wet processing facilities on-site; they do not require the use of silver, which is a non-renewable resource; and the archiving and retrieval of digital images is considerably easier with additional space-saving benefits.

Use of X-Rays in Clinical Practice

The body region to be imaged is positioned between the X-ray source and the image receptor, which captures a shadow image of internal body structures. X-rays may be blocked (attenuated) by dense tissues such as bone but pass more easily through soft tissues. On the X-ray, the areas where the image receptor is exposed to high X-ray energy will appear black. Soft tissue and bone will appear as shades of grey or white because some of the radiation energy is lost on its way from the source to the receptor.

X-rays are useful for identifying skeletal disease, as well as chest, lung and abdominal pathologies. Their use in some cases, such as in the imaging of muscle or brain structures, is debatable and alternative imaging methods such as computed tomography (CT), magnetic resonance imaging (MRI) or ultrasound might be more appropriate.

Radiopaque contrast agents are used to highlight organs or vessels, depending on the mode of their administration. They are often used in real-time procedures carried out with a so-called X-ray image intensifier, resulting in a sequence of images that are projected on to a fluorescent screen or a television-like monitor. Such producers include barium meal or enema, hysterosalpingography and uterine artery embolization for the treatment of uterine fibroids.

In gynaecology, hysterosalpingography is frequently used to assess tubal patency in subfertile women (Fig. 36.12). The procedure is usually performed in the first 10 days of the menstrual cycle to avoid inadvertent exposure of early pregnancy to radiation. There is no need for anaesthesia, although pain relief medications and antispasmodics are often given orally.

Hysterosalpingography has the following advantages:

- radiation does not persist after the procedure
- the procedure is minimally invasive
- complications are rare
- the procedure is relatively quick
- the procedure can provide valuable information on the appearance of the uterine cavity and the patency of the fallopian tube
- X-rays usually have no immediate adverse effects in the diagnostic range

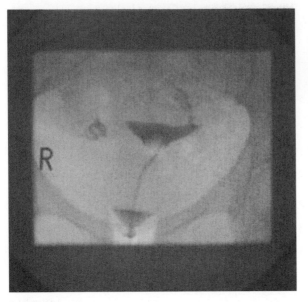

R = right side

Figure 36.12

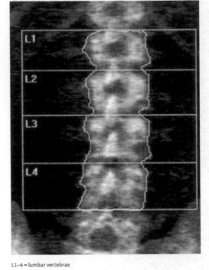

L1–4 = lumbar vertebrae

Figure 36.13

Dual Energy X-Ray Absorptiometry

Dual-energy X-ray absorptiometry (DXA) is the most widely used technology for measuring bone mineral density (BMD) in g/cm^2. It uses two beams of low-energy X-rays (approximately one-tenth that of a standard chest X-ray). These two beams of X-rays are absorbed by differing amounts depending on the type of tissue they are passing through enabling the calculation of BMD in the area of bone included in the acquired image by subtracting the soft tissue element. A DXA image of the lumbar spine is shown in Figure 36.13.

The results are presented both in graphical form where the patient's BMD and age are plotted with respect to a reference population (sex and ethnicity matched) provided by the manufacturer, and in the form of standard deviation (SD) scores: the T-score and the Z-score.

The T-score expresses how many SD the patient result differs from the mean value for a sex and ethnicity matched young adult reference mean and is used to divide patients into one of four categories defined by the World Health Organisation (WHO) as follows:

- T-score > –1 is considered to be normal

- T-score between –1 and –2.5 is classed as low bone mineral/osteopenic and the patient has a moderately increased risk of fracture
- T-score less than –2.5 is classed as osteoporosis, and these patients are at high risk of fracture
- T-score less than –2.5 with one or more fragility fractures are classed as established osteoporosis

The Z-score expresses how many SD the patient result differs from the mean value for an age, sex and ethnicity matched reference population and is used in children (where the use of T-score is inappropriate as peak bone mass hasn't been reached) and can be helpful in interpreting the results in the elderly.

The clinical interpretation of BMD results by DXA is a specialist area and is beyond the scope of this book.

Two types of DXA equipment are available. In central devices, the X-ray tank is positioned below an imaging couch and is joined to the detector by a C-arm such that the X-ray tank and detector are aligned and move simultaneously over the area to be measured (Fig. 36.14). Central devices can measure BMD at the lumbar spine, proximal femur and fore-arm and are considered the technique of choice to diagnose osteoporosis. Peripheral devices are much smaller and can measure BMD at the wrist, heel or fingers, depending on which device is being used.

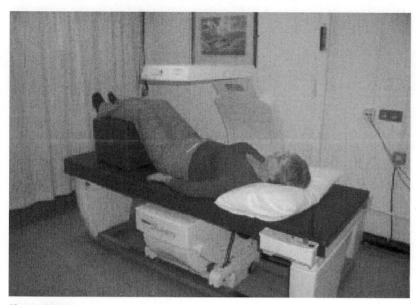

Figure 36.14

Computed Tomography

Ultrasound is usually the modality of first choice to assess female pelvic disease, but CT is also used as part of the assessment of pelvic tumours and other abdominal disease. CT scanning uses X-rays, and the principles of X-ray formation, detection and contrast outlined previously apply here as well. CT, however, produces transverse cross-sectional images of the body by reconstructing the attenuation of fine X-ray beams passed through the body. This gives images of higher contrast resolution than plain radiography does.

Software developments enable the reconstruction and display of three-dimensional images. These images are generated by stacking a series of two-dimensional planes on top of each other to generate a volumetric display of the area under examination. Advanced three-dimensional rendering techniques such as surface and volume rendering allow the construction of different three-dimensional models, with each anatomical structure being represented by a different colour. It is also possible to remove certain unwanted structures from the image through a process known as segmentation. The effective radiation dose is considerably higher with CT compared with plain film radiography (the typical abdominal and pelvic CT effective dose is 10mSv compared with 0.1mSv for a standard chest X-ray). However, in

general, fetal doses are unlikely to cause deterministic effects in and individual pregnancy, and women should be counselled that radiological exposure from a single diagnostic procedure is not likely to pose a radiation threat to the fetus (5).

Magnetic Resonance Imaging

MRI is another imaging technique used to visualise the structure and function of the body. Unlike CT, MRI does not use ionising radiation. Instead, a powerful magnetic field is created to align the H+ ions (protons) present in tissue molecules. A radiofrequency pulse is then used to disrupt the alignment of these protons with the main magnetic field. Following the pulse, the protons drift back into alignment with the magnetic field, emitting a detectable radiofrequency signal as they do so. Contrast agents may be injected directly into the area being examined or intravenously to enhance the appearance of vessels, tumours or inflammatory tissue.

In clinical practice, MRI is used to differentiate pathological tissue such as brain or ovarian tumours from normal tissue (Fig. 36.15). The spatial resolution (the ability to distinguish two structures that are very close to each other as separate) provided by MRI is comparable with that of CT, but its contrast resolution (the ability to distinguish between two similar but not identical tissues) is far better because modern

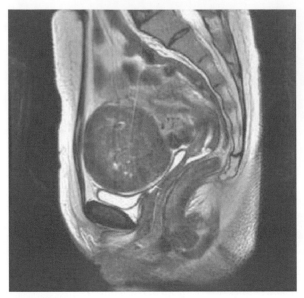

Figure 36.15

MRI scanners include a complex library of pulse sequences that can be employed to characterise different tissues on the basis of their interaction with the pulse signal.

Magnetic Resonance Imaging and Pregnancy

No harmful effects of MRI have been demonstrated on the fetus, especially as no ionising radiation is used. However, as a precaution, MRI in pregnant women should be undertaken only where necessary, especially in the first trimester. Contrast agents, for example gadolinium-based compounds, are known to cross the placenta, and their use during pregnancy is controversial. The Royal College of Radiologists current standards state: 'Use of gadolinium-containing contrast agent is not recommended unless absolutely necessary'(www.rcr.ac.uk/sites/default/files/docs/radiology/pdf/BFCR(10)4_Stand_contrast.pdf). However, contrast-enhanced MR imaging may be performed when essential to the diagnosis (e.g. in the absence of alternative imaging studies or when it is not possible to delay the MR imaging examination until after delivery).

Interventional Magnetic Resonance Imaging

In view of its safety record, MRI is well suited for interventional radiology, where the images produced by an MRI scanner are used to guide minimally invasive procedures. Such procedures, naturally, must be done in the absence of any ferromagnetic instruments. A subspecialty of interventional MRI is that of intraoperative MRI, where systems have been developed to allow imaging concurrent with the surgical procedure. More typical, however, is the temporary interruption of the surgical procedure so that MRI scans can be acquired to verify the success of the procedure or guide subsequent surgical work.

Radiation Therapy Simulation

MRI is used to locate tumours within the body before the initiation of radiation therapy. The person to be treated is placed in a specific, reproducible, body position and scanned. The MRI system then computes the precise location, shape and orientation of the tumour mass, correcting for any spatial distortion inherent in the system. The person is then marked with triangulation points that will permit the delivery of precise, targeted radiation therapy.

Magnetic-Resonance-Guided Focused Ultrasound

MRI is also used to guide ultrasound surgery, in which a high-energy ultrasound beam is focused on a small spot in a target tissue such as a uterine fibroid. The ultrasound beam heats the tissue to a temperature of more than 65 C, destroying it completely. The three-dimensional view of the target tissue offered by MRI allows accurate focusing of the ultrasound energy as well as monitoring of the treatment cycle, resulting in precise ablation of the diseased tissue.

Drawbacks of Magnetic Resonance Imaging

Claustrophobia is one of the most common reasons for people to refuse to undergo an MRI examination. Traditionally, owing to the construction of the original machines, the person under investigation had to be placed in the centre of the magnet and, coupled with a somewhat lengthy examination time, the experience was often unpleasant. Modern scanners have short bores and faster scan times, so the procedure is better tolerated. Certain groups of people, such as children, obese individuals and pregnant women, are difficult to accommodate within the machine without special provisions. Acoustic noise associated with the operation of an MRI scanner can also exacerbate the discomfort associated with the procedure.

Metal fragments in the eyes (welders), neurosurgical clips, pacing wires and other ferrous prostheses are contraindicated.

The latest guidance and safety notes on the use of MRI can be found at www.gov.uk/government/uploads/system/uploads/attachment_data/file/476931/MRI_guidance_2015_-_4-02d1.pdf.

Principles and Use of Electrosurgery

The use of thermal energy for therapy dates back many centuries. Hippocrates (460–370 BC) already recorded the use of heat for incising suprapubic abscesses. With the advent of electricity in the early 1800s, electrically heated surgical instruments became available. Surgical diathermy machines were first introduced in the late 1920s.

A diathermy machine converts the mains low-frequency current (230 V, 50 Hz) into a high-frequency current in the radiofrequency range (between 200 kHz and 3.3 MHz) to obtain a desired surgical effect, such as cutting, coagulation (clotting of blood), vaporisation and/or destruction.

Interactions of Electric Current with Tissue

Low-Frequency versus High-Frequency Currents

The effect of an electric current on tissues depends on the frequency of the current. A low-frequency current causes cyclic polarisation and depolarisation of cells owing to the transmembrane exchange of ions, resulting in neuromuscular stimulation. Depending on the actual frequency, this manifests as clonic or tetanic contraction.

By contrast, a high-frequency current changes direction so rapidly that ionic exchange at the cellular level does not happen because of the fixed time that such ions require to move through nerve tissue. Hence, no neuromuscular stimulation takes place. Nevertheless, the high energy delivered to tissue produces collision of intracellular ions and other materials, which manifests as heat.

Grounded versus Isolated Electrosurgery Systems

Earthed (grounded) diathermy systems allow the current to return back to the unit via earth. If the return electrode is faulty or poorly applied, an alternative return pathway such as the treated person's skin is used, resulting in severe burns. By contrast, in an isolated system, minimal or no current flows to earth and the circuit through the human body is isolated. Hence, should there be a faulty connection or appliance, the current does not return to the machine and there is no risk of burns.

The return electrode, or patient plate, in grounded diathermy systems provides a safe return pathway for the passage of the current from the active electrode through the human body. As the current that passes through the tissue produces a greater current density and heat intensity under a smaller electrode (Fig. 36.16), the surface area of the return electrode should be much larger than that of the active electrode.

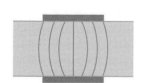

A Two electrodes of equal size: the heating effect is the same beneath each electrode

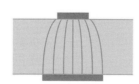

B Unequal electrodes: the heating effect is greater under the smaller electrode

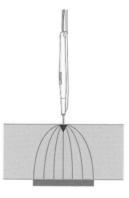

C Current density and thermal effects are highest when the electrode is pointed

Figure 36.16

Generally, a minimum surface area of 69 cm^2 or 10 inch^2 is recommended to maintain temperature increase at very low levels.

Monopolar versus Bipolar Electrosurgery

Surgical diathermy can be either monopolar or bipolar. During monopolar surgical diathermy, the electric current is transported through the human body and back to the generator. An electrode used in monopolar diathermy may be a blade, a ball, a needle tip or an open or closed loop. It is important to remember that the smaller the tip, the greater the heating effect will be because the current density will be concentrated at the smaller area (Fig. 36.17). The monopolar electrode is connected to the diathermy machine (Fig. 36.18), which in turn is connected to a return plate that is attached to another body part of the person undergoing the operation.

In bipolar diathermy, the current flows between the tips of a forceps' blades (Fig. 36.17), which are separated by an insulating material. One blade acts as an active electrode and the other as a return. The tissue in between the blades acts as the conducting medium for the current. Many bipolar diathermy generators incorporate a facility for autocoagulation (Fig. 36.19), where the degree of coagulation is sensed by the generator and the current is discontinued when the optimum effect has been achieved. Unlike monopolar diathermy, where cutting and coagulation modes are possible, bipolar diathermy only permits coagulation with no cutting. Several new bipolar electrodes are now available on the market.

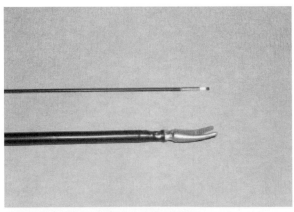

Bipolar electrode used in hysteroscopic surgery (top); a grasping bipolar electrode used in laparoscopic surgery (bottom).

Figure 36.17

Tissue Effects of Various Waveforms

Electrosurgical generators can produce current in several modes (Fig. 36.20), with distinct tissue effects for each modality.

A cutting current is produced with a continuous unmodulated sinusoidal waveform, with a relatively low voltage needed to produce the desired tissue vaporization effect (Fig. 36.20 A). The tip of the electrode is held just above the target tissue. Electric arcs are formed between the cutting electrode and the tissue, generating points of extremely high temperatures that vaporise cells in such a way that a clean tissue cut is achieved (Fig. 36.21). There is insufficient time for the heat to dissipate to adjacent tissue; hence there is less tissue trauma and cutting occurs without significant haemostasis.

A coagulation effect is produced with a higher voltage current than that used for cutting but the current is applied intermittently (Fig. 36.20B) and modulated with a duty cycle that is on for about 6% of the time, although this may vary depending on the desired effect. This modulation, or dampening, allows the tissue to cool between heating bursts. Thus no vaporisation occurs but the current causes coagulation, a complex process that is an important part of haemostasis. Higher voltage with longer modulation intervals results in great coagulation or haemostatic effect.

Desiccation is the process of extreme drying, whereby tissues are coagulated while being heated to 70–100 C. Soft coagulation uses a peak voltage of about 200 volts or less and the power output is precisely limited or minimal leading to minimal carbonisation, quick coagulation and as little sticking to the electrode as possible. Desiccation and soft coagulation both require contact by the active electrode with the tissue.

Monopolar or bipolar instruments can be used to desiccate tissues and the effect can be produced with either the cutting mode or the coagulation mode of the generator (Fig. 36.22), although the cutting mode is the preferred option. A blended waveform combines bursts of low-voltage (coagulation) currents (Fig. 36.20 C) and produces cutting with coagulation effects.

Other variables can impact the tissue effect, namely the duration of application, the power setting and the precise type of active electrode. Too long an activation should be avoided, as it may lead to adherence of the coagulum to the electrode and subsequent tearing of the coagulum from the vessels, resulting in

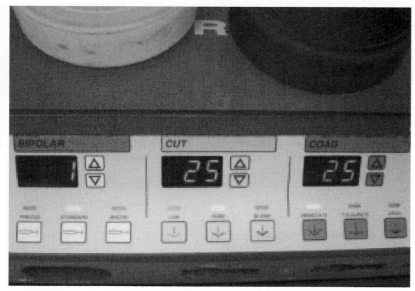

Figure 36.18

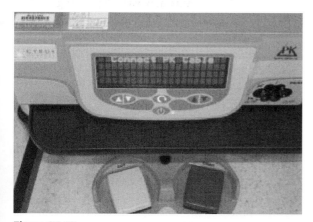

Figure 36.19

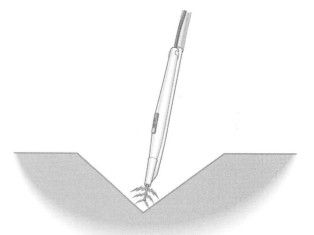

Figure 36.21

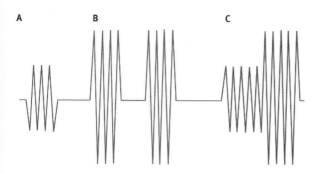

A Cutting mode I B Coagulation mode I C Blended mode

Figure 36.20

inadequate haemostasis. Modern generators may monitor the flow of current through the tissue to optimise the coagulation effect.

Fulguration (electrofulguration) or forced coagulation results when a high-powered current is used to produce a sparkling effect to coagulate a large bleeding area or to char tissue without touching the tissue with the electrode (Fig. 36.23). This effect produces deeper coagulation than can be achieved with soft coagulation and is used in specific circumstances only.

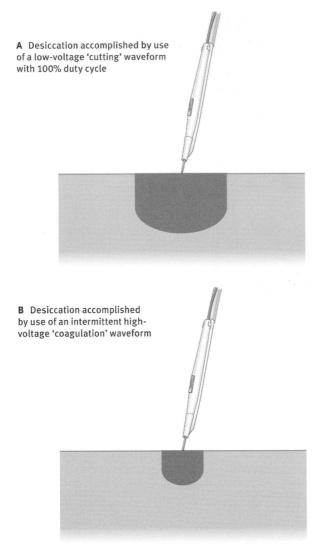

A Desiccation accomplished by use of a low-voltage 'cutting' waveform with 100% duty cycle

B Desiccation accomplished by use of an intermittent high-voltage 'coagulation' waveform

Figure 36.22

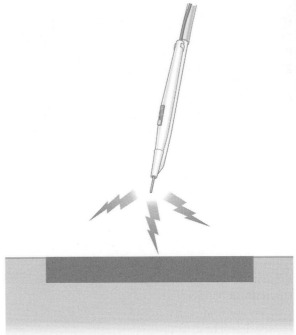

Figure 36.23

Argon-enhanced electrosurgery was introduced in the late 1980s. The inert, nonreactive argon gas wraps the electrosurgical current and concentrates and delivers the spark to the tissue in a beam-like fashion, creating a smoother, more malleable dry scab.

Safety of Electrosurgery

In the past 15 years, considerable improvements in electrosurgical safety have been achieved. Modern generators produce efficient and effective cutting and coagulation currents, automatically measure tissue impedance and adjust the output, monitor and warn of any potentially dangerous low-frequency leaks of current from the human body to earth and warn of incomplete application of the return electrode. These features reduce the risk of adverse effects to people undergoing electrosurgery. Additionally, modern generators have two separate return plates and the resistance is constantly measured in each. If for any reason there is a difference in the resistance of the return plates, the system will automatically be turned off. It is also important that the diathermy machine displays the power output and that the surgeon uses the lowest effective power setting, for example 30 W. Higher outputs are required when using diathermy with glycine, such as in transcervical resection or rollerball ablation of the endometrium.

Hazards associated with the use of active monopolar electrodes also include direct coupling, insulation failure and capacitive coupling, each of which may cause severe injury.

Direct coupling occurs when the electrode is activated in close proximity or direct contact with another conductive instrument within the body. This risk is avoidable or greatly minimised through the adoption of strict safety rules during surgery.

Insulation failure occurs when the coating that covers the active electrode is compromised. This may result from repeated use or incorrect handling of instruments and may not be detected by the surgeon or theatre staff.

Capacitive coupling may occur between two conductors that are separated by an insulator. For example, if an insulated active electrode is inserted down a metal cannula, the electric current can be transferred from the active electrode through its insulation and into the conductive metal cannula, which can discharge electrical energy if it comes into contact with body structures.

The following practices are recommended to ensure the safe use of electrical surgical instruments:

- Check the instrument's isolation before surgery.
- Use the lowest possible power and voltage settings to achieve the desired effect.
- Activate the electrode only when necessary.
- Never activate the electrode when in close proximity or direct contact with a metal or conductive object.

Consideration should also be given to the following points:

- Bipolar instruments are safer than monopolar devices.
- An all-metal or all-plastic cannula system is the safest option.
- Active-electrode monitoring systems reduce the risk of capacitive coupling.

Principles and Use of Microwave Energy

'Microwave' is a term that generally refers to the frequency of the electric signal. Microwave energy' is a form of non-ionizing electromagnetic energy that falls at the lower frequency end of the electromagnetic spectrum (range 300 MHz–300,000 MHz). Within this range, only molecular rotation is affected and not the molecular structure. In the medical field, systems have used frequencies such as 915 MHz, 2.45GHz and 9.2GHz. This equates with the signal oscillating its polarity ('+' and '–' sides) 915 million to 9 billion times every second. Water molecules are polar and will align to the opposite polarity and oscillate when exposed to high frequency. As a result of this high-speed movement, friction and heat are generated in the tissues. The zone of thermal lesion is generally superficial with a depth range of 1-4 cm and

is dependent on the frequency and time of exposure to the microwave energy.

The use of microwave energy has been shown to be effective in the management of heavy menstrual bleeding (7–9), benign prostatic hyperplasia and a variety of non-resectable hepatic tumours.

Principles and Use of Lasers in Endoscopic Surgery

The term *laser* is an acronym for 'light amplification by stimulated emission of radiation.' The laser device emits light photons (electromagnetic radiation) through a process called stimulated emission to vaporise, dissect and coagulate tissue. Laser beams additionally have a natural sterilisation effect as they evaporate bacteria, viruses and fungi and seal nerve endings, thus decreasing postoperative pain. Laser devices used in endoscopic surgery are either gas (CO_2 or argon ions) or solid-state lasers and are described as class 4 lasers with a capacity to cause fires, burns and retinal damage. Lasers can interact with tissues in four ways, namely photothermally (commonly employed in gynaecology), photochemically, photomechanically and photoablatively. The characteristics of lasers commonly used in endoscopic surgery are given in Table 36.1.

Carbon Dioxide Gas Lasers

CO_2 gas lasers have a wavelength of 10 600 nm and are absorbed to a high degree by soft tissues that contain water. This enables precise tissue cutting and dissection with minimal lateral damage. The vaporisation capability of CO_2 lasers is useful for the removal of endometriotic implants, especially near the ureters. However, the beam has to be transmitted from the generator to the endoscope by a system of articulated arms and mirrors, which are expensive and difficult to clean, and is then sent through a semiflexible fibre that runs down the endoscopic operating channel. As CO_2 lasers are invisible to the human eye, an additional visible aiming laser is needed to assist with treatment. Overall, the depth of the CO_2 laser is very limited making it unsuitable for laparoscopic surgery.

Solid-State Lasers

Solid-state lasers are commonly made by 'doping' a crystalline solid host with ions that provide the

Table 36.1 Lasers commonly used in endoscopic surgery

Type	Wavelength (nm)	Colour	Fibre	Depth of penetration
Argon	488–512	Blue-green	Yes	0.5 mm
KTP/532	532	Green	Yes	1–2 mm
Nd:YAG	1,064	Infrared	Yes	3–4 mm
CO_2	10,600	Infrared	No	0.1 mm

required energy states. Examples include the neodymium-doped yttrium aluminium garnet (Nd:YAG) laser, which can produce high-energy beams in the infrared spectrum at 1064 nm and can be transmitted down a fibreoptic cable to the operating site. The Nd:YAG laser provides good cutting and haemostatic effects as well as being able to vaporise tissue. When the beam is transmitted down a bare quartz fibre, it penetrates deeply into tissues, a property that may be useful for hysteroscopic surgery but may be unsafe in laparoscopic procedures. In laparoscopic procedures, the beam should be focused at the tip (the focal spot size varies from approximately 0.1 mm to 0.4 mm) to limit the amount of unintended tissue damage to 0.2–1.0 mm.

Passage of the Nd:YAG beam through a crystal of potassium titanyl phosphate (KTP) results in doubling of the original frequency and a wavelength that is half the original, with beam characteristics that are somewhere between those of the CO2 laser and the Nd:YAG laser. The KTP laser produces a visible beam at a wavelength, of 532 nm, is easily transmitted down flexible fibreoptic cables and penetrates tissue for about 1–2 mm. The beam can vaporise, cut and coagulate tissue with a single, bare and reusable quartz fibre.

During the use of Nd:YAG and KTP lasers, staff must wear protective goggles and the person undergoing laser surgery must be provided with suitable protection to prevent inadvertent exposure and injury to the retina by the beam.

Principles and Use of Radiotherapy

Radiation therapy or radiotherapy is the use of ionising radiation as a medical intervention, primarily for the treatment of cancer. The amount of radiation used is measured in gray (Gy). Use of radiotherapy for non-malignant conditions is very limited because of concerns about the risk of radiation-induced cancer.

Radiotherapy acts by damaging cellular DNA. This damage may be caused by photons, electrons, protons, neutrons or ion beams and may occur either directly or indirectly. The indirect effect is the most common mechanism of action and results from the ionisation of H_2O molecules, which generates H^+ and hydroxyl (OH^-) ions and free radicals ($H^\bullet$ and $OH^\bullet$) that damage the DNA. This can lead to the irreversible loss of the cells' reproductive integrity and their eventual death.

Radiotherapy also affects intracellular processes that are necessary for cellular growth, senescence and apoptosis and the intrinsic ability to repair damage. Cell survival curves depend on the dose of radiation, the position of the cell in the mitotic cycle, the O_2 tension, the intrinsic cellular radiosensitivity and the cellular environment. Tissue hypoxia increases resistance to the effects of radiation as O_2 makes the radiation damage to DNA permanent. Several strategies have been developed to increase tissue oxygenation and enhance the effectiveness of radiotherapy, including the practice of total dose fractionation (spreading the dose over time). Details of logarithmic survival curves and information on how manipulation of the cellular environment alters these curves are provided in the literature.

When protons (positively charged particles) are used, their biological effects are the same as those of other particles. However, unlike photons (soft X-rays), protons release their energy at the point of impact within the tumour, with a rapid fall-off in does in the healthy tissue beyond. Adverse effects are minimised and a higher dose can be used for treatment.

Radiotherapy may be used as primary therapy, in conjunction with either surgery, chemotherapy or endocrine therapy or in combination with one or more of these modalities.

When used as a primary therapeutic modality where there is survival benefit, it can be curative (resulting in the radical removal of disease) or palliative (where the aim of treatment is symptom control or the local control of disease).

When used as an adjuvant therapy, radiotherapy is usually given after the surgical removal of all detectable disease and its aim is to improve disease-specific and overall survival. Thus adjuvant radiotherapy is essentially administered to minimise the risk of recurrence, rather than for the treatment of a proven disease and a proportion of people who receive adjuvant therapy will already have been cured by their primary surgery.

When radiotherapy is given before the main treatment, it is described as neoadjuvant therapy and its aim is to reduce the size of the tumour so as to facilitate more effective surgery.

If administered at the same time as other therapies, it is described as concurrent therapy.

Delivery of Radiotherapy

External-Beam Radiotherapy

Linear accelerator (linac) machines deliver two-dimensional beams from several (one to four) directions to the area being treated. In conventional techniques, the treatment is first simulated on a specially calibrated diagnostic X-ray machine known as the simulator, which has the same geometry as the linear accelerator employed during treatment. Treatment simulation is used for tumour localisation, treatment plan verification and treatment monitoring.

An enhancement of virtual simulation in three-dimensional conformal radiotherapy (CRT), which uses a variable number of beams with the profile of each radiation beam being shaped to fit the profile of the target. As the shape of the treatment volume matches the shape of the tumour, the relative toxicity of radiation to the surrounding normal tissue is reduced, allowing a higher dose of radiation to be delivered to the tumour than possible with conventional techniques.

Intensity-modulated radiation therapy (IMRT) is the next generation of three-dimensional CRT. In this form of high-precision radiation therapy, the intensity of each radiation beam can be modulated so that a given treatment field may be targeted by beams of variable intensity. This allows for greater control of the distribution of the dose within the target, thereby creating limitless possibilities to sculpt the radiation dose to the tumour itself.

Despite such advances, the limitations of radiotherapy include the inability to identify microscopic disease with accuracy, the difficulty of immobilising the treated person/tumour for the duration of a treatment session (with IMRT this is typically 15–30 minutes) and problems arising from tumour shrinkage with treatment.

The next challenge in radiation oncology is therefore to accommodate changes in the position of the treated person and/or movement or shrinkage of the tumour during treatment. Incorporating real-time imaging with real-time adjustment of the therapeutic beams, an approach commonly called four-dimensional CRT, allows 'online' imaging of the individual during treatment and real-time reconstruction of the actual daily delivered dose on the basis of the individual's and the tumour's changing anatomies. This approach results in adaptive radiotherapy – the modulation of prescription and delivery on the basis of the actual daily delivered dose as opposed to the planned dose.

Internal-Beam Radiotherapy

Internally delivered radiotherapy may be in the form of:

- sealed-source radiotherapy (brachytherapy)
- unsealed-source radiotherapy (radioisotope therapy)

Both techniques utilize radioisotopes to deliver the radiation dose. An isotope is a form of the same element that contain equal numbers of protons but different numbers of neutrons in their nuclei, and hence differ in relative atomic mass but not in chemical properties. A radioisotope is simply a radioactive form of the element (Fig. 36.24). Most radioisotopes used in internal beam radiotherapy are gamma or beta emitters, although targeted alpha therapy is an emerging technology.

Brachytherapy involves the use of sealed sources, which are placed directly into, or adjacent to, the volume of tissue to be irradiated. The advantage is that it allows the tumour to be treated at very short distances and the radiation passes through less

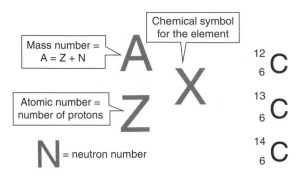

Figure 36.24 Schematic diagram of an atom showing the atomic number, mass number and the isotopes of carbon

healthy tissue. In addition, brachytherapy sources generally emit lower-energy radiation compared with external-beam radiotherapy. The proximity of the radiation source in brachytherapy allows the dose to be better localised to the tumour volume. The clinician can therefore treat the tumour with very high doses while the dose to the surrounding healthy tissue is minimised.

Brachytherapy is used to treat many gynaecological cancers including vaginal, cervical, ovarian and uterine cancer. The radioactive material, such as caesium-137 or iridium-192, is placed temporarily inside or near a tumour for a specific amount of time and then withdrawn. It may be administered at a low or high dose. Occasionally, radioactive seeds or pellets, such as iodine-125 seeds, are placed in or near the tumour and are left there permanently. After several weeks or months, the radioactivity level of the implants eventually diminishes to nothing. The seeds then remain in the body with no lasting effect.

Radioisotope therapy is an unsealed form of radiotherapy. It is delivered by injection, for example phosphorus-32 used to treat polycythaemia vera, or by ingestion, for example ingestion of iodine-131 to treat thyroid cancer or thyrotoxicosis.

An emerging field is targeted alpha therapy (TAT) or alpha radioimmunotherapy, especially for the control of dispersed cancers. The short range of very energetic alpha emissions in tissue means that a large fraction of that radiative energy goes into the targeted cancer cells, once a carrier such as a monoclonal antibody has taken the alpha-emitting radionuclide such as bismuth-213 to exactly the right places. Clinical trials for leukaemia, cystic glioma and melanoma are underway. TAT using lead-212 is increasingly important for treating pancreatic, ovarian and melanoma cancers.

Safety of Radiotherapy

Acute adverse effects of radiotherapy include:

- damage to epithelial surfaces (such as skin, oral and bowel mucosa)
- oedema and swelling of soft tissues as part of the inflammatory reaction, which may be ameliorated with steroids
- infertility caused by damage to the radiation-sensitive gonads
- generalised fatigue

Medium-term and long-term adverse effects depend on the particular area being treated and may be minimal. These include:

- fibrosis and diffuse scarring of the irradiated tissue hair loss
- dryness as a result of damage to the salivary and tear glands or vaginal dryness as a result of damage to the cervical glands
- fatigue and lethargy
- cancer secondary to irradiation
- death

Reirradiation may cause additional acute or intermediate adverse effects or exacerbation of already existing adverse effects, and people undergoing reirradiation must be monitored closely.

References

1   Lees C, Abramowicz J, Brezinka C, et al. *Ultrasound from Conception to 10⁺⁰ Weeks of Gestation*. Scientific impact paper No. 49. 2015; *RCOG*: 1–11

2   Martin E, Shaw A, Lees C. Survey of current practice in transvaginal ultrasound scanning in the UK. *Ultrasound* 2015; **23**: 138–148

3   Miller G. The safe use of contrast-enhanced diagnostic ultrasound. In: ter Haar G (ed.), *The Safe Use of Ultrasound in Medical Diagnosis*, 3rd ed. 2012. 105–124

4   Fowlkes JB. Non-thermal effects of diagnostic ultrasound. In: ter Haar G (ed.), *The Safe Use of Ultrasound in Medical Diagnosis*, 3rd ed. 2012. 69–80

5   Osama SE, Seumas DE, Watkinson T. Review. Safety of diagnostic imaging in pregnancy. Part 1: X-ray, nuclear medicine investigations, computed tomography and contrast media. *The Obstetrician & Gynaecologist* 2010; **12**: 71–78

6   Standards for Intravascular Contrast Administration to Adult Patients. www.rcr.ac.uk/sites/default/files/docs/radiology/pdf/BFCR(10)4_Stand_contrast.pdf.

7. Kanaoka Y, Hirai K, Ishiko O, Ogita S. Microwave endometrial ablation at a frequency of 2.45 GHz a pilot study. *Journal of Reproductive Medicine for the Obstetrician and Gynecologist* 2001; **46**(6): 559–563

8. Sambrook AM, Elders A, Cooper KG. Microwave endometrial ablation versus thermal balloon endometrial ablation (MEATBall): 5-year follow up of a randomised controlled trial. *BJOG: An International Journal of Obstetrics and Gynaecology* 2014; **121**(6): 747–753

9. Matsumoto N, Ikeda N, Takenaka T, Yazaki S, Sato Y. Clinical practice and short-term efficacy of 2.45-GHz microwave endometrial ablation to treat menorrhagia. *Gynaecology and Minimally Invasive Therapy* 2015; **4** (3): 76–80

Chapter 37

Statistics

Anthony N. Griffiths

Introduction

Statistics is often cited as one of the more difficult topics examined in the Part 1 MRCOG. Some candidates avoid the subject and hope to compensate by higher scoring in other subjects. This is unwise as the statistical component of the examination is significant and is also an easy way to gain substantial marks. While writing questions for the Part I examination and running Part I courses, it became obvious that the types of statistical questions asked were very limited with a repetitive nature (though, of course, the numbers are changed). This synoptic chapter will give you the appropriate level of knowledge of statistics required for the Part I examination.

What Is Statistics?

Statistics is a branch of mathematics that allows us to do three things:

1. *Describe* what is happening with numeric results. It can describe the basic features of data in a study, e.g. 70 % of candidates passed the Part I examination.

2. *Summarise* what is happening, e.g. the mean Caesarean section rate for my hospital is 21%, with a monthly range of 18–24%.

3. *Analyse* what is happening to aid in reaching a conclusion. This is the more difficult area, as it involves using tests, e.g. t test, etc. It is important to note that statistics never gives the answer and you must exercise caution and a degree of common sense. For example, a study suggests that chlamydia infection is more common in women with tattoos of blue dolphins (p<0.05). The mistake is to believe that having a tattoo increased your chance of chlamydia! This is an example of an association, not causation.

Hypothesis Testing (Table 37.1)

A hypothesis is simply an idea based on limited evidence that needs further investigation. In a clinical trial, you must try to disprove, rather than prove, your hypothesis. For example, if you carry out a randomised controlled trial of women treated with antibiotic or placebo after ventouse delivery, your hypothesis could be that antibiotics reduce the chance of perineal breakdown. There will always be some difference in the perineal breakdown rates between the two groups, but the question is whether this difference is due to chance or due to the antibiotic therapy.

To decide if the null or alternative hypothesis is more likely to be true, it is necessary to carry out an analytic test. It is also necessary to be able to interpret what a p value actually means in practice.

P Values, Type 1 and Type 2 Errors

Imagine the same trial design above for the use of antibiotics in the prevention of perineal breakdown. Either the null hypothesis or the alternative hypothesis is true (but not both). After the results are in, you can accept or reject the null hypothesis (i.e. that the difference seen is due to chance).

If you accept the null hypothesis (H0) when it is true = Correct decision

If you reject the null hypothesis (H0) when it is true = Wrong decision or a type I error

If you accept the null hypothesis (H0) when it is false (so the alternative hypothesis is true) = Wrong decision or a type II error

Table 37.1 Hypothesis testing

The null hypothesis (H0)	Suggests the difference seen is simply due to chance
The alternative hypothesis (H1)	Suggests the difference seen is not due to chance only

Table 37.2 Null hypothesis

	Null hypothesis (H0) is true (The difference seen is due to chance)	Alternative hypothesis is true (difference seen is not due to chance)
Accept null hypothesis	Right decision	Type II error
Reject null hypothesis	Type I error	Right decision

If you reject the null hypothesis when it is false (so the alternative is true) = Correct decision (Table 37.2).

The chance of a type I error (accepting that the alternative hypothesis is true when in fact the difference seen is actually due to chance) is the p value.

Type I error rate = alpha error = p value = false positive result.

Type II error rate = beta error.

Frequently trials are designed so that a p value <0.05 is accepted as significant evidence that the alternative hypothesis is true. This is the same as saying the type I error rate is <0.05.

If p=0.05 in a pharmaceutical trial, 1 in 20 trials will falsely accept the alternative hypothesis, i.e. the active works when in fact it is just chance.

The type II error rate is often set at 20%. In a pharmaceutical trial, this means that in 1 in 5 trials the alternative hypothesis will be incorrectly rejected.

What Is a p Value?

The p value is the probability, assuming that the null hypothesis is true, of observing a result at least as extreme as the test statistic.

What Is the Difference between Clinical Significance and Statistical Significance?

Imagine a new combined contraceptive pill that has been proven in a good quality randomised controlled trial to reduce body weight. In the trial results p<0.01, so the researchers accepted the alternative hypothesis as being true (the active agent was shown to be statistically significant in achieving weight loss). On further assessment of the methodology, the trial was powered to detect a difference of 200 grams over 12 months. The clinical difference is so small that it is practically irrelevant but still statistically significant. It is important to consider how much of an effect the drug really has before prescribing it.

Scales and Types of Variables

In order to select the right test for analyses or to summarise data appropriately, it is first important to define the type of variables being assessed.

A variable in statistics is any characteristic, number or quantity that can be measured or counted.

A variable may also be called a data item. Age, sex, business income and expenses, country of birth, capital expenditure, examination grades, eye colour and vehicle type are examples of variables.

Variables can be defined as quantitative or categorical.

Quantitative Variables

Quantitative variables can be measured or counted; essentially, if you can ask 'How much?', then it is a quantitative variable.

Examples of quantitative variables that can be measured include blood pressure, height, weight and body mass index. Quantitative variables that can be counted include number of children, number of attacks of genital herpes per annum or number of previous Caesarean sections, and so forth.

Quantitative variables can be continuous or discrete.

As the name suggests, continuous variables allow fractions between the complete units of the scales to be measured, e.g. body mass index could be 23.4 kg/m^2, whereas discrete variables can only sensibly be measured as whole units, e.g. number of children in a family.

Categorical Variables

Categorical variables take on values that are names or labels.

Categorical variables cannot be counted or measured but can be identified by asking the question 'What type?'. Examples include grades of cancer and degrees of placenta praevia. You cannot measure mean, mode or median for categorical variables. For example, it would be inappropriate to state that the average degree of placenta praevia is 2.5.

Categorical variables can be defined as ordered or unordered.

For example, grades of breast cancer have an order from grade 1 to grade 4 (4 is worse than 3, etc.).

Ordered categorical variables are also called ordinal variables.

Categorical variables tend to have an upper limit above which you cannot increase the range, for example there is no grade of placenta praevia above grade 4.

Some categorical variables are unordered, for example blood groups, male/female and alive/dead. Unordered categorical variables are called *nominal* variables.

If a nominal has only two options, for example alive or dead (you cannot really be half dead in research!), this is called a binary variable.

Summary Statistics for Continuous Variables

It is often useful to summarise quantitative variables. There are three common ways to do this, and they are frequently assessed in the MRCOG Part I examination.

Mean, Mode and Median

Mean

Mean is also known as the average. If you add up the sum of all the variables measured and divide this by the number of individual variables, you get the mean.

Mean = Sum of all the variables / Number of variables.

For example, a sample of five women who are all day 1 post hysterectomy were noted to have the following haemoglobin concentrations:

Hb (g/dl)				
10.2	9.8	10.0	12.0	8.0

Mean = Sum of all the variables / Number of variables.

Mean = 10.9 + 9.8 + 10.0 + 12.0 + 8.0 / 5.

Mean or average is a very simple way to summaries continuous variables. A major limitation with using means is that the mean is highly susceptible to outliers. For example, if in the example provided here there was one patient who was extremely anaemic with a haemoglobin concentration of 4 g/dl, this would significantly reduce the mean haemoglobin concentration for the whole sample.

Mode

The mode is also known as the modal frequency and is the number that is repeated most often in a series.

For example, five women day 1 post-Caesarean section were noted to have the following haemoglobin concentrations:

Hb (g/dl)				
10.2	9.8	9.8	11.0	8.0

In this case, there is one occurrence each of 10.2, 11.0 and 8.0 g/dl, but there are two cases of a haemoglobin concentration of 9.8 g/dl. This is the modal frequency. Unlike the mean, the modal frequency is not susceptible to outliers, but it is obvious from the example here that it is relatively limited in describing the real situation.

Median

The median is the middle point. Imagine you have a labour ward with 21 women and you are interested in describing the height of the women. You measure the height of all the women and order the sample from the shortest to the tallest. The median height would be the woman in position 11 in the sample, i.e. 10 patients on either side of her. If there was an even number of patients in the sample, it is appropriate to take an average of the middle two to derive the median height. A synonymous name for the median is the *second quartile*.

Although the mean, mode and median can all provide some information about a continuous variable, they do not tell us about the spread of the data. The individual heights of the women in the sample described here might all be close to the mean or might have a wide dispersion around the mean. To demonstrate dispersion around the mean, we must use another summary statistic. There are two common options for this:

1. To summarise the distribution around the *mean*, it is appropriate to use standard deviation (SD)
2. To summarise the distribution around the *median*, it is appropriate to use interquartile range (IQR)

Range, Standard Deviation and Interquartile Range

The range of a sample is defined from the lowest value to the highest value. In the case of the sample of women's heights, it would inform us of the heights of the shortest and tallest women. The range is dependent upon any outliers and does not really demonstrate the distribution.

Interquartile Range

The IQR demonstrates the distribution of a sample around the median. To calculate the IQR, first define the median value which is also called the second quartile. Then measure another median from the lowest figure in the sample to the second quartile. This median of the first half of the sample is also defined as the first quartile. Then measure the median from the second quartile to the highest figure in the sample. This median is called the *third quartile*. The interquartile (IQR) range extends from the first quartile to the third quartile.

Box and Whisker Plot

A box and whisker plot can demonstrate the median, IQR, range and any outliers. The box represents the IQR, the whiskers represent the range and the horizontal line is the median. Often in medical journals, one box and whisker plot is demonstrated next to another box and whisker plot. This allows a rapid comparison to be made between two continuous variables.

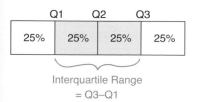

Figure 37.1 Interquartile range (IQR)

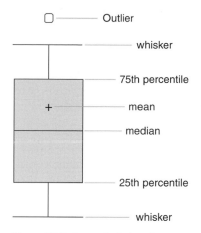

Figure 37.2 Box and whisker plot

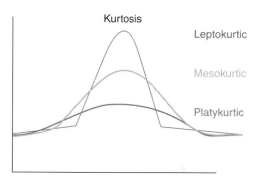

Figure 37.3 Leptokurtic and platykurtic bell-shaped curves

Standard Deviation

Standard deviation is a measure of distribution around the mean. Distribution around a mean can be described as normal distribution when the values reduce the further they lie from the mean in both a positive and negative direction. This distribution creates a bell-shaped curve. The bell can still be very 'pointy' with the distribution closely surrounding the mean or very flat. If the bell shape is very 'pointy', it is called a *leptokurtic shape*; if very flat, it is called a *platykurtic shape*.

How to Calculate Standard Deviation (SD)

To calculate SD, you must first calculate something known as *variance*.

Variance is defined as the average of the squared differences from the mean. The squaring avoids the cancelling out of the negative and positive figures created by summing up the differences from the mean.

Variance of a sample $= \sum(X - \overline{X})2$

Degrees of freedom = (n – 1).

Standard deviation = squared root (Variance of a sample / degrees of freedom).

Standard deviation $= \sqrt{\sum(X - \overline{X})2/n - 1}$

The n – 1 degrees of freedom often cause confusion. If you are studying a whole population, then you divide by n. Usually you are studying a small component of a whole population. This is called a *sample*. In the case of a sample, you have to divide by n – 1. To understand this concept, imagine a box of chocolates. If there are only two chocolates in the box, there is only one decision to be made, to have chocolate A or B first. Although there are two options, there is only one decision: N = 2 chocolates, where n – 1 in this case gives only one decision. Now imagine there is only chocolate; there is no decision required to determine which chocolate to eat first.

Standard Deviation and the Sample

SD allows you to say what proportion of a sample will fall within one standard deviation of the mean.

Mean +/– 1 standard deviation contains 68% of the sample population.

Mean +/– 2 standard deviations contains 95% of the sample population.

Mean +/– 3 standard deviations contains 99.7% of the sample population.

Standard Error of Mean (SEM)

Imagine you want to know the mean body mass index of a city with a population of 3 million people. If you measured the body mass index of the whole population, this would give you the answer, but of course this is impractical. If you measured the body mass index in a sample of 10 people from the population, you might expect this to be inaccurate. Standard error of the mean allows us to quantify the error in the sample mean compared to the whole population mean, depending upon the sample. You can imagine that the greater the sample size, the lower the error of the sample mean compared to the true population mean. Another factor that

affects the standard error of the mean is the spread of the variable being measured in the whole population. Imagine that the body mass index in the whole population is closely spread around the mean, i.e. the standard deviation is very small. When there is less spread around the mean in the whole population, there is less error in the standard error of the mean.

Standard error of the mean (SEM) = standard deviation (SD) / square root of the sample size

SEM = SD / $\sqrt{n}$

You can see from the equation above that you only need to know SD and the sample size to calculate the SEM.

You do not need to know the population size.

The SEM is always less than the SD.

SEM is completely different from the SD.

SD quantifies scatter, i.e. how much the values vary from one to another.

SEM quantifies how precisely you know the true mean of the population. It takes into account both the value of the SD and the sample size.

Confidence Intervals

Confidence intervals can be used to describe the amount of uncertainty associated with a sample estimate of a population. Imagine you used the same methods to obtain several samples from a larger population with the objective of looking at the body mass index. You would expect that by chance there will be differences in the mean BMI of the different samples, simply due to chance. It is important to remember that the true whole population parameters, i.e. mean BMI of the whole population, does not change; in statistical terms, this is called a *constant*.

Some of these sample populations will include the true population mean and others will not. A 95% confidence interval means that we would expect 95% of the sample estimate to include the true population mean.

Summary Statistics for Binary Variables

To summarise **binary variables**, we cannot use mean and SD or median and IQR. There are several options available, and each has its advantages and disadvantages. With many of these options, it is important to be able to define 'risk' in statistics.

Risk

Unlike the use of the term 'risk' in lay language, which is generally associated with a bad event, *risk* in statistical terms refers simply to the probability (usually statistical probability) that an event will occur, whether it be a good or a bad event, for example the risk of surviving 5 years after a particular malignancy diagnosis.

Absolute Risk

Absolute risk (AR) is the number of events (good or bad) in treated or control groups, divided by the number of people in that group.

Imagine a new drug for the treatment of ovarian cancer. The new drug is assessed in a placebo randomised controlled trial (ignore the ethics for a moment!). The primary outcome of the study is survival at 1 year post treatment. The following results are obtained. To make the statistics uncomplicated, there are exactly 100 patients in each arm of the study, there have been no patients dropping out of the study and no patients have been lost to follow-up.

In this case, you can rapidly assess which arm of the trial is better than the other. But imagine if the numbers you are dealing with are larger, for example if the sample sizes in the two groups were different, say 1345 in the new drug arm and 1411 in the placebo arm. In this scenario, you need to be able to compare the risks in the two groups.

The risk of an event happening = event happens / total sample size.

The 'risk' of dying at one year in the new drug arm of the trial is 35/100 = 0.35 (experimental risk) or the absolute risk treatment (ART).

The 'risk' of dying at one year in the placebo arm of the trial is 49/100 = 0.49 (control risk) or the absolute risk control (ARC).

Table 37.3 New treatment for ovarian cancer versus placebo and survival at one year

	Died	Alive	Total sample in each arm
New drug	35	65	100
Placebo	49	51	100

The probability of an event happening is the risk. To contrast the risk, you can use absolute risk reduction or absolute risk increase.

Absolute risk reduction (ARR) = control risk (ARC) – experimental risk (ART)

ARR = ARC – ART

ARR= 0.49 – 0.35

ARR = 0.16

The absolute risk reduction of dying compared to the placebo in the study provided previously is 0.16.

To express ARR as a percentage, multiply by 100.

Numbers Needed to Treat (NNT)

Numbers needed to treat (NNT) is a really useful and simple way to express how effective or not a treatment actually is.

Numbers needed to treat = 1 / Absolute risk reduction (ARR)

NNT = 1 / ARR

In the above case, ARR = 0.16

NTT = 1 / 0.16

NTT 6.25

In this case, you would need to treat 6.25 patients to prevent the death of one patient at one year compared to the placebo group.

Relative Risk (RR)

Relative risk (RR) = absolute risk in the treatment group / absolute risk in the control group

In the above example:

RR = ART / ARC

RR = 0.35 / 0.49

RR = 0.71

Relative Risk Reduction (RRR)

Relative risk reduction = (ARC – ART) / ARC

Note that (ARC – ART) is the same as the ARR.

The relative risk reduction is not affected by the prevalence of the condition, but the absolute risk and the NNT are greatly affected.

It is important to consider the absolute risk and the relative risk. For example, 'third generation contraceptive pills double the risk of a thromboembolic event' RR= 2 but the AR=0.0003.

Odds and Odds Ratio (OR)

Odds is a ratio of an event happening compared to the same event not happening.

Considering Table 37.3, showing the results of a new drug versus placebo and survival at one year:

The odds of dying in the new drug treatment arm is 35/65 = 0.54

The odds of dying in the placebo arm is 49/51 = 0.96

The odds ratio = odds of an event in the experimental arm / odds of an event in the control arm

OR = 0.54/0.96 = 0.56

To understand the difference between risk and odds, consider throwing a dice. The risk of throwing a six is 1/6 (one of the six available results) = 0.16. The odds of throwing a six, however, are 1/5 = 0.20.

Odds ratios are used as the outputs for case-controlled studies where it is inappropriate to use relative risk.

Diagnostic Tests

Diagnostic tests are frequently used in medicine and can include biochemical tests and biophysical tests such as ultrasound scans.

In general, diagnostic tests do not give an absolute answer as to whether a person has a disease or not but gives a probability that the person has or does not have the disease. This is known as a *post-test probability*.

For example, if a woman attends at 32 weeks' gestation with threatened preterm labour, you can estimate from the history the probability of her delivering. This would depend upon her previous obstetric history (has she had a previous preterm delivery, etc.). If she has a fetal fibronectin test, a positive or negative result does not mean that she will or will not go into labour. But positive and negative post-test probabilities can be generated from a combination of the test result and the pre-test probability.

Sensitivity and Specificity

Sensitivity and specificity are used to demonstrate the characteristics of a diagnostic test.

Sensitivity and specificity are related to the whole population.

The Truth

Test Score:	Has the disease	Does not have the disease	
Positive	True Positives (TP) a	False Positives (FP) b	$PPV = \dfrac{TP}{TP + FP}$
Negative	c False Negatives (FN)	d True Negatives (TN)	$NPV = \dfrac{TN}{TN + FN}$

Sensitivity $$\frac{TP}{TP + FN}$$

Specificity $$\frac{TN}{TN + FP}$$

Or, $$\frac{a}{a + c}$$ $$\frac{d}{d + b}$$

PPV = positive predictive values; NPV = negative predictive value.

PPV = positive predictive values; NPV = negative predictive value.

Sensitivity is the proportion of the population with the disease in question. The numerator represents the true positives (test positive and have the disease). The denominator represents the whole population with the disease (true positives and false negatives).

Specificity is the proportion of the population without the disease in question. The numerator represents the true negatives (test negative and do not have the disease). The denominator represents the whole population who do not have the disease (true negative and false positives).

Positive and Negative Predictive Values

It is useful to consider positive and negative predictive values as 'selfish statistics. If a patient has a positive test for HIV, the patient would not be interested in the sensitivity and specificity. The question that matters to the patient is: 'If the test is positive, what is the chance that I really have an HIV infection?' Equally, a negative test should result in the question: 'What is the probability that this patient does not have HIV when the test is negative?'

A positive predictive value (PPV) defines, in the case of a positive result, the chance the patient truly has the disease in question. In the case of PPV, the numerator is the true positives and the denominator is the whole population who had a positive test (true positives and false positives).

Sensitivity, specificity, positive and negative predictive values are often included in the MRCOG Part 1 examination. It is recommended to draw a 2 × 2 table like the one noted previously before answering the question.

Likelihood Ratios

Depending on whether a test result is positive or negative, the likelihood of the disease can be calculated with the aid of positive and negative likelihood ratios (LR).

Positive LR = probability that test is positive in a diseased person / probability that test is positive in non-diseased persons

Positive LR = Sensitivity / 1 – specificity

Negative LR = probability that test is negative in the diseased persons / probability that test is negative in non-diseased persons

Negative LR = 1 – Sensitivity / Specificity

The larger the value of the positive LR, the more conclusive the results of the test (the greater the post-test probability that the patient has the disease).

The smaller the value of the negative LR, the more conclusive the result of the test (the greater the post-test probability that the patient does not have the disease).

Likelihood Ratio and the Effect (Table 37.4)

Once the LRs, both positive and negative, have been calculated, it is possible to calculate the post-test probabilities from the pre-test probabilities with the aid of Fagan's nomogram.

Table 37.4 Which analytic test to use

Groups to compare	Parametric	Non-parametric
Difference between the means of *two independent* groups	Independent t test	Mann-Whitney U test
Differences between the means of *two matched* groups	Paired t test	Wilcoxon signed-rank test
Difference in the means of 3 or more independent groups for one variables	One way ANOVA	Kruskal-Wallis test
Difference in the means of 3 or more independent groups on the same subject	Repeated measured ANOVA	Friedman test
Comparison of relationships between variables		
	Parametric	**Non-parametric**
Strength of relationship between two continuous variables	Pearson's correlation co-efficient	Spearman's correlation co-efficient
Predicting the value of one variable given the value of a predictive variable	Simple linear regression	
Assessing the relationship between two categorical variables		Chi-squared test

Correlation

Correlation is a way of describing the relationship between two continuous variables. It is a way of measuring the strength of association between two continuous variables. If there is a perfect direct correlation between two variables, i.e. as one increases, so does the other in a linear way; this can be defined by a constant called 'r'. You do not need to know how to work out r collates but simply that r = +1 if there is a perfect correlate. If there is a perfect negative correlate, i.e. as one increase the other value decreases, then r = –1. If there is no correlation at all, then r = 0. Frequently there is a correlation that is not perfect, e.g. r = +0.6.

Analytical tests

In order to define which analytical test to apply in statistics, it is necessary to know what type of data you are dealing with, e.g. binary data, continuous date, nominal or categorical. It is also necessary to know whether the data are parametric or non-parametric, and paired or independent.

Parametric and Non-parametric Data

Parametric and non-parametric are two broad classifications of statistical procedures.

Parametric tests are based on assumptions about the distribution of the underlying population from which the sample was taken. The most common parametric assumption is that data are approximately normally distributed. For the MRCOG Part I examination, the question will state if the data are parametric or non-parametric, as it would be too difficult to perform this assessment on the data.

Non-parametric tests do not rely on assumptions about the shape or parameters of the underlying population distribution.

Parametric tests essentially compare the means of different samples, whereas non-parametric tests compare medians of different samples.

Paired and Independent Groups

Paired or matched data occurs when the same variable is measured in the same sample but at a different time, e.g. weight before and after a diet. With independent groups, the two groups sampled are completely different, e.g. comparing body mass index in women with and without pre-eclampsia.

Single Best Answer Questions

1. In a population of 100 women, the gold standard test (laparoscopy) is used to investigate whether or not they have rectovaginal endometriosis. Four are found to have rectovaginal endometriosis. A preoperative MRI has positive results for rectovaginal endometriosis in 3 of the 4 true positives and another 7 positives without rectovaginal endometriosis.
   Choose the best option that reflects the sensitivity of the test.

   a. 10 %
   b. 25 %
   c. 55 %
   d. 75 %
   e. 93 %

2. If p is set at <0.05 in a hypothesis testing trial, there will be an alpha error rate. Select the best option that reflects the average alpha error rate with the defined p value.

   a. 1 in 25 trials
   b. 1 in 20 trials
   c. 1 in 10 trials
   d. 1 in 5 trials
   e. 1 in 3 trials

3. In a population of 100 women after a gold standard test (laparoscopy), 4 are found to have rectovaginal endometriosis. A preoperative MRI has positive results for rectovaginal endometriosis in 3 of the 4 true positives and another 7 positives without rectovaginal endometriosis. Choose the option that best reflects the positive predictive value of the test.

   a. 10 %
   b. 20 %
   c. 30 %
   d. 40 %
   e. 50 %

4. A new antihypertensive drug is assessed by a randomised controlled trial in pregnant women. The main outcome is blood pressure 4 weeks after treatment is commenced.
   What test would you use to compare the mean blood pressures in the groups?

   a. Linear regression
   b. Two sample t test
   c. R squared co-efficient

d. Regression analysis

e. Chi-squared

5. With regard to a box plot, what does the box represent?

a. Inter-quartile range

b. Range

c. Variance

d. Confidence interval

e. The Z score +/− 2 standard errors

6. Considering the table below showing the results of a new analgesic in an RCT, what is the odds ratio for satisfactory pain control with the new drug?

	Total in each group	Satisfactory pain control	Failure of treatment
Experimental group	100	50	50
Control group	100	20	80

a. 1.5

b. 2

c. 4

d. 8

e. 10

7. You wish to analyse the induction to delivery time interval in women with and without pre-eclampsia. You have data for the two groups which is defined as non-parametric and unpaired. Choose the best option for the statistical test needed.

a. Student's t test

b. Kaiser Meyer Olkin measure of sampling adequacy

c. Pearson's r test

d. Chi-square test

e. Mann-Whitney U test

8. A study is designed to investigate the association between pregnant women's hair colour and post-partum blood loss. What type of scale is hair colour?

a. Interval

b. Linear ordinal

c. Nominal

d. Ordinal

e. Ratio

9. The table below demonstrates the duration of the second stage of labour in 5 women. What is the mode duration of the second stage of labour?

0.3 hours

0.5 hours

0.8 hours

1.7 hours

2.5 hours

10. With regard to calculating standard deviation (SD), if $SD = \sqrt{x/n - 1}$, what is x?

a. Mean

b. Mean / n − 1

c. Range/n

d. Standard error of the mean

e. Variance

Clinical Trials, Audit and Meta-analysis

Anthony N. Griffiths

Evidence-Based Medicine

Evidence-based medicine (EBM) is a process that allows the optimization of decisions in medicine through the analysis and application of evidence from research.

David Sackett defines EBM as 'the conscientious, explicit, and judicious use of current best evidence in making decisions about the care of individual patients'.

EBM should include:

- application of the best available evidence
- what treatments are available locally; this includes the skills and resources available
- what the patient's wishes are regarding the various treatment options

Quantitative and Qualitative Research

Research is a careful and detailed study into a specific problem, concern, or issue using the scientific method.

Research can be broadly defined as qualitative or quantitative.

Qualitative Research

Qualitative research is used to explore and understand patients' reasons, decision making, feeling and perceptions. Qualitative research tends to be used to answer 'why' questions.

There are several methods of data collection in qualitative research, including:

- interviews
- focus groups
- questionnaires
- online or paper surveys

Data are collected using several methods and recurrent themes emerge. The combining of data from several research methods in qualitative research is called *triangulation*.

Unlike quantitative research, there is no final numeric answer, P values or confidence intervals.

Quantitative Research

Quantitative research deals with questions that have numeric answers. If the question is 'how much', quantitative research is appropriate. The numeric data generated can be subjected to statistical analysis and a conclusion generated. Quantitative research can quantify attitudes, opinions and behaviours, as well as the more obvious medical research outputs. Quantitative research cannot be applied to gain an understanding of patients' underlying reasons, attitudes and feelings.

Quantitative data collection methods are more structured than qualitative data collection methods.

Primary and Secondary Quantitative Research Methods

Primary research reports results first hand. Primary research includes laboratory-based experiments, clinical trials and clinical surveys.

Primary research includes:

- laboratory-based experiments
- clinical trials
- surveys

Secondary research attempts to summarize or draw up conclusions from several sources of primary research.

Secondary research includes:

- systematic reviews
- non-systematic reviews
- meta-analysis
- guidelines

- economic analysis
- decision analysis

Clinical Trials

Clinical trials are research studies that aim to test whether a clinical strategy, screening test, diagnostic test, therapy, treatment or device is safe, effective and beneficial to a particular patient group or disease process.

Since clinical trials are research, they follow a strict scientific process. This allows reliability and reproducibility to be achieved.

A clinical trial may discover that a new therapy, treatment or device:

- causes unexpected harm to the patient
- has no beneficial effect for the patient
- improves patient outcomes

Types of clinical trials include:

- treatment trials
- diagnostic trials
- screening trials
- prevention trials
- quality of life studies
- genetic studies
- population studies

Phases of Clinical Trials

Clinical trials for pharmaceutical products occur well before human subjects are involved.

Pre-clinical Trials

Non-humans (animal or cell line) experiments are carried out in highly controlled environments. The aim of the study is to assess the toxicity, efficacy and pharmacokinetics of the drug.

Phase 0 Trials

Phase 0 trials are also known as the first in human studies. A very small group of healthy non-diseased humans volunteer to participate in these trials. The subjects are given sub-therapeutic doses of the drug being assessed. Since the drug is given in sub-therapeutic doses, these trials are also known as micro-dosing studies. Due to the very low dose used, the trial cannot assess the safety or efficacy of the drug.

The purpose of the trial is to assess the pharmacokinetics of the drug (what the body does to the drug).

Phase 1 Trials

Phase 1 trials are carried out on a small group of healthy volunteers (20–200). The volunteers are administered gradually increasing doses of the drug. The aim of phase 1 trials is to assess safety, tolerability, pharmacokinetics and pharmacodynamics (what the drug does to the body) of the drug. These trials are carried out in specialist research centres with strict safety and legislative controls in place. Phase 1 trials allow the assessment of the maximum tolerable dose of the drug and the correct dosing ranges.

Phase 2 Trials

Now that the drug has been defined as 'safe' from a phase 1 trial point of view and that the dosing has been assessed, phase 2 trials aim to evaluate whether the drug has an effective biological effect. These trials involve a larger number of volunteers (100–300). They can be case series or small randomised controlled studies.

Phase 3 Trials

These trials assess the effectiveness of the drug compared to the current gold standard treatment in large multi-centre randomized controlled trials. They are expensive and time-consuming. They involve a large number of subjects (1000–2000).

A large proportion of promising drugs in phase 2 trials fail to progress in a phase 3 trial. These trials are used as evidence to obtain a licence to bring the product to market.

Phase 4 Trials

These trials are essentially post-market surveillance. Harmful effects of a new drug may not be discovered until phase 4 trials, as only a relatively small number of patients have received the drug in phase 3 trials. Rarer but severe side effects can occur, resulting in the withdrawal of the drug from the market.

Types of Clinical Trials

Clinical trials can be divided into two groups, depending upon whether or not the investigator assigned the exposure (the intervention) being studied. If the investigator assigned the exposure, it is known as an *experimental study*; if not, it is an *observational study*.

Experimental Studies Can Be Randomized or Non-randomized

Observational studies can be simply reported upon or compared to another group. If groups are compared, it is known as an analytic study; if it simply provides a description, it is known as a descriptive study.

Descriptive studies can be further sub-classified depending upon when the study is carried out relative to the when the exposure occurred and when the outcome being studied occurred. For example, if a group of smokers is observed over 20 years in a prospective way (before the observed outcomes have occurred) and compared to a group of non-smokers, looking at health outcomes, the group of smokers can be also called a *cohort* of smokers, and this is known as a *prospective cohort study*.

If the same study was carried out after the exposures and outcomes had occurred, this is known as a *retrospective cohort study*.

A third type of descriptive study compares a group of people with a disease (or outcome) to a group as similar as possible but without the disease (or outcome), and looks for differences in exposures between the two groups. This is known as a *case-controlled study*.

Cohort Study

A group is subjected to an exposure and followed up over time. Outcomes are measured over this time period. An example of a cohort study in gynaecology is the 'Women's Health Initiative Observational study'. If the research looks forward in time to the outcomes, this is a prospective cohort study or longitudinal study. In a retrospective cohort study, the observer again looks at a cohort that has been subjected to an exposure but this time is looking back in time to observe outcomes. The prospective and retrospective nature is dependent on the perspective of the researcher's observations. Findings of cohort studies can be presented as a relative risk or odds ratio. Cohort studies take a long time to yield results and are expensive to carry out, and there is a risk of subject attrition. The results can be dangerously misleading, and it is important to remember that cohort studies report associations, not causation.

Case-Controlled Study

In a case-controlled study, the observer looks at a group that has an outcome and wishes to explore the potential exposures. An example of this would be to look at women with a history of ectopic pregnancy and explore risk-factors. Findings of case-controlled studies cannot be presented as relative risks, as the outcomes have already happened; they should be presented as odds ratios. Because the recording of exposure is often dependent upon the subject's recall, there is a high potential for bias to occur.

Randomized Controlled Trial (RCT)

A group of patients or subjects are randomised into an experimental and a control group. If there are only two groups, this is 1 to 1 randomization. It is possible to randomize to several groups, e.g. drug A or drug B or placebo control group. This is known as a *multi-arm parallel design*. About 80% of RCTs are of a parallel design. Other RCT trial designs include crossover study, cluster and factorial design.

Another type of trial design is when the study sets out to identify whether a new intervention is superior to another, or if it is non-inferior or equivalent. An RCT of a new drug may conclude that the new drug is equivalent to the currently used drug, but perhaps with a better side-effect profile.

Randomisation

With random allocation, each subject in the trial has a known probability of being assigned to each arm of the study, but the assigned intervention is determined simply by chance and cannot be predicted. This is often done with computer-generated random numbers. The randomisation should be carried out independent of the researcher, in order to avoid potential bias. Often the researcher contacts a remote study centre to randomise a subject.

In some trials, the balance of randomisation is not 1:1 but 2:1, for example. This can be used to gain more experience of a new procedure or to limit cost.

Blinding

One key advantage of randomization is that it allows blinding to be carried out. Blinding is where the subject does not know if he or she has been allocated to the experimental or control arm of the trial. This is known as *single blinding*. If the physician/researcher also does not know to which arm of the trial the subject is allocated, it allows the physician to give identical care to both groups of subjects. This is known as *double blinding*. It is important in an RCT that the only difference in care between the groups is the allocated randomized intervention. If the statistician analysing the results is also blinded, this is known as *triple blinding*.

The advantages of RCTs include the prevention of systematic bias, an unbiased distribution of confounders, and randomisation facilitating blinding and statistical analysis. Disadvantages of RCTs include being financially expensive and time-consuming to perform. There is also a volunteer bias in that subjects that agree to take part in an RCT may be different from the general population where the results are intended to be applied. There can also be ethical issues with RCTs.

Diagnostic Studies

A diagnostic test changes the pre-test probability of having a disease to a post-test probability, depending upon whether the test result is positive or negative. For a diagnostic test, the positive and negative likelihood ratios can be generated. Post-test probabilities can be demonstrated from the pre-test probabilities and the likelihood ratios with the aid of Fagan's nomograms (Fig. 38.1).

Validation Studies

A validation study is used to assess a diagnostic test. A population is subjected to a diagnostic test, for example an MRI. The population is subjected to a gold standard test, for example a laparoscopy. The results of the diagnostic test are compared to the results of the gold standard test. It is important that the results of the diagnostic test are looked at *after* the gold standard test and not before.

Systematic Review and Meta-analysis

A systematic review assesses the published evidence with an explicit statement of objectives, materials and methods. An example is in the Cochrane library, where RCTs are subjected to a pre-designed explicit assessment. Only RCTs that satisfy this assessment will be accepted for analysis. A review that is non-systematic is known as a narrative review.

A meta-analysis of a systematic review is a method that statistically combines the results of the studies in a systematic review and generates a conclusion about the overall effect of an intervention or treatment. A meta-analysis can show not only whether there is a significant effect and its direction, but also the magnitude of the effect. This is visually represented by a forest plot (Fig. 38.2).

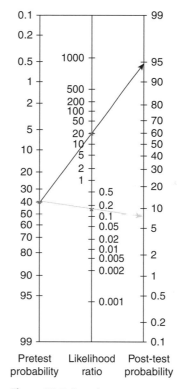

Figure 38.1 Fagan's nomogram

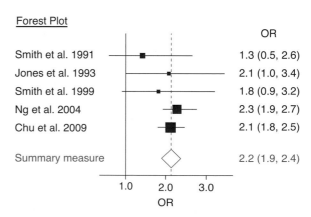

Figure 38.2 Forest plot

385

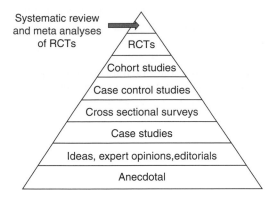

Figure 38.3 Pyramid of evidence

Levels of Evidence

The quality of evidence can be defined in a hierarchy, with the best being systematic reviews or meta-analyses (Fig. 38.3). Sadly, most decisions in medicine are still made on an anecdotal level.

Grading of Evidence

Ia: systematic review or meta-analysis of RCTs.
Ib: at least one RCT.
IIa: at least one well-designed controlled study without randomisation.
IIb: at least one well-designed quasi-experimental study, such as a cohort study.
III: well-designed non-experimental descriptive studies, such as comparative studies, correlation studies, case-control studies and case series.
IV: expert committee reports, opinions and/or clinical experience of respected authorities.

Audit

Clinical audit is a quality improvement process that seeks to improve patient care and outcomes through a systematic review of patient care against explicit criteria and the implementation of change (Fig. 38.3). Unlike research that aims to determine the best treatment or care for patients, clinical audit asks whether that treatment or care is actually taking place. Clinical audit can be carried out nationally or locally in hospitals, trusts or GP practices – essentially anywhere that healthcare is provided. It involves a process of first measuring what we do against either a gold standard that may have been defined nationally or by an expert group locally. Areas of change can be identified and new changes implemented. The process must undergo re-evaluation.

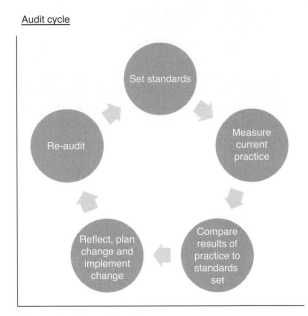

Audit cycle

Figure 38.4 The audit cycle

Single Best Answer Questions

1. You wish to understand why some women continue to smoke in pregnancy. What type of trial would be appropriate to carry out?

   a. Randomised controlled trial
   b. Controlled trial
   c. Qualitative study
   d. Prospective cohort
   e. Retrospective cohort

2. You wish to explore the genomic imprinting in placental tissue (exposure) and, over the next 5 years, to look at the growth outcome of children (outcome). What type of study would you carry out?

   a. Randomised controlled trial
   b. Prospective cohort study
   c. Retrospective cohort study
   d. Case-controlled study
   e. Sensitivity genetic loci analysis study

3. What is the most common method of group randomisation in published randomised controlled trials?

   a. Factorial
   b. Cross-over

c. Parallel
d. Cluster
e. 1:2:5 ratio

4 A woman presents with threatened preterm labour and has a negative fetal fibronectin test. You already know the pre-test probability of labour and also the negative likelihood ratio. Which of the following would you use to generate a post-test probability?

a. Forest plot
b. Box and whisker plot

c. ROC graph
d. Fagan's nomogram
e. Stem and leaf plot

5. You wish to visually represent the results of a meta-analysis of a systematic review. Which plot is appropriate to use?

a. Forest plot
b. Box and whisker plot
c. ROC graph
d. Fagan's nomogram
e. Stem and leaf plot

Appendix: Answers to SBA Questions

1 Physiology of Pregnancy and Labour

1 (b)
2 (e)
3 (d)
4 (e)
5 (e)
6 (c)
7 (b)

2 Fetal Physiology

1 (c)
2 (e)
3 (c)
4 (e)
5 (d)
6 (b)

4 Female Reproductive Physiology

1 (d)
2 (b)
3 (c)
4 (e)
5 (d)
6 (c)
7 (a)

5 Male Reproductive Physiology

1 (c)
2 (e)
3 (c)
4 (d)
5 (b)
6 (e)
7 (d)

6 The Pituitary, Adrenal, Thyroid and Pancreas

1 (b) Prolactinoma. It can cause headache due to its mass effect and can compress the optic chiasm to cause visual impairment. Excessive prolactin secretion stimulates milk secretion and has inhibitory effects on gonadotrophin releasing hormones from the hypothalamus.

2 (c) Sheehan's syndrome. It is usually associated with a history of postpartum haemorrhage and can present as total or partial pituitary gland failure. The investigations may show reduced levels of pituitary hormones. The insulin stress test shows impaired response of ACTH, GH and Prolactin to hypoglycaemia.

3 (a) Low aldosterone, Hyponatraemia, Hypoglycaemia, Hyperkalaemia. Low aldosterone levels in Addison's disease will cause all the above biochemical abnormalities.

4 (d) Pheochromocytoma. It causes episodes of very high blood pressure which is characteristically not sustained. It can be associated with family history of multiple endocrine neoplasia or neurofibromatosis.

5 (d) Hyperthyroidism. She has the characteristic clinical features of hyperthyroidism. You should include thyroid function tests in your baseline investigations to make the diagnosis.

6 (b) Increase Thyroxine. Increase thyroxine by 25 micrograms and recheck thyroid function tests in 4-6 weeks' time. The dose is adjusted to keep the serum TSH <3 mIU/L. Propylthiouracil and Carbimazole are used in hyperthyroidism.

7 (c) The diagnosis is Diabetic Ketoacidosis. She has high blood glucose along with ketonuria. Low levels of insulin, lead to increase secretion of hormones like growth hormone and cortisol, resulting in hyperglycaemia, volume depletion and subsequent dehydration. Free fatty acids are increased due to lipolysis and are converted to ketone bodies that can be measured in blood or urine.

8 Data Interpretation in Obstetrics

1 (b)
2 (e)
3 (a)

4 (c)
5 (b)
6 (d)
7 (b)
8 (d)
9 (b)
10 (c)
11 (b)
12 (b)
13 (d)
14 (a)
15 (c)

9 Clinical Management in Obstetrics

1 (d)
2 (c)
3 (a)
4 (d)
5 (b)
6 (d)
7 (a)
8 (c)
9 (a)
10 (d)
11 (d)
12 (c)

10 Concise Anatomy of the Urinary, Intestinal and Reproductive Tracts within the Pelvic Cavity

1 (a)
2 (a)
3 (e)
4 (c)
5 (d)

11 Concise Anatomy of the Pelvic Floor and Perineum

1 (a)
2 (b)
3 (c)
4 (d)
5 (d)

12 Concise Anatomy of the Pelvic Girdle

1 (d)

2 (e)
3 (d)
4 (c)
5 (c)

13 Concise Anatomy of the Abdominal Walls

1 (d)
2 (e)
3 (d)
4 (c)
5 (c)

16 Problems in Early Pregnancy

1 (a)
2 (a)
3 (d)
4 (a)
5 (a)
6 (d)
7 (d)
8 (b)

18 Pharmacokinetics, Pharmacodynamics and Teratogenesis

1 (d)
2 (c)
3 (c)
4 (c)
5 (b)
6 (e)

19 Non-hormonal Therapy in Obstetrics and Gynaecology

1 (d)
2 (d)
3 (e)
4 (c)
5 (d)
6 (d)

20 Drugs in Gynaecology and Contraception

1 (b), (b)
2 (d)
3 (c)
4 (e)
5 (b)

6 (e)
7 (b)
8 (a)
9 (c)
10 (a)
11 (a)

22 Data Interpretation in Gynaecology

1 (d) The woman probably has respiratory depression due to the effects of the morphine and has a mild respiratory acidosis.

2 (d) Acute vomiting tends to result in hypokalaemia. This ECG also shows features of hypokalaemia (ST depression, T wave inversion, Long QT interval, prominent U wave).

3 (b) The woman has a normal BMI. The average weight of a woman in the UK is 70 kg. Expected urine output would therefore be 35–70 ml/hour.

4 (b) This is the medial umbilical ligament which contains the obliterated umbilical artery.

5 (c) This is a typical appearance of a haemorrhagic cyst, with a 'lacy' appearance within the cyst. Most haemorrhagic cysts present in the luteal phase. The pain of a torsion would not settle with simple analgesia. An ovarian tumour would be very unusual at this age and would be unlikely to present with acute pain.

6 (e) This is the mid-luteal phase which corresponds to secretory endometrium.

7 (a) All parameters are normal, other than reduced progressive motility.

8 (a) The HCG level has fallen by more than 50% in 48 hours, so this is most likely to be a complete miscarriage.

9 (d) RMI = U × M × CA125; U = 1; M = 3; CA125 = 20

10 (a) Dispermic fertilisation of an 'empty' oocyte results in a complete hydatidiform mole.

24 Carbohydrate Metabolism

1 (c)
2 (d)
3 (b)
4 (b)
5 (a)

6 (e)
7 (d)
8 (a)
9 (b)

25 Fat Metabolism

1 (c)
2 (d)
3 (c)
4 (a)
5 (a)
6 (b)
7 (d)
8 (a)
9 (b)
10 (c)

26 Steroid Hormones and Prostaglandins

1 (b)
2 (c)
3 (e)
4 (a)
5 (e)
6 (a)
7 (e)
8 (b)
9 (d)
10 (a)
11 (d)
12 (c)
13 (d)
14 (c)

27 Calcium Homeostasis and Bone Health

1 (e)
2 (c)
3 (e)
4 (b)
5 (a)

29 Cellular Responses in Disease

1 (a)
2 (b)
3 (c)
4 (b)w
5 (e)

6 (a)

7 (d)

8 (d)

30 Pathology of Non-neoplastic and Neoplastic Gynaecological Diseases

1 (a)

2 (c)

3 (e)

4 (b)

31 Implantation and Placental Structure and Function

1 (b)

2 (b)

3 (a)

4 (c)

5 (d)

6 (e)

7 (e)

8 (b)

37 Statistics

1 (d)

2 (b) The p value is the probability of an observation occurring by chance. Alpha error is falsely rejecting the null hypothesis (no difference in the two groups).

3 (c) True test positives / total test positives.

4 (b)

5 (a)

6 (c)

7 (e)

8 (c)

9 (a)

10 (e)

38 Clinical Trials, Audit and Meta-analysis

1 (c)

2 (b)

3 (c)

4 (d)

5 (a)

Index

abdominal aorta, 107–8
abdominal wall
  anatomy
    anterior, 104–6
    external oblique muscle, 105
    femoral triangle and femoral ring, 106
    inguinal canal, 105–6
    internal oblique and transversus abdominis muscles, 105
    posterior, 106–7
  Caesarean section incision and repair, 78–9
ABG. *See* arterial blood gases
abruption, placental, 308
abscess, 213
absolute risk (AR), 377
absorption, drug, 6, 169
accuracy, diagnostic testing, 65–6
ACE inhibitors, 180
acetyl CoA, 251–2
aciclovir, 56, 150–1, 152
acid, 21, 22–3
acid-base balance
  ABG interpretation, 24–7
  ABG measurement, 24
  buffering systems, 23–4, 254–5
  homeostasis, 22–3
  postoperative care data interpretation, 216
  terminology, 21–2
  umbilical cord, 71
acidophils, 43, 44, 94
acidosis, 21. *See also* metabolic acidosis
  diabetic ketoacidosis, 254–5, 256
  respiratory, 25–6
acquired immunity, 310, 312
  antibodies, 313, 317
  APCs, 312
  B cells, 312
  MHC, 312, 315–16
  T cells, 313–14
  vaccination, 313
acquired Immunodeficiency syndrome (AIDS), 159–60, 161, 162. *See also* human immunodeficiency virus
acromegaly, 45
acrosome reaction, 40, 41

ACTH. *See* adrenocorticotrophic hormone
active transport, placental, 306–7
acute fatty liver of pregnancy (AFLP), 69
adaptation, cellular, 285
adaptive immunity. *See* acquired immunity
Addison's disease, 47
adenine, 318–19, 320
adenocarcinoma, cervix, 298–9
adeno-hypophysis, 43, 94
adenoma, pituitary, 94
adenomyosis, 293
adenylyl cyclase, 275–6
adipose tissue, 248, 249, 255
adrenal gland, 44
  dysfunction, 46–7
  hormones, 44
adrenocorticotrophic hormone (ACTH), 43, 44
AEDs. *See* antiepileptic drugs
aerobic metabolism, 238–41, 242, 243
AFLP. *See* acute fatty liver of pregnancy
agonists, 171, 172
AIDS. *See* acquired Immunodeficiency syndrome
aldosterone, 44
alkali, 21
alkaline phosphatase, 5, 69
alkalosis, 21
  metabolic, 22, 26–7
  respiratory, 26, 27
alkylating agents, 184
alopecia, 184
alpha radioimmunotherapy, 370
ambiguous genitalia, 338
ambulatory urodynamics, 235
amenorrhoea, 190–2, 195
aminoglycosides, 176
ammonia (NH$_3$), 23
amniotic fluid, 13, 14, 15
ampicillin, 172
Amsel's criteria, 141
anaemia, 5–6, 79–80
anaerobic metabolism, 238, 239, 240, 241
anaesthesia, 77–8, 94–5

anal sphincters, 79, 83, 90, 96
anal triangle, 96–7
analgesia, 181–2
androgens, 29, 44, 259, 260, 264
androstenedione, 262, 263
anion, 21
anion gap, 22
ano-coccygeal ligament, 96
anogenital warts, 155–6, 157, 158
ano-rectal junction, 89–90, 96
antacids, 182–3
antagonists, 171, 172
antenatal care, 79
  anaemia, 79–80
  gastric reflux, 80
  hyperemesis gravidarum, 79
antenatal screening
  congenital infection, 55, 56
  data interpretation, 67, 68
  hepatitis immunology and, 317
anterior pituitary, 43, 94
antibiotic-associated diarrhoea, 214
antibiotics, 171, 173
  anti-tumour, 184
  chlamydial infection treatment, 203
  COC interactions, 198–9
  gonococcal infection treatment, 203
  gonorrhoea resistance, 146, 147, 203
  PID treatment, 202–3
  surgical prophylaxis, 203, 205–7, 211–12
  teratogenesis, 176
  UTI treatment, 204
  vaginal and vulval infection treatment, 203–4
antibodies
  acquired immunity, 313, 317
  fetal, 317
  fetal protection against maternal, 316
  thyroid, 69, 80
anticoagulants, 172, 174, 176–7, 317
anti-D immunoglobulin, 136–7
antidepressants, 174
antiemetics, 182
antiepileptic drugs (AEDs), 6, 80–1, 171, 174, 175–6, 198–9
antifungals, 203–4, 231